Hereditary Colorectal Cancer

Laura Valle • Stephen B. Gruber
Gabriel Capellá
Editors

Hereditary Colorectal Cancer

Genetic Basis and Clinical Implications

Springer

Editors
Laura Valle
Hereditary Cancer Program
Catalan Institute of Oncology
IDIBELL and CIBERONC
Hospitalet de Llobregat
Barcelona, Spain

Stephen B. Gruber
University of Southern California
Norris Comprehensive Cancer Center
Los Angeles, CA, USA

Gabriel Capellá
Hereditary Cancer Program
Catalan Institute of Oncology
IDIBELL and CIBERONC
Hospitalet de Llobregat
Barcelona, Spain

ISBN 978-3-030-08948-1 ISBN 978-3-319-74259-5 (eBook)
https://doi.org/10.1007/978-3-319-74259-5

Softcover re-print of the Hardcover 1st edition 2018

Printed on acid-free paper

This Springer imprint is published by the registered company Springer International Publishing AG part of Springer Nature.
The registered company address is: Gewerbestrasse 11, 6330 Cham, Switzerland

Contents

About the Editors

Laura Valle is a Principal Investigator of the Hereditary Cancer Program at the Catalan Institute of Oncology, IDIBELL, Barcelona (Spain). She obtained her bachelor degrees in Biology (2000) and Biochemistry (2001) from the University of Navarra (Spain) and carried out her Ph.D. thesis about hereditary colon cancer at the Spanish National Cancer Research Center (CNIO) (2006, Extraordinary Doctorate Award). Her interest in the genetic susceptibility to cancer led her to a postdoctoral stay with Dr. Albert de la Chapelle at the Comprehensive Cancer Center of the Ohio State University. In 2009, Dr. Valle joined the Hereditary Cancer Program of the Catalan Institute of Oncology to develop a research line focused on hereditary colon cancer. In 2009, she obtained the prestigious and highly competitive Ramón y Cajal contract for young researchers, and in 2016, funding from the I3 program for the stabilization of doctors (both funded by the Spanish Government). In 2012, she obtained the accreditation in human genetics and the National Award for the most outstanding young researcher in human genetics, both awarded by the Spanish Association of Human Genetics, and in 2013, a L'Oréal-UNESCO "For Women in Science – Spain" Research Award. Since 2017, she is elected member of the Executive Board of the Spanish Association of Human Genetics. Dr. Valle has dedicated her scientific career to the identification of the genetic causes of cancer predisposition and the better characterization of new hereditary colorectal cancer syndromes, which have led to her consolidation as world expert in the subject. In the last years, she has been invited lecturer to prestigious conferences in the field, such as the ones organized by the European Society of Human Genetics, the International Society of Gastrointestinal Hereditary Tumors, or the Collaborative Group of the Americas on Inherited Colorectal Cancer.

Stephen B. Gruber is a board certified medical oncologist, cancer geneticist, and epidemiologist whose research and clinical practice focuse on clinical cancer genetics and the molecular genetic and environmental contributions to colorectal cancer. Dr. Gruber earned his bachelor's degree from the University of Pennsylvania in 1984. He subsequently graduated with a Master of Public Health Degree from Yale University in 1986 and a Doctor of Philosophy in epidemiology at Yale in 1988.

Dr. Gruber graduated from the University of Pennsylvania Medical School earning his medical degree in 1992, where he also completed his internship and residency in internal medicine. He completed fellowships in medical oncology at Johns Hopkins Hospital and in clinical medical genetics at the University of Michigan. Following 14 years on the faculty at the University of Michigan, where he was the H. Marvin Pollard Professor of Medicine, he was appointed director of the USC Norris Comprehensive Cancer Center, H. Leslie and Elaine S. Hoffman Cancer Research Chair, and Professor of Medicine and Professor of Preventive Medicine at the Keck School of Medicine of the University of Southern California. In 2017 Dr. Gruber was named the Jane & Kris Popovich Chair in Cancer Research. Dr. Gruber is an elected member of the American Society of Clinical Investigation and was honored with the Lifetime Achievement Award, Collaborative Group of the Americas on Inherited Colorectal Cancer.

Gabriel Capellá obtained his MD degree from the University of Barcelona in 1983. He trained as a general and digestive surgeon at the Hospital de Sant Pau, Barcelona. His interest in translational cancer research led him to a postdoctoral stay with Dr. Manuel Perucho during 1989 and 1990. Back to Spain he spent 8 years at the Gastrointestinal Research Laboratory at the Hospital de Sant Pau where he focused his research on the molecular basis of pancreatic and colorectal cancer. Since 1998 he worked at the Catalan Institute of Oncology where he was director of the Translational Research Laboratory until 2011. Since 2010 he is serving as Director of the Hereditary Cancer Program. His main interest is the study of the genetic basis of gastrointestinal cancer focusing on novel technologies for the clinical management of patient at risk of developing GI cancer. He is coauthor of more than 230 publications in international peer-reviewed journals. He has served as vice-director for Research and Innovation, Health Department, Catalan Government, and he is currently the Director of the Bellvitge Biomedical Research Institute. He is cofounder of VCN Biosciences a spin-off aimed at developing new cancer therapies based on oncolytic adenoviruses. Since 2014 he is member of the Council of the International Society for Gastrointestinal Hereditary Tumors (InSiGHT).

Part I
Genetic Causes and Associated Phenotypes: Hereditary Nonpolyposis CRC

Chapter 1
Lynch Syndrome

Elena M. Stoffel, Matthew B. Yurgelun, and C. Richard Boland

Abstract Lynch syndrome is a highly penetrant hereditary cancer syndrome caused by pathogenic germline variants in DNA mismatch repair (MMR) genes *MLH1*, *MSH2*, *MSH6*, *PMS2*, and *EPCAM*. Historically identified on the basis of family history of colorectal and endometrial cancers exhibiting autosomal dominant inheritance, universal screening of CRCs and endometrial cancers for features of MMR deficiency, together with cascade genetic testing in families, is at present the most effective approach for identifying individuals with Lynch syndrome. Here we review the history of Lynch syndrome, as well as the clinical and molecular investigations that have contributed to our understanding of Lynch syndrome and informed current approaches to diagnosis and clinical management.

Keywords Lynch syndrome · Genetic · Mismatch repair

1 Familial Colorectal Cancer: Polyposis or Nonpolyposis

Family history is one of the strongest determinants of colorectal cancer (CRC) risk [1], and one in three individuals diagnosed with CRC reports one or more affected relatives. The occurrence of CRC in multiple family members invokes the

E. M. Stoffel (✉)
Division of Gastroenterology, University of Michigan, Ann Arbor, MI, USA
e-mail: estoffel@med.umich.edu

M. B. Yurgelun
Dana-Farber Cancer Institute, Brigham & Women's Hospital and Harvard Medical School, Boston, MA, USA

C. R. Boland (✉)
Division of Gastroenterology, UCSD School of Medicine, University of California, San Diego, CA, USA
e-mail: crboland@ucsd.edu

L. Valle et al. (eds.), *Hereditary Colorectal Cancer*,
https://doi.org/10.1007/978-3-319-74259-5_1

possibility of shared environmental and/or inherited risk factors, and the presence of an autosomal dominant inheritance pattern strongly suggests genetic predisposition. Also, early onset of cancer and multiple cancers in individuals raises the specter of a constitutional predisposition to cancer. In some cases, an obvious clinical phenotype such as colorectal polyposis (classically seen in familial adenomatous polyposis or FAP) can prompt the identification of individuals needing genetic evaluation. However, most cases of familial CRC lack a distinctive adenomatous polyposis phenotype. These families were historically designated as "hereditary nonpolyposis colorectal cancer (HNPCC)" as a means of distinguishing them from FAP; however, the term HNPCC has proven problematic as these cases are now known to comprise heterogeneous conditions associated with differences in disease spectrum and mechanisms of pathogenesis.

Lynch syndrome is the disease caused by pathogenic germline variants in DNA mismatch repair (MMR) genes and is the most common of the hereditary colorectal cancer syndromes. Although the Amsterdam criteria (≥3 individuals with CRC, involving ≥2 generations, with ≥1 diagnosed at age < 50) [2] were originally developed as a means to identify affected families, family history affords limited sensitivity and specificity for identifying individuals with Lynch syndrome. Molecular profiling of CRCs has helped elucidate relationships between germline variants and pathogenesis of these cancers. Implementation of universal screening of CRCs and endometrial cancers for features of DNA mismatch repair (MMR) deficiency, together with cascade genetic testing in families, is at present the most effective approach for identifying individuals with Lynch syndrome (Fig. 1.1) [3, 4]. Here we review the history of Lynch syndrome, as well as the clinical and molecular investigations that have contributed to our understanding of Lynch syndrome and informed current approaches to diagnosis and clinical management.

1.1 Lynch Syndrome: A History

Lynch syndrome is a highly penetrant inherited cancer predisposition syndrome caused by pathogenic germline variants in DNA MMR genes (*MLH1*, *MSH2*, *MSH6*, *PMS2*) and *EPCAM*. Lynch syndrome is named for Dr. Henry Lynch, whose characterization of families affected with CRC was instrumental in characterizing the broad spectrum of hereditary cancer syndromes [5]. The first known description of Lynch syndrome, however, occurred more than a century ago by Dr. Aldred Scott Warthin, Chairman of Pathology at the University of Michigan. In his report of a family disproportionately affected with endometrial, gastric, and intestinal cancers occurring at early ages, affecting individuals in multiple generations, Warthin hypothesized that the cancers resulted from inherited susceptibility [6]. Decades later, Lynch recontacted descendants from the family described by Warthin (known as Family G) and recruited dozens of additional families with

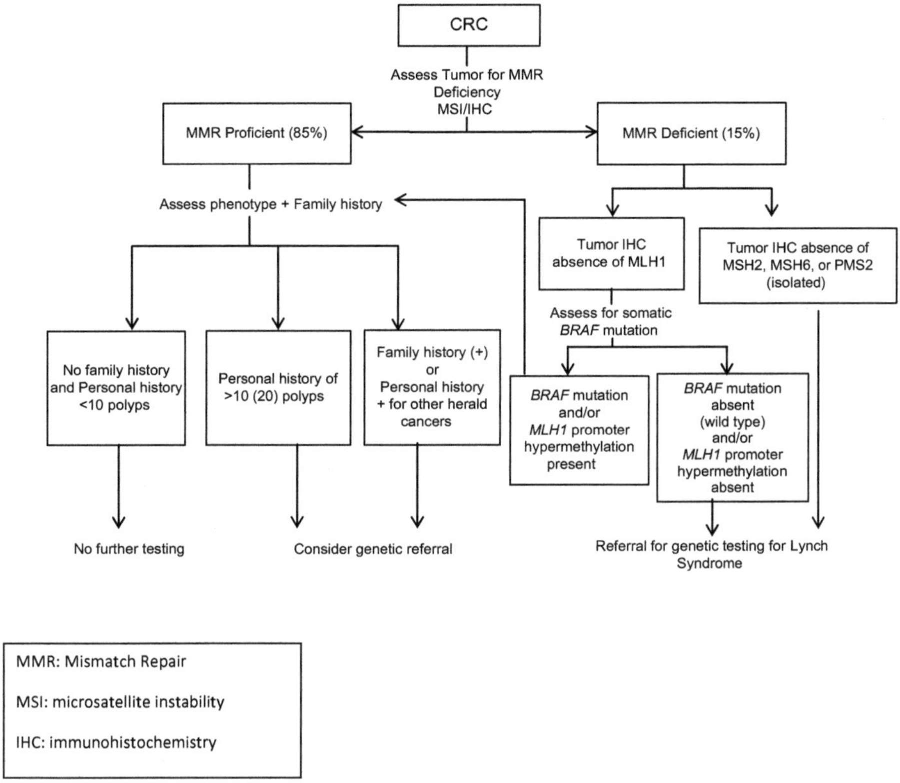

Fig. 1.1 Algorithm for assessing colorectal cancer patients for hereditary cancer syndromes

nonpolyposis colorectal cancer cases affecting multiple generations (Fig. 1.2). Collection of data and biospecimens from families identified in the United States and Europe made it possible to quantify increased incidence of not only colorectal but also gastric and endometrial cancers in these kindreds. Eventually, family history criteria (≥3 individuals with CRC, involving ≥2 generations, with ≥1 diagnosed at age < 50) were established as a means for identifying families to be recruited for study to ascertain biological basis of these familial cancers [7]. Examination of DNA from CRC tumors demonstrated an unusually large number of mutations in repetitive DNA sequences known as microsatellites, termed microsatellite instability-high (MSI-H), suggesting a novel mechanism of pathogenesis that differentiated these tumors from sporadic CRCs [8, 9]. Linkage analyses performed using germline DNA samples from affected families led investigators to chromosomes 2p and 3p, where germline variants in *MSH2* [10, 11] and *MLH1*

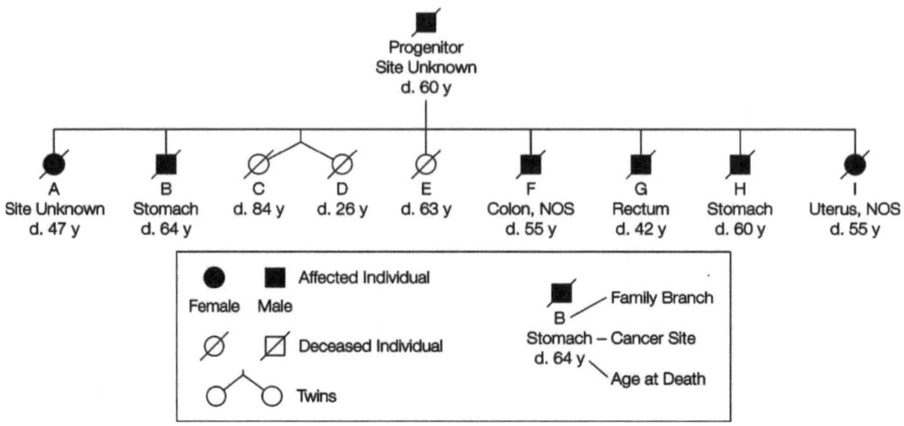

Fig. 1.2 Pedigree of Family G generations I and II (Fig. 2 reproduced from Douglas et al. [87])

[12–15], respectively, were identified. Shortly thereafter, germline variants in *PMS2* [16] and *MSH6* [17] were also discovered; later, deletions of the termination codon in *EPCAM* (also known as *TACSTD1*) associated with promoter methylation and epigenetic silencing of *MSH2*, which is immediately downstream of *EPCAM*, were implicated in a subset of affected families [18]. Today, clinical sequencing identifies pathogenic germline variants in *MLH1*, *MSH2*, *MSH6*, *PMS2*, *or EPCAM* in up to 90% of families with autosomal dominant MSI-H CRCs fulfilling clinical diagnostic criteria for Lynch syndrome.

1.2 Clinical Features and Epidemiology

Defining the biological basis of Lynch syndrome made it possible to identify affected families not only by clinical history but also by tumor molecular phenotype. Approximately 15% of all CRCs exhibit MSI-H phenotypes [19], with Lynch syndrome consistently implicated in 2.8–3.1% of all CRCs (roughly 20% of MSI-H CRCs) [20, 21], establishing it as the most common of the known hereditary colorectal cancer syndromes. Pathogenic variants in *MLH1* and *MSH2* account for the majority of germline pathogenic variants identified in Lynch syndrome families diagnosed in clinical settings. However germline variants in *MSH6* and *PMS2* are estimated to have higher prevalences in the general population, although lower disease penetrance and older ages at CRC diagnosis allow many *MSH6* and *PMS2* families to escape clinical diagnosis [22]. In a recent population-based study from Iceland, pathogenic germline DNA MMR variants were discovered in 0.442%, or 1 in 225 unselected individuals [23], with founder mutations in *MSH6* and *PMS2* accounting for >90%. Other recent population-based data from the United States, Canada, and Australia have estimated a 1 in 279 combined population prevalence of germline MMR mutations with *MSH6* and *PMS2* variants being far more common than those in *MLH1* and *MSH2* [24].

Although Lynch syndrome is best known as a hereditary colorectal cancer syndrome, pathogenic germline variants in DNA MMR genes are also associated with increased risks for other extracolonic cancers, particularly endometrial adenocarcinoma. Variability in age of onset, as well as the diversity of cancer types, has led to a better understanding of the disease spectrum. While some of the variability in cancer risks may be attributed to genotype (Table 1.1), the range of clinical phenotypes, along with differences in penetrance and expressivity among relatives harboring the same germline variant, suggests additional genetic and environmental factors may act as modifiers of cancer risk (see Chap. 5).

1.2.1 Colorectal Cancer

CRC is the predominant cancer in most Lynch syndrome families, and the diagnosis of a MMR-deficient (MMRd) tumor is often the "red flag" that prompts genetic evaluation. Approximately 15% of CRCs exhibit MMRd/MSI-H phenotypes [19], and while most are sporadic cancers (developing through the CIMP-epigenetic serrated neoplastic pathway), 3% arise in the setting of germline mutations in *MLH1*, *MSH2*, *MSH6*, *PMS2*, *or EPCAM*. The protein products of *MLH1*, *MSH2*, *MSH6*, and *PMS2* make up heterodimer complexes that have a critical role in DNA repair. The complex formed

Table 1.1 Estimated lifetime cancer risks (%) in Lynch syndrome, by gene [4, 26, 29, 30, 32–42]

Cancer type	Overall (%)	*MLH1* (%)	*MSH2* (%)	*MSH6* (%)	*PMS2* (%)	*EPCAM* (%)
Colorectal	10–75	25–70	30–60	10–22	10–20	70
Endometrial	14–71	14–54	20–52	34–71	15	12
Ovarian	1–20	4–15	5–17	1–15		
Gastric	1–13	4–11	2–14	1–10		
Small bowel	1–12	4–10	1–8	0–3		
Pancreatic	1–6					
Prostate	4–10					
Urinary tract	2–15	1–10	2–15	1–15		

between MSH2-MSH6 (MutSα) recognizes and binds to single nucleotide base pair mismatches, and small insertion-deletion abnormalities, after which a second heterodimer complex between MLH1-PMS2 (MutLα) binds to MutSα, and recruits exonuclease-1, triggering "long-patch excision" of newly synthesized DNA in the vicinity of the mismatched DNA. The DNA repair proteins quickly release from the DNA permitting resynthesis of the excised patch, usually correctly. Loss of DNA MMR activity results in the rapid accumulation of mutations and a hypermutated genome and eventually mutations in genes that are drivers of carcinogenesis [25]. Lynch-associated CRCs can be distinguished from sporadic MSI-H CRCs in that Lynch-associated tumors almost always lack the somatic *BRAF* mutations and *MLH1* promoter hypermethylation, which are hallmarks of serrated pathway neoplasms. Screening CRC tumors for MMRd, by PCR-based microsatellite analysis or immunohistochemistry (IHC) staining demonstrating loss of expression of MLH1, MSH2, MSH6, or PMS2 proteins, has been advocated as the most effective (and cost-effective) strategy for identifying individuals with Lynch syndrome [3, 4] (see Chap. 17).

Cumulative lifetime risk estimates for CRC in individuals with Lynch syndrome range from 10% to 75% [4, 26–42]. The variability may be explained in part by genotype, with risk for CRC highest for carriers of pathogenic germline variants in *MLH1* and *MSH2*, who also tend to be diagnosed at younger ages. Risk for CRC appears to be somewhat lower for carriers of pathogenic variants in *MSH6* and perhaps much lower for *PMS2* [33, 34, 43, 44]; however it is important to note that there remains significant variability and *MSH6*, *PMS2*, and *EPCAM* mutation carriers are underrepresented in published Lynch syndrome registries, resulting in lack of precision in cancer risk estimates. Consequently, it has been recommended that all Lynch syndrome mutation carriers adhere to intensive cancer surveillance recommendations, regardless of genotype [4, 32, 45].

Lynch-associated CRCs behave differently from sporadic CRCs, which has important implications for clinical management. With respect to oncologic treatment, the histopathologic and molecular characteristics of Lynch-associated CRCs are associated with differences in prognosis and therapeutic responses, in part because the DNA MMR system is involved in triggering cell death after chemotherapy-induced DNA damage, which is missing in CRCs with MSI (see Chaps. 23–25). Tumors arising as a result of defective mismatch repair are also hypermutated and generate neoantigenic peptides which can incite a brisk host immune response. Histopathologic examination of Lynch-associated CRCs often reveals abundant tumor infiltrating lymphocytes. Prognosis in patients with MMRd CRCs tends to be better, stage for stage, compared to MMR-proficient cancers [46]. With regard to oncologic therapies, patients with early-stage MMRd CRCs do not appear to benefit from adjuvant 5-FU monotherapy [47, 48]; however in some patients with metastatic MMRd CRCs, treatment with immune checkpoint inhibitors has been associated with excellent response [49, 50]. Clinical trials with other novel agents are underway and promise to provide additional insights for treatment of Lynch-associated CRC.

The diagnosis of Lynch syndrome also has implications for surgical management of patients with colorectal neoplasia (see Chap. 21). As metachronous primary CRC tumors are common in Lynch syndrome [51, 52], more extensive colonic resections (e.g., subtotal colectomy) should be considered for patients with colorectal neoplasia who require surgery [4, 32, 45].

With regard to CRC prevention, early and frequent colonoscopic surveillance has been shown to be effective in reducing CRC incidence and mortality [53–55] justifying recommendations for colonoscopy every 1–2 years beginning at age 20–25 [4, 32, 45]. However it is important to note that colonoscopy may not afford perfect protection, as interval CRCs have been reported in patients compliant with intensive surveillance [44, 54–57]. While rapid progression and flat morphology of Lynch-associated polyps likely play a role in development of these interval cancers, reports of hypermutated aberrant crypt foci raise the question of whether some Lynch-associated CRCs arise from flat dysplasia rather than from discrete polyps [58]. Enhanced endoscopic technologies (e.g., chromoendoscopy, narrow band imaging/NBI) may help improve visualization of these lesions [59], and additional strategies for early detection are being investigated.

Chemoprevention of Lynch-associated neoplasia remains an area of active research. The Colorectal Adenoma/Carcinoma Prevention Programme 2 (CAPP2) trial randomized subjects with Lynch syndrome to aspirin at a dose of 600 mg daily vs placebo and found approximately 60% reduction in incident CRCs and endometrial cancers in subjects randomized to aspirin, although the reductions were not detectable until a decade after the initial aspirin exposure [60]. Additional studies are currently underway to determine the optimum dose of aspirin and assess whether other nonsteroidal anti-inflammatory drugs may offer similar benefits (see Chap. 22).

1.2.2 Endometrial Cancer

Endometrial adenocarcinoma is the second most common cancer reported in families with Lynch syndrome. Lynch syndrome is implicated in approximately 3% of endometrial cancers, providing justification for screening all endometrial cancers diagnosed at age < 70 for MMRd phenotypes [32, 61, 62]. Approximately 20–30% of all endometrial cancers exhibit MMRd, and while most of these are sporadic tumors associated with somatic hypermethylation of the *MLH1* promoter, patients with MMRd endometrial cancers that do not exhibit *MLH1* promoter hypermethylation warrant referral for genetic evaluation for germline mutations in the MMR genes [62]. The cumulative lifetime risk for endometrial cancer in women with Lynch syndrome ranges from 14% to 71% [26–30, 34,

63]. While screening women for gynecologic cancers annually beginning at age 30–35 years using endometrial biopsy and/or transvaginal ultrasound has been endorsed by Lynch syndrome guidelines [4, 32, 45], prophylactic hysterectomy is the only intervention proven to be effective in reducing gynecologic cancer incidence [64] and should be discussed with women with Lynch syndrome who have completed childbearing.

1.2.3 Other Lynch Syndrome-Associated Cancers

Tumors other than CRC and endometrial cancer are overrepresented in families with Lynch syndrome (Table 1.1) [29, 30, 36, 65, 66]. Despite significant variability in disease penetrance and expressivity, risks for extracolonic tumors appear to be highest among *MSH2* mutation carriers [28, 35, 67]. While gastric cancers were among the most prominent tumors affecting Family G (when reported in 1913) and remain common in Lynch syndrome families in endemic areas such as Japan and Korea, the incidence of gastric cancer in families living in North America and Europe appears to be declining, with lifetime risk estimated between 5% and 13% [37]. Surveillance with upper endoscopy, with treatment for *Helicobacter pylori* infection if present, is recommended for MMR mutation carriers. With regard to ovarian cancer, lifetime risks range from 1% to 20%, and the lack of an effective screening test justifies consideration for prophylactic surgical oophorectomy at the time of hysterectomy. Although the absolute risk of cutaneous sebaceous neoplasms is small and likely varies widely family to family, routine dermatologic screening is recommended for Lynch syndrome carriers. Risks for small bowel, brain, urinary tract, hepatobiliary, and prostate cancers are also increased in Lynch syndrome; however, the benefit of surveillance for these cancers remains unproven and is not routinely recommended. Studies demonstrating a fourfold higher risk for pancreatic cancer in Lynch syndrome families compared with the general population [39] have led some to recommend MRI- and/or endoscopic ultrasound-based pancreatic cancer screening for MMR mutation carriers with a first degree relative affected with pancreatic cancer [68].

1.3 Approaches to Identifying Individuals at Risk for Lynch Syndrome

Strategies for identifying carriers of pathogenic germline variants in MMR genes include systematic assessment of family cancer history, molecular diagnostic testing of tumors, use of clinical prediction models, and germline DNA testing. While family history has historically been the cornerstone of genetic risk assessment, the variability in disease penetrance and expressivity can significantly limit its sensitivity. Fewer than half of families with genetically confirmed Lynch syndrome have histories that meet the Amsterdam criteria. As most Lynch-associated CRCs exhibit phenotypes of DNA MMRd, the Bethesda guidelines were developed in 1997 [69] and subsequently modified and revised [70] to select which patients with CRC who should undergo MSI testing. However, studies employing screening of unselected CRC tumors for MMRd have demonstrated that algorithms employing the Bethesda guidelines miss up to one third of Lynch syndrome cases [20]. As a result, universal testing of all CRC tumors for MMRd has been advocated as the most effective approach for identification of individuals with Lynch syndrome [4, 71] (see Chap. 17).

1.3.1 Molecular Tumor Profiling

Multiple studies have employed universal testing of CRC tumors for MMRd with IHC and/or PCR-based MSI testing, demonstrating high sensitivity (77–90%) for identifying individuals with Lynch syndrome [72], surpassing that of family history-based diagnostic algorithms such as Amsterdam criteria and Bethesda guidelines [20, 73]. While the efficacy for universal testing of endometrial cancers for MMRd has been shown to be similarly effective, the sensitivity of molecular testing in other tumor types has not been extensively studied. It is important to note that tumor molecular profiling of CRCs and endometrial cancers is neither perfectly sensitive nor specific for Lynch syndrome. Some individuals with germline mutations in MMR genes (in particular *MSH6* and *PMS2*) have tumors that are MMR proficient. There are also MMRd CRCs and endometrial cancers in which the cause of the MMRd cannot be identified. While it had been assumed that MMRd tumors lacking somatic *BRAF* mutations or *MLH1* promoter methylation must harbor a germline MMR gene mutation, recent findings from comprehensive molecular profiling of these tumors suggest that as many as half of these have biallelic somatic mutations in DNA MMR genes in the tumor that are not present in the germline DNA, which has bome to be referred to as Lynch-like syndrome (see Chap. 2) [74, 75].

1.3.2 Computational Risk Models

While universal tumor molecular profiling has been proposed to be the most cost-effective strategy for identifying patients with cancer who require genetic evaluation for Lynch syndrome [76], not every patient will have a tumor available for testing. A number of computational models (e.g., MMRPro [77], PREMM1,2,6 [78], PREMM5 [79]) have been developed that incorporate data from individuals' personal and family history to calculate a predicted probability of a MMR gene mutation, with germline sequencing for MMR genes recommended for patients when there is a predicted probability ≥5%. Modeling of a strategy screening asymptomatic young adults using PREMM1,2,6 model scores concluded this would be a cost-effective intervention for reducing morbidity and mortality related to Lynch-associated cancers [80]. The recently developed PREMM5 model, which is the only model to incorporate *PMS2* and *EPCAM* risk assessment, proposes lowering the threshold for germline sequencing to individuals with predicted probability of mutation of ≥2.5%; however the limited sensitivity of family history and/or computational models for identifying *PMS2* carriers remains a concern [79]. See Chap. 19 for detailed information on computational risk models.

1.4 Summary

While significant progress has been made over the past three decades in defining the biological basis of Lynch syndrome, there remains work to be done implementing clinical interventions to effectively diagnose and manage families affected with Lynch syndrome. The vast majority of at-risk individuals remain undiagnosed and operationalizing universal screening of CRCs and presymptomatic identification of individuals requiring intensive surveillance continue to present major challenges. Despite innovations in sequencing technologies, one in ten families with presumed Lynch syndrome undergoes germline genetic testing that yields clinical uninformative results. Sequencing of *PMS2* remains challenging due to the presence of 20 pseudogenes; series of *Alu* repeats in *MSH2* make the 5′ end of the gene and promoter region susceptible to large deletions that are difficult to detect. Germline variants of uncertain significance (VUS) are common in patients of non-European ancestry, and accurate reclassification of these has been challenging (see Chap. 29).

There are additional mechanisms that give rise to tumors with MMRd. Constitutional methylation of the *MLH1* promoter has been identified in individuals and in rare families may be caused by a single nucleotide variant near the transcriptional start site in the promoter of *MLH1* (c.-27C>A) which renders the promoter prone to methylation [81, 82]. The contributions of genetic, epigenetic, and/or environmental factors to modifying disease penetrance and expressivity both within and among families with Lynch syndrome remain to be elucidated.

Making the diagnosis of Lynch syndrome has immediate implications not only for the clinical management of cancer patients but also for care of their family members. While the importance of integrating cancer risk assessment for hereditary cancer syndromes into routine clinical care of patients (with and without cancer diagnoses) has been highlighted by many professional societies [4, 45, 62, 83–86], variability in genomic literacy among patients and providers and complexities of disease management present additional challenges. Cost-effectiveness models suggest the greatest benefit of genetic testing results from preventing cancers in the relatives of cancer patients [3]; however limited availability of genetics expertise and the costs of genetic testing continue to present barriers to implementation.

Translating genetic test results into improved health outcomes requires interdisciplinary collaboration between oncologists, surgeons, geneticists, gastroenterologists, gynecologists, and primary care providers. Assuring that information gained through genetic testing is shared with close as well as more distant relatives, facilitating so-called cascade testing of at-risk family members, and ensuring that MMR mutation carriers comply with recommended surveillance tests will continue to be areas for intervention. Finally, even though it is becoming apparent that germline mutations in DNA MMR genes are much more common than previously thought, Lynch syndrome remains unrecognized in many patients because of variations in disease penetrance and expressivity. More data are needed to understand the contributions of modifiable risk factors and to maximize effectiveness of primary and secondary cancer prevention strategies for at-risk families.

References

1. Fuchs CS, Giovannucci EL, Colditz GA, Hunter DJ, Speizer FE, Willett WC. A prospective study of family history and the risk of colorectal cancer. N Engl J Med. 1994;331(25):1669–74. https://doi.org/10.1056/NEJM199412223312501.
2. Vasen HF, Watson P, Mecklin JP, Lynch HT. New clinical criteria for hereditary nonpolyposis colorectal cancer (HNPCC, Lynch syndrome) proposed by the International Collaborative group on HNPCC. Gastroenterology. 1999;116(6):1453–6.
3. Evaluation of Genomic Applications in P, Prevention Working G. Recommendations from the EGAPP Working Group: genetic testing strategies in newly diagnosed individuals with colorectal cancer aimed at reducing morbidity and mortality from Lynch syndrome in relatives. Genet Med. 2009;11(1):35–41. https://doi.org/10.1097/GIM.0b013e31818fa2ff.
4. Giardiello FM, Allen JI, Axilbund JE, Boland CR, Burke CA, Burt RW, et al. Guidelines on genetic evaluation and management of Lynch syndrome: a consensus statement by the US Multi-Society Task Force on colorectal cancer. Gastroenterology. 2014;147(2):502–26. https://doi.org/10.1053/j.gastro.2014.04.001.
5. Boland CR, Lynch HT. The history of Lynch syndrome. Familial Cancer. 2013;12(2):145–57. https://doi.org/10.1007/s10689-013-9637-8.
6. Warthin AS. The further study of a cancer family. J Cancer Research. 1925;9:279–86.
7. Vasen HF, Mecklin JP, Khan PM, Lynch HT. The international collaborative group on hereditary non-polyposis colorectal cancer (ICG-HNPCC). Dis Colon Rectum. 1991;34(5):424–5.
8. Thibodeau SN, Bren G, Schaid D. Microsatellite instability in cancer of the proximal colon. Science. 1993;260(5109):816–9.
9. Ionov Y, Peinado MA, Malkhosyan S, Shibata D, Perucho M. Ubiquitous somatic mutations in simple repeated sequences reval a new mechanism for colonic carcinogenesis. Nature. 1993;363(6429):558–561.
10. Fishel R, Lescoe MK, Rao MR, Copeland NG, Jenkins NA, Garber J, et al. The human mutator gene homolog MSH2 and its association with hereditary nonpolyposis colon cancer. Cell. 1994;77(1):1. p following 166.

11. Leach FS, Nicolaides NC, Papadopoulos N, Liu B, Jen J, Parsons R, et al. Mutations of a mutS homolog in hereditary nonpolyposis colorectal cancer. Cell. 1993;75(6):1215–25.
12. Peltomaki P, Aaltonen LA, Sistonen P, Pylkkanen L, Mecklin JP, Jarvinen H, et al. Genetic mapping of a locus predisposing to human colorectal cancer. Science. 1993;260(5109):810–2.
13. Lindblom A, Tannergard P, Werelius B, Nordenskjold M. Genetic mapping of a second locus predisposing to hereditary non-polyposis colon cancer. Nat Genet. 1993;5(3):279–82. https://doi.org/10.1038/ng1193-279.
14. Bronner CE, Baker SM, Morrison PT et al. Mutation in the DNA Mismatch Repair gene homologue hMLH1 is associated with hereditary non-polyposis colon cancer. Nature. 1994; 368(6468): 258–261.
15. Papadopoulos N, Nicolaides NC, Wei YF et al. Mutation of a mutL homolog in hereditary colon cancer. Science. 1994;263(5153):1625–29.
16. Nicolaides NC, Papadopoulos N, Liu B, Wei YF, Carter KC, Ruben SM, et al. Mutations of two PMS homologues in hereditary nonpolyposis colon cancer. Nature. 1994;371(6492):75–80. https://doi.org/10.1038/371075a0.
17. Miyaki M, Konishi M, Tanaka K, Kikuchi-Yanoshita R, Muraoka M, Yasuno M, et al. Germline mutation of MSH6 as the cause of hereditary nonpolyposis colorectal cancer. Nat Genet. 1997;17(3):271–2. https://doi.org/10.1038/ng1197-271.
18. Ligtenberg MJ, Kuiper RP, Chan TL, Goossens M, Hebeda KM, Voorendt M, et al. Heritable somatic methylation and inactivation of MSH2 in families with Lynch syndrome due to deletion of the 3′ exons of TACSTD1. Nat Genet. 2009;41(1):112–7. https://doi.org/10.1038/ng.283.
19. Boland CR, Thibodeau SN, Hamilton SR, Sidransky D, Eshleman JR, Burt RW, et al. A National Cancer Institute Workshop on Microsatellite Instability for cancer detection and familial predisposition: development of international criteria for the determination of microsatellite instability in colorectal cancer. Cancer Res. 1998;58(22):5248–57.
20. Hampel H, Frankel WL, Martin E, Arnold M, Khanduja K, Kuebler P, et al. Screening for the Lynch syndrome (hereditary nonpolyposis colorectal cancer). N Engl J Med. 2005;352(18):1851–60.
21. Yurgelun MB, Kulke MH, Fuchs CS, Allen BA, Uno H, Hornick JL, et al. Cancer susceptibility gene mutations in individuals with colorectal cancer. J Clin Oncol. 2017;35(10):1086–95. https://doi.org/10.1200/JCO.2016.71.0012.
22. Goodenberger ML, Thomas BC, Riegert-Johnson D, Boland CR, Plon SE, Clendenning M, et al. PMS2 monoallelic mutation carriers: the known unknown. Genet Med. 2016;18(1):13–9. https://doi.org/10.1038/gim.2015.27.
23. Haraldsdottir S, Rafnar T, Frankel WL, Einarsdottir S, Sigurdsson A, Hampel H, et al. Comprehensive population-wide analysis of Lynch syndrome in Iceland reveals founder mutations in MSH6 and PMS2. Nat Commun. 2017;8:14755. https://doi.org/10.1038/ncomms14755.
24. Win AK, Jenkins MA, Dowty JG, Antoniou AC, Lee A, Giles GG, et al. Prevalence and penetrance of major genes and polygenes for colorectal cancer. Cancer Epidemiol Biomark Prev. 2017;26(3):404–12. https://doi.org/10.1158/1055-9965.EPI-16-0693.
25. Pinheiro M, Pinto C, Peixoto A, Veiga I, Lopes P, Henrique R, et al. Target gene mutational pattern in Lynch syndrome colorectal carcinomas according to tumour location and germline mutation. Br J Cancer. 2015;113(4):686–92. https://doi.org/10.1038/bjc.2015.281.
26. Quehenberger F, Vasen HF, van Houwelingen HC. Risk of colorectal and endometrial cancer for carriers of mutations of the hMLH1 and hMSH2 gene: correction for ascertainment. J Med Genet. 2005;42(6):491–6. 42/6/491 [pii]. https://doi.org/10.1136/jmg.2004.024299.
27. Jenkins MA, Baglietto L, Dowty JG, Van Vliet CM, Smith L, Mead LJ, et al. Cancer risks for mismatch repair gene mutation carriers: a population-based early onset case-family study. Clin

Gastroenterol Hepatol. 2006;4(4):489–98. https://doi.org/10.1016/j.cgh.2006.01.002. S1542-3565(06)00049-8 [pii].
28. Stoffel E, Mukherjee B, Raymond VM, Tayob N, Kastrinos F, Sparr J, et al. Calculation of risk of colorectal and endometrial cancer among patients with Lynch syndrome. Gastroenterology. 2009;137(5):1621–7. https://doi.org/10.1053/j.gastro.2009.07.039. S0016-5085(09)01158-5 [pii].
29. Aarnio M, Sankila R, Pukkala E, Salovaara R, Aaltonen LA, de la Chapelle A, et al. Cancer risk in mutation carriers of DNA-mismatch-repair genes. Int J Cancer. 1999;81(2): 214–8.
30. Moller P, Seppala TT, Bernstein I, Holinski-Feder E, Sala P, Gareth Evans D, et al. Cancer risk and survival in path_MMR carriers by gene and gender up to 75 years of age: a report from the Prospective Lynch Syndrome Database. Gut. 2017. https://doi.org/10.1136/gutjnl-2017-314057.
31. Win AK, Lindor NM, Winship I, Tucker KM, Buchanan DD, Young JP, et al. Risks of colorectal and other cancers after endometrial cancer for women with Lynch syndrome. J Natl Cancer Inst. 2013;105(4):274–9. https://doi.org/10.1093/jnci/djs525.
32. Vasen HF, Blanco I, Aktan-Collan K, Gopie JP, Alonso A, Aretz S, et al. Revised guidelines for the clinical management of Lynch syndrome (HNPCC): recommendations by a group of European experts. Gut. 2013;62(6):812–23. https://doi.org/10.1136/gutjnl-2012-304356.
33. Senter L, Clendenning M, Sotamaa K, Hampel H, Green J, Potter JD, et al. The clinical phenotype of Lynch syndrome due to germ-line PMS2 mutations. Gastroenterology. 2008;135(2):419–28. https://doi.org/10.1053/j.gastro.2008.04.026. S0016-5085(08)00737-3 [pii].
34. Baglietto L, Lindor NM, Dowty JG, White DM, Wagner A, Gomez Garcia EB, et al. Risks of Lynch syndrome cancers for MSH6 mutation carriers. J Natl Cancer Inst. 2010;102(3):193–201. https://doi.org/10.1093/jnci/djp473. djp473 [pii].
35. Vasen HF, Stormorken A, Menko FH, Nagengast FM, Kleibeuker JH, Griffioen G, et al. MSH2 mutation carriers are at higher risk of cancer than MLH1 mutation carriers: a study of hereditary nonpolyposis colorectal cancer families. J Clin Oncol. 2001;19(20):4074–80.
36. Engel C, Loeffler M, Steinke V, Rahner N, Holinski-Feder E, Dietmaier W, et al. Risks of less common cancers in proven mutation carriers with Lynch syndrome. J Clin Oncol. 2012;30(35):4409–15. https://doi.org/10.1200/JCO.2012.43.2278.
37. Capelle LG, Van Grieken NC, Lingsma HF, Steyerberg EW, Klokman WJ, Bruno MJ, et al. Risk and epidemiological time trends of gastric cancer in Lynch syndrome carriers in the Netherlands. Gastroenterology. 2010;138(2):487–92. https://doi.org/10.1053/j.gastro.2009.10.051. S0016-5085(09)01948-9 [pii].
38. van der Post RS, Kiemeney LA, Ligtenberg MJ, Witjes JA, Hulsbergen-van de Kaa CA, Bodmer D, et al. Risk of urothelial bladder cancer in Lynch syndrome is increased, in particular among MSH2 mutation carriers. J Med Genet. 2010;47(7):464–70. https://doi.org/10.1136/jmg.2010.076992.
39. Kastrinos F, Mukherjee B, Tayob N, Wang F, Sparr J, Raymond VM, et al. Risk of pancreatic cancer in families with Lynch syndrome. JAMA. 2009;302(16):1790–5. https://doi.org/10.1001/jama.2009.1529. 302/16/1790 [pii].
40. Win AK, Young JP, Lindor NM, Tucker KM, Ahnen DJ, Young GP, et al. Colorectal and other cancer risks for carriers and noncarriers from families with a DNA mismatch repair gene mutation: a prospective cohort study. J Clin Oncol. 2012;30(9):958–64. https://doi.org/10.1200/JCO.2011.39.5590.
41. Raymond VM, Mukherjee B, Wang F, Huang SC, Stoffel EM, Kastrinos F, et al. Elevated risk of prostate cancer among men with Lynch syndrome. J Clin Oncol. 2013;31(14):1713–8. https://doi.org/10.1200/JCO.2012.44.1238.

42. Kempers MJ, Kuiper RP, Ockeloen CW, Chappuis PO, Hutter P, Rahner N, et al. Risk of colorectal and endometrial cancers in EPCAM deletion-positive Lynch syndrome: a cohort study. Lancet Oncol. 2011;12(1):49–55. https://doi.org/10.1016/S1470-2045(10)70265-5. S1470-2045(10)70265-5 [pii].
43. Goodenberger ML, Thomas BC, Riegert-Johnson D, Boland CR, Plon SE, Clendenning M, et al. PMS2 monoallelic mutation carriers: the known unknown. Genet Med. 2015. https://doi.org/10.1038/gim.2015.27.
44. Moller P, Seppala T, Bernstein I, Holinski-Feder E, Sala P, Evans DG, et al. Cancer incidence and survival in Lynch syndrome patients receiving colonoscopic and gynaecological surveillance: first report from the prospective Lynch syndrome database. Gut. 2017;66(3):464–72. https://doi.org/10.1136/gutjnl-2015-309675.
45. Syngal S, Brand RE, Church JM, Giardiello FM, Hampel HL, Burt RW, et al. ACG clinical guideline: genetic testing and management of hereditary gastrointestinal cancer syndromes. Am J Gastroenterol. 2015;110(2):223–62.; quiz 63. https://doi.org/10.1038/ajg.2014.435.
46. Gryfe R, Kim H, Hsieh ET, Aronson MD, Holowaty EJ, Bull SB, et al. Tumor microsatellite instability and clinical outcome in young patients with colorectal cancer. N Engl J Med. 2000;342(2):69–77. https://doi.org/10.1056/NEJM200001133420201.
47. Carethers JM, Smith EJ, Behling CA, Nguyen L, Tajima A, Doctolero RT, et al. Use of 5-fluorouracil and survival in patients with microsatellite-unstable colorectal cancer. Gastroenterology. 2004;126(2):394–401.
48. Ribic CM, Sargent DJ, Moore MJ, Thibodeau SN, French AJ, Goldberg RM, et al. Tumor microsatellite-instability status as a predictor of benefit from fluorouracil-based adjuvant chemotherapy for colon cancer. N Engl J Med. 2003;349(3):247–57. https://doi.org/10.1056/NEJMoa022289.
49. Le DT, Uram JN, Wang H, Bartlett BR, Kemberling H, Eyring AD, et al. PD-1 blockade in tumors with mismatch-repair deficiency. N Engl J Med. 2015;372(26):2509–20. https://doi.org/10.1056/NEJMoa1500596.
50. Le DT, Durham JN, Smith KN, Wang H, Bartlett BR, Aulakh LK, et al. Mismatch repair deficiency predicts response of solid tumors to PD-1 blockade. Science. 2017;357(6349):409–13. https://doi.org/10.1126/science.aan6733.
51. Parry S, Win AK, Parry B, Macrae FA, Gurrin LC, Church JM, et al. Metachronous colorectal cancer risk for mismatch repair gene mutation carriers: the advantage of more extensive colon surgery. Gut. 2011;60(7):950–7. https://doi.org/10.1136/gut.2010.228056.
52. Win AK, Parry S, Parry B, Kalady MF, Macrae FA, Ahnen DJ, et al. Risk of metachronous colon cancer following surgery for rectal cancer in mismatch repair gene mutation carriers. Ann Surg Oncol. 2013;20(6):1829–36. https://doi.org/10.1245/s10434-012-2858-5.
53. Vasen HF, Abdirahman M, Brohet R, Langers AM, Kleibeuker JH, van Kouwen M, et al. One to 2-year surveillance intervals reduce risk of colorectal cancer in families with Lynch syndrome. Gastroenterology. 2010;138(7):2300–6. https://doi.org/10.1053/j.gastro.2010.02.053. S0016-5085(10)00326-4 [pii].
54. Jarvinen HJ, Renkonen-Sinisalo L, Aktan-Collan K, Peltomaki P, Aaltonen LA, Mecklin JP. Ten years after mutation testing for Lynch syndrome: cancer incidence and outcome in mutation-positive and mutation-negative family members. J Clin Oncol. 2009;27(28):4793–7. https://doi.org/10.1200/JCO.2009.23.7784.
55. Engel C, Rahner N, Schulmann K, Holinski-Feder E, Goecke TO, Schackert HK, et al. Efficacy of annual colonoscopic surveillance in individuals with hereditary nonpolyposis colorectal cancer. Clin Gastroenterol Hepatol. 2010;8(2):174–82. https://doi.org/10.1016/j.cgh.2009.10.003.
56. Edelstein DL, Axilbund J, Baxter M, Hylind LM, Romans K, Griffin CA, et al. Rapid development of colorectal neoplasia in patients with Lynch syndrome. Clin Gastroenterol Hepatol: Off Clin Pract J Am Gastroenterol Assoc. 2011;9(4):340–3. https://doi.org/10.1016/j.cgh.2010.10.033.

57. Lynch HT, de la Chapelle A. Hereditary colorectal cancer. N Engl J Med. 2003;348(10):919–32. https://doi.org/10.1056/NEJMra012242. 348/10/919 [pii].
58. Ahadova A, von Knebel Doeberitz M, Blaker H, Kloor M. CTNNB1-mutant colorectal carcinomas with immediate invasive growth: a model of interval cancers in Lynch syndrome. Familial Cancer. 2016;15(4):579–86. https://doi.org/10.1007/s10689-016-9899-z.
59. Kaminski MF, Hassan C, Bisschops R, Pohl J, Pellise M, Dekker E, et al. Advanced imaging for detection and differentiation of colorectal neoplasia: European Society of Gastrointestinal Endoscopy (ESGE) Guideline. Endoscopy. 2014;46(5):435–49. https://doi.org/10.1055/s-0034-1365348.
60. Burn J, Gerdes AM, Macrae F, Mecklin JP, Moeslein G, Olschwang S, et al. Long-term effect of aspirin on cancer risk in carriers of hereditary colorectal cancer: an analysis from the CAPP2 randomised controlled trial. Lancet. 2011;378(9809):2081–7. https://doi.org/10.1016/S0140-6736(11)61049-0.
61. Goverde A, Spaander MC, van Doorn HC, Dubbink HJ, van den Ouweland AM, Tops CM, et al. Cost-effectiveness of routine screening for Lynch syndrome in endometrial cancer patients up to 70years of age. Gynecol Oncol. 2016;143(3):453–9. https://doi.org/10.1016/j.ygyno.2016.10.008.
62. Committee on Practice B-G, Society of Gynecologic O. ACOG Practice Bulletin No. 147: Lynch syndrome. Obstet Gynecol. 2014;124(5):1042–54. https://doi.org/10.1097/01.AOG.0000456325.50739.72.
63. Bonadona V, Bonaiti B, Olschwang S, Grandjouan S, Huiart L, Longy M, et al. Cancer risks associated with germline mutations in MLH1, MSH2, and MSH6 genes in Lynch syndrome. JAMA. 2011;305(22):2304–10. https://doi.org/10.1001/jama.2011.743.
64. Schmeler KM, Lynch HT, Chen LM, Munsell MF, Soliman PT, Clark MB, et al. Prophylactic surgery to reduce the risk of gynecologic cancers in the Lynch syndrome. N Engl J Med. 2006;354(3):261–9. https://doi.org/10.1056/NEJMoa052627.
65. Win AK, Lindor NM, Young JP, Macrae FA, Young GP, Williamson E, et al. Risks of primary extracolonic cancers following colorectal cancer in Lynch syndrome. J Natl Cancer Inst. 2012;104(18):1363–72. https://doi.org/10.1093/jnci/djs351.
66. Watson P, Vasen HF, Mecklin JP, Bernstein I, Aarnio M, Jarvinen HJ, et al. The risk of extra-colonic, extra-endometrial cancer in the Lynch syndrome. Int J Cancer. 2008;123(2):444–9. https://doi.org/10.1002/ijc.23508.
67. Kastrinos F, Stoffel EM, Balmana J, Steyerberg EW, Mercado R, Syngal S. Phenotype comparison of MLH1 and MSH2 mutation carriers in a cohort of 1,914 individuals undergoing clinical genetic testing in the United States. Cancer Epidemiol Biomark Prev. 2008;17(8):2044–51. https://doi.org/10.1158/1055-9965.EPI-08-0301. 17/8/2044 [pii].
68. Canto MI, Harinck F, Hruban RH, Offerhaus GJ, Poley JW, Kamel I, et al. International Cancer of the Pancreas Screening (CAPS) Consortium summit on the management of patients with increased risk for familial pancreatic cancer. Gut. 2013;62(3):339–47. https://doi.org/10.1136/gutjnl-2012-303108.
69. Rodriguez-Bigas MA, Boland CR, Hamilton SR, Henson DE, Jass JR, Khan PM, et al. A National Cancer Institute Workshop on Hereditary Nonpolyposis Colorectal Cancer Syndrome: meeting highlights and Bethesda guidelines. J Natl Cancer Inst. 1997;89(23):1758–62.
70. Umar A, Boland CR, Terdiman JP, Syngal S, de la Chapelle A, Ruschoff J, et al. Revised Bethesda Guidelines for hereditary nonpolyposis colorectal cancer (Lynch syndrome) and microsatellite instability. J Natl Cancer Inst. 2004;96(4):261–8.
71. Moreira L, Balaguer F, Lindor N, de la Chapelle A, Hampel H, Aaltonen LA, et al. Identification of Lynch syndrome among patients with colorectal cancer. JAMA. 2012;308(15):1555–65. https://doi.org/10.1001/jama.2012.13088. 1383232 [pii].

72. Palomaki GE, McClain MR, Melillo S, Hampel HL, Thibodeau SN. EGAPP supplementary evidence review: DNA testing strategies aimed at reducing morbidity and mortality from Lynch syndrome. Genet Med. 2009;11(1):42–65. https://doi.org/10.1097/GIM.0b013e31818fa2db.
73. Hampel H, Frankel WL, Martin E, Arnold M, Khanduja K, Kuebler P, et al. Feasibility of screening for Lynch syndrome among patients with colorectal cancer. J Clin Oncol. 2008;26(35):5783–8. https://doi.org/10.1200/JCO.2008.17.5950. JCO.2008.17.5950 [pii].
74. Mensenkamp AR, Vogelaar IP, van Zelst-Stams WA, Goossens M, Ouchene H, Hendriks-Cornelissen SJ, et al. Somatic mutations in MLH1 and MSH2 are a frequent cause of mismatch-repair deficiency in Lynch syndrome-like tumors. Gastroenterology. 2014;146(3):643–6 e8. https://doi.org/10.1053/j.gastro.2013.12.002.
75. Haraldsdottir S, Hampel H, Tomsic J, Frankel WL, Pearlman R, de la Chapelle A, et al. Colon and endometrial cancers with mismatch repair deficiency can arise from somatic, rather than germline, mutations. Gastroenterology. 2014;147(6):1308–16 e1. https://doi.org/10.1053/j.gastro.2014.08.041.
76. Ladabaum U, Wang G, Terdiman J, Blanco A, Kuppermann M, Boland CR, et al. Strategies to identify the Lynch syndrome among patients with colorectal cancer: a cost-effectiveness analysis. Ann Intern Med. 2011;155(2):69–79. https://doi.org/10.1059/0003-4819-155-2-201107190-00002. 155/2/69 [pii].
77. Chen S, Wang W, Lee S, Nafa K, Lee J, Romans K, et al. Prediction of germline mutations and cancer risk in the Lynch syndrome. JAMA. 2006;296(12):1479–87. https://doi.org/10.1001/jama.296.12.1479.
78. Kastrinos F, Steyerberg EW, Mercado R, Balmana J, Holter S, Gallinger S, et al. The PREMM(1,2,6) model predicts risk of MLH1, MSH2, and MSH6 germline mutations based on cancer history. Gastroenterology. 2011;140(1):73–81. https://doi.org/10.1053/j.gastro.2010.08.021. S0016-5085(10)01239-4 [pii].
79. Kastrinos F, Uno H, Ukaegbu C, Alvero C, McFarland A, Yurgelun MB, et al. Development and validation of the PREMM5 model for comprehensive risk assessment of Lynch syndrome. J Clin Oncol. 2017;35(19):2165–72. https://doi.org/10.1200/JCO.2016.69.6120.
80. Dinh TA, Rosner BI, Atwood JC, Boland CR, Syngal S, Vasen HF, et al. Health benefits and cost-effectiveness of primary genetic screening for Lynch syndrome in the general population. Cancer Prev Res (Phila). 2011;4(1):9–22. https://doi.org/10.1158/1940-6207.CAPR-10-0262. 1940-6207.CAPR-10-0262 [pii].
81. Hitchins MP, Wong JJ, Suthers G, Suter CM, Martin DI, Hawkins NJ, et al. Inheritance of a cancer-associated MLH1 germ-line epimutation. N Engl J Med. 2007;356(7):697–705. https://doi.org/10.1056/NEJMoa064522.
82. Hitchins MP, Rapkins RW, Kwok CT, Srivastava S, Wong JJ, Khachigian LM, et al. Dominantly inherited constitutional epigenetic silencing of MLH1 in a cancer-affected family is linked to a single nucleotide variant within the 5'UTR. Cancer Cell. 2011;20(2):200–13. https://doi.org/10.1016/j.ccr.2011.07.003.
83. Robson ME, Storm CD, Weitzel J, Wollins DS, Offit K. American Society of Clinical O. American Society of Clinical Oncology policy statement update: genetic and genomic testing for cancer susceptibility. J Clin Oncol : Off J Am Soc Clin Oncol. 2010;28(5):893–901. https://doi.org/10.1200/JCO.2009.27.0660.
84. Hampel H, Bennett RL, Buchanan A, Pearlman R, Wiesner GL, Guideline Development Group ACoMG, et al. A practice guideline from the American College of Medical Genetics and Genomics and the National Society of Genetic Counselors: referral indications for cancer predisposition assessment. Genet Med. 2015;17(1):70–87. https://doi.org/10.1038/gim.2014.147.

85. Lu KH, Wood ME, Daniels M, Burke C, Ford J, Kauff ND, et al. American Society of Clinical Oncology expert statement: collection and use of a cancer family history for oncology providers. J Clin Oncol: Off J Am Soc Clin Oncol. 2014;32(8):833–40. https://doi.org/10.1200/JCO.2013.50.9257.
86. Balmana J, Balaguer F, Cervantes A, Arnold D, Group EGW. Familial risk-colorectal cancer: ESMO Clinical Practice Guidelines. Ann Oncol. 2013;24(Suppl 6):vi73–80. https://doi.org/10.1093/annonc/mdt209.
87. Douglas JA, et al. History and molecular genetics of Lynch syndrome in Family G. A century later. JAMA. 2005;294(17):2195–202.

Chapter 2
The Molecular Basis of Lynch-like Syndrome

Gardenia Vargas-Parra, Matilde Navarro, Marta Pineda, and Gabriel Capellá

Abstract Lynch-like syndrome (LLS) refers to individuals with MMR-deficient Lynch syndrome (LS) spectrum tumors (in the absence of *MLH1* methylation), in which no pathogenic germline mutation has been identified. Patients and their first-degree relatives are considered to have an intermediate risk of developing cancer between LS and the general population.

In this chapter, we aimed to review the most promising work in the area. Double somatic variants in MMR genes have been frequently reported (27–82% of LLS cases), while somatic promoter hypermethylation does not play a role. Carriers of germline MMR variants of unknown significance and missed mutations are part of LLS. Germline mutations in *POLE* and biallelic *MUTYH* mutations have been reported rarely. With the advent of NGS technologies, other genes like *FAN1*, *BUB1*, *MCM9*, and *SETD2* are emerging as candidate responsible genes for LLS.

Keywords Lynch syndrome · Lynch-like · Next-generation sequencing · Mismatch repair-deficiency · Methylation · Variant of unknown significance · Double somatic hit

Abbreviations

ASE	Allele-specific expression
CRC	Colorectal cancer
FFPE	Formalin-fixed paraffin embedded
IHC	Immunohistochemistry
LLS	Lynch-like syndrome
LOH	Loss of heterozygosity
LS	Lynch syndrome
MMR	Mismatch repair

G. Vargas-Parra · M. Navarro · M. Pineda · G. Capellá (✉)
Hereditary Cancer Program, Catalan Institute of Oncology, IDIBELL and CIBERONC, Hospitalet de Llobregat, Barcelona, Spain
e-mail: gcapella@iconcologia.net

L. Valle et al. (eds.), *Hereditary Colorectal Cancer*,
https://doi.org/10.1007/978-3-319-74259-5_2

MSI	Microsatellite instability
MS-MCA	Methylation-specific melting curve analysis
NGS	Next-generation sequencing
PBL	Peripheral blood leukocytes
VUS	Variant of unknown significance

1 Definition of Lynch-like Syndrome

Lynch syndrome (LS) is an inherited autosomal dominant cancer syndrome that accounts for 2–4% of all newly diagnosed colorectal and endometrial cancers [1–3]. It is caused by defective mismatch repair (MMR) activity due to germline (epi) mutations in MMR genes (*MLH1*, *MSH2*, *MSH6*, and *PMS2*). The diagnostic algorithm of LS is based on the identification of microsatellite instability (MSI) and/or loss of expression of MMR proteins by immunohistochemistry (IHC) in tumors. After identification of MMR deficiency (in the absence of *MLH1* promoter methylation and/or *BRAF* p.V600E mutation), germline MMR testing is performed.

However, about 50% of patients with MMR-deficient colorectal tumors from population-based studies lack identified pathogenic mutations by conventional analyses, thus hampering appropriate clinical management and risk assessment (Fig. 2.1 and Table 2.1a) [1, 4–12]. Individuals with MMR-deficient LS spectrum tumors

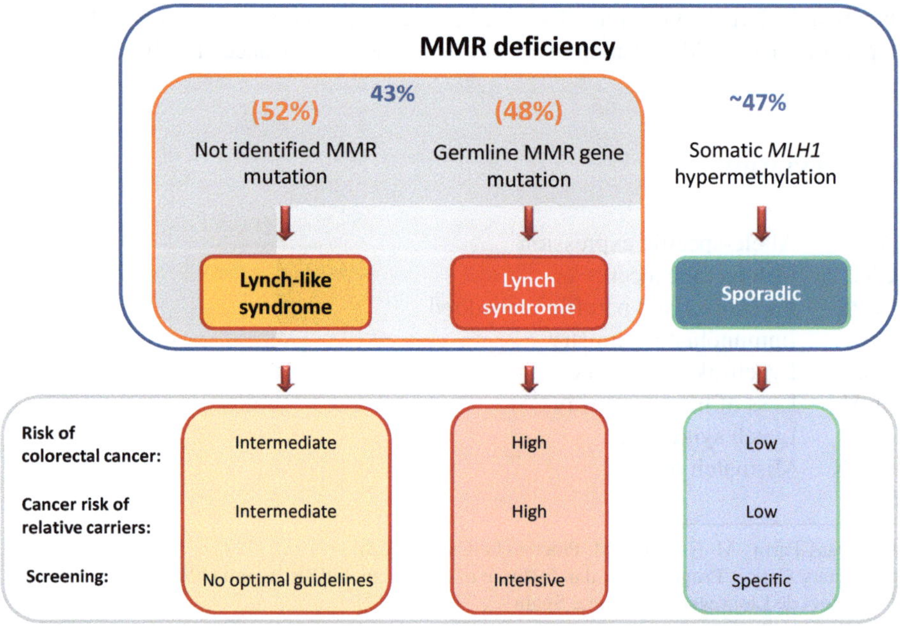

Fig. 2.1 Diagnostic yield and associated risk in MMR-deficient cases. Adapted from Buchanan et al. [12]

Table 2.1a Lynch-like syndrome in colorectal cancer (CRC) population-based studies: Prevalence of Lynch-like syndrome

Study	Hampel [3]	Rodríguez-Soler [5]	Win [6]	Mas-Moya [10]	Kang [8]	Chika [7]	O'Kane [11]	Combined
Country of origin	USA	Spain	Australia	USA	Korea	Japan	Ireland	
Cases screened (IHC, MSI), *n*	1066	1689	4853	3352	4765	1234	2426	19,385
MMR-deficient and germline tested, *n* (%)	85 (8)	135 (8)	592 (12)	356 (10,6)	312 (6,5)	61 (4,9)	62 (2,6)	1603 (8)
MLH1/PMS2 deficiency, *MLH1*-methylated/*BRAF*-mutated, *n*	50	79	250	238	69	22	43	751
MMR deficiency (in the absence of *MLH1*-methylation), *n*	35	56	342	61	124	11	62	691
MLH1/PMS2-deficient LLS (%)	15/19 (79)	21/25 (84)	104/153 (68)	6/14 (43)	42/75 (56)	1/2 (50)	NS	189/288 (66)
MSH2/MSH6-deficient LLS (%)	8/13 (62)	14/22 (64)	45/104 (43)	7/28 (25)	12/46 (26)	1/6 (17)	NS	87/219 (40)
MSH6-deficient LLS (%)	0/1 (0)	3/6 (50)	27/41 (66)	0/7 (0)	1/3 (33)	0/3 (0)	NS	31/84 (37)
PMS2-deficient LLS (%)	1/2 (50)	2/3 (67)	17/44 (39)	3/12 (25)	0/0 (0)	0/0 (0)	NS	23/61 (38)
Total Lynch-like syndrome cases/number tested	24/35	40/56	193/342	15/61	55/124	2/11	27/62	356/691
%LLS (95% confidence interval)	69 (51–83%)	71 (58–83%)	56 (51–62%)	25 (23–27%)	44 (36–52%)	18 (16–20%)	44	52 (50–60%)

(in the absence of *MLH1* methylation), in which no pathogenic germline mutation has been identified, are known as having “Lynch-like syndrome (LLS)” [1, 4–12], also called “suspected Lynch syndrome” [12]. Noteworthy, failure in the identification of pathogenic germline mutations in MMR genes among patients with MMR-deficient tumors does not exclude an inherited predisposition to cancer.

The mean age at colorectal cancer (CRC) diagnosis in LLS cases has been reported similar to LS or in-between LS and sporadic MMR-deficient individuals [1, 4–10] (Table 2.1b). Other clinical similarities amidst LS and LLS in comparison to sporadic CRC are predominance of proximal location, frequency of mucinous histology, and prevalence of synchronous or metachronous LS-associated tumors (Table 2.1b).

LLS patients together with their first-degree relatives are considered to have an intermediate risk of developing CRC [1, 4–10]. In 2007, a first approximation to cancer risk among Lynch-like cases was made. While 66% (50/75) of LS families fulfilled the Amsterdam II criteria, only 11% (2/18) of Lynch-like fulfilled them ($p = 0.001$) [4]. Similarly, Vargas et al. showed that cases meeting Bethesda criteria were overrepresented in LLS cases with MSH2 loss [7]. A study comprising 25 LLS families quantified the risk of CRC in their 177 first-degree relatives (FDRs) and found that MMR gene mutation carriers had the highest risk, LLS cases an intermediate risk, and the MMR-deficient cases due to *MLH1* promoter methylation the lowest [1, 4–12]. Recently, a bigger cohort comprising 271 LLS CRC cases and 1799 FDRs confirmed these findings [6]. The incidence of LS-associated tumors is about 11% in LLS patients, varying widely among series (Table 2.1b) [1, 5–10]. To date, there are no published data about the FDR risk of other tumors within the LS spectrum.

1.1 Current Clinical Management Recommendations

The inability to define evidence-based screening and management guidelines for LLS cases hampers the provision of clear-cut recommendations of their medical care. Therefore, LLS individuals and their relatives could be receiving different shades of cancer surveillance, ranging between low- and high-risk individuals, which mean that some of them are being subjected to unnecessarily over-screening and emotional distress, while others lack proper examination [13]. This is a problem that aggravates families and physicians and that also affects the healthcare system. Given the halfway risk of CRC observed among LLS, intermediate surveillance has been recommended as the best approach [5]. However, family history must be also taken into account. Of note, these LLS cases are most probably a heterogeneous group of different molecular and family backgrounds. Consequently, no optimal screening can be generalized until a specific diagnosis is made.

Table 2.1b Lynch-like syndrome in CRC population-based studies: Baseline characteristics and tumor pathology features of LLS, LS, and sporadic CRC patients

	LLS	LS	Sporadic		
Clinical and pathologic features	*n* (%)	*n* (%)	*n* (%)	*p*-value (LLS vs LS)	*p*-value (LLS vs sporadic)
Median age in years (range)[a]	**18–80 (59)**	**18–87 (52)**	**18–97 (69)**	0.27	0.21
Sex	**386**	**332**	**11,830**		
Female	172 (45)	142 (43)	5093 (43)		
Male	214 (55)	190 (57)	6737 (57)		
Amsterdam/Bethesda criteria[b]	**60** (69)	**121** (76)	**1263** (17)	0.65	**0.01**
Location	**387**	**345**	**8158**		
Right colon (proximal)	237 (61)	218 (63)	3190 (39)	0.73	**0.005**
Left colon/rectum (distal)	144 (37)	126 (37)	4968 (61)		
Missing	6 (2)	1 (0)	56 (1)		
Histologic grade	**291**	**242**	**5808**		
High grade (poorly differentiated)	83 (29)	52 (21)	947 (16)	0.60	**0.027**
Low grade (well/moderately differentiated)	156 (54)	152 (63)	4370 (75)		
Missing	52 (18)	38 (16)	491 (8)		
Histologic type	**301**	**230**	**5882**		
Adenocarcinoma	188 (62)	126 (55)	4829 (82)	1	0.10
Mucinous	89 (30)	69 (30)	778 (13)	1	0.078
Signet ring cells	3 (1)	5 (2)	5 (0)		
Medullary	4 (1)	5 (2)	18 (0)		
Other or missing	17 (6)	25 (11)	252 (4)		
TILs	**329**	**148**	**6243**		
Present	75 (23)	68 (46)	1779 (28)	0.85	0.13
Absent	59 (18)	80 (54)	1734 (28)		
Missing	195 (68)		2730 (44)		

(continued)

Table 2.1b (continued)

	LLS	LS	Sporadic		
Clinical and pathologic features	*n* (%)	*n* (%)	*n* (%)	*p*-value (LLS vs LS)	*p*-value (LLS vs sporadic)
MMR IHC pattern in tumor	**307**	**300**	**452**		
MLH1 and PMS2 loss	174 (57)	96 (32)	452 (100)		
MSH2 and MSH6 loss	77 (25)	120 (40)	0 (0)		
Isolated MSH6 loss	34 (11)	29 (10)	0 (0)		
Isolated PMS2 loss	22 (7)	39 (13)	0 (0)		
Unknown or normal	0 (0)	16 (5)	0 (0)		
LS-associated cancer (metachronous/ synchronous)	**350**	**269**	**5580**		
Present	39 (11)	64 (24)	323 (6)	0.07	**0.01**
Absent or missing	311 (89)	205 (76)	5257 (94)		

Summary of available data from Refs. [3, 5–8, 10]. Significant differences between groups were analyzed using the nonparametric Kruskal-Wallis test
P-values are two-sided. $P < 0.05$ was considered significant
LLS lynch-like syndrome, *LS* lynch syndrome, *TILs* tumor infiltrating lymphocytes, *MMR* mismatch repair, *IHC* immunohistochemistry
[a]Corresponds to the average (not the total) of the available data found in the literature
[b]The percentage is based on the total number of cases from the literature that reported this data (not the total number of included cases)

2 Potential Causes of MMR Deficiency in Lynch-like Syndrome

As stated above, failure in the identification of pathogenic germline mutations in MMR genes among patients with MMR-deficient tumors does not exclude either a lack of detection of germline and/or somatic MMR mutations or the involvement of other genes resulting in overlapping phenotypes. In this section, the evidence available on these issues is reviewed.

2.1 MMR Gene Mutations

Pathogenicity Assessment of MMR Gene Variants Up to 30% of detected MMR variants are classified as variants of unknown significance (VUS) [14], in which their clinical impact is not evident. In spite of systematic efforts such as those made by the InSiGHT LOVD database, there will always be a proportion of cases harboring variant class 3 (VUS) in one of the distinct MMR genes (Table 2.2) [15–26]. The carriers of those VUS will be classified as LLS. The final proportion of cases with VUS will depend both on the effort put in their functional characterization and the actual level of evidence that the scientific community will deem as acceptable to classify a variant as causal. Comprehensive approaches including cDNA splicing evaluation – focused on the generation of aberrant transcripts leading to premature stop codons or in-frame deletions disrupting functional domains – and multifactorial calculations of the posterior probability of pathogenicity offer a good performance, highlighting the benefit of applying quantitative and qualitative analyses for variant interpretation and classification [7].

Unidentified germline MMR Gene Mutations Current mutational analysis techniques could be missing complex or cryptic mutations in MMR genes [27–29]. An example of deep intronic mutations that could be overlooked with current strategies is the one found within the first intron of *MSH2*, at position c.212–553_c.212–479 [27]. This change creates a canonical donor splice site at the 3′ end of the insertion containing a stop codon, which is predicted to truncate the protein. Other examples of unidentified mutations are complex structural variations comprising MMR genes. A recurrent inversion of *MSH2* exons 1–7 has been identified in ten North American families [30–32], and an inversion of *MSH2* exons 2–6 has been recently reported in two Australian families [33]. Also, a fusion of *MLH1* with *LRRFIP2* after paracentric inversion on chromosome 3p22.2 has been described [29].

Besides, LLS individuals may be carriers of undetected mutations in regulatory regions of MMR genes, which are rarely screened in the mutational analysis of MMR genes. The 5′ and 3′ untranslated regions (UTRs) of most genes contain regulatory sequences that control mRNA processing and stability. On the one hand, germline variants in MMR promoter regions have been reported, some of them associated to allele-specific silencing or reduced promoter activity [34]. On the other hand, germline 3’UTR mutations in *MLH1* have been related to loss of protein

Table 2.2 Prevalence of pathogenic mutations and VUS identified in MMR genes when using gene panels in suspected hereditary CRC

					All genes analyzed				MMR genes	
References	*N* patients	Inclusion selection	Panel description	Guideline for variant classification	*N* pathogenic mutations	*N* of carriers (%)	*N* VUS	*N* VUS carriers (%)	*N* pathogenic mutations (% of carrier patients)	*N* VUS (% of carrier patients)
Susswein [26]	10,030	Suspected hereditary cancer patients	GeneDx, 29 genes, multigene panels	ACMG, insight	937	910 (9.0%)	2454	2454 (24.4%)	145 (1.5%)	NA
LaDuca [25]	2079	Suspected hereditary cancer patients	Ambry (14-22 genes)	Ambry, ACMG	173	141 (8.3%)	NA	NA	34 (1.6%)	NA
Yurgelun [23]	1260	Lynch syndrome suspected patients (NCCN criteria; MMR deficiency NA)	Myriad MyRisk (25 genes)	ACMG	185	182 (14.4%)	682	479 (38%)	114 (9.0%)	88 (6.9%)
Yurgelun [24]	1058	Consecutive CRC patients	Myriad MyRisk (25 genes)	ACMG	107	105 (9.9%)	408	330 (31.2%)	33 (3.1%)	74 (7.0%)
Chubb [15]	626	Early-onset CRC	Exome sequencing, analysis 9 CRC genes	Insight	89	89 (14.2%)	64	64 (10.2%)	68 (10.9%)	NA
Cragun [16]	586	CRC patients	ColoNext_Ambry (14 genes)	ACMG	62	61 (10.4%)	159	118 (20.1%)	23 (3.9%)	77 (13.1%)
Ricker [20]	475	Suspected hereditary cancer patients	Different multigene panels	ACMG	79	74 (15.6%)	268	268 (43.2%)	10 (2.1%)	NA
Pearlman [19]	450	CRC patients <50 years	Myriad MyRisk (25 genes)	ACMG	75	72 (16.0%)	178	178 (32.2%)	38 (8.4%)	NA
Slavin [22]	348	Suspected hereditary cancer patients	Different multigene panels	NA	69	69 (Na)	168	168 (Na)	7 (2.0%)	NA
Hermel [17]	227	Suspected hereditary cancer patients	Different multigene panels	Individual-lab	28	28 (12.3%)	44	44 (19.4%)	NA	NA
Rohlin [21]	91	Hereditary CRC suspected patients (previously tested negative)	19 CRC susceptibility genes	Insight, HGMD, LOVD, ClinVar	16	16 (17.6%)	30	30 (33.0%)	3 (3.3%)	8 (8.8%)
Howarth [18]	90	HBOC + HNPCC	Myriad MyRisk/Ambry BRCAplus	NA	9	9 (10.0%)	40	34 (37.8%)	1 (1%)	NA

NA not available information

expression as well [35]. Likewise, miRNA anomalous regulation has been proposed as possibly responsible for low expression of *MLH1* and *MSH2*, such as the case of miR-21 and miR-155 [36].

MMR Mosaicism It could be also a cause of misdiagnosis of LS although it has been reported only twice in LS-suspected cases. Sourrouille et al. described a CRC case with MSI and a frameshift mutation in *MSH2* (c.2541delA) in his blood lymphocyte DNA, whose mother had history of a colorectal tumor showing the same mutation in tumor tissue but not in peripheral blood lymphocyte DNA [37]. Mutational analysis at normal colon DNA from her mother revealed a weak signal for c.2541delA mutation, evidencing the presence of somatic mosaicism. The fact that she passed the mutation to her son formally demonstrates that she had germinal mosaicism. Also, somatic mosaicism was found in a woman with synchronous endometrioid adenocarcinomas of the ovary and endometrium at 44 years old [38]. Her family met Amsterdam II clinical criteria, and *MLH1* c.1050delA mutation was identified in her sister's blood, who had developed an endometrial cancer as well. The same mutation was found in the reported case but with a wild-type allele fraction of around 20% in normal tissue from different organs. Since their father had been affected with four tumors within the LS spectrum, this phenotype may be attributable to revertant somatic mosaicism [38].

Double Somatic MMR Gene (Epi)Mutations The accumulation of somatic alterations in DNA repair genes can certainly mimic germline-associated phenotypes. In fact, double somatic hits in MMR genes have been detected in a relevant proportion (27–82%) of LLS cases [7, 13, 37, 39–41] (summarized in Table 2.3). While somatic events appear to occur at the same frequencies in *MLH1* and *MSH2*, the general prevalence among different studies largely varies. The likely incorporation of subexome analysis at a high coverage in the evaluation of this type of tumors will certainly be useful for the identification and characterization of these cases.

MMR genes can also be targets of somatic methylation. MMR gene inactivation caused by promoter hypermethylation has been reported at somatic level usually for *MLH1* [42, 43]. In contrast, the relative contribution of somatic methylation in other MMR gene promoters in LLS has been poorly studied. Concerning *MSH2* gene, Vargas et al. did not detect *MSH2* promoter methylation in 13 samples from LLS patients harboring tumors lacking MSH2 expression [7]. This is in agreement with the low proportion of methylated tumors in MSH2-deficient LLS patients (1 of 40) previously reported [44, 45] (Table 2.4). Furthermore, Vargas et al. found no evidence

Table 2.3 Prevalence of double somatic hits among Lynch-like syndrome

	Sourrouille [37]	Geurts-Giele [13]	Haraldsdottir [39]	Mensenkamp [40]	Jansen [41]	Vargas-Parra [7]	Average (Range)
MLH1 deficient	1 of 7 14%	16 of 24 67%	7 of 8 88%	8 of 18 44%	3 of 7 43%	– –	**51%** (14–88%)
MSH2 deficient	3 of 8 38%	5 of 12 42%	16 of 20 80%	5 of 7 71%	5 of 13 33%	3 of 5 60%	**54%** (33–80%)
Total	**4 of 15** **27%**	**21 of 36** **58%**	**23 of 28** **82%**	**16 of 25** **64%**	**8 of 20** **40%**	**3 of 5** **60%**	**55%** (27–82%)

Table 2.4 Prevalence of somatic *MSH2* methylation among Lynch and Lynch-like syndrome

				Lynch-like syndrome				Lynch syndrome	
References	Methylation assay	Amplified *MSH2* region (GRCh38/hg38)	Cut-off	*MSH2* VUS carrier	*MSH6* VUS carrier	NI; MSH2 deficiency	NI; MSH6 deficiency	*MSH2* mutated	*EPCAM* mutated
Nagasaka [44]	COBRA	Chr2:47403017-47,403,154 (138 bp)	≥5% relative intensity of cut and uncut PCR band	0% (0 of 2)	–	0% (0 of 6)	–	24% (11 of 26)	100% (3 of 3)
Rumilla [45]	MSP	Chr2:47403104-47,403,218 (115 bp)	Untreated and bisulfite-treated DNA signal of 500 fluorescent units	–	–	2% (1 of 40)	–	–	100% (10 of 10)
Vargas-Parra [7]	MS-MCA	Chr2:47403257-47,403,380 (124 bp)	≥10% methylated	0% (0 of 5)	0% (0 of 3)	0% (0 of 8)	0% (0 of 1)	0% (0 of 8)	100% (1 of 1)

MS-MCA methylation-specific melting curve analysis, *COBRA* combined bisulfite restriction analysis, *MSP* methylation-specific PCR, *VUS* variant of unknown significance, *NI* not identified of methylation at the *MSH6* promoter in the nine MSH2-deficient tumors analyzed. Previously, *MSH6* methylation was studied in 99 sporadic tumors from LS spectrum with the same outcome [46, 47]. Finally, only one study has evaluated *PMS2* methylation status in 100 MLH1-/PMS2- and PMS2-deficient CRC samples, finding no methylation in the promoter of this gene [48]. Altogether, published observations reinforce the notion that somatic variants in *MLH1*, *MSH2*, or *MSH6* may be a frequent event in LLS cases, while somatic promoter hypermethylation does not apparently play a significant role.

2.2 *Overlapping Phenotypes*

Multiple and redundant mechanisms of DNA repair coexist within the cells. It is well known that DNA repair is the result of the coordinated action of many components that are organized in multimeric complexes. Components of the MMR pathway may cooperate with proteins involved in other DNA repair mechanisms. Because of this, it is likely that aberrations in other DNA repair genes may underlie MMR deficiency in LLS.

2.2.1 *MUTYH* Is a Bona Fide LLS Cancer Gene

Biallelic *MUTYH* mutations have been detected in 1–3% of LLS. Morak et al. reported a prevalence of 1.18% in a German-American cohort of 85 LLS cases [49]. More recently, a prevalence of biallelic *MUTYH* mutations of 3.1% in LLS was reported in a Spanish cohort [50]. The prevalence was similar (3.9%) when only cases fulfilling LS clinical criteria (Amsterdam or Bethesda) were considered. This percentage may be an underestimation due to the mutation detection strategy utilized, based on the prescreening of *MUTYH* hotspot mutations [51–53]. Of note, the prevalence of *MUTYH* mutations among LLS cases is significantly higher than the frequency observed in controls and unselected CRC from the Spanish population [54]. Recently, Yurgelun et al. identified 3 biallelic *MUTYH* carriers in a series of 1260 CRC patients for which neither clinical information nor tumor MSI status information was available [15–26].

To the best of our knowledge, 15 biallelic *MUTYH* carriers have been reported in patients with MMR-deficient tumors [49, 50, 55–58] (Table 2.5a). Interestingly, the LLS case with germline *MUTYH* biallelic mutations found in the Germanic-American series cohort from Morak et al. harbored double somatic *MSH2* transversions. These findings suggest that *MUTYH* deficiency could eventually cause somatic mutations in MMR genes, phenotypically mimicking LS. Of note, LS-suspected patients harboring *MLH1* methylated tumors were not included in the analysis of most of the series, and this may have led to the loss of some additional cases, as biallelic *MUTYH* mutations have been previously reported in *MLH1* methylated tumors [49, 50, 55–58].

Table 2.5a Variants in non-MMR genes identified in CRC-affected Lynch-like syndrome patients: Germline variants

Gene	cDNA change	Predicted aa change	Variant ID	References
Pathogenic variants				
MUTYH	c.494A>G	p.(Tyr165Cys)	rs34612342	Colebatch [56]; Cleary [55]; Morak [49]; Castillejo, Vargas [50]
	c.1187G>A	p.(Gly396Asp)	rs36053993	
	c.43A>G	p.(Met15Val)	Not reported	Seguí [58]
	c.1147delC	p.(Ala385Profs)	rs587778536	
	c.1227_1228dupGG	p.(Glu410Glyfs*43)	rs587780078	Lefevre [57]; Vargas-Parra [7]
POLE	c.1270C>G	p.(Leu424Val)	rs483352909	Palles [70]; Elsayed [72]
Variants of unknown significance				
POLE	c.861T>A	p.(Asp287Glu)	rs139075637	Jansen [73]
MCM9	c.911A>G	p.(Asn304Ser)	rs772909760	Liu [85]
	c.1592T>C	p.(Ile531Thr)	Not reported	
	c.1974G>T	p.(Gln658His)	rs78791427	
	c.1997G>A	p.(Arg666Trp)	rs759280235	
	c.3286A>G	p.(Met1096Val)	rs61742362	
FAN1	c.1856T>A	p.(Met619Lys)	Not reported	Vargas-Parra [7]
SETD2	c.1204C>T	p.(Arg402Trp)	rs779126757	Vargas-Parra [7]
	c.2508T>G	p.(Cys836Trp)	rs142668029	
	c.2798G>T	p.(Gly933Val)	rs202209141	

Table 2.5b Variants in non-MMR genes identified in CRC-affected Lynch-like syndrome patients: Somatic variants in proofreading polymerase genes

Gene	cDNA change	Predicted aa change	Variant ID	References
POLE	c.1100T>C	p.(Phe367Ser)	COSM5117983	Yoshida [74]
	c.847_846delinsTT	p.(Leu283Pro)	Not reported	Jansen [73]
	c.856C>T	p.(Pro286Ser)	COSM3688090	
	c.857C>G	p.(Pro286Arg)	COSM937333	
	c.1366G>C	p.(Ala456Pro)	COSM937319	
	c.1367C>T	p.(Ala456Val)	Not reported	
	c.1376C>T	p.(Ser459Pro)	COSM170809	
	c.2284C>T	p.(Arg762Trp)	Not reported	Vargas-Parra [7]
	c.2375A>G	p.(Lys792Arg)	Not reported	
POLD1	c.1003A>G	p.(Ile335Val)	Not reported	Jansen [73]
	c.1330C>T	p.(Arg444Trp)	Not reported	Vargas-Parra [7]

MUTYH biallelic mutations have been also described in large population-based CRC series in the absence of MAP phenotype [59–61] or in serrated polyposis cohorts [52]. Most of the LLS cases identified by Castillejo et al. had less than ten adenomatous polyps at the time of CRC diagnosis [50], thus not meeting the clinical criteria for MAP syndrome suspicion [62]. In fact, two of the five *MUTYH* biallelic cases developed more than ten adenomatous polyps in follow-up colonoscopies, after CRC diagnosis. Thus, the scarcity of adenomatous polyps, the presence of serrated polyps, or the presence of MSI in tumors should not exclude the *MUTYH* analysis. In all, current available evidence supports the existence of overlapping phenotypes between Lynch and MAP syndromes in the largest studies reported to date. Furthermore, our findings reinforce the need to systematically review surveillance reports in patients with hereditary CRC suspicion.

The role of germline *MUTYH* monoallelic mutations in cancer risk is a matter of controversy. Many researchers have found a modest increased susceptibility to cancer associated to monoallelic mutations [63–66], especially when codon 396 is affected [65]. However, larger studies have failed to replicate these findings [54, 67–69]. The lack of differences in the number of polyps between monoallelic carriers and wild-type group observed by Castillejo et al. is consistent with a weak susceptibility effect of these monoallelic mutations [50]. It may be speculated that *MUTYH* monoallelic carriers are predisposed to second hits. Further analyses are needed to elucidate the role of somatic second hits in *MUTYH* gene.

2.2.2 The Role of *POLE* and *POLD1*

Polymerase proofreading-associated polyposis (PPAP) has a dominant inheritance and high penetrance [70]. This syndrome is caused by missense mutations in the exonuclease domain of the polymerase proofreading genes, *POLE* and *POLD1*, conferring a predisposition to develop attenuated colorectal polyposis and CRC at an early age. Mutations in these enzymes promote the accumulation of somatic mutations due to misincorporation of bases during DNA replication and have been mainly related to hypermutated microsatellite-stable tumors [70, 71]. Noteworthy, germline mutations in polymerase proofreading genes may in some instance be associated with MMR deficiency in tumors [72, 73], probably associated to somatic MMR mutations due to hypermutability) [73, 74] (Table 2.5a).

2.2.3 The Putative Role of *FAN1* and *MCM9* Genes

FAN1 monoallelic mutations have recently been associated to hereditary MSS CRC [75] and hereditary pancreatic cancer [76]. Therefore, *FAN1* DNA repair gene (FANCD2/FANCI-associated nuclease 1) is emerging as a putative hereditary colorectal cancer gene. However, despite functional and cosegregation evidences [75], its role is currently a matter of controversy since no significant increase in the burden of *FAN1* mutations is detected in CRC cases versus controls [77].

Recently three missense variants in the *FAN1* gene have been identified among 30 LLS cases with MSH2-/MSH6-deficient tumors [[7] and unpublished data] (Table 2.5a). The c.1856T>A (p.M619K) variant was predicted probably pathogenic by in silico tools (at the functional and structural levels), and c.434G>A (p.R145H) and c.1129C>T (p.R377W) demonstrated cosegregation in CRC-affected relatives. As FAN1 interacts with MMR proteins MLH1, PMS2, and PMS1 [78] and has been related to maintenance of genome stability [79–81], the identification of germline *FAN1* variants in Lynch-like patients suggests that FAN1 deficiency might impair

MMR activity to a certain degree, leading to MMR-deficient tumors. This is the only study that has so far linked *FAN1* to Lynch-like syndrome. While suggestive, larger studies and robust functional analysis of identified variants are mandatory to refine the role of *FAN1* mutations in LLS.

MCM9 is a MutS-dependent DNA helicase that recruits MutL onto the mismatched base [82], involved in homologous recombination induced by interstrand cross-link repair [83]. In a recent study, the germline *MCM9* c.672_673delGGinsC was reported in a family with early-onset CRC, polyposis and ovarian failure [84], being postulated as a possible hereditary CRC gene. Moreover, MCM9 loss of function has been implicated in some MSI tumors [82]. Being the molecular relationship of this gene with MMR activity, Liu et al. sequenced *MCM9* gene in 109 Australian LS-suspected patients, finding 4 in silico predicted pathogenic missense variants out of 15 total variants [85] (Table 2.5a). Further functional and cosegregation studies are needed to guarantee MMR-deficient CRC causality among *MCM9* variant carriers.

2.2.4 Other CRC Genes Might Be Involved

Multiple genes have been associated to CRC development besides the abovementioned; however, little is known about their possible implication in LLS. Until recently, the picture was relatively simple as molecular characterization of patients and tumors was strictly guided by overall risk factors or population-based approaches. With the advent of NGS technologies and the progressive implementation of gene panels, a wider range of candidate genes are being studied in LS-suspected patients.

In a recent study, Yurgelun and colleagues used a 25-gene NGS panel to study 1260 patients who underwent LS genetic testing based on clinical criteria. They found germline *BRCA1*/*BRCA2* mutations in nine CRC cases, most of them meeting NCCN criteria for LS testing. Furthermore, they found three *APC* and one *STK11* mutated cases, as well as cases with MAP [15–26]. It has been reported that *BRCA* mutation carriers have a greater risk of developing CRC cancer at early age [86]. MMR deficiency was not formally tested, hampering the extrapolation of these observations to LLS.

Germline heterozygous mutations in *BUB1* and *BUB3*, components of the spindle checkpoint (SAC) responsible for correct chromosome segregation [87], have been identified in patients with early-onset and familial CRC [88, 89]. Recently Vargas et al. have identified a predicted pathogenic variant in *BUB1* in one endometrial cancer-affected LLS case. Also, germline variants of *SETD2*, a H3K36 trimethyltransferase necessary for recruiting MSH2/MSH6 to chromatin [90], have been detected in LLS cases [7] (Table 2.5a). Of note, this gene was included in the analysis after being frequently reported mutated in MSI CRC [91].

With the identification of rare and potentially pathogenic variants, *MCM9*, *FAN1*, *BUB1*, and *SETD2* are emerging as candidate genes responsible for LLS. Functional and cosegregation analysis will help in the elucidation of the pathogenicity of the identified variants.

2.2.5 Double Somatic Alterations in Other DNA Repair Genes

The in-depth analysis of tumors with selected gene panels is beginning to unravel a complex picture where putative loss of heterozygosity in MMR genes and double somatic mutations in other MMR genes and/or proofreading polymerases coexist [7, 73, 74, 92]. Somatic *POLE* driver mutations have been reported in a proportion of CRC, leading to an ultramutator phenotype with a predominance of C:G>T:A transitions [70] (Table 2.5b). Failure of both DNA repair mechanisms conveys a critical increase in the mutation rate and most surely a final polygenic effect. The exact hinder sequence remains unknown. The limited number of cases analyzed precludes drawing conclusions although it must be taken into account that pediatric tumors arising in CMMRD cases strongly associate with mutations in the exonuclease domain of proofreading polymerases [93]. Moreover, somatic mutations in other highly penetrant cancer genes (*APC, TP53, AXIN2, BMPR1A, PTEN*) are also present in tumors from LLS, making it difficult to understand the relative contribution of each alteration [7, 73].

3 Conclusions

Lynch-like syndrome cases are a set of highly heterogeneous cases in which the progressive availability of advanced sequencing technologies is continuously shedding light and refining its molecular classification. Being a syndrome defined by a MMR deficiency, the role of this DNA repair system is and will be relevant. Carriers of variants of unknown significance in MMR genes will be a prominent part of LLS, and a continuous effort will be necessary to more accurately classify these variants. Also, missed MMR alterations encompassing regions not usually included in the analysis (deep intronic regions, regulatory regions) or complex rearrangements will reclassify LLS into LS in some cases.

The spectrum of germline alterations present in these cases is expanding to other members of the complex DNA repair systems. Germline biallelic *MUTYH* mutations and polymerase proofreading mutations are responsible of a small proportion of LLS being this observation confirmed as subexome panels are being introduced in the clinical setting. Using this methodology, several candidate genes – i.e., *FAN1*, *BUB1*, *MCM9*, and *SETD2*, among others – are emerging as likely drivers of a proportion of these cases. Of note, candidate genes identified so far are cancer genes, mostly involved in DNA repair as these genes are overrepresented in the panels used so far. The use of WES approaches will clarify whether the spectrum of alterations expands. Furthermore, the presence of double somatic hits in MMR genes accounts for a proportion of LLS cases although a detailed analysis of the clonal architecture of these alterations will be critical to convincingly show its impact.

The combined germline and somatic assessment of the mutational status of cancer genes by means of a subexome panel – that opens the scope of the genes tested – has proved useful for the elucidation of the molecular basis in a higher proportion of LLS cases. Further studies of larger series and more in-depth functional characterization of variants detected will be critical to establish the true clinical validity of observed findings both at the germline and somatic level. Altogether, germline and somatic subexome analyses are emerging at the standard of care in the analysis of these LLS cases paving the way to a change in the molecular testing algorithms used so far.

Grant Support This work was funded by the Spanish Ministry of Economy and Competitiveness (grant SAF2015–68016-R) and co-funded by FEDER (A Way to Build Europe) funds, the Spanish Association Against Cancer, the government of Catalonia (grant 2014SGR338), Fundación Mutua Madrileña (grant AP114252013), and RTICC MINECO Network RD12/0036/0031. This work is also supported by the Mexican National Council for Science and Technology (CONACyT) fellowship grant awarded to GV.

Disclosures The authors declare no conflict of interest.

References

1. Hampel H, Frankel WL, Martin E, Arnold M, Khanduja K, Kuebler P, et al. Screening for the Lynch syndrome (hereditary nonpolyposis colorectal cancer). N Engl J Med. 2005;352:1851–60.
2. Moreira L, Balaguer F, Lindor N, de la Chapelle A, Hampel H, Aaltonen LA, et al. Identification of Lynch syndrome among patients with colorectal cancer. JAMA. 2012;308:1555–65. https://doi.org/10.1001/jama.2012.13088.
3. Hampel H, Frankel W, Panescu J, Lockman J, Sotamaa K, Fix D, et al. Screening for Lynch syndrome (hereditary nonpolyposis colorectal cancer) among endometrial cancer patients. Cancer Res. 2006;66:7810–7.
4. Overbeek LIH, Kets CM, Hebeda KM, Bodmer D, van der Looij E, Willems R, et al. Patients with an unexplained microsatellite instable tumour have a low risk of familial cancer. Br J Cancer. 2007;96:1605–12. https://doi.org/10.1038/sj.bjc.6603754.
5. Rodriguez-Soler M, Perez-Carbonell L, Guarinos C, Zapater P, Castillejo A, Barbera VM, et al. Risk of cancer in cases of suspected lynch syndrome without germline mutation. Gastroenterology. 2013;144:924–6. https://doi.org/10.1053/j.gastro.2013.01.044.
6. Win AK, Buchanan DD, Rosty C, MacInnis RJ, Dowty JG, Dite GS, et al. Role of tumour molecular and pathology features to estimate colorectal cancer risk for first-degree relatives. Gut. 2015;64(1):101–10. https://doi.org/10.1136/gutjnl-2013-306567.
7. Vargas-Parra GM, Gonzalez-Acosta M, Thompson BA, Gomez C, Fernandez A, Damaso E, et al. Elucidating the molecular basis of MSH2-deficient tumors by combined germline and somatic analysis. Int J Cancer. 2017. https://doi.org/10.1002/ijc.30820.
8. Kang SY, Park CK, Chang DK, Kim JW, Son HJ, Cho YB, et al. Lynch-like syndrome : characterization and comparison with EPCAM deletion carriers. Int J Cancer. 2015;136:1568–78. https://doi.org/10.1002/ijc.29133.
9. Chika N, Eguchi H, Kumamoto K, Suzuki O, Ishibashi K, Tachikawa T, et al. Prevalence of Lynch syndrome and lynch-like syndrome among patients with colorectal cancer in a Japanese hospital-based population. Jpn J Clin Oncol. 2017;47(2):108–17. https://doi.org/10.1093/jjco/hyw178.
10. Mas-Moya J, Dudley B, Brand RE, Thull D, Bahary N, Nikiforova MN, et al. Clinicopathological comparison of colorectal and endometrial carcinomas in patients with lynch-like syndrome versus patients with Lynch syndrome. Hum Pathol. 2015;46(11):1616–25. https://doi.org/10.1016/j.humpath.2015.06.022.

11. O'Kane GM, Ryan E, McVeigh TP, Creavin B, Hyland JM, O'Donoghue DP, et al. Screening for mismatch repair deficiency in colorectal cancer: data from three academic medical centers. Cancer Med. 2017;6(6):1465–72. https://doi.org/10.1002/cam4.1025.
12. Buchanan DD, Rosty C, Clendenning M, Win AK. Clinical problems of colorectal cancer and endometrial cancer cases with unknown cause of tumor mismatch repair deficiency (suspected Lynch syndrome). Appl Clin Genet. 2014;7:183–93.
13. Geurts-Giele WR, Leenen CH, Dubbink HJ, Meijssen IC, Post E, Sleddens HF, et al. Somatic aberrations of mismatch repair genes as a cause of microsatellite-unstable cancers. J Pathol. 2014;234:548–59. https://doi.org/10.1002/path.4419.
14. Thompson BA, Spurdle AB, Plazzer J-P, Greenblatt MS, Akagi K, Al-Mulla F, et al. Application of a 5-tiered scheme for standardized classification of 2,360 unique mismatch repair gene variants in the InSiGHT locus-specific database. Nat Genet. 2014;46:107–15. https://doi.org/10.1038/ng.2854.
15. Chubb D, Broderick P, Frampton M, Kinnersley B, Sherborne A, Penegar S, et al. Genetic diagnosis of high-penetrance susceptibility for colorectal cancer (CRC) is achievable for a high proportion of familial CRC by exome sequencing. J Clin Oncol Off J Am Soc Clin Oncol. 2015;33(5):426–32. https://doi.org/10.1200/JCO.2014.56.5689.
16. Cragun D, Radford C, Dolinsky JS, Caldwell M, Chao E, Pal T. Panel-based testing for inherited colorectal cancer: a descriptive study of clinical testing performed by a US laboratory. Clin Genet. 2014;86(6):510–20. https://doi.org/10.1111/cge.12359.
17. Hermel DJ, McKinnon WC, Wood ME, Greenblatt MS. Multi-gene panel testing for hereditary cancer susceptibility in a rural Familial Cancer Program. Familial Cancer. 2017;16(1):159–66. https://doi.org/10.1007/s10689-016-9913-5.
18. Howarth DR, Lum SS, Esquivel P, Garberoglio CA, Senthil M, Solomon NL. Initial results of multigene panel testing for hereditary breast and ovarian cancer and Lynch syndrome. Am Surg. 2015;81(10):941–4.
19. Pearlman R, Frankel WL, Swanson B, Zhao W, Yilmaz A, Miller K, et al. Prevalence and Spectrum of germline cancer susceptibility gene mutations among patients with early-onset colorectal cancer. JAMA Oncol. 2017;3(4):464–71. https://doi.org/10.1001/jamaoncol.2016.5194.
20. Ricker C, Culver JO, Lowstuter K, Sturgeon D, Sturgeon JD, Chanock CR, et al. Increased yield of actionable mutations using multi-gene panels to assess hereditary cancer susceptibility in an ethnically diverse clinical cohort. Cancer Genet. 2016;209(4):130–7. https://doi.org/10.1016/j.cancergen.2015.12.013.
21. Rohlin A, Rambech E, Kvist A, Torngren T, Eiengard F, Lundstam U, et al. Expanding the genotype-phenotype spectrum in hereditary colorectal cancer by gene panel testing. Familial Cancer. 2017;16(2):195–203. https://doi.org/10.1007/s10689-016-9934-0.
22. Slavin TP, Neuhausen SL, Nehoray B, Niell-Swiller M, Solomon I, Rybak C, et al. The spectrum of genetic variants in hereditary pancreatic cancer includes Fanconi anemia genes. Familial Cancer. 2017. https://doi.org/10.1007/s10689-017-0019-5.
23. Yurgelun MB, Allen B, Kaldate RR, Bowles KR, Judkins T, Kaushik P, et al. Identification of a variety of mutations in cancer predisposition genes in patients with suspected Lynch syndrome. Gastroenterology. 2015;149(3):604–13 e20. https://doi.org/10.1053/j.gastro.2015.05.006.
24. Yurgelun MB, Kulke MH, Fuchs CS, Allen BA, Uno H, Hornick JL, et al. Cancer susceptibility gene mutations in individuals with colorectal cancer. J Clin Oncol Off J Am Soc Clin Oncol. 2017;35(10):1086–95. https://doi.org/10.1200/JCO.2016.71.0012.
25. LaDuca H, Stuenkel AJ, Dolinsky JS, Keiles S, Tandy S, Pesaran T, et al. Utilization of multigene panels in hereditary cancer predisposition testing: analysis of more than 2,000 patients. Genet Med Off J Am Coll Med Genet. 2014;16(11):830–7. https://doi.org/10.1038/gim.2014.40.
26. Susswein LR, Marshall ML, Nusbaum R, Vogel Postula KJ, Weissman SM, Yackowski L, et al. Pathogenic and likely pathogenic variant prevalence among the first 10,000 patients referred for next-generation cancer panel testing. Genet Med Off J Am Coll Med Genet. 2016;18(8):823–32. https://doi.org/10.1038/gim.2015.166.

27. Clendenning M, Buchanan DD, Walsh MD, Nagler B, Rosty C, Thompson B, et al. Mutation deep within an intron of MSH2 causes Lynch syndrome. Familial Cancer. 2011;10:297–301. https://doi.org/10.1007/s10689-011-9427-0.
28. Ligtenberg MJ, Kuiper RP, Chan TL, Goossens M, Hebeda KM, Voorendt M, et al. Heritable somatic methylation and inactivation of MSH2 in families with Lynch syndrome due to deletion of the 3′ exons of TACSTD1. Nat Genet. 2009;41:112–7. https://doi.org/10.1038/ng.283.
29. Morak M, Koehler U, Schackert HK, Steinke V, Royer-Pokora B, Schulmann K, et al. Biallelic MLH1 SNP cDNA expression or constitutional promoter methylation can hide genomic rearrangements causing Lynch syndrome. J Med Genet. 2011;48:513–9. https://doi.org/10.1136/jmedgenet-2011-100050.
30. Wagner A, van der Klift H, Franken P, Wijnen J, Breukel C, Bezrookove V, et al. A 10-Mb paracentric inversion of chromosome arm 2p inactivates MSH2 and is responsible for hereditary nonpolyposis colorectal cancer in a North-American kindred. Genes Chromosomes Cancer. 2002;35(1):49–57. https://doi.org/10.1002/gcc.10094.
31. Mork ME, Rodriguez A, Taggart MW, Rodriguez-Bigas MA, Lynch PM, Bannon SA, et al. Identification of MSH2 inversion of exons 1-7 in clinical evaluation of families with suspected Lynch syndrome. Familial Cancer. 2016. https://doi.org/10.1007/s10689-016-9960-y.
32. Rhees J, Arnold M, Boland CR. Inversion of exons 1-7 of the MSH2 gene is a frequent cause of unexplained Lynch syndrome in one local population. Familial Cancer. 2014;13:219–25. https://doi.org/10.1007/s10689-013-9688-x.
33. Liu Q, Hesson LB, Nunez AC, Packham D, Williams R, Ward RL, et al. A cryptic paracentric inversion of MSH2 exons 2-6 causes Lynch syndrome. Carcinogenesis. 2016;37(1):10–7. https://doi.org/10.1093/carcin/bgv154.
34. Liu Q, Thompson BA, Ward RL, Hesson LB, Sloane MA. Understanding the pathogenicity of noncoding mismatch repair gene promoter variants in Lynch syndrome. Hum Mutat. 2016;37(5):417–26. https://doi.org/10.1002/humu.22971.
35. Wilding JL, McGowan S, Liu Y, Bodmer WF. Replication error deficient and proficient colorectal cancer gene expression differences caused by 3'UTR polyT sequence deletions. Proc Natl Acad Sci U S A. 2010;107(49):21058–63. https://doi.org/10.1073/pnas.1015604107.
36. Valeri N, Gasparini P, Braconi C, Paone A, Lovat F, Fabbri M, et al. MicroRNA-21 induces resistance to 5-fluorouracil by down-regulating human DNA MutS homolog 2 (hMSH2). Proc Natl Acad Sci. 2010;107:21098–103. https://doi.org/10.1073/pnas.1015541107.
37. Sourrouille I, Coulet F, Lefevre JH, Colas C, Eyries M, Svrcek M, et al. Somatic mosaicism and double somatic hits can lead to MSI colorectal tumors. Familial Cancer. 2013;12:27–33.
38. Pastrello C, Fornasarig M, Pin E, Berto E, Pivetta B, Viel A. Somatic mosaicism in a patient with Lynch syndrome. Am J Med Genet A. 2009;149:212–5. https://doi.org/10.1002/ajmg.a.32620.
39. Haraldsdottir S, Hampel H, Tomsic J, Frankel WL, Pearlman R, de la Chapelle A, et al. Colon and endometrial cancers with mismatch repair deficiency can arise from somatic, rather than germline, mutations. Gastroenterology. 2014;147:1308–16.e1. https://doi.org/10.1053/j.gastro.2014.08.041.
40. Mensenkamp AR, Vogelaar IP, van Zelst–Stams WAG, Goossens M, Ouchene H, Hendriks–Cornelissen SJB, et al. Somatic mutations in MLH1 and MSH2 are a frequent cause of mismatch-repair deficiency in Lynch syndrome-like tumors. Gastroenterology. 2014;146:643–6.e8. https://doi.org/10.1053/j.gastro.2013.12.002.
41. Jansen AM, Geilenkirchen MA, van Wezel T, Jagmohan-Changur SC, Ruano D, van der Klift HM, et al. Whole gene capture analysis of 15 CRC susceptibility genes in suspected Lynch syndrome patients. PLoS One. 2016;11(6):e0157381. https://doi.org/10.1371/journal.pone.0157381.
42. Herman JG, Umar A, Polyak K, Graff JR, Ahuja N, Issa JP, et al. Incidence and functional consequences of hMLH1 promoter hypermethylation in colorectal carcinoma. Proc Natl Acad Sci U S A. 1998;95(12):6870–5.
43. Yamamoto H, Imai K. Microsatellite instability: an update. Arch Toxicol. 2015;89:899–921. https://doi.org/10.1007/s00204-015-1474-0.

44. Nagasaka T, Rhees J, Kloor M, Gebert J, Naomoto Y, Boland CR, et al. Somatic hypermethylation of MSH2 is a frequent event in Lynch syndrome colorectal cancers. Cancer Res. 2010;70:3098–108. https://doi.org/10.1158/0008-5472.CAN-09-3290.
45. Rumilla K, Schowalter KV, Lindor NM, Thomas BC, Mensink KA, Gallinger S, et al. Frequency of deletions of EPCAM (TACSTD1) in MSH2-associated Lynch syndrome cases. J Mol Diagn. 2011;13:93–9.
46. Lima EM. DNA mismatch repair gene methylation in gastric cancer in individuals from northern Brazil. Biocell. 2008;32:237–43.
47. Vymetalkova VP, Slyskova J, Korenkova V, Bielik L, Langerova L, Prochazka P, et al. Molecular characteristics of mismatch repair genes in sporadic colorectal tumors in Czech patients. BMC Med Genet. 2014;15:17. https://doi.org/10.1186/1471-2350-15-17.
48. Truninger K, Menigatti M, Luz J, Russell A, Haider R, Gebbers J-O, et al. Immunohistochemical analysis reveals high frequency of PMS2 defects in colorectal cancer. Gastroenterology. 2005;128:1160–71. https://doi.org/10.1053/j.gastro.2005.01.056.
49. Morak M, Heidenreich B, Keller G, Hampel H, Laner A, de la Chapelle A, et al. Biallelic MUTYH mutations can mimic Lynch syndrome. Eur J Hum Genet. 2014;22:1334–7. https://doi.org/10.1038/ejhg.2014.15.
50. Castillejo A, Vargas G, Castillejo I, Navarro M, Barbera VM, Gonzalez S, et al. Prevalence of germline MUTYH mutations among lynch-like syndrome patients. European. J Cancer. 2014;50:2241–50. https://doi.org/10.1016/j.ejca.2014.05.022.
51. Gomez-Fernandez N, Castellvi-Bel S, Fernandez-Rozadilla C, Balaguer F, Munoz J, Madrigal I, et al. Molecular analysis of the APC and MUTYH genes in Galician and Catalonian FAP families: a different spectrum of mutations? BMC Med Genet. 2009;10:57.
52. Guarinos C, Juárez M, Egoavil C, Rodríguez-Soler M, Pérez-Carbonell L, Salas R, et al. Prevalence and characteristics of MUTYH-associated polyposis in patients with multiple adenomatous and serrated polyps. Clin Cancer Res Off J Am Assoc Cancer Res. 2014;20:1158–68. https://doi.org/10.1158/1078-0432.CCR-13-1490.
53. Nielsen M, Morreau H, Vasen HF, Hes FJ. MUTYH-associated polyposis (MAP). Crit Rev Oncol Hematol. 2011;79:1–16. https://doi.org/10.1016/j.critrevonc.2010.05.011.
54. Balaguer F, Castellvi-Bel S, Castells A, Andreu M, Munoz J, Gisbert JP, et al. Identification of MYH mutation carriers in colorectal cancer: a multicenter, case-control, population-based study. Clin Gastroenterol Hepatol Off Clin Pract J Am Gastroenterol Assoc. 2007;5:379–87. https://doi.org/10.1016/j.cgh.2006.12.025.
55. Cleary SP, Cotterchio M, Jenkins MA, Kim H, Bristow R, Green R, et al. Germline MutY human homologue mutations and colorectal cancer: a multisite case-control study. Gastroenterology. 2009;136(4):1251–60.
56. Colebatch A, Hitchins M, Williams R, Meagher a, Hawkins NJ, Ward RL. The role of MYH and microsatellite instability in the development of sporadic colorectal cancer. Br J Cancer. 2006;95:1239–43. https://doi.org/10.1038/sj.bjc.6603421.
57. Lefevre JH, Colas C, Coulet F, Bonilla C, Mourra N, Flejou JF, et al. MYH biallelic mutation can inactivate the two genetic pathways of colorectal cancer by APC or MLH1 transversions. Familial Cancer. 2010;9(4):589–94.
58. Seguí N, Navarro M, Pineda M, Köger N, Bellido F, González S, et al. Exome sequencing identifies MUTYH mutations in a family with colorectal cancer and an atypical phenotype. Gut. 2015;64:355–6. https://doi.org/10.1136/gutjnl-2014-307084.
59. Giráldez MD, Balaguer F, Bujanda L, Cuatrecasas M, Muñoz J, Alonso-Espinaco V, et al. MSH6 and MUTYH deficiency is a frequent event in early-onset colorectal cancer. Clin Cancer Res Off J Am Assoc Cancer Res. 2010;16:5402–13. https://doi.org/10.1158/1078-0432.CCR-10-1491.
60. Knopperts AP, Nielsen M, Niessen RC, Tops CMJ, Jorritsma B, Varkevisser J, et al. Contribution of bi-allelic germline MUTYH mutations to early-onset and familial colorectal cancer and to low number of adenomatous polyps: case-series and literature review. Familial Cancer. 2013;12:43–50. https://doi.org/10.1007/s10689-012-9570-2.

61. Wang L, Baudhuin LM, Boardman LA, Steenblock KJ, Petersen GM, Halling KC, et al. MYH mutations in patients with attenuated and classic polyposis and with young-onset colorectal cancer without polyps. Gastroenterology. 2004;127:9–16.
62. Syngal S, Brand RE, Church JM, Giardiello FM, Hampel HL, Burt RW, et al. ACG clinical guideline: Genetic testing and management of hereditary gastrointestinal cancer syndromes. Am J Gastroenterol. 2015;110:223–62.
63. Croitoru ME, Cleary SP, Berk T, Nicola NDI, Kopolovic I, Bapat B, et al. Germline MYH mutations in a clinic-based series of Canadian multiple colorectal adenoma patients. J Surg Oncol. 2007:499–506. https://doi.org/10.1002/jso.
64. Jones N, Vogt S, Nielsen M, Christian D, Wark PA, Eccles D, et al. Increased colorectal cancer incidence in obligate carriers of heterozygous mutations in MUTYH. Gastroenterology. 2009;137:489–94., 94.e1; quiz 725–6. https://doi.org/10.1053/j.gastro.2009.04.047.
65. Khalaf R, Jones C, Strutt W, Williamson P. Colorectal cancer in a monoallelic MYH mutation carrier. J Gastrointest Surg Off J Soc Surg Aliment Tract. 2013;17:1500–2. https://doi.org/10.1007/s11605-013-2206-5.
66. Win AK, Dowty JG, Cleary SP, Kim H, Buchanan DD, Young JP, et al. Risk of colorectal cancer for carriers of mutations in MUTYH, with and without a family history of cancer. Gastroenterology. 2014;146(5):1208–11 e1–5. https://doi.org/10.1053/j.gastro.2014.01.022.
67. Lubbe SJ, Di Bernardo MC, Chandler IP, Houlston RS. Clinical implications of the colorectal cancer risk associated with MUTYH mutation. J Clin Oncol Off J Am Soc Clin Oncol. 2009;27:3975–80. https://doi.org/10.1200/JCO.2008.21.6853.
68. Ma X, Zhang B, Zheng W. Genetic variants associated with colorectal cancer risk: comprehensive research synopsis, meta-analysis, and epidemiological evidence. Gut. 2014;63:326–36. https://doi.org/10.1136/gutjnl-2012-304121.
69. Theodoratou E, Campbell H, Tenesa A, Houlston R, Webb E, Lubbe S, et al. A large-scale meta-analysis to refine colorectal cancer risk estimates associated with MUTYH variants. Br J Cancer. 2010;103:1875–84. https://doi.org/10.1038/sj.bjc.6605966.
70. Palles C, Cazier J-B, Howarth KM, Domingo E, Jones AM, Broderick P, et al. Germline mutations affecting the proofreading domains of POLE and POLD1 predispose to colorectal adenomas and carcinomas. Nat Genet. 2012;45:136–44. https://doi.org/10.1038/ng.2503.
71. Valle L, Hernandez-Illan E, Bellido F, Aiza G, Castillejo A, Castillejo M-I, et al. New insights into POLE and POLD1 germline mutations in familial colorectal cancer and polyposis. Hum Mol Genet. 2014;23:3506–12. https://doi.org/10.1093/hmg/ddu058.
72. Elsayed FA, Kets CM, Ruano D, van den Akker B, Mensenkamp AR, Schrumpf M, et al. Germline variants in POLE are associated with early onset mismatch repair deficient colorectal cancer. Eur J Hum Genet EJHG. 2014:1–5. https://doi.org/10.1038/ejhg.2014.242.
73. Jansen AM, van Wezel T, van den Akker BE, Ventayol Garcia M, Ruano D, Tops CM, et al. Combined mismatch repair and POLE/POLD1 defects explain unresolved suspected Lynch syndrome cancers. Eur J Hum Genet. 2016;24(7):1089–92. https://doi.org/10.1038/ejhg.2015.252.
74. Yoshida R, Miyashita K, Inoue M, Shimamoto A, Yan Z, Egashira A, et al. Concurrent genetic alterations in DNA polymerase proofreading and mismatch repair in human colorectal cancer. Eur J Hum Genet. 2011;19(3):320–5. https://doi.org/10.1038/ejhg.2010.216.
75. Seguí N, Mina LB, Lázaro C, Sanz-Pamplona R, Pons T, Navarro M, et al. Germline mutations in FAN1 cause hereditary colorectal cancer by impairing DNA repair. Gastroenterology. 2015:1–4. https://doi.org/10.1053/j.gastro.2015.05.056.
76. Smith AL, Alirezaie N, Connor A, Chan-Seng-Yue M, Grant R, Selander I, et al. Candidate DNA repair susceptibility genes identified by exome sequencing in high-risk pancreatic cancer. Cancer Lett. 2016;370(2):302–12. https://doi.org/10.1016/j.canlet.2015.10.030.
77. Broderick P, Dobbins SE, Chubb D, Kinnersley B, Dunlop MG, Tomlinson I, et al. Validation of recently proposed colorectal cancer susceptibility gene variants in an analysis of families and patients-a systematic review. Gastroenterology. 2017;152(1):75–7 e4. https://doi.org/10.1053/j.gastro.2016.09.041.

78. Cannavo E, Gerrits B, Marra G, Schlapbach R, Jiricny J. Characterization of the interactome of the human MutL homologues MLH1, PMS1, and PMS2. J Biol Chem. 2007;282:2976–86. https://doi.org/10.1074/jbc.M609989200.
79. Kinch LN, Ginalski K, Rychlewski L, Grishin NV. Identification of novel restriction endonuclease-like fold families among hypothetical proteins. Nucleic Acids Res. 2005;33:3598–605. https://doi.org/10.1093/nar/gki676.
80. MacKay C, Déclais A-C, Lundin C, Agostinho A, Deans AJ, MacArtney TJ, et al. Identification of KIAA1018/FAN1, a DNA repair nuclease recruited to DNA damage by monoubiquitinated FANCD2. Cell. 2010;142:65–76. https://doi.org/10.1016/j.cell.2010.06.021.
81. O'Donnell L, Durocher D. DNA repair has a new FAN1 club. Mol Cell. 2010;39:167–9. https://doi.org/10.1016/j.molcel.2010.07.010.
82. Traver S, Coulombe P, Peiffer I, Hutchins JR, Kitzmann M, Latreille D, et al. MCM9 is required for mammalian DNA mismatch repair. Mol Cell. 2015;59(5):831–9. https://doi.org/10.1016/j.molcel.2015.07.010.
83. Nishimura K, Ishiai M, Horikawa K, Fukagawa T, Takata M, Takisawa H, et al. Mcm8 and Mcm9 form a complex that functions in homologous recombination repair induced by DNA interstrand crosslinks. Mol Cell. 2012;47(4):511–22. https://doi.org/10.1016/j.molcel.2012.05.047.
84. Goldberg Y, Halpern N, Hubert A, Adler SN, Cohen S, Plesser-Duvdevani M, et al. Mutated MCM9 is associated with predisposition to hereditary mixed polyposis and colorectal cancer in addition to primary ovarian failure. Cancer Genet. 2015;208(12):621–4. https://doi.org/10.1016/j.cancergen.2015.10.001.
85. Liu Q, Hesson LB, Nunez AC, Packham D, Hawkins NJ, Ward RL, et al. Pathogenic germline MCM9 variants are rare in Australian lynch-like syndrome patients. Cancer Genet. 2016;209(11):497–500. https://doi.org/10.1016/j.cancergen.2016.10.001.
86. Phelan CM, Iqbal J, Lynch HT, Lubinski J, Gronwald J, Moller P, et al. Incidence of colorectal cancer in BRCA1 and BRCA2 mutation carriers: results from a follow-up study. Br J Cancer. 2014;110(2):530–4. https://doi.org/10.1038/bjc.2013.741.
87. Leland S, Nagarajan P, Polyzos A, Thomas S, Samaan G, Donnell R, et al. Heterozygosity for a Bub1 mutation causes female-specific germ cell aneuploidy in mice. Proc Natl Acad Sci U S A. 2009;106:12776–81. https://doi.org/10.1073/pnas.0903075106.
88. de Voer RM, Geurts van Kessel A, Weren RD, Ligtenberg MJL, Smeets D, Fu L, et al. Germline mutations in the spindle assembly checkpoint genes BUB1 and BUB3 are risk factors for colorectal cancer. Gastroenterology. 2013;145:544–7. https://doi.org/10.1053/j.gastro.2013.06.001.
89. Hanks S, Coleman K, Reid S, Plaja A, Firth H, FitzPatrick D, et al. Constitutional aneuploidy and cancer predisposition caused by biallelic mutations in BUB1B. Nat Genet. 2004;36:1159–61. https://doi.org/10.1038/ng1449.
90. Li F, Mao G, Tong D, Huang J, Gu L, Yang W, et al. The histone mark H3K36me3 regulates human DNA mismatch repair through its interaction with MutSα. Cell. 2013;153:590–600. https://doi.org/10.1016/j.cell.2013.03.025.
91. Choi YJ, Oh HR, Choi MR, Gwak M, An CH, Chung YJ, et al. Frameshift mutation of a histone methylation-related gene SETD1B and its regional heterogeneity in gastric and colorectal cancers with high microsatellite instability. Hum Pathol. 2014;45:1674–81. https://doi.org/10.1016/j.humpath.2014.04.013.
92. Billingsley CC, Cohn DE, Mutch DG, Stephens JA, Suarez AA, Goodfellow PJ. Polymerase ε (POLE) mutations in endometrial cancer: clinical outcomes and implications for Lynch syndrome testing. Cancer. 2015;121:386–94. https://doi.org/10.1002/cncr.29046.
93. Shlien A, Campbell BB, de Borja R, Alexandrov LB, Merico D, Wedge D, et al. Combined hereditary and somatic mutations of replication error repair genes result in rapid onset of ultra-hypermutated cancers. Nat Genet. 2015;47:257–62. https://doi.org/10.1038/ng.3202.

Chapter 3
Constitutional Mismatch Repair Deficiency

Chrystelle Colas, Laurence Brugières, and Katharina Wimmer

Abstract Inherited heterozygous mutations in the MMR genes result in Lynch syndrome (LS). Individuals with biallelic mutation of one of the MMR genes developed malignancies in childhood. This recessively inherited condition is named CMMRD for constitutional mismatch repair deficiency. The spectrum of tumours is distinct from LS. Malignant brain tumours are at least as frequent as gastrointestinal tumours, and in more than a third of cases, haematological malignancies were also reported. Patients also displayed clinical features of neurofibromatosis type 1. The most commonly involved genes in CMMRD are *PMS2* and *MSH6*, while biallelic *MLH1* and *MSH2* mutations are rare.

Because of variable clinical presentation, lack of unequivocal diagnostic features and phenotypical overlap with other cancer syndromes, CMMRD syndrome is frequently unrecognised by clinicians, and its incidence is almost certainly underestimated. A better knowledge of clinical criteria and diagnosis methods for CMMRD syndrome will increase the number of patients being identified at the time when they develop their first tumour. This will allow to adjust treatment modalities and to offer surveillance strategies to detect other malignancies not only to the patient but also to his/her family.

Keywords Biallelic mutations · Paediatric cancers · Constitutional mismatch repair deficiency · Cerebral tumours · Lymphoma · Colorectal cancer · NF1 · MMR

C. Colas (✉)
Department of Genetics, Curie Institute, Paris, France
e-mail: chrystelle.colas@curie.fr

L. Brugières
Department of Children and Adolescents Oncology, Gustave Roussy Cancer Campus, Villejuif, France

K. Wimmer
Division of Human Genetics, Medical University Innsbruck, Innsbruck, Austria

L. Valle et al. (eds.), *Hereditary Colorectal Cancer*,
https://doi.org/10.1007/978-3-319-74259-5_3

Inherited heterozygous mutations in the DNA mismatch repair (MMR) genes result in Lynch syndrome (LS), characterised by gastrointestinal and genitourinary cancers in adulthood. In 1999, two reports described the phenotype of the offspring from consanguineous unions within LS families who carried homozygous *MLH1* germline mutations. These individuals developed haematological malignancies (and one individual a cerebral tumour) in early childhood [1, 2]. They also displayed clinical features reminiscent of neurofibromatosis type 1 (NF1). Since then, nearly 200 paediatric and young adults have been reported carrying biallelic germline mutations in one of the four MMR genes involved in LS [3–5]. This recessively inherited condition is now recognised as a distinct childhood cancer predisposition syndrome (OMIM #276300) named CMMRD for constitutional mismatch repair deficiency (other names used include bMMRD for biallelic mismatch repair deficiency or mismatch repair cancer syndrome). Although molecularly not proven, it is retrospectively most likely that Jacques Turcot in 1959 described the first cases of CMMRD when he reported on two siblings with numerous colorectal adenomatous polyps, colorectal carcinoma and malignant brain tumours [6]. However, during the following years, not only patients who should retrospectively be considered CMMRD patients but also polyposis patients with brain tumours who carry *APC* gene germline mutations were reported under the term Turcot syndrome [7]. Hence, CMMRD and Turcot syndrome essentially overlap.

1 Clinical Characteristics

Children with CMMRD are affected by a large variety of cancer types most of which occurring during childhood (Fig. 3.1). The median age of onset of the first tumour is 7.5 years with a wide range observed (0.4–39) [4]. The median survival time after diagnosis of the primary tumour is below 30 months, and most patients do not reach adulthood [3]. CMMRD patients may present with synchronous or metachronous malignancies of different types [3].

The spectrum of tumours in CMMRD is distinct from Lynch syndrome (LS). Malignant brain tumours are at least as frequent as gastrointestinal tract carcinomas, and in more than a third of CMMRD patients, also haematological malignancies were reported. The median age at diagnosis of haematological malignancies and brain tumours has been estimated to 6.6 and 10.3 years, respectively [3]. Brain tumours are mostly high-grade gliomas, although low-grade lesions also have been observed. These lower-grade lesions are at high risk of transformation to high-grade lesions [5]. CNS primitive neuroectodermal tumours (CNS-PNET) and medulloblastomas are the second frequent CNS tumours. Recent molecular findings suggest that CMMRD-associated CNS tumours have an exceptionally high rate of somatic mutations resulting from complete replication repair deficiency due to the combination of the constitutional MMR deficiency with somatic mutations inactivating the proofreading capacity of the replicative polymerases [8].

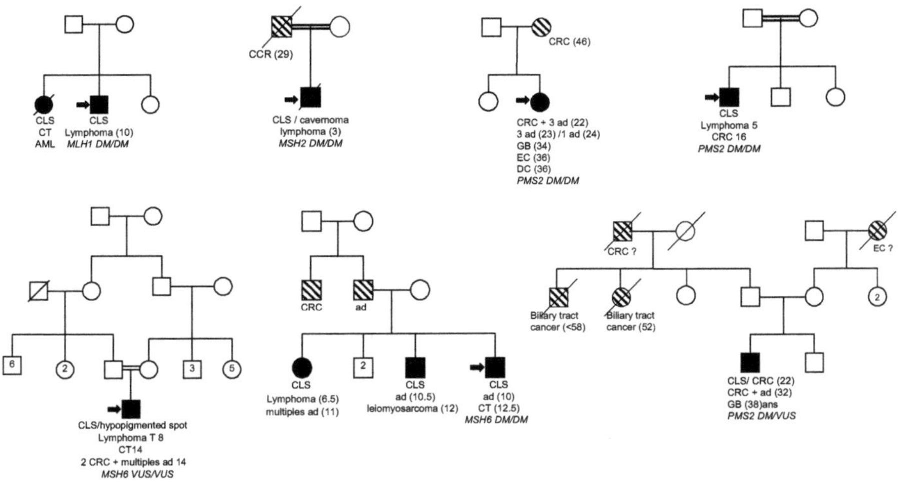

Fig. 3.1 Example of pedigrees of CMMRD patients (authors' unpublished data). Abbreviations: Ad colonic adenoma, AML acute myeloid leukaemia, CRC colorectal cancer, CLS café au lait spots, CT cerebral tumour, DC duodenal cancer, EC endometrial cancer, GB glioblastoma, DM deleterious mutation, VUS variant of unknown significance. Between brackets; age at diagnosis

The most commonly observed haematopoietic malignancies are non-Hodgkin's lymphomas (NHL) and in particular T-lymphoblastic NHL. T-cell acute lymphoblastic leukaemia (T-ALL), acute myeloid leukaemia (AML) and B-cell lymphomas have also been observed [3, 4, 9]. The predisposition of MMR-deficient individuals to haematological malignancy phenotypically recapitulates the MMR-deficient mouse models [10, 11] supporting the notion that the MMR mouse models are an effective tool for expanding our knowledge of the effects of MMR deficiency.

Colorectal cancers (CRC) are the most prevalent LS-associated tumours seen in CMMRD patients, but also cancers of the small bowel, endometrium cancer, ovary and urinary tract have been reported [3, 4]. CRC develops in childhood, with the youngest patients reported to be 8 years, whereas the youngest age of adenoma was reported in a 6-year-old girl. Metachronous cancers of the large and small bowel have been reported frequently. Development of small bowel cancer was observed at a strikingly young age (median of 18 years, range 7–33 years) [10].

A high percentage of the published CMMRD patients developed adenomas of the gastrointestinal tract often associated with high-grade dysplasia developing rapidly into early-onset cancer. Adenomas of the colon and rectum were found in 67% of individuals at baseline colonoscopy and 100% of the cohort who underwent follow-up surveillance [10]. Almost all patients will have polyposis by the third decade of life, and many of them will develop multiple synchronous adenomas ranging from a few to up to 100 polyps, reminiscent of familial adenomatous polyposis (FAP) or polymerase proofreading-associated polyposis (PPAP) which might be a differential diagnosis to patients with a CMMRD phenotype that lack MMR mutations [11]. Adenomas of the small bowel were also reported [3, 10].

A variety of other malignancies were seen only in a few CMMRD patients. Neuroblastoma, Wilms tumour, occurs in the first decade of life, although sarcomas (osteosarcoma, rhabdomyosarcoma, dermatofibrosarcoma) and genitourinary cancers and renal cell carcinoma are observed in the second decade [3]. Several patients have been described with multiple pilomatricomas, a usually benign skin neoplasm that arises from hair follicle matrix cells [3, 12].

Non-neoplastic manifestations include features of NF1, in particular café au lait macules (CALMS). The borders are reported to be more irregular than in classic CALM lesions, but also classical CALM as seen in NF1 patients have been reported. The vast majority of these patients had multiple (two or more) CALMs, but they did not always reach the critical number of 6, needed to be a diagnostic criteria of NF1 [13]. Several patients showed other features diagnostic for NF1 as freckling, benign cutaneous or plexiform neurofibromas, Lisch nodules and tibia pseudarthrosis, and one patient had an optic glioma [13]. Other features include areas of skin hypopigmentation, developmental venous anomalies, agenesis of the corpus callosum and mild immunodeficiency with decreased level of immunoglobulin (Ig) [4]. Indeed, the MMR deficiency leads to impaired Ig class switch recombination characterised by a decrease or absence of IgG2, IgG4 and IgA concomitant with increased IgM levels, that is, hyper-IgM syndrome [14, 15].

2 Genetics

The mode of inheritance is autosomal recessive. Biallelic mutations have been reported in all LS-associated MMR genes, *MSH2*, *MLH1*, *MSH6* and *PMS2*. But, the distribution of mutations among these four genes is strikingly different from that in LS. The most commonly involved genes in CMMRD are *PMS2* and *MSH6*, while biallelic *MLH1* and especially *MSH2* mutations are rare [3–5]. This distribution of biallelic mutations fits with the frequency of the mutations in these genes in the general population, while the distribution of heterozygous mutations in LS patients may be subject to ascertainment bias due to the lower penetrance and clinical severity of *PMS2* and *MSH6* heterozygous mutations [16]. Furthermore, it might be speculated that a possible lethality of homozygous mutations in *MSH2* or *MLH1* may account for the distribution difference.

Most of the mutations found in CMMRD patients are trucating expected to cause complete expression and, consequently, function loss of the corresponding MMR protein. But almost 30% of those mutations have been described as variant of uncertain significance (VUS) (more frequently in *MSH2* and *MLH1* than in *PMS2* and *MSH6*) [17] and which may have some residual function of the MMR corresponding protein [3, 4, 18].

In addition to the rarity of the syndrome, this high rate of potentially hypomorphic mutations among CMMRD patients complicates the assessment of genotype-phenotype correlations. Nevertheless, it is noteworthy that haematological malignancies are significantly more prevalent in patients with biallelic *MLH1/*

MSH2 than *PMS2* mutations and brain tumours were significantly more prevalent in *PMS2* mutation carriers [3, 18]. Looking at the mean age at diagnosis of the malignancy, *MLH1/MSH2* biallelic mutation carriers tend to develop each tumour entity at lower age than those with *MSH6* and *PMS2* mutations. The percentage of biallelic mutation carriers with more than one malignancy was lowest in *MLH1/MSH2* and highest in *PMS2* biallelics [3]. This may indicate that the chance to survive the first tumour and develop a second metachronous malignancy is higher in *PMS2* biallelic mutation carriers than in *MLH1/MSH2* biallelic carriers. This observation would be in agreement with the notion that patients with biallelic *MLH1/MSH2* mutations show a more severe phenotype than those with biallelic *MSH6* and *PMS2* mutations.

In contrast to LS, family history is often non-contributory, although both parents are usually obligate carriers (Fig. 3.1) [3]. Penetrance of monoallelic *MSH6* and *PMS2* mutations is lower than that of *MSH2* and *MLH1*, and therefore it is common for affected children to have unaffected parents. The rate of consanguinity varies according to the countries of origin. A high rate of consanguinity is observed especially among homozygous cases, whereas in western countries, most of the cases are associated with compound heterozygous mutation in non-consanguineous families [3].

The penetrance of cancers in CMMRD is one of the highest among childhood cancer syndromes. It is extremely uncommon for a patient not to be affected by the third decade [3, 4]. Existing data support the existence of a clinical continuum that spans the less severe CMMRD phenotypes that mimic LS to more severe and early-onset LS phenotypes that mimic CMMRD [3, 19, 20].

3 Diagnosis

Diagnosis of CMMRD in a paediatric or young adult patient has important implications for the management not only of the patient but also of the entire family. However, diagnosis may often be delayed or even not stated.

A rapid diagnosis of the syndrome is necessary due to the aggressiveness of CMMRD and the need to adjust treatment to the MMR defect and to adapt follow-up considering the high risk of second malignancy. Despite the wide range of clinical presentations, a few symptoms are highly suggestive of CMMRD and especially the combination of tumours belonging to the spectrum (high-grade gliomas, T-lymphoblastic lymphoma or colorectal carcinomas) associated with café au lait and/or depigmented spots. Since CMMRD may often be associated with frequent clinical signs and abnormalities, a clinical score for the suspect diagnosis of CMMRD was developed by the care for CMMRD (C4CMMRD) consortium (Table 3.1) [4]. This score is highly sensitive for CMMRD and suggests genetic counselling and testing for patients who reach a score of three or more points.

Table 3.1 Indication for CMMRD testing in cancer patients is recommended when the patient fulfils ≥3 points

Indication for CMMRD testing in cancer patients	≥ 3 points
Malignancies/premalignancies: One is mandatory; if more than one is present in the patient, add the points	
Carcinoma from the LS spectrum[a] at age < 25 years	3 points
Multiple bowel adenomas at age < 25 years and absence of APC/MUTYH mutation(s) or a single high-grade dysplasia adenoma at age < 25 years	3 points
WHO grade III or IV glioma at age < 25 years	2 points
NHL of T-cell lineage or sPNET at age < 18 years	2 points
Any malignancy at age < 18 years	1 point
Additional features: Optional; if more than one of the following is present, add the points	
Clinical sign of NF1 and/or ≥2 hyperpigmented and/or Hypopigmented skin alterations Ø > 1 cm in the patient	2 points
Diagnosis of LS in a first-degree or second-degree relative	2 points
Carcinoma from LS spectrum[a] before the age of 60 in first-degree, second-degree or third-degree relative	1 point
A sibling with carcinoma from the LS spectrum[a], high-grade glioma, sPNET or NHL	2 points
A sibling with any type of childhood malignancy	1 point
Multiple pilomatricomas in the patient	2 points
One pilomatricoma in the patient	1 point
Agenesis of the corpus callosum or non-therapy-induced cavernoma in the patient	1 point
Consanguineous parents	1 point
Deficiency/reduced levels of IgG2/4 and/or IgA	1 point

From Wimmer et al. [4] (with author's permission)

[a]Colorectal, endometrial, small bowel, ureter, renal pelvis, biliary tract, stomach, bladder carcinoma

Abbreviations: *CMMRD* constitutional mismatch repair deficiency, *LS* Lynch syndrome, *NHL* non-Hodgkin's lymphomas, *sPNET* supratentorial primitive neuroectodermal tumour

It is highly recommended to test for CMMRD in any case of childhood gastrointestinal cancer and to apply the clinical score to all cases of T-cell malignancies and malignant gliomas from countries of origins where consanguinity is high as the frequency of the syndrome is extremely high in these specific cancers.

3.1 Molecular Constitutional Analysis

Genetic confirmation of biallelic mutation in one of the four MMR genes is the only validated tool to diagnose CMMRD. This is complicated by the large number of variants of unknown significance in these genes and the difficulties to sequence *PMS2* which has multiple pseudogenes [21–23]. Since the diagnosis is urgent and will affect both surveillance and therapeutic decisions, several diagnostic screening algorithms and tests were developed.

3.2 Immunochemistry

Loss of the corresponding MMR protein in both normal and malignant cells by immunochemistry is highly concordant with a diagnosis of CMMRD [4, 5]. In contrast to LS, where expression loss is observed only in neoplastic cells, most of the time, IHC in CMMRD patients shows expression loss of one (or two) of the MMR proteins in both neoplastic and non-neoplastic tissues. Hence, negative IHC staining in surrounding normal cells should not be interpreted as a failure of proper staining, and care should be taken to use a staining control from a different individual. By doing so, IHC can distinguish between the two syndromes in most of the cases. Furthermore, it guides subsequent mutation analysis in the four MMR genes.

As in LS, biallelic truncating mutations in *PMS2* or *MSH6* will result in isolated loss of these proteins, whereas mutations in *MLH1* or *MSH2* will lead to concurrent loss of MLH1/PMS2 or MSH2/MSH6, respectively, since MLH1 and MSH2 are the obligatory partners in the formation of MLH1/PMS2 and MSH2/MSH6 heterodimers. Of note, in the case of an underlying missense mutation, IHC may show normal expression of the affected MMR gene, which may be a possible pitfall when using IHC analysis to confirm suspected CMMRD.

In the cases in which no tumour tissue is available for immunostaining such as haematologic malignancies or in a healthy individual suspected of CMMRD, immunostaining for MMR can be performed on a skin biopsy [5].

3.3 Microsatellite Instability

MSI analysis following the current protocols for LS uses a panel of dinucleotide and/or mononucleotide repeat markers. This approach is a reliable tool to diagnose MMR deficiency in gastrointestinal and other LS-associated tumours of CMMRD patients. However, MSI analysis in tumours cannot differentiate between CMMRD and LS. Moreover, standard MSI analysis frequently fails to show MSI in brain tumours and other malignancies [3, 5]. A MSS result especially in cerebral tumour cannot exclude the diagnosis.

In principle, MSI is present also in DNA from normal cells of CMMRD patients, but altered microsatellite alleles are present only in a small proportion of the cells from normal tissue. A simple method to detect MSI in non-neoplastic tissue is germline MSI (gMSI) [24]. This assay relies on the analysis of 'stutter' peaks typically associated with microsatellite PCR products. Its main limitation is that it uses dinucleotide microsatellites and, therefore, is insensitive to a MSH6 deficiency [20, 24].

3.4 Other Screening Methods

The current diagnosis of CMMRD requires identification of biallelic, deleterious germline MMR defects. Unfortunately, mutation analysis leads to non-informative results when variants of unknown functional significance (VUS) are detected, as observed in around 30% of patients. Moreover, the detection of *PMS2* alterations responsible for most of CMMRD families is complicated by the presence of numerous pseudogenes, requiring sophisticated mutation analysis protocols to reach high mutation detection rates [21–23, 25]. Assays based on lymphocytes from patients with CMMRD have been developed as tools for diagnosis in problematic cases where mutation analysis may not come to a final conclusion [20]. Two functional assays, the evaluation of MSI and methylation tolerance in immortalised lymphoblastoid cells, gave unequivocal results in CMMRD patients. With abnormal results for both assays confirming the diagnosis of CMMRD and normal results for both assays rule this out, the method was 100% sensitive and 100% specific. These assays could be useful for confirmation or rejection of CMMRD diagnosis in patients with VUS or where the mutation analysis failed to detect biallelic MMR mutations despite an evocative CMMRD clinical phenotype. It can also be used in the absence of available tumours or to test the siblings if genetic testing is not possible because both mutations were not identified.

Recently, high mutational burden in the tumour with a mutation rate of 100/MB as compared to <10/MB in most childhood cancers has been described to be extremely specific to CMMRDD and may play a role in future diagnostic algorithms [8]. Assays are also needed to evaluate response to treatment and repair of specific mutations.

Taken together, IHC staining of the MMR genes, (g)MSI analysis on tumour and normal tissues, functional tests and determination of the mutation rate in tumours are diagnostic methods to substantiate the suspected diagnosis. Since IHC will also guide target-gene mutation analysis and has been shown to render reliable results in most solid tumours, it is considered the preferred method. However, all methods have potential pitfalls and may fail to confirm the suspected diagnosis. Therefore, combining several assays is recommended if needed.

4 Genetic Counselling

Genetic counselling must be offered to the patients and/or their parents prior to performing mutation analysis in the affected child. Patients and/or their parents should be informed by a team of paediatric oncologists and medical geneticists about the suspected diagnosis if this is substantiated by MSI and/or IHC analysis. Considering the burden of this syndrome, psychological support should systematically be proposed to families. The family has to be informed of potential therapeutic implications of the test result and also of the high risk for a second malignancy in a patient with a positive test result. Genetic counselling must also include information on the potential 25% recurrence risk in siblings and on the risks for LS-associated cancer in heterozygous mutation carriers, particularly both parents. A definite molecular diagnosis is needed to offer the families of CMMRD patients appropriate counselling and discuss with them the options of predictive testing as well as prenatal/preimplantation diagnostics if this is desired.

5 Implications for Management

5.1 Screening

The two major international groups (European Consortium Care for CMMRD (C4CMMRD) and International bMMRD Consortium) have designed surveillance protocols based on available data on tumour frequency at specific ages [5, 26, 27]. Specific surveillance of the gastrointestinal tract, the central nervous system (CNS) and haematopoietic system is performed from early childhood, while additional surveillance of the genitourinary tract starts from age 20.

Brain MRI is suggested to be implemented at diagnosis or from 2 years old, every 6 months and upon any clinical warning sign. Gastrointestinal surveillance with colonoscopy is effective in identification and resection of polyps. The International bMMRD Consortium published screening guidelines in 2012, recommending annual colonoscopy screening to begin at age 3 years, which is 5 years earlier than the youngest diagnosis of CRC observed in CMMRD. Other groups have suggested that colonoscopy screening begins at age 6 due to reports of colonic polyps at this age [26]. Annual colonoscopy is recommended until polyps are identified and every 6 months once polyps are identified. Patients with polyps with high-grade dysplasia are at significant risk of carcinoma. Dependent on the polyps localisation and their degree of dysplasia, surgical intervention may be required with consideration of a subtotal colectomy with ileo-rectal anastomosis after endoscopic evaluation of the rectum or proctocolectomy if the rectal polyps are not manageable, in the same way than in other polyposis syndromes. These considerations are complicated by the high prevalence of upper gastrointestinal or small bowel polyps and cancers. Age of onset of small bowel polyps is later than for colonic adenoma, in the second decade of life. Upper endoscopy and video capsule endoscopy are recommended starting at least at 8 years of age.

Although lymphoid and other haematological malignancies are the third most common malignancies observed in children with CMMRD and can be observed in early childhood, lack of current effective tools limits the screening recommendation. Nevertheless, both repeated CBC and abdominal ultrasounds may be considered at a frequency of every 6 months.

A current suggestion is to implement whole body MRI once a year at age 6 or when anaesthesia is not needed anymore [5]. This method should not replace the brain MRI which is more sensitive for detection of CNS lesions.

The efficacy of these screening modalities is unknown, and prospective studies are needed for their evaluation.

5.2 Treatment

The role of chemotherapy and radiotherapy in the occurrence of second malignancies is difficult to assess. Mismatch repair deficiency affects replication. Currently there is no information of extensive toxicity to these CMMRD patients as a result of chemo-radiation therapies.

Several common chemotherapeutic agents require adequate mismatch repair to exert their tumour damage. These include mercaptopurine and temozolomide which are commonly used in haematopoietic and glioma treatment. MMR-deficient cells have been shown to be more tolerant to temozolomide and radiotherapy than MMR-proficient cells, and CMMRD tumour resistance to therapy has been reported [28–30]. Importantly, there is no obvious lack of efficacy of other therapeutic agents such as alkylating agents or anthracyclines. This should prompt us to design specific protocols for those cases of CMMRD-associated tumours.

Finally, the hypermutation phenotype which is described for some CMMRD malignant cancers offers opportunities for novel approaches to the treatment of these patients. Specifically, immune checkpoint inhibition which has been reported to have a significant efficacy in LS has been shown to have significant effect in inducing tumour response and prolonging survival for two patients with CMMRD recurrent glioblastoma [31]. This underlines the need of early diagnosis of CMMRD which may lead to include patients in trials aiming to evaluate the efficacy of these drugs. Specific trials for tumours associated with this syndrome should be open to inclusions in the next future. Tumour sequencing commonly identifies mutations in targetable genes for available compounds and can potentially offer precision medicine approach to these patients.

Chemoprevention may potentially be the most effective intervention for this highly penetrant cancer syndrome. Several compounds have been suggested including anti-inflammatory agents such as aspirin which has been shown to reduce the risk of cancer in LS [32]. Tumour maturing agents such as retinoids and more recently checkpoint inhibitors can be considered as potential 'tumour preventive tools' [31, 33]. These promising therapies should be assessed through prospective trials.

6 Conclusion

Because of variable clinical presentation, lack of unequivocal diagnostic features and phenotypical overlap with other cancer syndromes (e.g. NF1, Li-Fraumeni syndrome, FAP or PPAP), CMMRD syndrome is frequently unrecognised by clinicians, and its incidence is almost certainly underestimated. A better knowledge of clinical criteria and diagnosis methods for CMMRD syndrome will increase the number of patients being identified at the time when they develop their first tumour. This will allow to adjust treatment modalities and to offer surveillance strategies to detect other malignancies not only to the patient but also to siblings who carry also a biallelic MMR gene mutation. Still many of these patients will die from cancer. A systematic collection and evaluation of all clinical data will help to improve the management in CMMRD. Therefore, patients, their siblings and parents should be asked to be included in a registry such as the one established by the European C4CMMRD consortium.

References

1. Wang Q, Lasset C, Desseigne F, Frappaz D, Bergeron C, Navarro C, et al. Neurofibromatosis and early onset of cancers in hMLH1-deficient children. Cancer Res. 1999;59(2):294–7.
2. Ricciardone MD, Ozçelik T, Cevher B, Ozdağ H, Tuncer M, Gürgey A, et al. Human MLH1 deficiency predisposes to hematological malignancy and neurofibromatosis type 1. Cancer Res. 1999;59(2):290–3.
3. Lavoine N, Colas C, Muleris M, Bodo S, Duval A, Entz-Werle N, et al. Constitutional mismatch repair deficiency syndrome: clinical description in a French cohort. J Med Genet. 2015;52(11):770–8.
4. Wimmer K, Kratz CP, Vasen HFA, Caron O, Colas C, Entz-Werle N, et al. Diagnostic criteria for constitutional mismatch repair deficiency syndrome: suggestions of the European consortium 'care for CMMRD' (C4CMMRD). J Med Genet. 2014;51(6):355–65.
5. Bakry D, Aronson M, Durno C, Rimawi H, Farah R, Alharbi QK, et al. Genetic and clinical determinants of constitutional mismatch repair deficiency syndrome: report from the constitutional mismatch repair deficiency consortium. Eur J Cancer Oxf Engl 1990. 2014;50(5):987–96.
6. Turcot J, Despres JP, St Pierre F. Malignant tumors of the central nervous system associated with familial polyposis of the colon: report of two cases. Dis Colon Rectum. 1959;2:465–8.
7. Hamilton SR, Liu B, Parsons RE, Papadopoulos N, Jen J, Powell SM, et al. The molecular basis of Turcot's syndrome. N Engl J Med. 1995;332(13):839–47.
8. Shlien A, Campbell BB, de Borja R, Alexandrov LB, Merico D, Wedge D, et al. Combined hereditary and somatic mutations of replication error repair genes result in rapid onset of ultra-hypermutated cancers. Nat Genet. 2015;47(3):257–62.
9. Ripperger T, Schlegelberger B. Acute lymphoblastic leukemia and lymphoma in the context of constitutional mismatch repair deficiency syndrome. Eur J Med Genet. 2016;59(3):133–42.
10. Aronson M, Gallinger S, Cohen Z, Cohen S, Dvir R, Elhasid R, et al. Gastrointestinal findings in the largest series of patients with hereditary biallelic mismatch repair deficiency syndrome: report from the International Consortium. Am J Gastroenterol. 2016;111(2):275–84.
11. Wimmer K, Beilken A, Nustede R, Ripperger T, Lamottke B, Ure B, et al. A novel germline POLE mutation causes an early onset cancer prone syndrome mimicking constitutional mismatch repair deficiency. Familial Cancer. 2017;16(1):67–71.
12. Chmara M, Wernstedt A, Wasag B, Peeters H, Renard M, Beert E, et al. Multiple pilomatricomas with somatic CTNNB1 mutations in children with constitutive mismatch repair deficiency. Genes Chromosomes Cancer. 2013;52(7):656–64.
13. Wimmer K, Rosenbaum T, Messiaen L. Connections between constitutional mismatch repair deficiency syndrome and neurofibromatosis type 1. Clin Genet. 2017;91(4):507–19.
14. Gardès P, Forveille M, Alyanakian M-A, Aucouturier P, Ilencikova D, Leroux D, et al. Human MSH6 deficiency is associated with impaired antibody maturation. J Immunol Baltim Md 1950. 2012;188(4):2023–9.
15. Crouse GF. Non-canonical actions of mismatch repair. DNA Repair. 2016;38:102–9.
16. Win AK, Jenkins MA, Dowty JG, Antoniou AC, Lee A, Giles GG, et al. Prevalence and penetrance of major genes and polygenes for colorectal cancer. Cancer Epidemiol Biomark Prev Publ Am Assoc Cancer Res Cosponsored Am Soc Prev Oncol. 2017;26(3):404–12.

17. Colas C. Clinical and biological consequences of constitutional mismatch repair deficiency in human [Thèse de doctorat en Génétique des tumeurs]. Paris 6. 2011.
18. Felton KEA, Gilchrist DM, Andrew SE. Constitutive deficiency in DNA mismatch repair. Clin Genet. 2007;71(6):483–98.
19. Li L, Hamel N, Baker K, McGuffin MJ, Couillard M, Gologan A, et al. A homozygous PMS2 founder mutation with an attenuated constitutional mismatch repair deficiency phenotype. J Med Genet. 2015;52(5):348–52.
20. Bodo S, Colas C, Buhard O, Collura A, Tinat J, Lavoine N, et al. Diagnosis of constitutional mismatch repair-deficiency syndrome based on microsatellite instability and lymphocyte tolerance to methylating agents. Gastroenterology. 2015;149(4):1017–1029.e3.
21. Wimmer K, Wernstedt A. PMS2 gene mutational analysis: direct cDNA sequencing to circumvent pseudogene interference. Methods Mol Biol Clifton NJ. 2014;1167:289–302.
22. Vaughn CP, Hart KJ, Samowitz WS, Swensen JJ. Avoidance of pseudogene interference in the detection of 3′ deletions in PMS2. Hum Mutat. 2011;32(9):1063–71.
23. van der Klift HM, Mensenkamp AR, Drost M, Bik EC, Vos YJ, Gille HJJP, et al. Comprehensive mutation analysis of PMS2 in a large cohort of probands suspected of lynch syndrome or constitutional mismatch repair deficiency syndrome. Hum Mutat. 2016;37(11):1162–79.
24. Ingham D, Diggle CP, Berry I, Bristow CA, Hayward BE, Rahman N, et al. Simple detection of germline microsatellite instability for diagnosis of constitutional mismatch repair cancer syndrome. Hum Mutat. 2013;34(6):847–52.
25. Vogt J, Wernstedt A, Ripperger T, Pabst B, Zschocke J, Kratz C, et al. PMS2 inactivation by a complex rearrangement involving an HERV retroelement and the inverted 100-kb duplicon on 7p22.1. Eur J Hum Genet EJHG. 2016;24(11):1598–604.
26. Vasen HFA, Ghorbanoghli Z, Bourdeaut F, Cabaret O, Caron O, Duval A, et al. Guidelines for surveillance of individuals with constitutional mismatch repair-deficiency proposed by the European Consortium 'Care for CMMR-D' (C4CMMR-D). J Med Genet. 2014;51(5):283–93.
27. Durno CA, Aronson M, Tabori U, Malkin D, Gallinger S, Chan HSL. Oncologic surveillance for subjects with biallelic mismatch repair gene mutations: 10 year follow-up of a kindred. Pediatr Blood Cancer. 2012;59(4):652–6.
28. Karran P, Attard N. Thiopurines in current medical practice: molecular mechanisms and contributions to therapy-related cancer. Nat Rev Cancer. 2008;8(1):24–36.
29. Ilencikova D, Sejnova D, Jindrova J, Babal P. High-grade brain tumors in siblings with biallelic MSH6 mutations. Pediatr Blood Cancer. 2011;57(6):1067–70.
30. Hunter C, Smith R, Cahill DP, Stephens P, Stevens C, Teague J, et al. A hypermutation phenotype and somatic MSH6 mutations in recurrent human malignant gliomas after alkylator chemotherapy. Cancer Res. 2006;66(8):3987–91.
31. Bouffet E, Larouche V, Campbell BB, Merico D, de Borja R, Aronson M, et al. Immune checkpoint inhibition for hypermutant glioblastoma multiforme resulting from germline biallelic mismatch repair deficiency. J Clin Oncol Off J Am Soc Clin Oncol. 2016;34(19):2206–11.
32. Burn J, Gerdes A-M, Macrae F, Mecklin J-P, Moeslein G, Olschwang S, et al. Long-term effect of aspirin on cancer risk in carriers of hereditary colorectal cancer: an analysis from the CAPP2 randomised controlled trial. Lancet Lond Engl. 2011;378(9809):2081–7.
33. Gottschling S, Reinhard H, Pagenstecher C, Krüger S, Raedle J, Plotz G, et al. Hypothesis: possible role of retinoic acid therapy in patients with biallelic mismatch repair gene defects. Eur J Pediatr. 2008;167(2):225–9.

Chapter 4
Mismatch Repair-Proficient Hereditary Nonpolyposis Colorectal Cancer

Laura Valle

Abstract Approximately 40% of the families meeting the Amsterdam criteria for a diagnosis of hereditary nonpolyposis colorectal cancer lack evidence of heritable defects in the DNA mismatch repair (MMR) system; more specifically, these patients have no germline mutations in the MMR genes and, therefore, no tumor microsatellite instability or loss of immunohistochemical staining of MMR proteins. The proportion of nonpolyposis CRC families without MMR defects further increases when less stringent criteria for hereditary CRC are considered. As has been the case for other hereditary cancer syndromes, the identification of the genes associated with hereditary colorectal cancer would facilitate the molecular diagnosis of the disease and the development of appropriate surveillance guidelines and clinical management protocols for these patients. However, as will be discussed in this chapter, the identification of causal genes has not proven easy.

Keywords Familial colorectal cancer type X · MMR-proficient · Hereditary cancer · Colorectal cancer predisposition · Novel genes

Between 21 and 73% of the families meeting the Amsterdam criteria for a diagnosis of hereditary nonpolyposis colorectal cancer (CRC) lack evidence of heritable defects in the DNA mismatch repair (MMR) system [1, 2]. Because the genetic etiology of this entity is unknown, these families are grouped as familial colorectal cancer type X (FCCTX), being this designation a temporary one until the cause of the familial aggregation is identified.

L. Valle (✉)
Hereditary Cancer Program, Catalan Institute of Oncology, IDIBELL and CIBERONC, Hospitalet de Llobregat, Barcelona, Spain
e-mail: lvalle@iconcologia.net

L. Valle et al. (eds.), *Hereditary Colorectal Cancer*,
https://doi.org/10.1007/978-3-319-74259-5_4

1 Clinical Characteristics

MMR-proficient hereditary nonpolyposis colorectal cancer or FCCTX is not a single syndrome and should not be considered as such. Nevertheless, from the moment FCCTX was described, researchers and clinicians tried to define the clinical features that differentiate this entity from the well-characterized Lynch syndrome; by definition, the only difference is the absence or presence of mismatch repair deficiency.

Analysis of FCCTX patients and associated tumors revealed that the tumor spectrum, penetrance, and age of onset were different for this group compared to Lynch syndrome. In particular, CRC risk among FCCTX patients is increased approximately two fold over the general population (compared to > six fold for Lynch syndrome patients), CRC is diagnosed later in life (>10 years later than in Lynch syndrome), FCCTX families usually lack extracolonic and multiple primary tumors, and the diagnosed colorectal tumors mainly appear in the distal/left or rectum colon [1–7]. Several studies have observed a high adenoma/carcinoma ratio in FCCTX [3, 6], which might suggest a slower adenoma-carcinoma progression rate than in Lynch syndrome [8, 9].

While CRCs linked to Lynch syndrome are characterized by poorly differentiated tumors, mucinous differentiation, an expanding growth pattern, and lymphocytic reaction (e.g., tumor-infiltrating lymphocytes, peritumoral lymphocytes, and Crohn-like reactions), FCCTX tumors show medium/high differentiation, glandular and infiltrative growth patterns, and frequent dirty necrosis, similar to sporadic MMR-proficient tumors [3, 10].

2 Tumor Molecular Characteristics

Compared to MMR-deficient hereditary cases, i.e., Lynch syndrome, FCCTX shows drastic molecular differences, mostly secondary to the status of the DNA mismatch repair machinery. Overall, FCCTX tumors are characterized by the absence of microsatellite instability (MMR proficiency), presence of chromosomal instability, and lack of high CpG methylator phenotype (CIMP), which overlaps with the characteristics of most sporadic MMR-proficient tumors [11–13]. The differences between hereditary (FCCTX) and sporadic MMR-proficient tumors are very subtle but probably the most relevant to elucidate the molecular characteristics of FCCTX.

Hereditary MMR-proficient colorectal tumors show the lowest methylation indices when compared to sporadic MSS, sporadic MSI, and Lynch syndrome tumors. In fact FCCTX tumors have an excess of LINE-1 (long interspersed nucleotide element-1) hypomethylation, a marker for genome-wide hypomethylation [12]. LINE-1 hypomethylation is thought to interfere with chromosomal segregation, thus promoting chromosomal instability [14, 15]. Interestingly, LINE-1 hypomethylation also occurs in MMR-proficient early-onset CRC in the absence of familial history of cancer, which suggests common genetic characteristics [16]. The presence of LINE-1 hypomethylation has been associated with poor prognosis and shorter survival in several tumor types, including CRC [15–21].

The genomic profiles obtained for FCCTX tumors largely resemble those of sporadic MMR-proficient CRCs. Even several changes at first linked to FCCTX were later identified at similar frequencies in sporadic tumors, as was the case of the gain of chromosome 20q or the loss of chromosome 18 [11, 13, 22–24]. Other changes identified in small-sized studies will require validation in larger cohorts to be confirmed, as it is the case of the overrepresentation of chromosome 2p and 2q gains and of 10q loss identified in 16 FCCTX compared to 328 MMR-proficient sporadic CRCs [24].

As occurs for copy number alterations, no differences in the mutation frequencies in known CRC genes, such as *BRAF*, *KRAS*, or *PIK3CA*, are observed between FCCTX and sporadic MMR-proficient tumors [12, 22, 24]. Nevertheless, some evidence indicates that *TP53* mutations might be rarer in FCCTX tumors [11, 24].

3 Attempts to Identify Causal Genes

Before the development of high-throughput sequence capture methods and next-generation sequencing technologies, hereditary cancer studies were mainly based on genome-wide linkage analysis of large individual pedigrees or multiple pedigrees, followed by positional cloning and study of somatic analysis of mutations, which lead to the identification of the main hereditary colorectal cancer genes (e.g., Leppert et al. and Nishisho et al. [25, 26]). However, despite the enormous efforts made after the identification of the most prominent hereditary CRC genes, i.e., *MLH1*, *MSH2*, *MSH6*, and *PMS2*, linkage analyses followed by positional cloning and/or sequencing of the genes (coding regions) located within the candidate linkage peaks seemed to be unable to identify additional causal genes for hereditary nonpolyposis CRC, implying large heterogeneity, oligo- or polygenic modes of inheritance, or unconventional mechanisms of gene inactivation, among other possibilities. Using genome-wide linkage studies in families with CRC, several dominant predisposition loci were mapped to different chromosomal regions such as 3q13.31–q27.1, 3q22, 4q21.1, 5q14–q22, 7q31, 8q13.2, 9q22.2–31.2, 10p15.3–p15.1, 12q24.32, 13q22.1–13q31.3, and others; however, so far no causal genes have been identified in those regions [27–39].

In the last decade, the rapid development of massively parallel sequencing-based approaches and genome-wide copy number techniques, associated to the decrease in their economic cost, restored hope for the identification of additional hereditary CRC genes. Among the approaches most commonly used for the identification of causal mutations in a genome-wide manner are whole-genome sequencing (WGS), whole-exome sequencing (WES), and genome-wide – usually array-based – scanning of copy number alterations. These approaches may be used for the study of isolated high-risk families (large pedigrees) or of multiple families or probands (often with specific phenotypes such an early age of onset) to identify a shared causal gene. Moreover, in some instances, combination of the abovementioned methodologies, such as WES/WGS and linkage data, and/or combination of germline and somatic analyses are used to optimize the process.

Despite the ability of WES and WGS to uncover numerous novel causal mutations and genes in Mendelian disorders, and even in several inherited cancer syndromes, including polyposis CRC, the success in MMR-proficient hereditary CRC has been very limited, almost insignificant (reviewed by Valle [40]). Nevertheless, several novel genes have been proposed as responsible for hereditary nonpolyposis CRC cases, with more or less strong supporting evidence of causality.

In addition to the abovementioned – in principle – agnostic approaches for the identification of novel hereditary CRC genes, the study of genes involved in DNA repair or in well-known relevant pathways for colorectal carcinogenesis has been, and still is, a main line of research for the identification of the causes of FCCTX.

4 Candidate Genes

In the case of MMR-proficient hereditary nonpolyposis CRC, for none or very few of the candidate genes identified by using WGS, WES, or genome-wide scanning of copy number alterations, the evidence gathered to date is robust enough to include their testing in routine genetic diagnosis. Indeed, for most of the proposed genes, the identification of additional pathogenic mutations in high-risk families and/or stronger functional evidence is needed to consider the study of the gene in the clinical setting. Table 4.1 shows the candidate genes proposed to date and the supporting evidence for their causal role in CRC predisposition.

Considering the evidence gathered in the original studies, including functional and co-segregation evidence, together with the identification of (possibly) deleterious mutations in other hereditary CRC cases, the genes with the strongest evidence of association with hereditary CRC were *RPS20* [41], *FAN1* [43], *SEMA4A* [46], *BRF1* [48], *PTPN12* [50], *LRP6* [50], *BUB1*, and *BUB3* [45] and the constitutional epigenetic silencing of *PTPRJ* [49]. *FAN1*, *BUB1*, and *BUB3* encode proteins involved in DNA damage response and genetic instability and *LRP6*, a component of the Wnt-Fzd-LRP5-LRP6 complex that triggers beta-catenin signaling. *RPS20* encodes a ribosomal protein and *PTPN12* and *PTPRJ*, protein tyrosine phosphatases (source: GeneCards; www.genecards.org).

Despite the supporting evidence as hereditary CRC genes in the corresponding original articles, a large study that included the analysis of the exomes of 1006 early-onset unrelated CRC patients (<55 y/o at diagnosis) with at least one first-degree relative affected with CRC and of 1609 healthy controls showed that for all the candidate genes, except for *RPS20*, the frequency of mutations in controls did not differ from the frequency observed in familial cases [42, 47, 62]. Nevertheless, these results should be cautiously interpreted because of the extremely low frequency of mutations identified in the genes together with the fact that, if causal, the

Table 4.1 Novel genes and candidate genes for nonpolyposis CRC predisposition identified through whole-exome/whole-genome sequencing or genome-wide copy number approaches

Gene	Phenotype	Original study	Evidence in favor	Evidence against
Nonpolyposis CRC				
RSP20	HNPCC	Nieminen et al. 2014 [41]	Broderick et al. 2016 [42]	
FAN1	HNPCC	Segui et al. 2015 [43]	Smith et al. 2016 (hereditary pancreatic cancer) [44]	Broderick et al. 2016 [42]
BUB1, *BUB3*	Early-onset, familial CRC	De Voer et al. 2013 [45]		Broderick et al. 2016 [42]
SEMA4A	HNPCC	Schulz et al. 2014 [46]		Kinnersley et al. 2016 [47]
BRF1	HNPCC	Bellido et al. 2018 [48]		
PTPRJ (epimutation)	Early-onset CRC	Venkatachalam et al. 2010 [49]		
PTPN12, *LRP6*	Early-onset CRC	De Voer et al. 2016 [50]		Broderick et al. 2016 [42]
POLE2, *POT1*, *MRE11*, *IL12RB1*, *LIMK2*	Early-onset CRC	Chubb et al. 2016 [61]	Spier et al. 2015 [51] (*POLE2*)	
ROBO1	HBOC, early-onset CRC	Villacis et al. 2016 [52]		
HNRNPA0, *WIF1*	CRC, multiple tumors	Wei et al. 2015 [53]		
UACA, *SFXN4*, *TWSG1*, *PSPH*, *NUDT7*, *ZNF490*, *PRSS37*, *CCDC18*, *PRADC1*, *MRPL3*, *AKR1C4*.	HNPCC	Gylfe et al. 2013 [54]		
CDKN1B, *XRCC4*, *EPHX1*, *NFKBIZ*, *SMARCA4*, *BARD1*	HNPCC	Esteban-Jurado et al. 2014 [55]		
ADAMTS4, *CYTL1*, *SYNE1*, *MCTP2*, *ARHGAP12*, *ATM*, *DONSON*, *ROS1*, *MCTP2*	Early-onset, familial CRC	Tanskanen et al. 2015 [56]		

(continued)

Table 4.1 (continued)

Gene	Phenotype	Original study	Evidence in favor	Evidence against
BRCA2/FANCD1, BRIP1/FANCJ, FANCC, FANCE, REV3L/POLZ	HNPCC	Esteban-Jurado et al. 2016 [57]	Garre et al. 2015 [58] (*BRCA2*) Yurgelun et al. 2015 [59] (*BRCA2, BRIP1*)	
ZRANB1, CDC27, CENPE, DDX12, HAUS6/FAM29A, HIST1H2BE, KIF23, TACC2, ZC3HC1, CTBP2, IRF5, MED12, RNF111, SF1, TLE1, TLE4, TRIP4, BTNL2, BAGE, CARD8, FANK1, KIR2DL1, KIR2DS4, KIR3DL3, MASP1, NLRP8	HNPCC	DeRycke et al. 2013 [60]	–	
FANCM, LAMB4, PTCHD3, LAMC3, TREX, NOTCH3	CRC	Smith et al. 2013 [61]		

Abbreviations: *CRC* colorectal cancer, *HBOC* hereditary breast and ovarian cancer, *HNPCC* hereditary nonpolyposis colorectal cancer

penetrance of the candidate genes possibly corresponds to a relatively moderate risk, probably dependent on the genomic and environmental contexts (see correspondence for *SEMA4A* by Sill et al. [63]). In fact, in the ">1000 familial CRC exomes" study, no significant association (T1 burden test) was detected for *MSH6* or *PMS2* when considering disruptive and predictive damaging variants [62]. Therefore, the identification and reporting in the next years of additional families with comprehensive co-segregation data and evidence of the functional effect of the identified mutations will be crucial to finally confirm or discard the implication of the identified candidate genes in the predisposition to MMR-proficient CRC.

In addition to those genes, the study of relatively large numbers of families/probands has allowed the identification of additional candidate genes [54–57, 60–62, 64] (Table 4.1), for which additional evidence needs to be gathered in order to elucidate their real role in the contribution to hereditary CRC.

With regard to the genes identified through candidate gene approaches, mostly based on the implication of known hereditary cancer genes in different DNA repair pathways, we face the same issues as with the genes identified through agnostic approaches: the evidence gathered to date is still insufficient, even contradictory in some instances, to include their study in routine genetic testing, being this the case for *OGG1* [65–67], *NUDT1* [65, 66], *BMP4* [68], and *EPHB* [69]. On the other hand, some genes first identified as potential candidates, such as *UNC5C* [70] and *GALNT12* [71, 72], have been discarded as causal genes for hereditary CRC [73, 74].

5 Pleiotropism: Genetic Overlap with Other Hereditary Cancer Syndromes

The prevalence of pathogenic mutations in the novel (candidate) genes identified is almost insignificant when considering the entire burden of unexplained hereditary cases. The use of next-generation sequencing-based approaches, either for the discovery of novel genes (WGS or WES) or for genetic testing (WES or multigene panels), has allowed the identification of hereditary CRC families with germline pathogenic mutations in genes classically associated with other cancer syndromes, such as *BRCA1* and *BRCA2* [57–59, 75], *TP53* [76], *BARD1* [55], or *BRIP1* [57, 59], or associated with other – very distinct – CRC/polyposis syndromes. This has been the case for the adenomatous polyposis genes, *MUTYH* and *POLD1*, and the juvenile polyposis gene, *BMPR1A*, which have been found mutated in hereditary nonpolyposis CRC families [77–82].

In order to clarify the contribution of non-CRC susceptibility genes to undefined familial CRC, Houlston and colleagues performed a mutational screen of 114 cancer susceptibility genes in ~850 early-onset/familial CRC patients and 1609 controls, analyzing whole-exome sequencing data [62, 83]. Overall, 6.7% of the unexplained familial CRC patients and 5.3% of the controls carried a pathogenic or likely pathogenic mutation in one of the 114 genes analyzed. Despite the non-significant difference in the frequency between cases and controls, mutations were identified in interesting candidates such as *FLCN*, *BLM*, *ERCC*, and *BRCA1/2*, although no significant enrichment was identified in cases.

In 2017, 450 prospectively accrued CRC patients (~85% self-reported their race as white) diagnosed with CRC before age 50 were tested for mutations in 25 cancer susceptibility genes using next-generation sequencing (multigene panel) [75]. A total of 89% had MMR-proficient tumors. Seventy-five pathogenic or likely pathogenic mutations were identified in 72 patients (16%); however, only 61 patients (13.6%) had mutations in high- or moderate-penetrance genes: 8% of the total had Lynch syndrome only; 0.4% had Lynch syndrome and another hereditary cancer syndrome; and 7.6% had a different hereditary cancer syndrome. Among the patients with MMR-proficient tumors (n = 402), 5.5% carried at least one mutation in a high- or moderate-penetrance cancer gene; 2.2% had mutations in high-penetrance CRC genes: five in *APC*, one in *APC* and *PMS2*, two being carriers of biallelic mutations in *MUTYH*, and one in *SMAD4*. Overall, 3.2% had mutations in other high- or moderate-penetrance cancer genes: three in *ATM*, one in *ATM* and *CHEK2*, two in *BRCA1*, four in *BRCA2*, one in *CDKN2A*, and two in *PALB2*.

Similarly, 1058 CRC patients prospectively recruited without preselection for age at diagnosis or personal/family history were tested for mutations in 25 genes associated with inherited cancer risk [84]. While 3.1% (n = 33) had Lynch syndrome, 2.3% (n = 25) carried mutations in non-Lynch syndrome high- or moderate-penetrance cancer genes, including 5 in *APC*, 11 in *BRCA1/2*, 2 in *PALB2*, 2 in *CHEK2*, 1 in *CDKN2A*, 1 in *TP53*, and 3 being carriers of biallelic mutations in *MUTYH*. Neither proband age at CRC diagnosis nor family history of CRC and personal history of other cancers significantly predicted the presence of pathogenic mutations in non-Lynch syndrome genes.

References

1. Lindor NM, Rabe K, Petersen GM, Haile R, Casey G, Baron J, et al. Lower cancer incidence in Amsterdam-I criteria families without mismatch repair deficiency: familial colorectal cancer type X. JAMA. 2005;293(16):1979–85.
2. Dominguez-Valentin M, Therkildsen C, Da Silva S, Nilbert M. Familial colorectal cancer type X: genetic profiles and phenotypic features. Mod Pathol. 2014;28(1):30–6.
3. Llor X, Pons E, Xicola RM, Castells A, Alenda C, Pinol V, et al. Differential features of colorectal cancers fulfilling Amsterdam criteria without involvement of the mutator pathway. Clin Cancer Res. 2005;11(20):7304–10.
4. Mueller-Koch Y, Vogelsang H, Kopp R, Lohse P, Keller G, Aust D, et al. Hereditary non-polyposis colorectal cancer: clinical and molecular evidence for a new entity of hereditary colorectal cancer. Gut. 2005;54(12):1733–40.
5. Valle L, Perea J, Carbonell P, Fernandez V, Dotor AM, Benitez J, et al. Clinicopathologic and pedigree differences in amsterdam I-positive hereditary nonpolyposis colorectal cancer families according to tumor microsatellite instability status. J Clin Oncol. 2007;25(7):781–6.
6. Francisco I, Albuquerque C, Lage P, Belo H, Vitoriano I, Filipe B, et al. Familial colorectal cancer type X syndrome: two distinct molecular entities? Familial Cancer. 2011;10(4):623–31.
7. Shiovitz S, Copeland WK, Passarelli MN, Burnett-Hartman AN, Grady WM, Potter JD, et al. Characterisation of familial colorectal cancer Type X, Lynch syndrome, and non-familial colorectal cancer. Br J Cancer. 2014;111(3):598–602.
8. Jass JR. Hereditary non-polyposis colorectal cancer: the rise and fall of a confusing term. World J Gastroenterol. 2006;12(31):4943–50.
9. Lindor NM. Familial colorectal cancer type X: the other half of hereditary nonpolyposis colon cancer syndrome. Surg Oncol Clin N Am. 2009;18(4):637–45.
10. Klarskov L, Holck S, Bernstein I, Nilbert M. Hereditary colorectal cancer diagnostics: morphological features of familial colorectal cancer type X versus Lynch syndrome. J Clin Pathol. 2012;65(4):352–6.
11. Abdel-Rahman WM, Ollikainen M, Kariola R, Jarvinen HJ, Mecklin JP, Nystrom-Lahti M, et al. Comprehensive characterization of HNPCC-related colorectal cancers reveals striking molecular features in families with no germline mismatch repair gene mutations. Oncogene. 2005;24(9):1542–51.
12. Goel A, Xicola RM, Nguyen TP, Doyle BJ, Sohn VR, Bandipalliam P, et al. Aberrant DNA methylation in hereditary nonpolyposis colorectal cancer without mismatch repair deficiency. Gastroenterology. 2010;138(5):1854–62.
13. Therkildsen C, Jonsson G, Dominguez-Valentin M, Nissen A, Rambech E, Halvarsson B, et al. Gain of chromosomal region 20q and loss of 18 discriminates between Lynch syndrome and familial colorectal cancer. Eur J Cancer. 2013;49(6):1226–35.
14. Ogino S, Kawasaki T, Nosho K, Ohnishi M, Suemoto Y, Kirkner GJ, et al. LINE-1 hypomethylation is inversely associated with microsatellite instability and CpG island methylator phenotype in colorectal cancer. Int J Cancer. 2008;122(12):2767–73.
15. Igarashi S, Suzuki H, Niinuma T, Shimizu H, Nojima M, Iwaki H, et al. A novel correlation between LINE-1 hypomethylation and the malignancy of gastrointestinal stromal tumors. Clin Cancer Res. 2010;16(21):5114–23.
16. Antelo M, Balaguer F, Shia J, Shen Y, Hur K, Moreira L, et al. A high degree of LINE-1 hypomethylation is a unique feature of early-onset colorectal cancer. PLoS One. 2012;7(9):e45357.
17. Ogino S, Nosho K, Kirkner GJ, Kawasaki T, Chan AT, Schernhammer ES, et al. A cohort study of tumoral LINE-1 hypomethylation and prognosis in colon cancer. J Natl Cancer Inst. 2008;100(23):1734–8.
18. Boland CR. Recent discoveries in the molecular genetics of Lynch syndrome. Familial Cancer. 2016;15(3):395–403.

19. Ikeda K, Shiraishi K, Eguchi A, Shibata H, Yoshimoto K, Mori T, et al. Long interspersed nucleotide element 1 hypomethylation is associated with poor prognosis of lung adenocarcinoma. Ann Thorac Surg. 2013;96(5):1790–4.
20. Iwagami S, Baba Y, Watanabe M, Shigaki H, Miyake K, Ishimoto T, et al. LINE-1 hypomethylation is associated with a poor prognosis among patients with curatively resected esophageal squamous cell carcinoma. Ann Surg. 2013;257(3):449–55.
21. Shigaki H, Baba Y, Watanabe M, Murata A, Iwagami S, Miyake K, et al. LINE-1 hypomethylation in gastric cancer, detected by bisulfite pyrosequencing, is associated with poor prognosis. Gastric Cancer. 2013;16(4):480–7.
22. Sanchez-de-Abajo A, de la Hoya M, van Puijenbroek M, Tosar A, Lopez-Asenjo JA, Diaz-Rubio E, et al. Molecular analysis of colorectal cancer tumors from patients with mismatch repair proficient hereditary nonpolyposis colorectal cancer suggests novel carcinogenic pathways. Clin Cancer Res. 2007;13(19):5729–35.
23. Middeldorp A, van Eijk R, Oosting J, Forte GI, van Puijenbroek M, van Nieuwenhuizen M, et al. Increased frequency of 20q gain and copy-neutral loss of heterozygosity in mismatch repair proficient familial colorectal carcinomas. Int J Cancer. 2012;130(4):837–46.
24. Bellido F, Pineda M, Sanz-Pamplona R, Navarro M, Nadal M, Lazaro C, et al. Comprehensive molecular characterisation of hereditary non-polyposis colorectal tumours with mismatch repair proficiency. Eur J Cancer. 2014;50(11):1964–72.
25. Leppert M, Dobbs M, Scambler P, O'Connell P, Nakamura Y, Stauffer D, et al. The gene for familial polyposis coli maps to the long arm of chromosome 5. Science (New York, NY). 1987;238(4832):1411–3.
26. Nishisho I, Nakamura Y, Miyoshi Y, Miki Y, Ando H, Horii A, et al. Mutations of chromosome 5q21 genes in FAP and colorectal cancer patients. Science (New York, NY). 1991;253(5020):665–9.
27. Wiesner GL, Daley D, Lewis S, Ticknor C, Platzer P, Lutterbaugh J, et al. A subset of familial colorectal neoplasia kindreds linked to chromosome 9q22.2-31.2. Proc Natl Acad Sci U S A. 2003;100(22):12961–5.
28. Kemp ZE, Carvajal-Carmona LG, Barclay E, Gorman M, Martin L, Wood W, et al. Evidence of linkage to chromosome 9q22.33 in colorectal cancer kindreds from the United Kingdom. Cancer Res. 2006;66(10):5003–6.
29. Skoglund J, Djureinovic T, Zhou XL, Vandrovcova J, Renkonen E, Iselius L, et al. Linkage analysis in a large Swedish family supports the presence of a susceptibility locus for adenoma and colorectal cancer on chromosome 9q22.32-31.1. J Med Genet. 2006;43(2):e7.
30. Neklason DW, Kerber RA, Nilson DB, Anton-Culver H, Schwartz AG, Griffin CA, et al. Common familial colorectal cancer linked to chromosome 7q31: a genome-wide analysis. Cancer Res. 2008;68(21):8993–7.
31. Papaemmanuil E, Carvajal-Carmona L, Sellick GS, Kemp Z, Webb E, Spain S, et al. Deciphering the genetics of hereditary non-syndromic colorectal cancer. Eur J Hum Genet. 2008;16(12):1477–86.
32. Picelli S, Vandrovcova J, Jones S, Djureinovic T, Skoglund J, Zhou XL, et al. Genome-wide linkage scan for colorectal cancer susceptibility genes supports linkage to chromosome 3q. BMC Cancer. 2008;8:87.
33. Gray-McGuire C, Guda K, Adrianto I, Lin CP, Natale L, Potter JD, et al. Confirmation of linkage to and localization of familial colon cancer risk haplotype on chromosome 9q22. Cancer Res. 2010;70(13):5409–18.
34. Neklason DW, Tuohy TM, Stevens J, Otterud B, Baird L, Kerber RA, et al. Colorectal adenomas and cancer link to chromosome 13q22.1-13q31.3 in a large family with excess colorectal cancer. J Med Genet. 2010;47(10):692–9.
35. Saunders IW, Ross J, Macrae F, Young GP, Blanco I, Brohede J, et al. Evidence of linkage to chromosomes 10p15.3-p15.1, 14q24.3-q31.1 and 9q33.3-q34.3 in non-syndromic colorectal cancer families. Eur J Hum Genet. 2012;20(1):91–6.

36. Kontham V, von Holst S, Lindblom A. Linkage analysis in familial non-Lynch syndrome colorectal cancer families from Sweden. PLoS One. 2013;8(12):e83936.
37. Teerlink C, Nelson Q, Burt R, Cannon-Albright L. Significant evidence of linkage for a gene predisposing to colorectal cancer and multiple primary cancers on 22q11. Clin Transl Gastroenterol. 2014;5:e50.
38. Rudkjobing LA, Eiberg H, Mikkelsen HB, Binderup ML, Bisgaard ML. The analysis of a large Danish family supports the presence of a susceptibility locus for adenoma and colorectal cancer on chromosome 11q24. Familial Cancer. 2015;14(3):393–400.
39. Sanchez-Tome E, Rivera B, Perea J, Pita G, Rueda D, Mercadillo F, et al. Genome-wide linkage analysis and tumoral characterization reveal heterogeneity in familial colorectal cancer type X. J Gastroenterol. 2015;50(6):657–66.
40. Valle L. Recent discoveries in the genetics of familial colorectal cancer and polyposis. Clin Gastroenterol Hepatol. 2017;15(3):461–462.
41. Nieminen TT, O'Donohue MF, Wu Y, Lohi H, Scherer SW, Paterson AD, et al. Germline mutation of RPS20, encoding a ribosomal protein, causes predisposition to hereditary nonpolyposis colorectal carcinoma without DNA mismatch repair deficiency. Gastroenterology. 2014;147(3):595–8 e5.
42. Broderick P, Dobbins SE, Chubb D, Kinnersley B, Dunlop MG, Tomlinson I, et al. Validation of recently proposed colorectal cancer susceptibility gene variants in an analysis of families and patients-a systematic review. Gastroenterology. 2016;152(1):75–7 e4.
43. Segui N, Mina LB, Lazaro C, Sanz-Pamplona R, Pons T, Navarro M, et al. Germline mutations in FAN1 cause hereditary colorectal cancer by impairing DNA repair. Gastroenterology. 2015;149(3):563–6.
44. Smith AL, Alirezaie N, Connor A, Chan-Seng-Yue M, Grant R, Selander I, et al. Candidate DNA repair susceptibility genes identified by exome sequencing in high-risk pancreatic cancer. Cancer Lett. 2016;370(2):302–12.
45. de Voer RM, Geurts van Kessel A, Weren RD, Ligtenberg MJ, Smeets D, Fu L, et al. Germline mutations in the spindle assembly checkpoint genes BUB1 and BUB3 are risk factors for colorectal cancer. Gastroenterology. 2013;145(3):544–7.
46. Schulz E, Klampfl P, Holzapfel S, Janecke AR, Ulz P, Renner W, et al. Germline variants in the SEMA4A gene predispose to familial colorectal cancer type X. Nat Commun. 2004;5:5191.
47. Kinnersley B, Chubb D, Dobbins SE, Frampton M, Buch S, Timofeeva MN, et al. Correspondence: SEMA4A variation and risk of colorectal cancer. Nat Commun. 2016;7:10611.
48. Bellido F, Sowada N, Mur P, Lázaro C, Pons T, Valdés-Mas R, et al. Association Between Germline Mutations in BRF1, a Subunit of the RNA Polymerase III Transcription Complex, and Hereditary Colorectal Cancer. Gastroenterology. 2018;154(1):181–194. doi:10.1053/j.gastro.2017.09.005
49. Venkatachalam R, Ligtenberg MJ, Hoogerbrugge N, Schackert HK, Gorgens H, Hahn MM, et al. Germline epigenetic silencing of the tumor suppressor gene PTPRJ in early-onset familial colorectal cancer. Gastroenterology. 2010;139(6):2221–4.
50. de Voer RM, Hahn MM, Weren RD, Mensenkamp AR, Gilissen C, van Zelst-Stams WA, et al. Identification of novel candidate genes for early-onset colorectal cancer susceptibility. PLoS Genet. 2016;12(2):e1005880.
51. Spier I, Holzapfel S, Altmuller J, Zhao B, Horpaopan S, Vogt S, et al. Frequency and phenotypic spectrum of germline mutations in POLE and seven other polymerase genes in 266 patients with colorectal adenomas and carcinomas. Int J Cancer. 2015;137(2):320–31.
52. Villacis RA, Abreu FB, Miranda PM, Domingues MA, Carraro DM, Santos EM, et al. ROBO1 deletion as a novel germline alteration in breast and colorectal cancer patients. Tumour Biol. 2016;37(3):3145–53.
53. Wei C, Peng B, Han Y, Chen WV, Rother J, Tomlinson GE, et al. Mutations of HNRNPA0 and WIF1 predispose members of a large family to multiple cancers. Familial Cancer. 2015;14(2):297–306.

54. Gylfe AE, Katainen R, Kondelin J, Tanskanen T, Cajuso T, Hanninen U, et al. Eleven candidate susceptibility genes for common familial colorectal cancer. PLoS Genet. 2013;9(10):e1003876.
55. Esteban-Jurado C, Vila-Casadesus M, Garre P, Lozano JJ, Pristoupilova A, Beltran S, et al. Whole-exome sequencing identifies rare pathogenic variants in new predisposition genes for familial colorectal cancer. Genet Med. 2014;17(2):131–42.
56. Tanskanen T, Gylfe AE, Katainen R, Taipale M, Renkonen-Sinisalo L, Jarvinen H, et al. Systematic search for rare variants in Finnish early-onset colorectal cancer patients. Cancer Genet. 2015;208(1–2):35–40.
57. Esteban-Jurado C, Franch-Exposito S, Munoz J, Ocana T, Carballal S, Lopez-Ceron M, et al. The Fanconi anemia DNA damage repair pathway in the spotlight for germline predisposition to colorectal cancer. Eur J Hum Genet. 2016;24(10):1501–5.
58. Garre P, Martin L, Sanz J, Romero A, Tosar A, Bando I, et al. BRCA2 gene: a candidate for clinical testing in familial colorectal cancer type X. Clin Genet. 2015;87(6):582–7.
59. Yurgelun MB, Allen B, Kaldate RR, Bowles KR, Judkins T, Kaushik P, et al. Identification of a variety of mutations in cancer predisposition genes in patients with suspected Lynch syndrome. Gastroenterology. 2015;149(3):604–13 e20.
60. DeRycke MS, Gunawardena SR, Middha S, Asmann YW, Schaid DJ, McDonnell SK, et al. Identification of novel variants in colorectal cancer families by high-throughput exome sequencing. Cancer Epidemiol Biomark Prev. 2013;22(7):1239–51.
61. Smith CG, Naven M, Harris R, Colley J, West H, Li N, et al. Exome resequencing identifies potential tumor-suppressor genes that predispose to colorectal cancer. Hum Mutat. 2013;34(7):1026–34.
62. Chubb D, Broderick P, Dobbins SE, Frampton M, Kinnersley B, Penegar S, et al. Rare disruptive mutations and their contribution to the heritable risk of colorectal cancer. Nat Commun. 2016;7:11883.
63. Sill H, Schulz E, Steinke-Lange V, Boland CR. Correspondence: reply to 'SEMA4A variation and risk of colorectal cancer'. Nat Commun. 2016;7:10695.
64. Spier I, Kerick M, Drichel D, Horpaopan S, Altmuller J, Laner A, et al. Exome sequencing identifies potential novel candidate genes in patients with unexplained colorectal adenomatous polyposis. Familial Cancer. 2016;15(2):281–8.
65. Garre P, Briceno V, Xicola RM, Doyle BJ, de la Hoya M, Sanz J, et al. Analysis of the oxidative damage repair genes NUDT1, OGG1, and MUTYH in patients from mismatch repair proficient HNPCC families (MSS-HNPCC). Clin Cancer Res. 2011;17(7):1701–12.
66. Dallosso AR, Dolwani S, Jones N, Jones S, Colley J, Maynard J, et al. Inherited predisposition to colorectal adenomas caused by multiple rare alleles of MUTYH but not OGG1, NUDT1, NTH1 or NEIL 1, 2 or 3. Gut. 2008;57(9):1252–5.
67. Kinnersley B, Buch S, Castellvi-Bel S, Farrington SM, Forsti A, Hampe J, et al. Re: role of the oxidative DNA damage repair gene OGG1 in colorectal tumorigenesis. J Natl Cancer Inst. 2014;106(5):dju086.
68. Lubbe SJ, Pittman AM, Matijssen C, Twiss P, Olver B, Lloyd A, et al. Evaluation of germline BMP4 mutation as a cause of colorectal cancer. Hum Mutat. 2011;32(1):E1928–38.
69. Zogopoulos G, Jorgensen C, Bacani J, Montpetit A, Lepage P, Ferretti V, et al. Germline EPHB2 receptor variants in familial colorectal cancer. PLoS One. 2008;3(8):e2885.
70. Coissieux MM, Tomsic J, Castets M, Hampel H, Tuupanen S, Andrieu N, et al. Variants in the netrin-1 receptor UNC5C prevent apoptosis and increase risk of familial colorectal cancer. Gastroenterology. 2011;141(6):2039–46.
71. Guda K, Moinova H, He J, Jamison O, Ravi L, Natale L, et al. Inactivating germ-line and somatic mutations in polypeptide N-acetylgalactosaminyltransferase 12 in human colon cancers. Proc Natl Acad Sci U S A. 2009;106(31):12921–5.
72. Clarke E, Green RC, Green JS, Mahoney K, Parfrey PS, Younghusband HB, et al. Inherited deleterious variants in GALNT12 are associated with CRC susceptibility. Hum Mutat. 2012;33(7):1056–8.

73. Mur P, Elena SC, Ausso S, Aiza G, Rafael VM, Pineda M, et al. Scarce evidence of the causal role of germline mutations in UNC5C in hereditary colorectal cancer and polyposis. Sci Rep. 2016;6:20697.
74. Segui N, Pineda M, Navarro M, Lazaro C, Brunet J, Infante M, et al. GALNT12 is not a major contributor of familial colorectal cancer type X. Hum Mutat. 2014;35(1):50–2.
75. Pearlman R, Frankel WL, Swanson B, Zhao W, Yilmaz A, Miller K, et al. Prevalence and Spectrum of germline cancer susceptibility gene mutations among patients with early-onset colorectal cancer. JAMA Oncol. 2017;3(4):464–71.
76. Yurgelun MB, Masciari S, Joshi VA, Mercado RC, Lindor NM, Gallinger S, et al. Germline TP53 mutations in patients with early-onset colorectal cancer in the colon cancer family registry. JAMA Oncol. 2015;1(2):214–21.
77. Wang L, Baudhuin LM, Boardman LA, Steenblock KJ, Petersen GM, Halling KC, et al. MYH mutations in patients with attenuated and classic polyposis and with young-onset colorectal cancer without polyps. Gastroenterology. 2004;127(1):9–16.
78. Knopperts AP, Nielsen M, Niessen RC, Tops CM, Jorritsma B, Varkevisser J, et al. Contribution of bi-allelic germline MUTYH mutations to early-onset and familial colorectal cancer and to low number of adenomatous polyps: case-series and literature review. Familial Cancer. 2013;12(1):43–50.
79. Castillejo A, Vargas G, Castillejo MI, Navarro M, Barbera VM, Gonzalez S, et al. Prevalence of germline MUTYH mutations among Lynch-like syndrome patients. Eur J Cancer. 2014;50(13):2241–50.
80. Segui N, Navarro M, Pineda M, Koger N, Bellido F, Gonzalez S, et al. Exome sequencing identifies MUTYH mutations in a family with colorectal cancer and an atypical phenotype. Gut. 2015;64(2):355–6.
81. Valle L, Hernandez-Illan E, Bellido F, Aiza G, Castillejo A, Castillejo MI, et al. New insights into POLE and POLD1 germline mutations in familial colorectal cancer and polyposis. Hum Mol Genet. 2014;23(13):3506–12.
82. Bellido F, Pineda M, Aiza G, Valdes-Mas R, Navarro M, Puente DA, et al. POLE and POLD1 mutations in 529 kindred with familial colorectal cancer and/or polyposis: review of reported cases and recommendations for genetic testing and surveillance. Genet Med. 2016;18(4):325–32.
83. Dobbins SE, Broderick P, Chubb D, Kinnersley B, Sherborne AL, Houlston RS. Undefined familial colorectal cancer and the role of pleiotropism in cancer susceptibility genes. Familial Cancer. 2016;15(4):593–9.
84. Yurgelun MB, Kulke MH, Fuchs CS, Allen BA, Uno H, Hornick JL, et al. Cancer susceptibility gene mutations in individuals with colorectal cancer. J Clin Oncol. 2017;35(10):1086–95.

Chapter 5
Genetic and Environmental Modifiers of Cancer Risk in Lynch Syndrome

Aung K. Win and Rodney J. Scott

Abstract Lynch syndrome, caused by pathogenic mutations in DNA mismatch repair genes, is associated with high risks of colorectal and endometrial cancer. Approximately 1 in 280 (0.35%) of the population are estimated to carry a pathogenic mutation in one of these genes. However, penetrance (age-specific cancer risk) estimates for mutation carriers have been found to vary substantially depending on person's sex and which gene is mutated. Further, penetrance is also highly variable across carriers with mutations in the same gene. These observed differences in risk are consistent with that genetic and environmental factors are likely to modify cancer risks for people with Lynch syndrome. Identifying and characterising these risk-modifying factors are essential to enable targeted risk-based screening/treatment and risk-reduction strategies on the basis of 'individual' risk estimates rather than 'average' risk estimates. In this chapter, we review the latest evidence on genetic and environmental factors that have been investigated in association with cancer risk, primarily colorectal cancer, for people with Lynch syndrome.

Keywords Lynch syndrome · Colorectal cancer · Endometrial cancer · Modifiers Penetrance

A. K. Win (✉)
Centre for Epidemiology and Biostatistics, Melbourne School of Population and Global Health, The University of Melbourne, Melbourne, VIC, Australia

Genetic Medicine and Familial Cancer Centre, The Royal Melbourne Hospital, Parkville, VIC, Australia
e-mail: awin@unimelb.edu.au

R. J. Scott (✉)
School of Biomedical Sciences and Pharmacy, University of Newcastle, Newcastle, NSW, Australia

Department of Molecular Medicine, NSW Health Pathology, Newcastle, NSW, Australia
e-mail: rodney.scott@newcastle.edu.au

L. Valle et al. (eds.), *Hereditary Colorectal Cancer*,
https://doi.org/10.1007/978-3-319-74259-5_5

1 Introduction

Lynch syndrome is associated with increased risks of developing epithelial malignancies, primarily colorectal cancer and endometrial cancer, at unusually early ages [1]. Since the risk is not uniform across the four DNA mismatch repair (MMR) genes (*MSH2, MLH1, MSH6* or *PMS2)* or *EPCAM* deletion known to be associated with the syndrome, it is also highly variable across individuals with the same mutated gene [2, 3]. Approximately 1 in 280 (0.35%) of the population are estimated to carry a pathogenic mutation in one of these genes [4]. People with Lynch syndrome are not born with any apparent premalignant change that precedes malignant disease suggesting that other factors may be involved in promoting disease development or indeed inhibiting it.

There is substantial evidence for a wide variation in age-specific risks of cancer (penetrance) in Lynch syndrome by which gene is mutated [3, 5–16]. For example, people who have inherited a germline variant in *MLH1* or *MSH2* have a higher risk of developing colorectal cancer compared with those who have inherited a *PMS2* mutation [7, 13–16]. Cancer risk in Lynch syndrome might also vary by the type of mutation [17] or the person's race/ethnicity [18] or the geographic location where they live [19]. Further, there is evidence for a wide variation in risk even across people with mutations in the same gene—the majority of carriers are either at only modestly increased risk or at very high risk rather than being clustered around the 'average' risk [3]. This observation is consistent with the existence of factors modifying disease penetrance ranging from the genetic through to the environment or a combination of both. This needs to be considered when providing people who have been diagnosed with a germline pathogenic variant as disease risk will be a function of the actual variant and will need to include disease penetrance conferred by the gene in question.

To enable comprehensive counselling and provide targeted risk-based screening and risk-reduction strategies, we need accurate risk estimates based on a wide range of factors including personal particulars (age, sex, ethnicity and geographic location), the MMR gene mutated and the position and functional effect of the mutation, family history of cancer as well as all genetic and environmental/lifestyle/dietary factors that modify cancer risk for mutation carriers. In this review, we focus on the latest evidence on genetic and environmental factors that have been investigated in association with cancer risk for people with Lynch syndrome.

2 Genetic Modifiers

Since the identification of the genetic basis of Lynch syndrome, the question has been asked as to why some persons within the same family or indeed persons carrying the same variant from different families develop disease at vastly different ages. Furthermore, disease risk is also a function of which gene happens to be associated with the inherited variant. Locus-specific disease penetrance is one aspect that has been examined, and the results clearly indicate that *MSH6* variant carriers have a different disease risk profile compared with *MSH2* or *MLH1* variant carriers [6] as do *PMS2* variant carriers [7, 14–16]. For the purposes of this section of the chapter, there will be a focus on colorectal cancer risk due primarily to the frequency of this malignancy and the number of studies that have examined genetic modifiers of risk in the context of this malignancy.

2.1 Cell Cycle Control

DNA repair is integrally associated with cell cycle control, and functional polymorphisms in genes associated with this aspect of genomic integrity are attractive candidates for modifier gene studies. The gene *TP53* is well recognised for its association with tumour development as well as its role in Li-Fraumeni syndrome [20]. *TP53* is involved in the maintenance of genomic integrity, blocking cell proliferation after DNA damage and initiating apoptosis if it is too extensive, and has been termed a master regulator [21]. With respect to disease risk in Lynch syndrome, there appears to be little evidence for an association between a functional polymorphism p.R72P in *TP53* and the age of onset of colorectal cancer [22–26].

Other cell cycle-related genes that have been investigated in Lynch syndrome include *CCND1*, *AURKA*, *MDM2* and *IGF1,* but no unequivocal results have been forthcoming [25, 27–37]. In a study conducted in the MD Anderson Cancer Centre, single nucleotide polymorphisms or SNPs in 128 cell cycle genes have been examined from which 10 (*PPP2R2B, KIF20A, TGFB1, XRCC5, TNF, BCL2, TTC28, CHFR, CDC25C, ATM*) were found to have an association with colorectal cancer risk in Lynch syndrome [32]. There has been no large replication study undertaken in Lynch syndrome to confirm or otherwise the results of these studies. Nevertheless, the results are suggestive of an effect that warrants further investigation.

2.2 DNA Repair

DNA is the only macromolecule that is repaired; all others are removed. The repair processes that have evolved are uniquely adapted to deal with the various types of DNA damage and synthesis error that occur. DNA repair comprises nucleotide excision repair, base excision repair, double-strand break repair, non-homologous end joining and mismatch repair. When considered together, DNA repair comprises over 130 genes that function in this process. All of these genes have significant roles in this process in maintaining genomic integrity [38]. The DNA repair pathways of MMR and base excision repair (BER) are involved in the identification, removal and repair of replication-induced DNA errors. MMR involves correcting mismatched bases that occur during DNA replication [39], whereas BER is specific for oxidative DNA damage repair [40]. Double-strand breaks (DSBs) in DNA are repaired by either homologous recombination, or non-homologous end joining (NHEJ), which is error prone. Functional polymorphisms in DNA repair genes have been implicated in colorectal cancer susceptibility in the general population, suggesting that altered repair function could explain some of the phenotypic differences observed in Lynch syndrome. There have been only limited reports examining DNA repair gene polymorphisms and their effects on disease risk in Lynch syndrome and they include the genes *ATM, MSH3, OGG1, XRCC1, XRCC2, XRCC3, BRCA2* and *Lig4*. None of the functional polymorphisms examined in these DNA repair genes could be shown to influence disease risk [41–44]. The failure to reveal a modifying effect from any of these genes does not rule out the possibility that there exist other DNA repair gene polymorphisms that influence disease risk. Further studies are required before DNA repair gene polymorphisms are shown not to be associated with disease expression in Lynch syndrome.

Telomerase is an enzyme involved in maintaining telomere length after cell division. Telomere shortening has been linked to the initiation of epithelial malignancies and chromosomal instability [45, 46]. A polymorphism in *hTERT* has been associated with cancer risk, and one report tentatively linked this polymorphism to an earlier age of cancer and/or polyp development in people with Lynch syndrome [47]. Of interest in this report is the absence of effect in people older than 45 years of age, suggesting that this modifier may no longer be effective when telomere shortening has already occurred in ageing populations [48]. But, another study reported that there was no evidence of association between any of the *hTERT* SNPs and colorectal risk in Lynch syndrome [49].

2.3 Xenobiotic Clearance and Micronutrient Metabolism

Carcinogens encompass both naturally occurring agents found primarily in plants and xenobiotic agents that are man-made. Exposures to carcinogens result in either DNA damage or DNA adduct formation, both of which can alter gene expression via a variety of pathways that culminate in uncontrolled cellular proliferation. The removal of many carcinogens is controlled by a complex process involving phase I enzymes such as cytochrome P450 (CYP) and phase II enzymes that include the glutathione S-transferases (GSTs) and N-acetyl transferases (NATs) [50]. Many of the genes involved in phase I and phase II clearance are polymorphic and confer different enzymatic activities that can be associated with the rates of carcinogen clearance. There have been, for example, many studies examining the presence of functional polymorphisms in these genes and their association with colorectal cancer risk [51–55]. Due to their polymorphic nature, genes involved in xenobiotic metabolism have been considered as modifier genes, as a result of their association with the risk of malignancy.

With respect to Lynch syndrome, relatively few reports exist describing disease-modifying effects of polymorphisms in the xenobiotic metabolising genes *NAT1*,

NAT2, *GST* and *CYP* and have been published [56–66]. A study on people with Lynch syndrome examining the association between disease and polymorphisms in *NAT2* suggested an association [56] that was replicated in an independent cohort [57]. Further investigation of this potential association in two other unrelated cohorts did not confirm any association [58, 59]. Other phase I and phase II enzymes have been examined with equivocal results [60–66].

Thus far, the relationship between polymorphic variants in xenobiotic clearance enzymes is complex and is likely to reflect the underlying genetic structure of the population. This is evident from studies undertaken in European populations compared with those from Asia where particular polymorphisms in GST show an association in the Korean population but not Australian or European [56, 60, 66] ones. Of particular note from all of these studies is the relatively small sample sizes used to assess risk. If the effects of xenobiotic clearance enzymes on disease risk are to be fully understood, much larger studies will be required to dissect apart which of the phase I and phase II enzymes are truly associated with disease risk in Lynch syndrome.

2.4 Variants from Colorectal Cancer Genome-Wide Association Studies

Genome-wide association studies (GWAS) have revealed a number of genetic variants that are associated with the risk of colorectal cancer [67–81]. Many of the loci represent novel regions within the genome where little, if any, information is known about the functional aspects of these associated loci. Given that the genetic associations linked to colorectal cancer risk in the general population suggests that they might also influence disease risk in Lynch syndrome. A Dutch study reported two SNPs, rs16892766 (8q23.3) and rs3802842 (11q23.1), to be associated with colorectal cancer risk in Lynch syndrome [82]. Another study using Australian and Polish samples partially replicated these findings but only in people carrying *MLH1* germline variants [83]. In a combined analysis of these two studies, authors observed that as the number of risk alleles increased in an individual, the age of disease onset decreased [84]. The functional effects of rs3802842 remain to be determined as the regions where it resides harbour four open reading frames and do not result in any amino acid coding change signifying that it may be involved in some regulatory activity [85]. The SNP located on chromosome 8q23.3 maps to UTP23 [85] where it is presumed to alter the functional activity of the encoded protein. However, other two large studies did not observe any such associations overall or separately for male and female carriers or each of the MMR gene mutated [36, 86]. Using 11 independent SNPs reported to be associated with colorectal cancer in GWAS for the general population, Win et al. [86] reported that there was no evidence of an association between the total number of risk alleles of these 11 SNPs and colorectal cancer risk for Lynch syndrome. A Dutch study of 507 *PMS2* mutation carriers has reported no evidence of association between 24 GWAS SNPs, including SNPs at 11q23.1 and 8q23.3, and colorectal cancer risk for *PMS2*-associated Lynch syndrome [87].

2.5 Searching for Modifier Genes

There is some evidence that colorectal cancer risk in Lynch syndrome is modified by functional polymorphisms in genes. Most studies to date have taken a candidate gene approach which has revealed some associations or has chosen SNPs a priori based on the GWAS associations with colorectal cancer from the general population. It is unclear whether any of the millions of other SNPs tested, but not associated with colorectal cancer in the general population, may predict disease risk for people with Lynch syndrome. The use of genome-wide approaches is likely to reveal modifier loci similar to that undertaken for women carrying germline *BRCA1* variants that impact on disease risk [88].

3 Environmental Modifiers

Environmental and lifestyle factors may modify cancer risks for people with Lynch syndrome. Identifying modifiers of disease risk for these high-risk people is important for understanding carcinogenesis, as it may indicate potential initiators or promoters of the disease. In addition, identifying potentially protective factors or, conversely, harmful and avoidable risk factors could provide opportunities to reduce their risk of cancer. In this section of the chapter, the findings from published studies that investigated the environmental factors associated with colorectal cancer (Table 5.1) and endometrial cancer (Table 5.2) for Lynch syndrome are summarised and discussed.

Current evidence of environmental modifiers in Lynch syndrome have been provided mainly from three resources: Colon Cancer Family Registry (CCFR) [89–95]; Genetic, Environmental and Other influences among persons with Lynch syndrome (GEOLynch) [96–99]; and Colorectal Adenoma/Carcinoma Prevention Programme 2 (CAAP2) [100, 101] and some others [102–106] including two from Asia [18, 107]. There has been inconsistence or null in majority of findings for environmental modifiers in Lynch syndrome because of the substantial methodological challenges in investigating modifiers of disease for rare mutation carriers [108]. Of the studies investigating modifiers in Lynch syndrome, there are noticeable differences in terms of study design (prospective vs. retrospective/weighted cohort [109]), the definition of study participants (e.g. people who were tested and confirmed for having a pathogenic MMR variant vs. people who met Amsterdam Criteria [110, 111] for hereditary nonpolyposis colorectal cancer [HNPCC]), ascertainment of study participants (e.g. through genetics clinics or population cancer registries), the country or area

Table 5.1 Environmental or lifestyle factors associated with colorectal cancer risk in Lynch syndrome

Exposure	Author	Country of study	Study design	No. of participants*	Study participants	Outcome	Comparison	Strength for association HR or OR (95% CI)
BMI at age 20	Win et al. [89]	Australia, New Zealand, Canada, USA (CCFR)	Weighted cohort	659/1324	*MLH1*, *MSH2*, *MSH6*, *PMS2* carriers	CRC	Obese vs. normal	2.35 (1.30–4.23): Overall
	Campbell et al. [102]	Canada	Case-control	461/1465 men 466/1203 women	Members of AC-I or RBG families	CRC	Obese vs. normal	1.92 (1.33–3.63): Men 0.81 (0.38–1.72): Women
Current BMI	Movahedi et al. [100]	16 countries (CAPP2)	Prospective cohort (mean follow-up 55.7 months)	55/937	*MLH1*, *MSH2*, *MSH6* carriers, Members of AC-I families	CRC	Obese vs. normal/ underweight	2.34 (1.17–4.67): Overall 2.41 (0.85–6.81): Men 2.36 (0.91–6.20): Women 2.75 (1.12–6.75): Placebo 2.00 (0.61–6.70): Aspirin
	Botma A. [96]	Netherlands (GEOLynch)	Prospective cohort (median follow-up 20.0 months)	22/243	*MLH1*, *MSH2*, *MSH6*, *PMS2* carriers	CRA	Overweight/ obese vs. normal	8.72 (2.06–36.9): Men 0.75 (0.19–3.07): Women
	Campbell et al. [102]	Canada	Case-control	461/1465 men 466/1203 women	Members of AC-I or RBG families	CRC	Obese vs. normal	1.83 (1.33–2.51): Men 0.85 (0.62–1.16): Women
	Diergaarde et al. [103]	Netherlands	Case-control	145/103	MMR carriers or members of AC-I or AC-II families	CRC/ CRA	>25.5 vs. <23.2 kg/m^2	0.9 (0.4–1.8): Overall
Height	Botma A. [96].	Netherlands (GEOLynch)	Prospective cohort (median follow-up 20.0 months)	22/243	*MLH1*, *MSH2*, *MSH6*, *PMS2* carriers	CRA	Per 5 cm	0.43 (0.23–0.83): Men 1.09 (0.70–1.68): Women
	Campbell et al. [102]	Canada	Case-control	461/1465 men 466/1203 women	Members of AC-I or RBG families	CRC	≥1.85 m vs. <1.65 m ≥1.75 m vs. <1.55 m	0.97 (0.52–1.81): Men 2.81 (1.61–4.90): Women

(continued)

Table 5.1 (continued)

Exposure	Author	Country of study	Study design	No. of participants*	Study participants	Outcome	Comparison	Strength for association HR or OR (95% CI)
Smoking	Winkels et al. [97]	Netherlands (GEOLynch)	Prospective cohort (median follow-up 10.0 months)	58/386	*MLH1*, *MSH2*, *MSH6*, *PMS2* carriers	CRA	Former vs. never Current vs. never	3.03 (1.49–6.16) 6.13 (2.84–13.2)
	Pande et al. [90]	Australia, New Zealand, Canada, USA (CCFR, MDA)	Weighted cohort	426/752	*MLH1*, *MSH2*, *MSH6* carriers	CRC	Ever vs. never Former vs. never Current vs. never	0.89 (0.61–1.31) 0.54 (0.35–0.83) 1.77 (1.11–2.81)
	Brand et al. [105]	USA	Retrospective cohort	NR/340	*MLH1*, *MSH2* carriers	CRC	Ever vs. never	2.4 ($p < 0.05$): *MSH2* men 1.3: *MSH1* men 1.4: *MSH2* women 1.3: *MLH1* women
	Watson et al. [104]	USA	Retrospective cohort	NR/360	*MLH1*, *MSH2* carriers	CRC	Ever vs. never	1.43 ($p = 0.04$)
	Diergaarde et al. [103]	Netherlands	Case-control	145/103	MMR carriers or members of AC-I or AC-II families	CRC/CRA	Ever vs. never Former vs. never Current vs. never	1.5 (0.8–2.8) 1.1 (0.6–2.3) 2.4 (1.1–5.3)
	Kamiza et al. [18]	Taiwan	Retrospective cohort	147/301	*MLH1*, *MSH2* carriers	CRC	Ever vs. never	1.06 (0.73–1.52): Overall 0.98 (0.65–1.48): *MLH1* 1.28 (0.58–2.83): *MSH2*
	Tanakaya et al. [107]	Japan	Cross-sectional	63 CRC cases	29 male and 34 female MMR carriers	Multiple CRC	Ever vs. never	58.8% vs. 10.0% ($p = 0.02$)
Alcohol consumption	Dashti et al. [91]	Australia, New Zealand, Canada, USA (CCFR)	Weighted cohort	769/1925	*MLH1*, *MSH2*, *MSH6*, *PMS2* carriers	CRC	>28 vs. ≤14 g/day	1.69 (1.07–2.65)

	Winkels et al. [97]	Netherlands (GEOLynch)	Prospective cohort (median follow-up 10.0 months)	58/386	*MLH1*, *MSH2*, *MSH6*, *PMS2* carriers	CRA	>13 vs. <3 g/day	1.56 (0.71–3.43)
	Diergaarde et al. [103]	Netherlands	Case-control	145/103	MMR carriers or members of AC-I or AC-II families	CRC/CRA	≥12.8 vs. ≤2.6 g/day	1.0 (0.5–2.0)
	Watson et al. [104]	USA	Retrospective cohort	NR/271	*MLH1*, *MSH2* carriers	CRC	Ever vs. never	NR (p > 0.4)
	Kamiza et al. [18]	Taiwan	Retrospective cohort	147/301	*MLH1*, *MSH2* carriers	CRC	Ever vs. never	0.92 (0.62–1.36): Overall 0.73 (0.45–1.16): *MLH1* 2.33 (1.04–5.21): *MSH2*
NSAIDs	Burn et al. [101]	16 countries (CAPP2)	Randomised control trial (mean follow-up 55.7 months)	18/427 aspirin vs. 30/434 placebo	*MLH1*, *MSH2*, *MSH6* carriers, members of AC-I families	CRC	600 mg aspirin/day vs. placebo	0.56 (0.32–0.99)
	Ait Ouakrim et al. [92]	Australia, New Zealand, Canada, USA (CCFR)	Weighted cohort	714/1858	*MLH1*, *MSH2*, *MSH6*, *PMS2* carriers	CRC	≥5 years vs. <1 month	0.25 (0.10–0.62): Aspirin 0.26 (0.10–0.69): Ibuprofen
Dietary supplements	Chau et al. [93]	Australia, New Zealand, Canada, USA (CCFR)	Weighted cohort	744/1966	*MLH1*, *MSH2*, *MSH6*, *PMS2* carriers	CRC	≥3 years vs. <1 month	0.47 (0.32–0.69): Multivitamin 0.42 (0.23–0.74): Calcium 0.87 (0.36–2.08): Folic acid
	Heine-Broring et al. [98]	Netherlands (GEOLynch)	Prospective cohort (median follow-up 39.1 months)	122/470	*MLH1*, *MSH2*, *MSH6*, *PMS2* carriers	CRA	Ever vs. never use during last month	1.15 (0.72–1.84): Multivitamin 0.69 (0.25–1.92): Calcium

(continued)

Table 5.1 (continued)

Exposure	Author	Country of study	Study design	No. of participants*	Study participants	Outcome	Comparison	Strength for association HR or OR (95% CI)
Dietary nutrients	Diergaarde et al. [103]	Netherlands	Case-control	145/103	MMR carriers or members of AC-I or AC-II families	CRC/CRA	Highest vs. lowest tertile	0.5 (0.2–1.3): Fat 1.1 (0.5–2.7): Protein 1.4 (0.5–4.2): Carbohydrates 0.5 (0.2–1.0): Dietary fibre 0.8 (0.4–1.6): Calcium 0.8 (0.4–1.6): Vitamin C 1.0 (0.5–2.0): Beta-carotene 0.9 (0.4–1.9): Folate
Fruits and vegetables	Diergaarde et al. [103]	Netherlands	Case-control	145/103	MMR carriers or members of AC-I or AC-II families	CRC/CRA	Highest vs. lowest tertile	0.4 (0.2–0.9): Fruits 1.2 (0.6–2.4): Vegetables
	Kamiza et al. [18]	Taiwan	Retrospective cohort	147/301	*MLH1*, *MSH2* carriers	CRC	Highest vs. lowest tertile	0.60 (0.38–0.94): Fruits 0.93 (0.63–1.73): Vegetables
Meat	Diergaarde et al. [103]	Netherlands	Case-control	145/103	MMR carriers or members of AC-I or AC-II families	CRC/CRA	Highest vs. lowest tertile	1.0 (0.5–2.1): Total meat 0.8 (0.4–1.6): Red meat 0.8 (0.4–1.5): Poultry 1.2 (0.6–2.4): Fish
	Kamiza et al. [18]	Taiwan	Retrospective cohort	147/301	*MLH1*, *MSH2* carriers	CRC	Highest vs. lowest tertile	0.99 (0.65–1.52): Meat 0.93 (0.57–1.53): Seafood 0.86 (0.55–1.33): Staple food

Tea/coffee	Kamiza et al. [18]	Taiwan	Retrospective cohort	147/301	*MLH1, MSH2* carriers	CRC	Highest vs. lowest tertile	0.68 (0.48–0.96): Tea 0.62 (0.42–0.91): Tea *MLH1* 1.30 (0.48–3.58): Tea *MSH2* 0.96 (0.65–1.41): Coffee 0.83 (0.52–1.32): Coffee *MLH1* 1.56 (0.69–3.51): Coffee *MSH2*
Diet patterns	Botma et al. [99]	Netherlands (GEOLynch)	Prospective cohort (median follow-up 20.0 months)	58/486	*MLH1, MSH2, MSH6, PMS2* carriers	CRA	Highest vs. lowest tertile	0.73 (0.32–1.66): Prudent 1.70 (0.83–3.52): Meat 2.16 (1.03–4.49): Snack 1.25 (0.61–2.55): Cosmopolitan
Regular physical activity	Kamiza et al. [18]	Taiwan	Retrospective cohort	147/301	*MLH1, MSH2* carriers	CRC	Yes vs. no	0.58 (0.40–0.86): Overall 0.55 (0.35–0.86): *MLH1* 0.64 (0.26–1.59): *MSH2*
Occupation	Kamiza et al. [18]	Taiwan	Retrospective cohort	147/301	*MLH1, MSH2* carriers	CRC	Manual vs. skilled	1.75 (1.20–2.55): Overall 1.63 (1.07–2.47): *MLH1* 2.60 (0.88–7.73): *MSH2*

CRC colorectal cancer, *CRA* colorectal adenoma/polyp, *HR* hazards ratio, *OR* odds ratio, *CI* confidence interval, *NR* not reported, *CAAP2* Colorectal Adenoma/Carcinoma Prevention Programme 2, *CCFR* Colon Cancer Family Registry, *GEOLynch* Genetic, Environmental and Other influences among persons with Lynch syndrome, *AC-I* Amsterdam Criteria-I for hereditary nonpolyposis colorectal cancer [110], *AC-II* Amsterdam Criteria-II for hereditary nonpolyposis colorectal cancer [111], *RBG* revised Bethesda guidelines for hereditary nonpolyposis colorectal cancer [112], *MMR* mismatch repair, *MDA* University of Texas M.D. Anderson Cancer Center

*No. of participants: no. of colorectal cancer/total no. of participants for cohort studies; no. of cases/no. of controls for case-control studies

Table 5.2 Environmental or lifestyle factors associated with endometrial cancer risk in Lynch syndrome

Author	Country of study	Study design	No. of participants*	Study participants	Risk factor	Strength for association HR (95% CI)
Win et al. [94]	Australia, New Zealand, Canada, USA (CCFR)	Weighted cohort	126/601	*MLH1*, *MSH2*, *MSH6*, *PMS2* carriers	BMI at age 20: Per 5 kg/m^2	0.73 (0.40–1.34)
Dashti et al. [95]	Australia, New Zealand, Canada, USA (CCFR)	Weighted cohort	133/1128	*MLH1*, *MSH2*, *MSH6*, *PMS2* carriers	Parity: ≥1 vs. 0 HC: ≥1 vs. <1 year PMH: ≥1 vs. <1 year Age at menarche: ≥13 vs. <13 years Age at menopause: ≥50 vs. <50 years	0.21 (0.10–0.42) 0.39 (0.23–0.64) 0.81 (0.40–1.67) 0.70 (0.44–1.11) 1.64 (0.53–5.05)
Staff et al. [106]	Finland	Retrospective cohort	50/136	*MLH1*, *MSH2*, *MSH6* carriers	BMI at age 18: ≥20.8 vs. <20.8 kg/m^2 Current BMI: ≥25.4 vs. <25.4 Smoking: Ever vs. never Alcohol: Ever vs. never Diabetes: Yes vs. no Parity: ≥1 vs. 0 HC: Ever vs. never PMH: Per year Age at menarche: ≥13 vs. <13 years	1.55 (0.86–2.79) 1.20 (0.68–2.11) 0.74 (0.40–1.35) 0.83 (0.47–1.48) 4.18 (1.52–11.5) 0.74 (0.36–1.52) 1.06 (0.59–1.90) 1.07 (1.02–1.13) 1.08 (0.59–1.96)

HC hormonal contraceptive, *PMH* postmenopausal hormone, *BMI* body mass index, *HR* hazards ratio, *CI* confidence interval, *CCFR* Colon Cancer Family Registry where study conducted (e.g. European vs. Asian), the definition of environmental exposure (e.g. use of multivitamin supplements during the last month vs. at least twice a week for at least 1 month) or outcome definition (e.g. colorectal cancer vs. adenoma [benign precursor of colorectal cancer]).

3.1 Environmental Modifiers of Colorectal Cancer Risk in Lynch Syndrome

3.1.1 Body Mass and Height

A prospective cohort study from the Netherlands (GEOLynch) has reported that compared with normal weight, overweight/obese (body mass index [BMI] $\geq$ 25 kg/m^2) is associated with an increased risk of colorectal adenoma for men with Lynch syndrome but not for women [96]. Similarly, a case-control study from Canada has reported that compared with normal weight, overweight (BMI $\geq$ 25 kg/m^2) or obese (BMI $\geq$ 30 kg/m^2) is associated with an increased risk of colorectal cancer for men who met Amsterdam Criteria-I [110] or revised Bethesda guidelines [112] for HNPCC but not for women [102], although a small case-control study reported a null association [103]. In addition, a prospective analysis from the CAPP2 trial has shown that obesity is associated with an increased risk of colorectal cancer in Lynch syndrome [100]. This association is not different either between men and women or between aspirin intervention and placebo group.

A weighted cohort analysis from the CCFR has shown that BMI at age 20 years was positively associated with colorectal cancer risk for people with Lynch syndrome [89]. Consistent with this, Canadian case-control study has reported that obesity or overweight at age 20 years is associated with an increased risk of colorectal cancer for men but not for women [102]. This study has also reported that tall height is associated with an increased risk of colorectal cancer risk for women. However, GEOLynch study has showed no evidence of association between height and colorectal adenoma risk for both men and women with Lynch syndrome [96].

3.1.2 Smoking

The association between smoking and colorectal cancer or adenoma in Lynch syndrome has been investigated in seven studies (Table 5.1). A prospective analysis from the GEOLynch has reported both current and former smoking are associated with an increased risk of colorectal adenoma in Lynch syndrome [97]. A case-control study from the Netherlands has reported a positive association between current smoking and colorectal tumours but no evidence for association with former smoking [103]. Similarly, a weighted cohort analysis of data from the CCFR and the University of Texas M.D. Anderson Cancer Center has found an increased risk of colorectal cancer associated with current smoking but not with former smoking [90].

Using data from the Creighton University HNPCC registry in the USA, both retrospective cohort analysis [104] and fuzzy clustering analysis [105] showed that ever smokers had a higher risk of colorectal cancer than never smokers. Of the two Asian studies, a cross-sectional study of Japanese men with Lynch syndrome reported that multiple colorectal cancers were more common in smokers than non-smokers [107], while a Taiwanese study showed no evidence for an association between smoking and colorectal cancer [18].

3.1.3 Alcohol Consumption

For Lynch syndrome, five studies [18, 91, 97, 103, 104] have investigated the association between alcohol consumption and the risk of colorectal cancer or adenoma, and their findings have been inconclusive (Table 5.1). Two studies showed no evidence for an association between alcohol consumption and colorectal cancer [104] or colorectal tumours [103]. A weighted cohort analysis from the CCFR has shown that alcohol consumption, particularly more than 28 g/day of ethanol (~2 standard drinks of alcohol in the USA), is associated with an increased risk of colorectal cancer [91]. A trend of alcohol consumption associated with increasing risk of colorectal adenoma was observed in a GEOLynch study [97]. In addition, Taiwanese study reported an association between alcohol consumption and an increased risk of colorectal cancer for *MSH2* mutation carriers but not for *MLH1* mutation carriers.

3.1.4 Aspirin

A two-by-two factorial, randomised, double-blind, placebo-controlled trial of CAPP2 investigated the effect of aspirin at a daily dose of 600 mg in 937 confirmed carriers of a pathologic MMR gene mutation or members of a family that met the Amsterdam Criteria [110] and had a personal history of a Lynch syndrome-associated cancer but an intact colon from 43 international sites in 16 countries. At a mean follow-up period of 29 months, there was no evidence of aspirin effect on the development of colorectal neoplasia, with most being adenomas [113]. However, an analysis at a mean follow-up period of 55.7 months has shown that a daily intake of 600 mg aspirin reduces approximately 40% incidence of colorectal cancer [101]. In consistence with this, a weighted cohort analysis from the CCFR has shown a substantial reduction of colorectal cancer risk for aspirin users [92]. Further, this observational study reported the potential chemopreventive effect of ibuprofen on colorectal cancer for people with Lynch syndrome. To provide for recommendation of aspirin chemoprevention in Lynch syndrome as a standard care, the optimum dose and duration of aspirin treatment is not yet informed. CAPP3, a double-blind dose non-inferiority trial, is now under way of recruiting 3000 people with Lynch syndrome to compare the effect of 100, 300 or 600 mg daily aspirin.

3.1.5 Diet and Supplements

Two studies from the Netherlands and Taiwan reported fruit consumption to be associated with a risk reduction in colorectal cancer or adenoma in Lynch syndrome [18, 103]. Taiwanese study also reported that tea consumption was inversely associated with colorectal cancer for *MLH1* mutation carriers [18]. These studies investigated many other dietary factors including meat, fish and vegetables, and they did not observe evidence for association with colorectal cancer or adenoma in Lynch syndrome. GEOLynch study from the Netherlands investigated associations between diet patterns and the risk of colorectal adenoma in Lynch syndrome, and 'snack' pattern was observed to be associated with an increased risk of colorectal adenoma [99].

With regard to dietary supplements, a prospective cohort analysis from the GEOLynch of 470 MMR gene mutation carriers over a median follow-up of 39 months reported no evidence of associations between multivitamin and calcium supplement intake and the risk of colorectal adenoma [98]. However, a weighted cohort study from the CCFR of 1966 mutation carriers reported that regular intake of multivitamin and/or calcium supplements for at least 3 years is associated with an approximate halving of colorectal cancer risk [93]. There is no evidence for an association between folic acid supplement intake or dietary folate and colorectal cancer risk in Lynch syndrome [93, 103].

3.1.6 Physical Activity

A study from the Taiwan Hereditary Nonpolyposis Colorectal Cancer Consortium has reported that regular physical activity is associated with a decreased risk of colorectal cancer for *MLH1* mutation carriers [18].

3.2 *Environmental Modifiers of Endometrial Cancer Risk in Lynch Syndrome*

There are only three published studies investigating environmental risk factors associated with endometrial cancer in Lynch syndrome [94, 95, 106] (Table 5.2). Weighted cohort analyses from the CCFR have reported that later age at menarche, parity ($\geq$1 live births) and hormonal contraceptive use ($\geq$1 year) are associated with a lower risk of endometrial cancer [95], and there is no evidence of association between BMI at age 20 years and the risk of endometrial cancer in Lynch syndrome [94]. However, a Finnish study did not replicate these findings regarding female hormonal factors although they observed no evidence of association between adult BMI or BMI at age 18 years and endometrial cancer risk in Lynch syndrome [106]. This Finnish study has further reported that history of diabetes is associated with an increased risk of endometrial cancer in Lynch syndrome [106]. An intervention study of oral contraceptive and medroxyprogesterone acetate in 51 women with Lynch syndrome has shown a reduction in endometrial epithelial proliferation associated with a short-term exposure to exogenous progesterone [114]. For women with Lynch syndrome, some endogenous and exogenous hormonal factors appear to be associated with the risk of endometrial cancer.

3.3 Searching for Environmental Modifiers

From the current literature, there is strong evidence that regular use of aspirin substantially reduces the risk of colorectal cancer in Lynch syndrome, but there is still lack of information on the optimum dose and duration of aspirin use as well as from which age it should be started. There is accumulating evidence that a high body mass and cigarette smoking increase the risk of colorectal cancer or adenoma in Lynch syndrome. The direction and strength of observed associations are similar to those for the general population. There are only few published studies investigating other lifestyle and environmental factors including dietary factors associated with cancer risk in Lynch syndrome. Large prospective studies and clinical trials are required to further elucidate the role of environmental and lifestyle factors in colorectal, endometrial and other types of cancer for people with Lynch syndrome, as it could provide important options to reduce cancer risk for these high-risk people.

References

1. Lynch HT, Snyder CL, Shaw TG, Heinen CD, Hitchins MP. Milestones of Lynch syndrome: 1895-2015. Nat Rev Cancer. 2015;15(3):181–94. https://doi.org/10.1038/nrc3878.
2. Scott RJ, McPhillips M, Meldrum CJ, Fitzgerald PE, Adams K, Spigelman AD, et al. Hereditary nonpolyposis colorectal cancer in 95 families: differences and similarities between mutation-positive and mutation-negative kindreds. Am J Hum Genet. 2001;68(1):118–27. https://doi.org/10.1086/316942.
3. Dowty JG, Win AK, Buchanan DD, Lindor NM, Macrae FA, Clendenning M, et al. Cancer risks for MLH1 and MSH2 mutation carriers. Hum Mutat. 2013;34(3):490–7. https://doi.org/10.1002/humu.22262.
4. Win AK, Jenkins MA, Dowty JG, Antoniou AC, Lee A, Giles GG, et al. Prevalence and penetrance of major genes and polygenes for colorectal cancer. Cancer Epidemiol Biomark Prev. 2017;26(3):404–12. https://doi.org/10.1158/1055-9965.epi-16-0693.
5. Quehenberger F, Vasen HFA, van Houwelingen HC. Risk of colorectal and endometrial cancer for carriers of mutations of the hMLH1 and hMSH2 gene: correction for ascertainment. J Med Genet. 2005;42(6):491–6. https://doi.org/10.1136/jmg.2004.024299.
6. Bonadona V, Bonaiti B, Olschwang S, Grandjouan S, Huiart L, Longy M, et al. Cancer risks associated with germline mutations in *MLH1*, *MSH2*, and *MSH6* genes in Lynch syndrome. JAMA. 2011;305(22):2304–10. https://doi.org/10.1001/jama.2011.743.

7. Senter L, Clendenning M, Sotamaa K, Hampel H, Green J, Potter JD, et al. The clinical phenotype of Lynch syndrome due to germ-line *PMS2* mutations. Gastroenterology. 2008;135(2):419–28. https://doi.org/10.1053/j.gastro.2008.04.026.
8. Stoffel E, Mukherjee B, Raymond VM, Tayob N, Kastrinos F, Sparr J, et al. Calculation of risk of colorectal and endometrial cancer among patients with Lynch syndrome. Gastroenterology. 2009;137(5):1621–7. https://doi.org/10.1053/j.gastro.2009.07.039.
9. Choi YH, Cotterchio M, McKeown-Eyssen G, Neerav M, Bapat B, Boyd K, et al. Penetrance of colorectal cancer among *MLH1*/*MSH2* carriers participating in the colorectal cancer familial registry in Ontario. Hered Cancer Clin Pract. 2009;7(1):14. https://doi.org/10.1186/1897-4287-7-14.
10. Dunlop MG, Farrington SM, Carothers AD, Wyllie AH, Sharp L, Burn J, et al. Cancer risk associated with germline DNA mismatch repair gene mutations. Hum Mol Genet. 1997;6(1):105–10. https://doi.org/10.1093/hmg/6.1.105.
11. Hampel H, Stephens JA, Pukkala E, Sankila R, Aaltonen LA, Mecklin JP, et al. Cancer risk in hereditary nonpolyposis colorectal cancer syndrome: later age of onset. Gastroenterology. 2005;129(2):415–21. https://doi.org/10.1016/j.gastro.2005.05.011.
12. Win AK, Young JP, Lindor NM, Tucker KM, Ahnen DJ, Young GP, et al. Colorectal and other cancer risks for carriers and noncarriers from families with a DNA mismatch repair gene mutation: a prospective cohort study. J Clin Oncol. 2012;30(9):958–64. https://doi.org/10.1200/JCO.2011.39.5590.
13. ten Broeke SW, Brohet RM, Tops CM, van der Klift HM, Velthuizen ME, Bernstein I, et al. Lynch syndrome caused by germline PMS2 mutations: delineating the cancer risk. J Clin Oncol. 2015;33(4):319–25. https://doi.org/10.1200/jco.2014.57.8088.
14. Moller P, Seppala T, Bernstein I, Holinski-Feder E, Sala P, Evans DG, et al. Cancer incidence and survival in Lynch syndrome patients receiving colonoscopic and gynaecological surveillance: first report from the prospective Lynch syndrome database. Gut. 2017;66(3):464–72. https://doi.org/10.1136/gutjnl-2015-309675.
15. Moller P, Seppala T, Bernstein I, Holinski-Feder E, Sala P, Evans DG, et al. Incidence of and survival after subsequent cancers in carriers of pathogenic MMR variants with previous cancer: a report from the prospective Lynch syndrome database. Gut. 2017;66(9):1657–64. https://doi.org/10.1136/gutjnl-2016-311403.
16. Moller P, Seppala TT, Bernstein I, Holinski-Feder E, Sala P, Gareth Evans D, et al. Cancer risk and survival in path_MMR carriers by gene and gender up to 75 years of age: a report from the prospective Lynch syndrome database. Gut. 2017. https://doi.org/10.1136/gutjnl-2017-314057.
17. Stuckless S, Parfrey PS, Woods MO, Cox J, Fitzgerald GW, Green JS, et al. The phenotypic expression of three *MSH2* mutations in large Newfoundland families with Lynch syndrome. Fam Cancer. 2007;6(1):1–12. https://doi.org/10.1007/s10689-006-0014-8.
18. Kamiza AB, Hsieh LL, Tang R, Chien HT, Lai CH, Chiu LL, et al. Risk factors associated with colorectal cancer in a subset of patients with mutations in MLH1 and MSH2 in Taiwan fulfilling the Amsterdam II criteria for Lynch syndrome. PLoS One. 2015;10(6):e0130018. https://doi.org/10.1371/journal.pone.0130018.
19. Park J-G, Park YJ, Wijnen JT, Vasen HFA. Gene-environment interaction in hereditary nonpolyposis colorectal cancer with implications for diagnosis and genetic testing. Int J Cancer. 1999;82(4):516–9. https://doi.org/10.1002/(SICI)1097-0215(19990812)82:4<516::AID-IJC8>3.0.CO;2-U.
20. Levine AJ, Oren M. The first 30 years of p53: growing ever more complex. Nat Rev Cancer. 2009;9(10):749–58. https://doi.org/10.1038/nrc2723.
21. Levine AJ. p53, the cellular gatekeeper for growth and division. Cell. 1997;88(3):323–31. https://doi.org/10.1016/S0092-8674(00)81871-1.
22. Jones JS, Chi X, Gu X, Lynch PM, Amos CI, Frazier ML. p53 polymorphism and age of onset of hereditary nonpolyposis colorectal cancer in a Caucasian population. Clin Cancer Res. 2004;10(17):5845–9. https://doi.org/10.1158/1078-0432.ccr-03-0590.

23. Kruger S, Engel C, Bier A, Silber AS, Gorgens H, Mangold E, et al. The additive effect of p53 Arg72Pro and RNASEL Arg462Gln genotypes on age of disease onset in Lynch syndrome patients with pathogenic germline mutations in MSH2 or MLH1. Cancer Lett. 2007;252(1):55–64. https://doi.org/10.1016/j.canlet.2006.12.006.
24. Kruger S, Silber AS, Engel C, Gorgens H, Mangold E, Pagenstecher C, et al. Arg462Gln sequence variation in the prostate-cancer-susceptibility gene RNASEL and age of onset of hereditary non-polyposis colorectal cancer: a case-control study. Lancet Oncol. 2005;6(8):566–72. https://doi.org/10.1016/s1470-2045(05)70253-9.
25. Sotamaa K, Liyanarachchi S, Mecklin JP, Jarvinen H, Aaltonen LA, Peltomaki P, et al. p53 codon 72 and MDM2 SNP309 polymorphisms and age of colorectal cancer onset in Lynch syndrome. Clin Cancer Res. 2005;11(19 Pt 1):6840–4. https://doi.org/10.1158/1078-0432.ccr-05-1139.
26. Talseth BA, Meldrum C, Suchy J, Kurzawski G, Lubinski J, Scott RJ. Age of diagnosis of colorectal cancer in HNPCC patients is more complex than that predicted by R72P polymorphism in TP53. Int J Cancer. 2006;118(10):2479–84. https://doi.org/10.1002/ijc.21661.
27. Kong S, Amos CI, Luthra R, Lynch PM, Levin B, Frazier ML. Effects of cyclin D1 polymorphism on age of onset of hereditary nonpolyposis colorectal cancer. Cancer Res. 2000;60(2):249–52.
28. Bala S, Peltomaki P. CYCLIN D1 as a genetic modifier in hereditary nonpolyposis colorectal cancer. Cancer Res. 2001;61(16):6042–5.
29. Kruger S, Engel C, Bier A, Mangold E, Pagenstecher C, Doeberitz M, et al. Absence of association between cyclin D1 (CCND1) G870A polymorphism and age of onset in hereditary nonpolyposis colorectal cancer. Cancer Lett. 2006;236(2):191–7. https://doi.org/10.1016/j.canlet.2005.05.013.
30. Talseth BA, Ashton KA, Meldrum C, Suchy J, Kurzawski G, Lubinski J, et al. Aurora-A and Cyclin D1 polymorphisms and the age of onset of colorectal cancer in hereditary nonpolyposis colorectal cancer. Int J Cancer. 2008;122(6):1273–7. https://doi.org/10.1002/ijc.23177.
31. Chen J, Sen S, Amos CI, Wei C, Jones JS, Lynch P, et al. Association between Aurora-A kinase polymorphisms and age of onset of hereditary nonpolyposis colorectal cancer in a Caucasian population. Mol Carcinog. 2007;46(4):249–56. https://doi.org/10.1002/mc.20283.
32. Chen J, Pande M, Huang YJ, Wei C, Amos CI, Talseth-Palmer BA, et al. Cell cycle-related genes as modifiers of age of onset of colorectal cancer in Lynch syndrome: a large-scale study in non-Hispanic white patients. Carcinogenesis. 2013;34(2):299–306. https://doi.org/10.1093/carcin/bgs344.
33. Talseth BA, Meldrum C, Suchy J, Kurzawski G, Lubinski J, Scott RJ. MDM2 SNP309 T>G alone or in combination with the TP53 R72P polymorphism does not appear to influence disease expression and age of diagnosis of colorectal cancer in HNPCC patients. Int J Cancer. 2007;120(3):563–5. https://doi.org/10.1002/ijc.22339.
34. Zecevic M, Amos CI, Gu X, Campos IM, Jones JS, Lynch PM, et al. IGF1 gene polymorphism and risk for hereditary nonpolyposis colorectal cancer. J Natl Cancer Inst. 2006;98(2):139–43. https://doi.org/10.1093/jnci/djj016.
35. Reeves SG, Rich D, Meldrum CJ, Colyvas K, Kurzawski G, Suchy J, et al. IGF1 is a modifier of disease risk in hereditary non-polyposis colorectal cancer. Int J Cancer. 2008;123(6):1339–43. https://doi.org/10.1002/ijc.23668.
36. Houlle S, Charbonnier F, Houivet E, Tinat J, Buisine MP, Caron O, et al. Evaluation of Lynch syndrome modifier genes in 748 MMR mutation carriers. Eur J Hum Genet. 2011;19(8):887–92. https://doi.org/10.1038/ejhg.2011.44.
37. Chen J, Etzel CJ, Amos CI, Zhang Q, Viscofsky N, Lindor NM, et al. Genetic variants in the cell cycle control pathways contribute to early onset colorectal cancer in Lynch syndrome. Cancer Causes Control. 2009;20(9):1769–77. https://doi.org/10.1007/s10552-009-9416-x.
38. Wood NJ, Quinton NA, Burdall S, Sheridan E, Duffy SR. Exploring the potential chemopreventative effect of aspirin and rofecoxib on hereditary nonpolyposis colorectal cancer-like endometrial cancer cells in vitro through mechanisms involving apoptosis, the cell cycle,

and mismatch repair gene expression. Int J Gynecol Cancer. 2007;17(2):447–54. https://doi.org/10.1111/j.1525-1438.2007.00867.x
39. Kunkel TA, Erie DA. DNA mismatch repair. Annu Rev Biochem. 2005;74:681–710. https://doi.org/10.1146/annurev.biochem.74.082803.133243.
40. David SS, O'Shea VL, Kundu S. Base-excision repair of oxidative DNA damage. Nature. 2007;447(7147):941–50. https://doi.org/10.1038/nature05978.
41. Maillet P, Chappuis PO, Vaudan G, Dobbie Z, Muller H, Hutter P, et al. A polymorphism in the ATM gene modulates the penetrance of hereditary non-polyposis colorectal cancer. Int J Cancer. 2000;88(6):928–31. https://doi.org/10.1002/1097-0215(20001215)88:6<928::AID-IJC14>3.0.CO;2-P.
42. Jones JS, Gu X, Lynch PM, Rodriguez-Bigas M, Amos CI, Frazier ML. ATM polymorphism and hereditary nonpolyposis colorectal cancer (HNPCC) age of onset (United States). Cancer Causes Control. 2005;16(6):749–53. https://doi.org/10.1007/s10552-005-1540-7.
43. Kim IJ, Ku JL, Kang HC, Park JH, Yoon KA, Shin Y, et al. Mutational analysis of *OGG1, MYH, MTH1* in FAP, HNPCC and sporadic colorectal cancer patients: R154H *OGG1* polymorphism is associated with sporadic colorectal cancer patients. Hum Genet. 2004;115(6):498–503. https://doi.org/10.1007/s00439-004-1186-7.
44. Reeves SG, Meldrum C, Groombridge C, Spigelman A, Suchy J, Kurzawski G, et al. DNA repair gene polymorphisms and risk of early onset colorectal cancer in Lynch syndrome. Cancer Epidemiol. 2012;36(2):183–9. https://doi.org/10.1016/j.canep.2011.09.003.
45. Meeker AK, Argani P. Telomere shortening occurs early during breast tumorigenesis: a cause of chromosome destabilization underlying malignant transformation? J Mammary Gland Biol Neoplasia. 2004;9(3):285–96. https://doi.org/10.1023/B:JOMG.0000048775.04140.92.
46. Londono-Vallejo JA, Der-Sarkissian H, Cazes L, Bacchetti S, Reddel RR. Alternative lengthening of telomeres is characterized by high rates of telomeric exchange. Cancer Res. 2004;64(7):2324–7. https://doi.org/10.1158/0008-5472.CAN-03-4035.
47. Bellido F, Guino E, Jagmohan-Changur S, Segui N, Pineda M, Navarro M, et al. Genetic variant in the telomerase gene modifies cancer risk in Lynch syndrome. Eur J Hum Genet. 2013;21(5):511–6. https://doi.org/10.1038/ejhg.2012.204.
48. Djojosubroto MW, Choi YS, Lee HW, Rudolph KL. Telomeres and telomerase in aging, regeneration and cancer. Mol Cells. 2003;15(2):164–75.
49. Win AK, Clendenning M, Crawford W, Rosty C, Preston SG, Southey MC, et al. Genetic variants within the *hTERT* gene and the risk of colorectal cancer in Lynch syndrome. Genes Cancer. 2015;6(11–12):445–51. https://doi.org/10.18632/genesandcancer.85.
50. Smith G, Stanley LA, Sim E, Strange RC, Wolf CR. Metabolic polymorphisms and cancer susceptibility. Cancer Surv. 1995;25:27–65.
51. Slattery ML, Potter JD, Samowitz W, Bigler J, Caan B, Leppert M. NAT2, GSTM-1, cigarette smoking, and risk of colon cancer. Cancer Epidemiol Biomark Prev. 1998;7(12):1079–84.
52. Brockton N, Little J, Sharp L, Cotton SC. N-acetyltransferase polymorphisms and colorectal cancer: a HuGE review. Am J Epidemiol. 2000;151(9):846–61.
53. Loktionov A, Watson MA, Gunter M, Stebbings WS, Speakman CT, Bingham SA. Glutathione-S-transferase gene polymorphisms in colorectal cancer patients: interaction between GSTM1 and GSTM3 allele variants as a risk-modulating factor. Carcinogenesis. 2001;22(7):1053–60. https://doi.org/10.1093/carcin/22.7.1053.
54. Ye Z, Parry JM. Genetic polymorphisms in the cytochrome P450 1A1, glutathione S-transferase M1 and T1, and susceptibility to colon cancer. Teratog Carcinog Mutagen. 2002;22(5):385–92. https://doi.org/10.1002/tcm.10035.
55. He LJ, Yu YM, Qiao F, Liu JS, Sun XF, Jiang LL. Genetic polymorphisms of N-acetyltransferase 2 and colorectal cancer risk. World J Gastroenterol. 2005;11(27):4268–71. https://doi.org/10.3748/wjg.v11.i27.4268.
56. Heinimann K, Scott RJ, Chappuis P, Weber W, Muller H, Dobbie Z, et al. N-acetyltransferase 2 influences cancer prevalence in hMLH1/hMSH2 mutation carriers. Cancer Res. 1999;59(13):3038–40.

57. Frazier ML, O'Donnell FT, Kong S, Gu X, Campos I, Luthra R, et al. Age-associated risk of cancer among individuals with N-acetyltransferase 2 (NAT2) mutations and mutations in DNA mismatch repair genes. Cancer Res. 2001;61(4):1269–71.
58. Talseth BA, Meldrum C, Suchy J, Kurzawski G, Lubinski J, Scott RJ. Genetic polymorphisms in xenobiotic clearance genes and their influence on disease expression in hereditary nonpolyposis colorectal cancer patients. Cancer Epidemiol Biomark Prev. 2006;15(11):2307–10. https://doi.org/10.1158/1055-9965.EPI-06-0040.
59. Pistorius S, Gorgens H, Kruger S, Engel C, Mangold E, Pagenstecher C, et al. N-acetyltransferase (NAT) 2 acetylator status and age of onset in patients with hereditary nonpolyposis colorectal cancer (HNPCC). Cancer Lett. 2006;241(1):150–7. https://doi.org/10.1016/j.canlet.2005.10.018.
60. Felix R, Bodmer W, Fearnhead NS, van der Merwe L, Goldberg P, Ramesar RS. GSTM1 and GSTT1 polymorphisms as modifiers of age at diagnosis of hereditary nonpolyposis colorectal cancer (HNPCC) in a homogeneous cohort of individuals carrying a single predisposing mutation. Mutat Res. 2006;602(1–2):175–81. https://doi.org/10.1016/j.mrfmmm.2006.09.004.
61. Pande M, Amos CI, Osterwisch DR, Chen J, Lynch PM, Broaddus R, et al. Genetic variation in genes for the xenobiotic-metabolizing enzymes CYP1A1, EPHX1, GSTM1, GSTT1, and GSTP1 and susceptibility to colorectal cancer in Lynch syndrome. Cancer Epidemiol Biomark Prev. 2008;17(9):2393–401. https://doi.org/10.1158/1055-9965.EPI-08-0326.
62. Moisio AL, Sistonen P, Mecklin JP, Jarvinen H, Peltomaki P. Genetic polymorphisms in carcinogen metabolism and their association to hereditary nonpolyposis colon cancer. Gastroenterology. 1998;115(6):1387–94.
63. Jones JS, Gu X, Campos IM, Lynch PM, Amos CI, Frazier ML. GSTM1 polymorphism does not affect hereditary nonpolyposis colorectal cancer age of onset. Cancer Epidemiol Biomark Prev. 2004;13(4):676–8.
64. Campbell PT, Edwards L, McLaughlin JR, Green J, Younghusband HB, Woods MO. Cytochrome P450 17A1 and catechol O-methyltransferase polymorphisms and age at Lynch syndrome colon cancer onset in Newfoundland. Clin Cancer Res. 2007;13(13):3783–8. https://doi.org/10.1158/1078-0432.CCR-06-2987.
65. Pande M, Chen J, Amos CI, Lynch PM, Broaddus R, Frazier ML. Influence of methylenetetrahydrofolate reductase gene polymorphisms C677T and A1298C on age-associated risk for colorectal cancer in a caucasian Lynch syndrome population. Cancer Epidemiol Biomark Prev. 2007;16(9):1753–9. https://doi.org/10.1158/1055-9965.epi-07-0384.
66. Shin JH, JL K, Shin KH, Shin YK, Kang SB, Park JG. Glutathione S-transferase M1 associated with cancer occurrence in Korean HNPCC families carrying the hMLH1/hMSH2 mutation. Oncol Rep. 2003;10(2):483–6. https://doi.org/10.3892/or.10.2.483.
67. Tomlinson I, Webb E, Carvajal-Carmona L, Broderick P, Kemp Z, Spain S, et al. A genome-wide association scan of tag SNPs identifies a susceptibility variant for colorectal cancer at 8q24.21. Nat Genet. 2007;39(8):984–8. https://doi.org/10.1038/ng2085.
68. Broderick P, Carvajal-Carmona L, Pittman AM, Webb E, Howarth K, Rowan A, et al. A genome-wide association study shows that common alleles of *SMAD7* influence colorectal cancer risk. Nat Genet. 2007;39(11):1315–7. https://doi.org/10.1038/ng.2007.18.
69. Zanke BW, Greenwood CMT, Rangrej J, Kustra R, Tenesa A, Farrington SM, et al. Genome-wide association scan identifies a colorectal cancer susceptibility locus on chromosome 8q24. Nat Genet. 2007;39(8):989–94. https://doi.org/10.1038/ng2089.
70. Tomlinson IPM, Webb E, Carvajal-Carmona L, Broderick P, Howarth K, Pittman AM, et al. A genome-wide association study identifies colorectal cancer susceptibility loci on chromosomes 10p14 and 8q23.3. Nat Genet. 2008;40(5):623–30. https://doi.org/10.1038/ng.111.
71. Houlston RS, Webb E, Broderick P, Pittman AM, Di Bernardo MC, Lubbe S, et al. Meta-analysis of genome-wide association data identifies four new susceptibility loci for colorectal cancer. Nat Genet. 2008;40(12):1426–35. https://doi.org/10.1038/ng.262.
72. Tenesa A, Farrington SM, Prendergast JGD, Porteous ME, Walker M, Haq N, et al. Genome-wide association scan identifies a colorectal cancer susceptibility locus on 11q23 and

replicates risk loci at 8q24 and 18q21. Nat Genet. 2008;40(5):631–7. https://doi.org/10.1038/ng.133.
73. Houlston RS, Cheadle J, Dobbins SE, Tenesa A, Jones AM, Howarth K, et al. Meta-analysis of three genome-wide association studies identifies susceptibility loci for colorectal cancer at 1q41, 3q26.2, 12q13.13 and 20q13.33. Nat Genet. 2010;42(11):973–7. https://doi.org/10.1038/ng.670.
74. Dunlop MG, Dobbins SE, Farrington SM, Jones AM, Palles C, Whiffin N, et al. Common variation near CDKN1A, POLD3 and SHROOM2 influences colorectal cancer risk. Nat Genet. 2012;44(7):770–6. https://doi.org/10.1038/ng.2293.
75. Peters U, Jiao S, Schumacher FR, Hutter CM, Aragaki AK, Baron JA, et al. Identification of genetic susceptibility loci for colorectal tumors in a genome-wide meta-analysis. Gastroenterology. 2013;144(4):799–807.e24. https://doi.org/10.1053/j.gastro.2012.12.020.
76. Jia WH, Zhang B, Matsuo K, Shin A, Xiang YB, Jee SH, et al. Genome-wide association analyses in East Asians identify new susceptibility loci for colorectal cancer. Nat Genet. 2013;45(2):191–6. https://doi.org/10.1038/ng.2505.
77. Whiffin N, Hosking FJ, Farrington SM, Palles C, Dobbins SE, Zgaga L, et al. Identification of susceptibility loci for colorectal cancer in a genome-wide meta-analysis. Hum Mol Genet. 2014;23(17):4729–37. https://doi.org/10.1093/hmg/ddu177.
78. Real LM, Ruiz A, Gayan J, Gonzalez-Perez A, Saez ME, Ramirez-Lorca R, et al. A colorectal cancer susceptibility new variant at 4q26 in the Spanish population identified by genome-wide association analysis. PLoS One. 2014;9(6):e101178. https://doi.org/10.1371/journal.pone.0101178.
79. Schmit SL, Schumacher FR, Edlund CK, Conti DV, Raskin L, Lejbkowicz F, et al. A novel colorectal cancer risk locus at 4q32.2 identified from an international genome-wide association study. Carcinogenesis. 2014;35(11):2512–9. https://doi.org/10.1093/carcin/bgu148.
80. Schumacher FR, Schmit SL, Jiao S, Edlund CK, Wang H, Zhang B, et al. Genome-wide association study of colorectal cancer identifies six new susceptibility loci. Nat Commun. 2015;6:7138. https://doi.org/10.1038/ncomms8138.
81. Peters U, Hutter CM, Hsu L, Schumacher FR, Conti DV, Carlson CS, et al. Meta-analysis of new genome-wide association studies of colorectal cancer risk. Hum Genet. 2012;131(2):217–34. https://doi.org/10.1007/s00439-011-1055-0.
82. Wijnen JT, Brohet RM, van Eijk R, Jagmohan-Changur S, Middeldorp A, Tops CM, et al. Chromosome 8q23.3 and 11q23.1 variants modify colorectal cancer risk in Lynch syndrome. Gastroenterology. 2009;136(1):131–7. https://doi.org/10.1053/j.gastro.2008.09.033.
83. Talseth-Palmer BA, Brenne IS, Ashton KA, Evans TJ, McPhillips M, Groombridge C, et al. Colorectal cancer susceptibility loci on chromosome 8q23.3 and 11q23.1 as modifiers for disease expression in Lynch syndrome. J Med Genet. 2011;48(4):279–84. https://doi.org/10.1136/jmg.2010.079962.
84. Talseth-Palmer BA, Wijnen JT, Brenne IS, Jagmohan-Changur S, Barker D, Ashton KA, et al. Combined analysis of three Lynch syndrome cohorts confirms the modifying effects of 8q23.3 and 11q23.1 in *MLH1* mutation carriers. Int J Cancer. 2013;132(7):1556–64. https://doi.org/10.1002/ijc.27843.
85. Carvajal-Carmona LG, Cazier JB, Jones AM, Howarth K, Broderick P, Pittman A, et al. Fine-mapping of colorectal cancer susceptibility loci at 8q23.3, 16q22.1 and 19q13.11: refinement of association signals and use of in silico analysis to suggest functional variation and unexpected candidate target genes. Hum Mol Genet. 2011;20(14):2879–88. https://doi.org/10.1093/hmg/ddr190.
86. Win AK, Hopper JL, Buchanan DD, Young JP, Tenesa A, Dowty JG, et al. Are the common genetic variants associated with colorectal cancer risk for DNA mismatch repair gene mutation carriers? Eur J Cancer. 2013;49(7):1578–87. https://doi.org/10.1016/j.ejca.2013.01.029.
87. ten Broeke SW, Elsayed FA, Pagan L, Olderode-Berends MJW, Garcia EG, Gille HJP et al. SNP association study in *PMS2*-associated Lynch syndrome. Fam Cancer. 2017. https://doi.org/10.1007/s10689-017-0061-3.

88. Couch FJ, Wang X, McGuffog L, Lee A, Olswold C, Kuchenbaecker KB, et al. Genome-wide association study in BRCA1 mutation carriers identifies novel loci associated with breast and ovarian cancer risk. PLoS Genet. 2013;9(3):e1003212. https://doi.org/10.1371/journal.pgen.1003212.
89. Win AK, Dowty JG, English DR, Campbell PT, Young JP, Winship I, et al. Body mass index in early adulthood and colorectal cancer risk for carriers and non-carriers of germline mutations in DNA mismatch repair genes. Br J Cancer. 2011;105(1):162–9. https://doi.org/10.1038/bjc.2011.172.
90. Pande M, Lynch PM, Hopper JL, Jenkins MA, Gallinger S, Haile RW, et al. Smoking and colorectal cancer in Lynch syndrome: results from the colon cancer family registry and The University of Texas M.D. Anderson Cancer Center. Clin Cancer Res. 2010;16(4):1331–9. https://doi.org/10.1158/1078-0432.ccr-09-1877.
91. Dashti SG, Buchanan DD, Jayasekara H, Ait Ouakrim D, Clendenning M, Rosty C, et al. Alcohol consumption and the risk of colorectal cancer for mismatch repair gene mutation carriers. Cancer Epidemiol Biomark Prev. 2017;26(3):366–75. https://doi.org/10.1158/1055-9965.epi-16-0496.
92. Ait Ouakrim D, Dashti SG, Chau R, Buchanan DD, Clendenning M, Rosty C, et al. Aspirin, ibuprofen, and the risk of colorectal cancer in Lynch syndrome. J Natl Cancer Inst. 2015;107(9):djv170. https://doi.org/10.1093/jnci/djv170.
93. Chau R, Dashti SG, Ait Ouakrim D, Buchanan DD, Clendenning M, Rosty C, et al. Multivitamin, calcium and folic acid supplements and the risk of colorectal cancer in Lynch syndrome. Int J Epidemiol. 2016;45(3):940–53. https://doi.org/10.1093/ije/dyw036.
94. Win AK, Dowty JG, Antill YC, English DR, Baron JA, Young JP, et al. Body mass index in early adulthood and endometrial cancer risk for mismatch repair gene mutation carriers. Obstet Gynecol. 2011;117(4):899–905. https://doi.org/10.1097/AOG.0b013e3182110ea3.
95. Dashti SG, Chau R, Ouakrim DA, Buchanan DD, Clendenning M, Young JP, et al. Female hormonal factors and the risk of endometrial cancer in Lynch syndrome. JAMA. 2015;314(1):61–71. https://doi.org/10.1001/jama.2015.6789.
96. Botma A, Nagengast FM, Braem MGM, Hendriks JCM, Kleibeuker JH, Vasen HFA, et al. Body mass index increases risk of colorectal adenomas in men with Lynch syndrome: the GEOLynch cohort study. J Clin Oncol. 2010;28(28):4346–53. https://doi.org/10.1200/jco.2010.28.0453.
97. Winkels RM, Botma A, Van Duijnhoven FJ, Nagengast FM, Kleibeuker JH, Vasen HF, et al. Smoking increases the risk for colorectal adenomas in patients with Lynch syndrome. Gastroenterology. 2012;142(2):241–7. https://doi.org/10.1053/j.gastro.2011.10.033.
98. Heine-Broring RC, Winkels RM, Botma A, van Duijnhoven FJ, Jung AY, Kleibeuker JH, et al. Dietary supplement use and colorectal adenoma risk in individuals with Lynch syndrome: the GEOLynch cohort study. PLoS One. 2013;8(6):e66819. https://doi.org/10.1371/journal.pone.0066819.
99. Botma A, Vasen HF, van Duijnhoven FJ, Kleibeuker JH, Nagengast FM, Kampman E. Dietary patterns and colorectal adenomas in Lynch syndrome: the GEOLynch cohort study. Cancer. 2013;119(3):512–21. https://doi.org/10.1002/cncr.27726.
100. Movahedi M, Bishop DT, Macrae F, Mecklin JP, Moeslein G, Olschwang S, et al. Obesity, aspirin, and risk of colorectal cancer in carriers of hereditary colorectal cancer: a prospective investigation in the CAPP2 study. J Clin Oncol. 2015;33(31):3591–7. https://doi.org/10.1200/jco.2014.58.9952.
101. Burn J, Gerdes AM, Macrae F, Mecklin JP, Moeslein G, Olschwang S, et al. Long-term effect of aspirin on cancer risk in carriers of hereditary colorectal cancer: an analysis from the CAPP2 randomised controlled trial. Lancet. 2011;378(9809):2081–7. https://doi.org/10.1016/S0140-6736(11)61049-0.
102. Campbell PT, Cotterchio M, Dicks E, Parfrey P, Gallinger S, McLaughlin JR. Excess body weight and colorectal cancer risk in Canada: associations in subgroups of clinically defined familial risk of cancer. Cancer Epidemiol Biomark Prev. 2007;16(9):1735–44. https://doi.org/10.1158/1055-9965.epi-06-1059.

103. Diergaarde B, Braam H, Vasen HF, Nagengast FM, GNPv M, Kok FJ, et al. Environmental factors and colorectal tumor risk in individuals with hereditary nonpolyposis colorectal cancer. Clin Gastroenterol Hepatol. 2007;5(6):736–42. https://doi.org/10.1016/j.cgh.2007.02.019.
104. Watson P, Ashwathnarayan R, Lynch HT, Roy HK. Tobacco use and increased colorectal cancer risk in patients with hereditary nonpolyposis colorectal cancer (Lynch syndrome). Arch Intern Med. 2004;164(22):2429–31. https://doi.org/10.1001/archinte.164.22.2429.
105. Brand RM, Jones DD, Lynch HT, Brand RE, Watson P, Ashwathnayaran R, et al. Risk of colon cancer in hereditary non-polyposis colorectal cancer patients as predicted by fuzzy modeling: influence of smoking. World J Gastroenterol. 2006;12(28):4485–91. https://doi.org/10.3748/wjg.v12.i28.4485.
106. Staff S, Aaltonen M, Huhtala H, Pylvanainen K, Mecklin JP, Maenpaa J. Endometrial cancer risk factors among Lynch syndrome women: a retrospective cohort study. Br J Cancer. 2016;115(3):375–81. https://doi.org/10.1038/bjc.2016.193.
107. Tanakaya K, Furukawa Y, Nakamura Y, Hirata K, Tomita N, Tamura K, et al. Relationship between smoking and multiple colorectal cancers in patients with Japanese Lynch syndrome: a cross-sectional study conducted by the Japanese Society for Cancer of the Colon and Rectum. Jpn J Clin Oncol. 2015. 2015;45(3):307–10. https://doi.org/10.1093/jjco/hyu218.
108. Milne RL, Antoniou AC. Modifiers of breast and ovarian cancer risks for BRCA1 and BRCA2 mutation carriers. Endocr Relat Cancer. 2016;23(10):T69–84. https://doi.org/10.1530/erc-16-0277.
109. Antoniou AC, Goldgar DE, Andrieu N, Chang-Claude J, Brohet R, Rookus MA, et al. A weighted cohort approach for analysing factors modifying disease risks in carriers of high-risk susceptibility genes. Genet Epidemiol. 2005;29(1):1–11. https://doi.org/10.1002/gepi.20074.
110. Vasen HF, Mecklin JP, Khan PM, Lynch HT. The International Collaborative Group on Hereditary Non-Polyposis Colorectal Cancer (ICG-HNPCC). Dis Colon Rectum. 1991;34(5):424–5. http://dx.doi.org/10.1007/BF02053699.
111. Vasen HFA, Watson P, Mecklin JP, Lynch HT. New clinical criteria for hereditary nonpolyposis colorectal cancer (HNPCC, Lynch syndrome) proposed by the International Collaborative Group on HNPCC. Gastroenterology. 1999;116(6):1453–6. https://doi.org/10.1016/S0016-5085(99)70510-X.
112. Umar A, Boland CR, Terdiman JP, Syngal S, Adl C, Ruschoff J, et al. Revised Bethesda Guidelines for hereditary nonpolyposis colorectal cancer (Lynch syndrome) and microsatellite instability. J Natl Cancer Inst. 2004;96(4):261–8. https://doi.org/10.1093/jnci/djh034.
113. Burn J, Bishop DT, Mecklin J-P, Macrae F, Moslein G, Olschwang S, et al. Effect of aspirin or resistant starch on colorectal neoplasia in the Lynch syndrome. N Engl J Med. 2008;359(24):2567–78. https://doi.org/10.1056/NEJMoa0801297.
114. Lu KH, Loose DS, Yates MS, Nogueras-Gonzalez GM, Munsell MF, Chen LM, et al. Prospective multicenter randomized intermediate biomarker study of oral contraceptive versus depo-provera for prevention of endometrial cancer in women with Lynch syndrome. Cancer Prev Res (Phila). 2013;6(8):774–81. https://doi.org/10.1158/1940-6207.capr-13-0020.

Part II
Genetic Causes and Associated Phenotypes: Gastrointestinal Polyposis Syndromes

Chapter 6
Adenomatous Polyposis Syndromes: Introduction

Stefan Aretz

Abstract The adenomatous polyposis of the colorectum is the most frequent polyposis type and a precancerous condition with a high lifetime risk of colorectal cancer (CRC), unless detected early. Currently, at least five different inherited forms can be delineated by molecular genetic analyses. Although all types are defined by multiple adenomas which result in a similar diagnostic and therapeutic approach, a significant clinical variability in terms of number and age at onset and the presence of benign and malignant extraintestinal lesions can be observed.

Keywords Polyposis coli · FAP · Gastrointestinal polyposis

The occurrence of single colorectal polyps including adenomas is a common and age-related phenomenon [1, 2]. The minimum number of adenomas to diagnose an adenomatous polyposis is not clearly defined and also depends on the localisation, the age at onset, and the family history; however, at least ten synchronous, histologically confirmed colorectal adenomas are usually required [3]. The adenomatous polyposis of the colorectum is the most frequent polyposis type and a precancerous condition characterised by the presence of dozens to thousands of adenomas, which, unless detected early and removed, result in a high lifetime risk of colorectal cancer (CRC).

Even to date, the differential diagnosis of the various types of gastrointestinal polyposis syndromes is primarily made by endoscopy and histologic examination of polyps, complemented by gathering extraintestinal manifestations (see infobox) and the family history. To identify the predominant polyp type, a sufficient number of polyps have to be examined; nonetheless, in a substantial portion of cases, there is a broad phenotypic overlap between different polyposis types that makes a clinical diagnosis challenging.

S. Aretz (✉)
Institute of Human Genetics, Center for Hereditary Tumor Syndromes, University of Bonn, Bonn, Germany
e-mail: Stefan.Aretz@uni-bonn.de

L. Valle et al. (eds.), *Hereditary Colorectal Cancer*,
https://doi.org/10.1007/978-3-319-74259-5_6

Currently, at least five different inherited forms of adenomatous polyposis can be delineated by molecular genetic analyses which are described in detail below (Table 6.1, Fig. 6.1). The *APC*-related familial adenomatous polyposis (FAP) is the most common and best known form; all the other conditions which include both dominantly and recessively inherited types have been identified in recent years so that the characterisation of the full phenotype has not yet been finished. However, also in unexplained cases, a hereditary basis is likely.

Although all types are defined by the presence of multiple adenomas, which result in a similar diagnostic and therapeutic approach, a significant clinical variability in terms of number and age at onset can be observed, even within families. In addition, the upper gastrointestinal tract is frequently affected, and most syndromes are accompanied by a more or less syndrome-specific spectrum of benign and malignant extraintestinal lesions. The likelihood to identify a causative germline mutation by routine diagnostics strongly depends on the clinical presentation with higher detection rates in those cases with a more pronounced and early-onset phenotype.

Extraintestinal lesions which may point to a gastrointestinal adenomatous polyposis

- Congenital hypertrophy of the retinal pigment epithelium (CHRPE)
- Jaw osteomas
- Multiple epidermoid cysts
- Sebaceous gland neoplasias (adenomas, epitheliomas, carcinomas)
- Hepatoblastoma, Medulloblastoma

Table 6.1 Adenomatous polyposis syndromes

Disease	Gene(s)	Incidence	Number colorectal adenomas	Age at onset polyposis	Distribution of adenomas	Histology polyps	Lifetime risk CRC (untreated)	Mean age CRC (untreated)	Extraintestinal lesions	Comments
Autosomal dominant (heterozygous germline mutations)										
Classical familial adenomatous polyposis (FAP)	*APC*	1:10,000	100 till >5000	Second decade	Colon, duodenum	Adenomas, rarely HP, SA	100%	~ 40 y	Desmoids, osteomas, CHPRE, epidermoid cysts, fibromas, fundic gland polyps, papillary thyroid carcinomas hepatoblastoma, medulloblastoma, adrenal tumours	Mutation detection rate increases with severity of disease (age at onset, number of colorectal adenomas; high frequency of mosaic cases
Attenuated familial adenomatous polyposis (AFAP)	*APC*	?	10–100	≥ third decade	Colon, duodenum	Adenomas, rarely HP, SA	70–80%	50–60 y	High risk of desmoid tumours, osteomas, and epidermoid cysts when pathogenic variants located in codons 1395–1493	Phenotypic continuum with classical FAP
Gastric adenocarcinoma and proximal polyposis of the stomach (GAPPS)	*APC promoter 1B*	?	None or a few	14–75	Gastric body and fundus	FGP with/ without dysplasia, rarely HP + adenomas	Low	?	≥ 100 gastric FGP (body and fundus) with and without dysplasia, intestinal-type gastric adenocarcinoma, non or few colon adenomas	Only limited phenotypic information so far
Polymerase proofreading-associated polyposis (PPAP)	*POLE, POLD1*	Very rare	20–several hundreds		Colon, duodenum	Adenomas	Unknown		High risk for endometrial cancer	

(continued)

Table 6.1 (continued)

Disease	Gene(s)	Incidence	Number colorectal adenomas	Age at onset polyposis	Distribution of adenomas	Histology polyps	Lifetime risk CRC (untreated)	Mean age CRC (untreated)	Extraintestinal lesions	Comments
Autosomal recessive (biallelic germline mutations)										
MUTYH-associated polyposis (MAP)	*MUTYH*	1:20–40,000	0–>500		Colon, duodenum	Adenomas, HP	80–100%	40–50 y	Increased risk for extraintestinal malignancies (ovary, bladder skin, probably breast and endometrium), sebaceous gland tumours	Low recurrence risk for offspring
NTHL1-associated polyposis (NAP)	*NTHL1*	Very rare	~ 5 to hundred		Colon, duodenum	Adenomas	Unknown		Tumour spectrum yet unknown, multiple primary tumours, high risk for endometrial cancer	Low recurrence risk for offspring
Constitutional Mismatch-repair deficiency (CMMRD)	*MLH1, MSH2, MSH6, PMS2*	Very rare	Multiple - hundred	First–fourth decade	Colon, duodenum, jejunum	Adenomas			Early-onset brain tumours, haematological malignancies, cafe au lait skin macules, embryonic tumours; multiple primary tumours	MSI-H in tumour tissue; IHC: nuclear loss of the respective MMR protein in tumour and normal tissue; rapid progression from adenoma to carcinoma; paucity of LS-associated cancers in parents/ family history

MSH3-associated polyposis	*MSH3*	Very rare	Multiple		Colon, duodenum	Adenomas	Unknown	No or late-onset GI cancer	Not known yet; potential broad and overlapping tumour spectrum with CMMRD	Limited phenotypic information so far; attenuated gastrointestinal phenotype, EMAST in tumour tissue, IHC: nuclear loss of MSH3 in tumour and normal tissue; low recurrence risk for offspring

Abbreviations: *CHRPE* congenital hypertrophy of the retinal pigment epithelium, *EMAST* elevated microsatellite alterations at selected tetranucleotide repeats, *FGP* fundic gland polyp, HP hyperplastic polyps, *IHC* immunohistochemistry, LS Lynch syndrome, *MMR* DNA mismatch repair, *MSI-H* high microsatellite instability, y years old

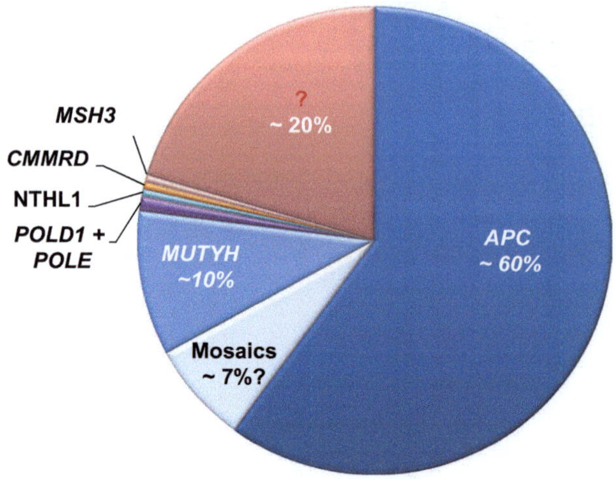

Fig. 6.1 Spectrum and frequency of causative germline mutations in adenomatous polyposis

References

1. Clark JC, Collan Y, Eide TJ, Esteve J, Ewen S, Gibbs NM, Jensen OM, Koskela E, MacLennan R, Simpson JG, et al. Prevalence of polyps in an autopsy series from areas with varying incidence of large-bowel cancer. Int J Cancer. 1985;36:179–86.
2. Rex DK, Lehman GA, Ulbright TM, Smith JJ, Pound DC, Hawes RH, Helper DJ, Wiersema MJ, Langefeld CD, Li W. Colonic neoplasia in asymptomatic persons with negative fecal occult blood tests: influence of age, gender, and family history. Am J Gastroenterol. 1993;88:825–31.
3. Tomlinson I, Jaeger E, Leedham S, Thomas H. The classification of intestinal polyposis. Nat Genet. 2013;45(1):2.

Chapter 7
Familial Adenomatous Polyposis or APC-Associated Polyposis

Maartje Nielsen and Stephan Aretz

Abstract Familial adenomatous polyposis (FAP) or APC-associated polyposis is an autosomal dominant inherited syndrome caused by APC germline mutations. Most patients will develop hundreds of adenomatous polyps and thereby have a 100% risk of developing CRC during lifetime. Depending on the location of the mutation in the APC gene, a milder phenotype with usually less than 100 adenomas is also possible, called attenuated FAP (AFAP). Patients with AFAP also have a high risk of developing mostly benign, extracolonic manifestations. This chapter will discuss the genetic and clinical aspects, detection, extracolonic manifestations, and tumour characteristics of this polyposis syndrome.

Keywords Familial adenomatous polyposis · APC-associated polyposis · APC Polyposis · AFAP

Familial adenomatous polyposis (FAP, OMIM 175100) is an autosomal dominant inherited polyposis syndrome caused by germline mutations in the tumour suppressor gene *APC*; it affects approximately 2–3 in 100,000 individuals [1–3]. The incidence is 1:6850 to 1:23,700 born living, irrespective of gender and ethnic background [2–6]. Classic FAP is associated with hundreds of adenomatous polyps and a CRC lifetime risk of 100% at an average age of 35–40 years. A milder phenotype, with a lower polyp number, is named *attenuated* FAP. Mutations in *APC* can be found in 10–80% of patient with more than 20 adenomatous polyps [7], and less than 1% of all CRC cases, irrespective of polyp number, are ascribed to FAP [8].

M. Nielsen (✉)
Department of Clinical Genetics, Leiden University Medical Centre, Leiden, The Netherlands
e-mail: m.nielsen@lumc.nl

S. Aretz
Institute of Human Genetics, Center for Hereditary Tumor Syndromes, University of Bonn, Bonn, Germany

L. Valle et al. (eds.), *Hereditary Colorectal Cancer*,
https://doi.org/10.1007/978-3-319-74259-5_7

Originally, the term familial adenomatous polyposis was used to describe *APC* mutation-positive and mutation-negative patients, based on the clinical phenotype of more than a hundred polyps. Since it became clear that patients with a colorectal adenomatous polyposis can also have germline mutations in other genes, like the *MUTYH* gene discovered in 2002, the term *APC-associated polyposis* (*AAP*) for patients with proven *APC* mutations might be more appropriate. Since the term FAP is so embedded in the clinical practice, it will be difficult to replace it, and therefore it is relevant to realize that a diagnosis of FAP can be based on a clinical phenotype, a proven *APC*, or other germline gene mutation. In general, it is more appropriate to describe the phenotype as (colorectal) adenomatous polyposis unless a genetic cause is identified.

1 Genetics

The *APC* gene is a relatively large gene; its main three transcripts encompass 15 coding exons and 18 exons altogether (NCBI, LRG_130), encoding a protein of 2843 amino acids and located in chromosome 5q22.2. Exon 15 is by far the largest exon, containing over three-quarters of the coding sequence. The *APC* gene codes for a multifunctional protein that comprises several motifs and domains, allowing it to bind and/or interact with multiple molecules that include β-catenin, α-catenin, GSK3β, axin, conductin, and tubulin [9]. The APC protein is involved in the Wnt signal cascade, where it is part of a complex involved in downregulating β-catenin. When the APC function is lost, β-catenin accumulates and migrates to the nucleus [10]. This leads to repression of apoptosis, induction of cell cycle progression and proliferation, and control of cell growth.

Over 700 different disease-causing mutations have been reported throughout the *APC* gene, but most mutations occur in the 5′ half of the coding region of exon 15, otherwise referred to as the mutation cluster region. Hotspot mutations are found at codon 1061 and 1309. Differences in phenotype may relate to the location of the mutation within the *APC* gene.

Depending on clinical features and mutation detection techniques applied, mutations in the *APC* gene can be identified in approximately 70% of patients with more than a 100 polyps (Fig. 7.1). A list of mutations is available online at the *Leiden Open Variation Database* (LOVD): http://chromium.liacs.nl/LOVD2/colon_cancer/home.php?select_db=*APC*. The most common germline mutations involve the introduction of a premature stop codon, either by a nonsense or frameshift mutation. With multiplex ligation-dependent probe amplification (MLPA), partial and whole gene deletions have been found in a substantial proportion (4–33%) of patients previously tested negative for *APC* mutations [11–13]. Approximately 75% of germline *APC* mutations are inherited and 10–25% are de novo [14]. With more sensitive techniques, it has been shown that in 11–21% of these de novo cases, *APC* mosaicism is present in a parent or the patient [15, 16].

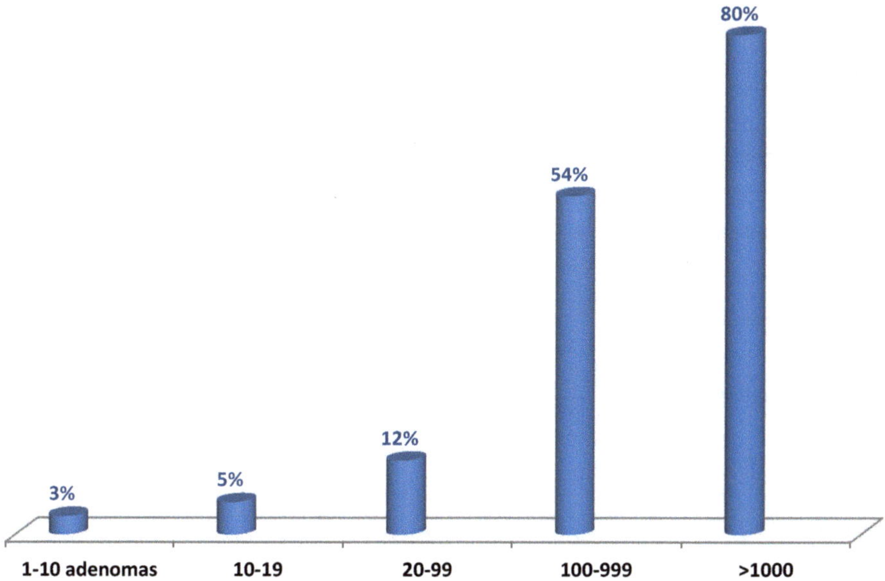

Fig. 7.1 Detection rate of APC mutations (Adapted from Grover et al. [7])

Furthermore, recent studies have shown that in unexplained cases with more than 20 adenomas, pathogenic *APC* mosaic mutations are present in about 25–50% if DNA from two or more adenomas was analysed [17, 18] (Fig. 7.2).

Finally, a small fraction of cases can have a deep intronic *APC* mutation or a rare missense mutation of the *APC* gene [19, 20].

2 Clinical Characteristics

Germline *APC* mutations lead to a broad clinical spectrum regarding colorectal presentation with polyp count ranging between tens and thousand and a high risk of developing extracolonic tumours. These phenotypic extremes are part of a clinical continuum that depends partly on the location of the germline *APC* mutation, although this is without clear thresholds.

Classic FAP patients have already developed numerous adenomatous polyps in their colon in their 20s making a colectomy at a relative young age necessary. These patients usually have mutations occurring between codon 1250 and 1464 but particularly at codon 1309 [21]. This region is also called the mutation cluster region (MCR), since most somatic mutation in tumours also occur between these codons [22]. Without surgical intervention, FAP patients almost inevitably develop CRC by the mean age of 40–50 years [23]. In 70–80% of patients CRC is left sided [24–26].

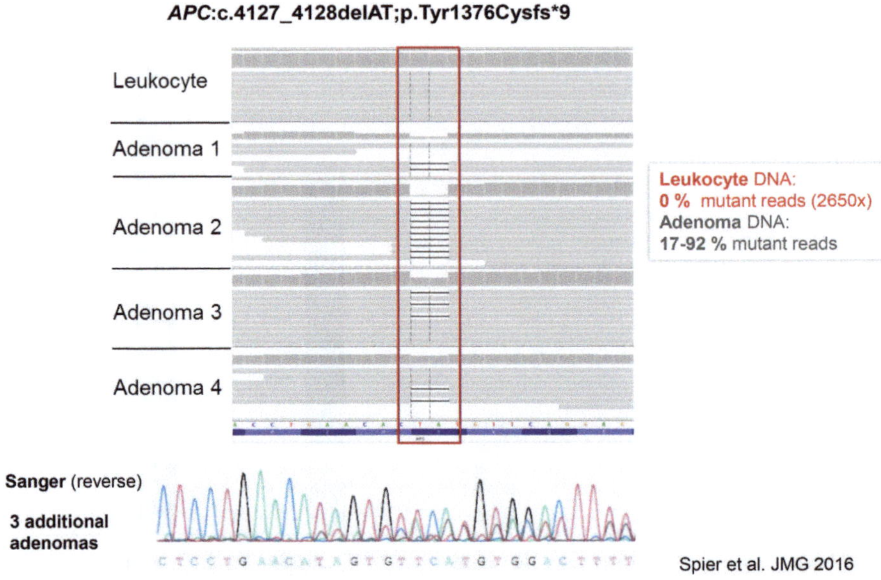

Fig. 7.2 APC mosaicism as shown with 1) exome sequencing data (Integrative Genomics Viewer) of leucocyte and adenoma DNA, the same APC mutation is present in four adenomas but not in leucocyte DNA and 2) Sanger sequencing of the corresponding region (DNA of adenoma 4, reverse sequence). Figure depicted from Spier et al, JMG 2016

The duodenum and the periampullary region are the second most common parts where adenomas will develop, and the prevalence varies between 33 and 92% [27–30]. In a recent Dutch follow-up study, duodenal adenomatous polyposis was documented in 191 of the 565 patients initially enrolled in the study (33.8%). Fundic gland polyposis was reported in 102 (18.1%) patients, and 24 (4.2%) patients had at least one gastric adenoma, all located in the antrum [31].

Duodenal carcinoma is the second most common malignancy after CRC, with a lifetime risk of at least 3–5% [32, 33]. During follow-up, it was the second most common cause of cancer death (7/33, 21%), after CRC [31]. In a Dutch cohort compared to the general population, the risks of developing a duodenal adenocarcinoma or ampullary carcinoma (in whom duodenal carcinoma is rare) are 331 and 124 times higher, respectively, in FAP patients [34].

A somewhat less severe, intermediate phenotype (i.e. hundreds to thousands of polyps) is associated with mutations within codons 157–1595, excluding the mutation cluster region. Finally, part of patients with *APC* mutations have an even milder phenotype with less than a hundred adenomas and a later onset of both adenomas and CRC, called attenuated FAP (AFAP). On average, CRC will develop 12 years later compared with classic FAP. Most of these patients have a mutation in the 5′ part, alternative spliced region in exon 9 or in the extreme 3′ site of the *APC* gene [21].

However, it is important to realize that although correlations between genotype and phenotype have been shown in groups of patients, the exact phenotype in patients cannot be predicted based on the location of the germline mutation alone. Even within families and patients with the same mutation, differences in adenoma count and CRC risk exist [35–37].

It is likely that other factors, external factors or genetic modifiers, influence adenoma count and (extra) colonic tumour risk in FAP patients.

Recently, in a study of 419 proven APC germline mutation carriers, two CRC-associated SNPs (single-nucleotide polymorphisms) previously found in genome-wide association studies for CRC, rs16892766 (8q23.3) and rs3802842 (11q23.1), were found to be associated with higher adenoma count [38]. Another study did not find an effect of CRC SNPs (including rs16892766 and rs3802842) on the number of colorectal adenomas in 142 analysed FAP patients. In a third study, an association of two SNPs and CRC risk and age of diagnosis in a FAP cohort was found first, but this could not be reproduced in a second independent cohort, and authors emphasized the need of large sample sizes when searching for modifier genes in the future [39].

More recently, a phenotype with a high risk of gastric adenocarcinoma and occurrence of predominantly proximal polyposis of the stomach (GAPPS) has been described [40]. More precise, the diagnosis of GAPPS should be considered in individuals that have the following features: (1) gastric polyps restricted to the body and fundus; (2) more than 100 polyps in the proximal stomach or more than 30 polyps in a first-degree relative of an individual with GAPPS; (3) predominantly fundic gland polyps (FGPs), some having regions of dysplasia; (4) an autosomal dominant pattern of inheritance; and (5) no evidence of colorectal or duodenal polyposis [41]. In 2016 it was found that these patients have germline mutations in promoter 1B of *APC* [42]. Notably, in some patients with a proven disease-associated variant in promoter 1B, colonic polyposis has also been shown [41, 42] and colonoscopic screening might be warranted in these patients too. Interestingly, the colonic adenomas in GAPPS patients show similarities in histochemical profile to fundic gland polyposis [43].

3 Extracolonic Manifestations

The majority (70%) of FAP patients develop extracolonic manifestations [21]. Besides CRC and duodenal cancer, other malignant lesions that can occur in FAP are thyroid carcinoma (papillary, the cribriform-morular variant; Fig. 7.3) and brain (usually medulloblastoma), liver (hepatoblastoma), and pancreas (pancreatoblastoma) tumours [33, 41, 44]. A recent follow-up study in the Netherlands with a mean age at last follow-up of 40 years, reported extracolonic malignancies, including duodenal cancer, in 74 (12.7%) of 582 APC mutation carriers [31]. Thyroid cancer (papillary) was present in 9 of the 582 Dutch FAP patients (1.5%, 7 females/2 males), during follow-up with a mean age of 33.5 years. One patient died because

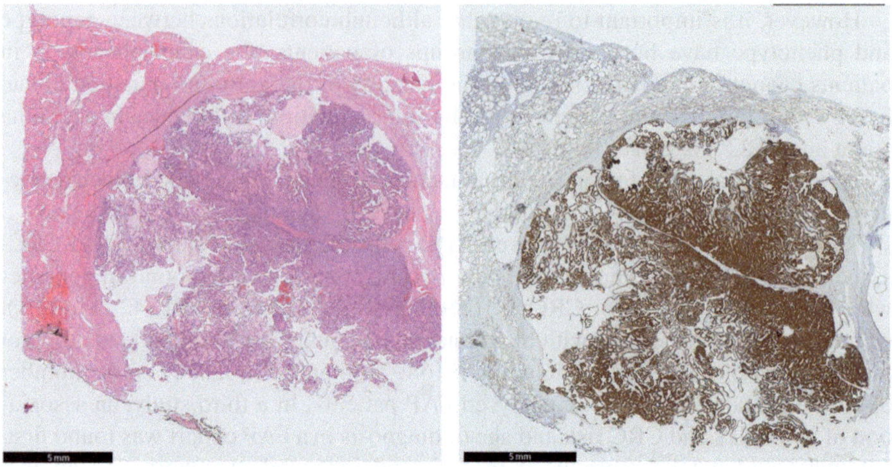

Fig. 7.3 Cribriform-morular variant of papillary thyroid carcinoma in an FAP patient with proven APC mutation. Left panel, HE staining, and right panel, positive β-catenin nucleic staining due to WNT pathway upregulation (Obtained from: http://www.hereditarypathology.org, under courtesy of prof. dr. Hans Morreau, LUMC)

of thyroid cancer at the age of 78 years. In the same cohort, hepatoblastoma was reported in 4 (0.7%) carriers, bladder cancer in 4 (0.7%), and pancreatic malignancy, malignant brain tumour, and meningioma were each observed in two patients [31]. Thyroid screening and extending surveillance for other cancers based in these prevalences were not advised by authors, because they will unlikely contribute in a significant manner to the survival of FAP patients [31].

Approximately 10–25% of FAP patients develop another potentially deadly complication, namely, desmoid tumours. A high risk of recurrence and local infiltration make desmoid tumours the most common cause of death amongst FAP patients after they receive prophylactic colectomy [45]. In the Dutch follow-up study, desmoid tumours were the third most common cause of death in general (11% of all deaths, $n = 6/56$ deaths in the total cohort), after colon cancer (25%) and cardiovascular disease (12%) [31]. The mean age at death due to a desmoid tumour was 40.5 years.

Desmoid tumours are mostly seen in the abdomen and small bowel mesentery and are usually initiated by traumatic events, in particular surgery [46], but it's also seen in shoulder girdle, chest wall, and inguinal regions [47, 48]. Independent risk factors include a germline mutation distal to codon 1444, abdominal surgery, and a family history of desmoids [49].

Extracolonic manifestations with less clinical significance include lesions such as congenital hypertrophy of retinal pigment epithelium (CHRPE), present in over 90% of FAP patients), dental abnormalities (absences of teeth amongst others), fundic gland polyps, osteomas, Gardner fibromas (a benign tumour of the connective tissue), adrenal masses (mostly adrenocortical adenomas without endocrinopathy), and epidermoid cysts or lipomas on any part of the body [9, 12, 21, 41, 50]. Lipomas and osteomas were documented in 11 (1.9%) and 7 (1.2%) patients during follow-up in the Dutch cohort, respectively.

Two phenotypic subgroups of FAP in which patients have a specific clustering of extracolonic tumours besides their polyposis have been defined in the past, before it became clear that these were actually allelic variants of the APC-associated polyposis spectrum. Patients with the so-called Gardner syndrome show a clustering of epidermoid cysts, Gardner fibromas, lipomas, and desmoid tumours, and patients with Turcot syndrome are characterized by the presence of thyroid tumours and central nervous system (CNS) tumours [51]. Because these terms do not refer to genetically distinct conditions they should not be used any longer.

4 *APC* Mutation Detection

In general, the detection rate of an *APC* germline mutation strongly depends on the number of colorectal adenomas, age at onset, and family history. In patients with more than 100 adenomas, an *APC* germline mutation can be found in 56–82%, irrespective of the family history, and the detection rate rises to 76–80% in patients with more than a thousand adenomas [7, 52] (Fig. 1) [7]. In patients with between 20 and 100 adenomas, the percentage of *APC* mutations is still a significant 12%, but in patients with less than 20 adenomas, the percentage falls to 5%, although this highly depends on the age of diagnosis. In a patient aged 20 years with between 10 and 19 adenomas, there is a 38% chance of finding an *APC* mutation, dropping to only 2% in patients aged 50 years. The presence of an affected family member with CRC do not influence outcomes in patients with more than a hundred polyps, but increases the mutation rate in patients aged 50 with between 10 and 19 adenomas (11% *APC* mutations detected) [7].

Sometimes patients, especially children, can present with extracolonic features before colorectal adenomas are diagnosed in themselves or their parents. Several studies have analysed (single cases or small groups) whether patients with extracolonic manifestations have underlying FAP or not.

In a group of seven patients with apparently sporadic Gardner fibroma (GAF), a germline *APC* mutation was detected in 3 (43%) of them. These GAFs had a worse phenotype than the *APC* negative tested, multifocal (1) or large unresectable (2) GAFs [53]. One study found a higher prevalence of β-catenin staining in Gardner fibromas in FAP patients as compared to the total group analysed, including sporadic cases (90% versus 64%) [54]. Single cases presenting with Gardner fibroma before the age of 1 year—with previously unrecognized FAP families—with constitutional *APC* mutations have also been reported [55–57].

A Dutch study performed immunohistochemistry of β-catenin and mutation analysis of *CTNNB1* in 18 paediatric desmoid tumours, diagnosed between 1990 and 2009 [48]. After selection based on nuclear β-catenin staining, a germline *APC* mutation was identified in two tumours, 11% of the total. These two cases, aged 1.5

and 15 years at diagnosis, were the only ones with a family history of FAP or polyposis in one of the parents and sibling.

For CHRPE no evidence exists momentarily that this can be a first sign of an underlying germline *APC* mutation. A total of 25 CHRPEs were found in 21 of the 1745 (1.2%) patients from the general population whose fundus images were examined [58]. Age is not a factor relevant to the presence of CHRPE as it is a congenital condition, and ages of detection in this cohort ranged between 11 months and 87 years. In these 21 patients, no evidence was found from patients' clinical records to suggest the presence of FAP and Gardner and Turcot syndromes. Previously four cases of CHRPE (aged 4, 14, 16, and 39 years) without polyposis were send in for *APC* analysis to the diagnostic laboratory of the Leiden University Medical Hospital. No *APC* mutation was detected (own data). CHRPE or pigmented ocular fundus lesions in FAP do present differently than in sporadic CHRPE, in that they are more often multiple and bilateral [59]. Larger studies are needed in patients with young bilateral CHRPE to see if there is a relevant chance of detecting an underlying germline *APC* mutation.

In one child with an osteoma and no colorectal phenotype at time of diagnosis, a de novo frameshift *APC* mutation was found [52].

Lastly, in a study of 50 young patients with apparently sporadic hepatoblastoma, germline mutations in the *APC* gene were identified in up to 10%. Authors thus concluded that in a substantial fraction of sporadic hepatoblastoma, the disease is the first manifestation of a de novo FAP [60]. However, another study did not find this association, no APC germline mutation was found in 29 children with apparently sporadic hepatoblastoma [61].

Concluding, it is possible that a patient with a de novo or familial occurring *APC* mutation might present first with a Gardner fibroma, osteoma, desmoid tumour, or hepatoblastoma, but larger studies on this subject are needed.

5 Tumour Characteristics

Alterations in the *APC* gene are present in about 80% of sporadic colorectal carcinoma, and loss of heterozygosity (LOH) of chromosome 5q is reported in 30–40% of CRC cases [62]. It is therefore assumed that a mutated *APC* gene is an early and likely initiating event in colon tumorigenesis. This probably explains why patients with a germline APC mutation develop mainly colon tumours and less tumours elsewhere. Before tumorigenesis can start, a second and sometimes even third hit in the other *APC* allele is needed [63, 64]. APC normally binds to GSK3β as part of a complex which regulates β-catenin stability, and disruption of this complex leads to elevated levels of β-catenin. This then activates proteins that participate in cell cycle, growth, and regulation of cell death, such as CCND1, AXIN2, and BIRC5, called the WNT signalling pathway [65]. For adenomas to grow, WNT activation is beneficial, but too much activation will lead to apoptosis or evoking cell death [13], and retention of some functional APC protein is therefore required.

The so-called seven 20-amino-acid repeats (20 aa repeats) of the APC protein play a central role in the degradation of β-catenin [66]. It has been shown in an adenoma study that indeed the second hit in *APC* does not occur randomly but rather depends on the location of the first hit or underlying *APC* germline mutation, resulting in retention of one or two of the seven 20 aa repeats [67]. This retention of one or two aa repeats is thought to lead to a signalling activity that is sufficient to confer proliferation advantage without inducing cell death and is labelled as the 'just-right hypothesis' [67].

Relevance of the *APC*/β-catenin signalling pathway has also been shown to be strongly involved in the pathogenesis of other tumours associated with FAP, such as desmoid tumours and thyroid cancer [68, 69] (Fig. 7.3).

Another study, focused on the early evolution of adenomas of polyposis patients, performed whole exome sequencing and targeted analysis of colorectal adenoma in FAP and MAP patients [70]. Overall it was shown that FAP adenomas have less coding somatic mutations (0.16 mutations/Mb) compared to MAP adenomas (0.65 mutation/Mb, $p < 0.014$). Possibly, tumour suppressor genes undergo allelic loss in FAP rather than being disrupted by point mutations as compared to MAP, as has been shown previously [71].

In FAP adenomas, mutations were seen in several genes. Another frequently mutated gene, besides *APC* was the *WTX* gene, mutated in 9% of FAP adenomas (6/69). The *WTX* gene also has a role in the regulation of the WNT pathway [72].

A hallmark of most FAP-associated tumours is nuclear β-catenin staining, and this can be used as a prescreening tool, for example, in extracolonic tumours, to select (young) patients that might not have developed adenomas yet, for *APC* germline analysis. When nuclear β-catenin staining is present, this is due to a somatic *CTNNB1* mutation in most sporadic cases. In the absence of such a mutation, *APC* germline testing should be considered [73].

References

1. Burn J, Chapman P, Delhanty J, Wood C, Lalloo F, Cachon-Gonzalez MB, et al. The UK Northern region genetic register for familial adenomatous polyposis coli: use of age of onset, congenital hypertrophy of the retinal pigment epithelium, and DNA markers in risk calculations. J Med Genet. 1991;28(5):289–96.
2. Bulow S, Faurschou NT, Bulow C, Bisgaard ML, Karlsen L, Moesgaard F. The incidence rate of familial adenomatous polyposis. Results from the Danish Polyposis Register. Int J Color Dis. 1996;11(2):88–91.
3. Bjork J, Akerbrant H, Iselius L, Alm T, Hultcrantz R. Epidemiology of familial adenomatous polyposis in Sweden: changes over time and differences in phenotype between males and females. Scand J Gastroenterol. 1999;34(12):1230–5.
4. Bussey HJ. Familial polyposis coli. Pathol Annu. 1979;14(Pt 1):61–81.
5. Jarvinen HJ. Epidemiology of familial adenomatous polyposis in Finland: impact of family screening on the colorectal cancer rate and survival. Gut. 1992;33(3):357–60.
6. Bisgaard ML, Fenger K, Bulow S, Niebuhr E, Mohr J. Familial adenomatous polyposis (FAP): frequency, penetrance, and mutation rate. Hum Mutat. 1994;3(2):121–5.

7. Grover S, Kastrinos F, Steyerberg EW, Cook EF, Dewanwala A, Burbidge LA, et al. Prevalence and phenotypes of APC and MUTYH mutations in patients with multiple colorectal adenomas. JAMA. 2012;308(5):485–92. https://doi.org/10.1001/jama.2012.8780.
8. Pearlman R, Frankel WL, Swanson B, Zhao W, Yilmaz A, Miller K, et al. Prevalence and spectrum of germline cancer susceptibility gene mutations among patients with early-onset colorectal cancer. JAMA Oncol. 2016. https://doi.org/10.1001/jamaoncol.2016.5194.
9. Lipton L, Tomlinson I. The genetics of FAP and FAP-like syndromes. Familial Cancer. 2006;5(3):221–6.
10. Zhang L, Shay JW. Multiple roles of APC and its therapeutic implications in colorectal cancer. J Natl Cancer Inst. 2017;109(8). https://doi.org/10.1093/jnci/djw332.
11. Nielsen M, Bik E, Hes FJ, Breuning MH, Vasen HF, Bakker E, et al. Genotype-phenotype correlations in 19 Dutch cases with APC gene deletions and a literature review. Eur J Hum Genet: EJHG. 2007;15(10):1034–42. https://doi.org/10.1038/sj.ejhg.5201871.
12. Sieber OM, Lamlum H, Crabtree MD, Rowan AJ, Barclay E, Lipton L, et al. Whole-gene APC deletions cause classical familial adenomatous polyposis, but not attenuated polyposis or "multiple" colorectal adenomas. Proc Natl Acad Sci U S A. 2002;99(5):2954–8.
13. Aretz S, Stienen D, Uhlhaas S, Pagenstecher C, Mangold E, Caspari R, et al. Large submicroscopic genomic APC deletions are a common cause of typical familial adenomatous polyposis. J Med Genet. 2005;42(2):185–92. https://doi.org/10.1136/jmg.2004.022822.
14. Aretz S, Uhlhaas S, Caspari R, Mangold E, Pagenstecher C, Propping P, et al. Frequency and parental origin of de novo APC mutations in familial adenomatous polyposis. Eur J Hum Genet: EJHG. 2004;12(1):52–8. https://doi.org/10.1038/sj.ejhg.5201088.
15. Hes FJ, Nielsen M, Bik EC, Konvalinka D, Wijnen JT, Bakker E, et al. Somatic APC mosaicism: an underestimated cause of polyposis coli. Gut. 2008;57(1):71–6. https://doi.org/10.1136/gut.2006.117796.
16. Aretz S, Stienen D, Friedrichs N, Stemmler S, Uhlhaas S, Rahner N, et al. Somatic APC mosaicism: a frequent cause of familial adenomatous polyposis (FAP). Hum Mutat. 2007;28(10):985–92. https://doi.org/10.1002/humu.20549.
17. Jansen AM, Crobach S, Geurts-Giele WR, van den Akker BE, Garcia MV, Ruano D, et al. Distinct patterns of somatic mosaicism in the APC gene in neoplasms from patients with unexplained adenomatous polyposis. Gastroenterology. 2017;152(3):546–9 e3. https://doi.org/10.1053/j.gastro.2016.10.040.
18. Spier I, Drichel D, Kerick M, Kirfel J, Horpaopan S, Laner A, et al. Low-level APC mutational mosaicism is the underlying cause in a substantial fraction of unexplained colorectal adenomatous polyposis cases. J Med Genet. 2016;53(3):172–9. https://doi.org/10.1136/jmedgenet-2015-103468.
19. Spier I, Horpaopan S, Vogt S, Uhlhaas S, Morak M, Stienen D, et al. Deep intronic APC mutations explain a substantial proportion of patients with familial or early-onset adenomatous polyposis. Hum Mutat. 2012;33(7):1045–50. https://doi.org/10.1002/humu.22082.
20. Azzopardi D, Dallosso AR, Eliason K, Hendrickson BC, Jones N, Rawstorne E, et al. Multiple rare nonsynonymous variants in the adenomatous polyposis coli gene predispose to colorectal adenomas. Cancer Res. 2008;68(2):358–63.
21. Nieuwenhuis MH, Vasen HF. Correlations between mutation site in APC and phenotype of familial adenomatous polyposis (FAP): a review of the literature. Crit Rev Oncol Hematol. 2007;61(2):153–61.
22. Miyoshi Y, Nagase H, Ando H, Horii A, Ichii S, Nakatsuru S, et al. Somatic mutations of the APC gene in colorectal tumors: mutation cluster region in the APC gene. Hum Mol Genet. 1992;1(4):229–33.
23. Bussey HJR. Familial polyposis coli: family studies, histopathology, differential diagnosis, and results of treatment. Baltimore: Johns Hopkins University Press; 1975.
24. Atkin WS, Morson BC, Cuzick J. Long-term risk of colorectal cancer after excision of rectosigmoid adenomas. N Engl J Med. 1992;326(10):658–62.
25. Ponder BA. Cancer genetics. Nature. 2001;411(6835):336–41.

26. Lichtenstein P, Holm NV, Verkasalo PK, Iliadou A, Kaprio J, Koskenvuo M, et al. Environmental and heritable factors in the causation of cancer–analyses of cohorts of twins from Sweden, Denmark, and Finland. N Engl J Med. 2000;343(2):78–85.
27. Bulow S, Bjork J, Christensen IJ, Fausa O, Jarvinen H, Moesgaard F, et al. Duodenal adenomatosis in familial adenomatous polyposis. Gut. 2004;53(3):381–6.
28. Campos FG, Sulbaran M, Safatle-Ribeiro AV, Martinez CAR. Duodenal adenoma surveillance in patients with familial adenomatous polyposis. World J Gastrointest Endosc. 2015;7(10):950–9. https://doi.org/10.4253/wjge.v7.i10.950.
29. Hashimoto T, Ogawa R, Matsubara A, Taniguchi H, Sugano K, Ushiama M, et al. Familial adenomatous polyposis-associated and sporadic pyloric gland adenomas of the upper gastrointestinal tract share common genetic features. Histopathology. 2015;67(5):689–98. https://doi.org/10.1111/his.12705.
30. Bjork J, Akerbrant H, Iselius L, Bergman A, Engwall Y, Wahlstrom J, et al. Periampullary adenomas and adenocarcinomas in familial adenomatous polyposis: cumulative risks and APC gene mutations. Gastroenterology. 2001;121(5):1127–35.
31. Ghorbanoghli Z, Bastiaansen BA, Langers AM, Nagengast FM, Poley JW, Hardwick JC, et al. Extracolonic cancer risk in Dutch patients with APC (adenomatous polyposis coli)-associated polyposis. J Med Genet. 2017. https://doi.org/10.1136/jmedgenet-2017-104545.
32. Latchford AR, Neale KF, Spigelman AD, Phillips RK, Clark SK. Features of duodenal cancer in patients with familial adenomatous polyposis. Clin Gastroenterol Hepatol Off Clin Pract J Am Gastroenterol Assoc. 2009;7(6):659–63. https://doi.org/10.1016/j.cgh.2009.02.028.
33. Groves CJ, Saunders BP, Spigelman AD, Phillips RK. Duodenal cancer in patients with familial adenomatous polyposis (FAP): results of a 10 year prospective study. Gut. 2002;50(5):636–41.
34. Offerhaus GJ, Giardiello FM, Krush AJ, Booker SV, Tersmette AC, Kelley NC, et al. The risk of upper gastrointestinal cancer in familial adenomatous polyposis. Gastroenterology. 1992;102(6):1980–2.
35. Giardiello FM, Krush AJ, Petersen GM, Booker SV, Kerr M, Tong LL, et al. Phenotypic variability of familial adenomatous polyposis in 11 unrelated families with identical APC gene mutation. Gastroenterology. 1994;106(6):1542–7.
36. Nugent KP, Phillips RK, Hodgson SV, Cottrell S, Smith-Ravin J, Pack K, et al. Phenotypic expression in familial adenomatous polyposis: partial prediction by mutation analysis. Gut. 1994;35(11):1622–3.
37. Rozen P, Samuel Z, Shomrat R, Legum C. Notable intrafamilial phenotypic variability in a kindred with familial adenomatous polyposis and an APC mutation in exon 9. Gut. 1999;45(6):829–33.
38. Ghorbanoghli Z, Nieuwenhuis MH, Houwing-Duistermaat JJ, Jagmohan-Changur S, Hes FJ, Tops CM, et al. Colorectal cancer risk variants at 8q23.3 and 11q23.1 are associated with disease phenotype in APC mutation carriers. Familial Cancer. 2016;15(4):563–70. https://doi.org/10.1007/s10689-016-9877-5.
39. Talseth-Palmer BA, Wijnen JT, Andreassen EK, Barker D, Jagmohan-Changur S, Tops CM, et al. The importance of a large sample cohort for studies on modifier genes influencing disease severity in FAP patients. Hered Cancer Clin Pract. 2013;11(1):20. https://doi.org/10.1186/1897-4287-11-20.
40. Worthley DL, Phillips KD, Wayte N, Schrader KA, Healey S, Kaurah P, et al. Gastric adenocarcinoma and proximal polyposis of the stomach (GAPPS): a new autosomal dominant syndrome. Gut. 2012;61(5):774–9. https://doi.org/10.1136/gutjnl-2011-300348.
41. Jasperson KW, Patel SG, Ahnen DJ. APC-associated polyposis conditions. In: Pagon RA, Adam MP, Ardinger HH, Wallace SE, Amemiya A, LJH B, et al., editors. GeneReviews(R). Seattle: University of Washington; 1993.
42. Li J, Woods SL, Healey S, Beesley J, Chen X, Lee JS, et al. Point mutations in exon 1B of APC reveal gastric adenocarcinoma and proximal polyposis of the stomach as a familial adenomatous polyposis variant. Am J Hum Genet. 2016;98(5):830–42. https://doi.org/10.1016/j.ajhg.2016.03.001.

43. McDuffie LA, Sabesan A, Allgaeuer M, Xin L, Koh C, Heller T, et al. Beta-Catenin activation in fundic gland polyps, gastric cancer and colonic polyps in families afflicted by 'gastric adenocarcinoma and proximal polyposis of the stomach' (GAPPS). J Clin Pathol. 2016;69(9):826–33. https://doi.org/10.1136/jclinpath-2016-203746.
44. Uchino S, Ishikawa H, Miyauchi A, Hirokawa M, Noguchi S, Ushiama M, et al. Age- and gender-specific risk of thyroid cancer in patients with familial adenomatous polyposis. J Clin Endocrinol Metab. 2016;101(12):4611–7. https://doi.org/10.1210/jc.2016-2043.
45. Clark SK, Phillips RK. Desmoids in familial adenomatous polyposis. Br J Surg. 1996;83(11):1494–504.
46. Lips DJ, Barker N, Clevers H, Hennipman A. The role of APC and beta-catenin in the aetiology of aggressive fibromatosis (desmoid tumors). Eur J Surg Oncol. 2009;35(1):3–10. https://doi.org/10.1016/j.ejso.2008.07.003.
47. Fallen T, Wilson M, Morlan B, Lindor NM. Desmoid tumors – a characterization of patients seen at Mayo Clinic 1976–1999. Familial Cancer. 2006;5(2):191–4. https://doi.org/10.1007/s10689-005-5959-5.
48. Kattentidt Mouravieva AA, Geurts-Giele IR, de Krijger RR, van Noesel MM, van de Ven CP, van den Ouweland AM, et al. Identification of Familial Adenomatous Polyposis carriers among children with desmoid tumours. Eur J Cancer (Oxford, England: 1990). 2012;48(12):1867–74. https://doi.org/10.1016/j.ejca.2012.01.004.
49. Nieuwenhuis MH, Lefevre JH, Bulow S, Jarvinen H, Bertario L, Kerneis S, et al. Family history, surgery, and APC mutation are risk factors for desmoid tumors in familial adenomatous polyposis: an international cohort study. Dis Colon Rectum. 2011;54(10):1229–34. https://doi.org/10.1097/DCR.0b013e318227e4e8.
50. Smith TG, Clark SK, Katz DE, Reznek RH, Phillips RK. Adrenal masses are associated with familial adenomatous polyposis. Dis Colon Rectum. 2000;43(12):1739–42.
51. Galiatsatos P, Foulkes WD. Familial adenomatous polyposis. Am J Gastroenterol. 2006;101(2):385–98.
52. Friedl W, Aretz S. Familial adenomatous polyposis: experience from a study of 1164 unrelated german polyposis patients. Hered Cancer Clin Pract. 2005;3(3):95–114. https://doi.org/10.1186/1897-4287-3-3-95.
53. Coffin CM, Hornick JL, Zhou H, Fletcher CD. Gardner fibroma: a clinicopathologic and immunohistochemical analysis of 45 patients with 57 fibromas. Am J Surg Pathol. 2007;31(3):410–6. https://doi.org/10.1097/01.pas.0000213348.65014.0a.
54. Dahl NA, Sheil A, Knapke S, Geller JI. Gardner fibroma: clinical and histopathologic implications of germline APC mutation association. J Pediatr Hematol Oncol. 2016;38(5):e154–7. https://doi.org/10.1097/MPH.0000000000000493.
55. Levesque S, Ahmed N, Nguyen VH, Nahal A, Blumenkrantz M, Puligandla P, et al. Neonatal Gardner fibroma: a sentinel presentation of severe familial adenomatous polyposis. Pediatrics. 2010;126(6):e1599–602. https://doi.org/10.1542/peds.2010-1045.
56. Vieira J, Pinto C, Afonso M, do Bom Sucesso M, Lopes P, Pinheiro M, et al. Identification of previously unrecognized FAP in children with Gardner fibroma. Eur J Hum Genet EJHG. 2015;23(5):715–8. https://doi.org/10.1038/ejhg.2014.144.
57. Schafer M, Kadmon M, Schmidt W, Treiber I, Moog U, Sutter C, et al. Neonatal Gardner fibroma leads to detection of familial adenomatous polyposis: two case reports. Eur J Pediatr Surg Rep. 2016;4(1):17–21. https://doi.org/10.1055/s-0036-1582443.
58. Coleman P, Barnard NA. Congenital hypertrophy of the retinal pigment epithelium: prevalence and ocular features in the optometric population. Ophthalmic Physiol Opt. 2007;27(6):547–55. https://doi.org/10.1111/j.1475-1313.2007.00513.x.
59. Nusliha A, Dalpatadu U, Amarasinghe B, Chandrasinghe PC, Deen KI. Congenital hypertrophy of retinal pigment epithelium (CHRPE) in patients with familial adenomatous polyposis (FAP); a polyposis registry experience. BMC Res Notes. 2014;7:734. https://doi.org/10.1186/1756-0500-7-734.

60. Aretz S, Koch A, Uhlhaas S, Friedl W, Propping P, von Schweinitz D, et al. Should children at risk for familial adenomatous polyposis be screened for hepatoblastoma and children with apparently sporadic hepatoblastoma be screened for APC germline mutations? Pediatr Blood Cancer. 2006;47(6):811–8. https://doi.org/10.1002/pbc.20698.
61. Harvey J, Clark S, Hyer W, Hadzic N, Tomlinson I, Hinds R. Germline APC mutations are not commonly seen in children with sporadic hepatoblastoma. J Pediatr Gastroenterol Nutr. 2008;47(5):675–7. https://doi.org/10.1097/MPG.0b013e318174e808.
62. Fearnhead NS, Britton MP, Bodmer WF. The ABC of APC. Hum Mol Genet. 2001;10(7):721–33.
63. Segditsas S, Rowan AJ, Howarth K, Jones A, Leedham S, Wright NA, Gorman P, Chambers W, Domingo E, Roylance RR, Sawyer EJ, Sieber OM, Tomlinson IP. APC and the three-hit hypothesis. Oncogene. 2009 Jan 8;28(1):146–55. https://doi.org/10.1038/onc.2008.361. Epub 2008 Oct 6.
64. Sieber O, Segditsas S, Knudsen A, Zhang J, Luz J, Rowan A, et al. Disease severity and genetic pathways in attenuated familial adenomatous polyposis vary greatly, but depend on the site of the germline mutation. Gut. 2006;55:1440.
65. Clevers H, Loh KM, Nusse R. Stem cell signaling. An integral program for tissue renewal and regeneration: Wnt signaling and stem cell control. Science. 2014;346(6205):1248012. https://doi.org/10.1126/science.1248012.
66. Albuquerque C, Breukel C, van der Luijt R, Fidalgo P, Lage P, Slors FJ, et al. The 'just-right' signaling model: APC somatic mutations are selected based on a specific level of activation of the beta-catenin signaling cascade. Hum Mol Genet. 2002;11(13):1549–60.
67. Cheadle JP, Krawczak M, Thomas MW, Hodges AK, Al-Tassan N, Fleming N, et al. Different combinations of biallelic APC mutation confer different growth advantages in colorectal tumours. Cancer Res. 2002;62(2):363–6.
68. Kumamoto K, Ishida H, Ohsawa T, Ishibashi K, Ushiama M, Yoshida T, et al. Germline and somatic mutations of the APC gene in papillary thyroid carcinoma associated with familial adenomatous polyposis: analysis of three cases and a review of the literature. Oncol Lett. 2015;10(4):2239–43. https://doi.org/10.3892/ol.2015.3578.
69. Latchford A, Volikos E, Johnson V, Rogers P, Suraweera N, Tomlinson I, et al. APC mutations in FAP-associated desmoid tumours are non-random but not 'just right'. Hum Mol Genet. 2007;16(1):78–82. https://doi.org/10.1093/hmg/ddl442.
70. Rashid M, Fischer A, Wilson CH, Tiffen J, Rust AG, Stevens P, et al. Adenoma development in familial adenomatous polyposis and MUTYH-associated polyposis: somatic landscape and driver genes. J Pathol. 2016;238(1):98–108. https://doi.org/10.1002/path.4643.
71. Cardoso J, Molenaar L, de Menezes RX, van Leerdam M, Rosenberg C, Moslein G, et al. Chromosomal instability in MYH- and APC-mutant adenomatous polyps. Cancer Res. 2006;66(5):2514–9.
72. Major MB, Camp ND, Berndt JD, Yi XH, Goldenberg SJ, Hubbert C, et al. Wilms tumor suppressor WTX negatively regulates WNT/beta-catenin signaling. Science. 2007;316(5827):1043–6. https://doi.org/10.1126/science/1141515.
73. Wang WL, Nero C, Pappo A, Lev D, Lazar AJ, Lopez-Terrada D. CTNNB1 genotyping and APC screening in pediatric desmoid tumors: a proposed algorithm. Pediatr Dev Pathol Off J Soc Pediatr Pathol Paediatr Pathol Soc. 2012;15(5):361–7. https://doi.org/10.2350/11-07-1064-OA.1.

Chapter 8
Adenomatous Polyposis Syndromes: Polymerase Proofreading-Associated Polyposis

Claire Palles, Andrew Latchford, and Laura Valle

Abstract *POLE* and *POLD1* encode the major subunits of polymerase ε and polymerase δ, respectively. Missense germline mutations in the exonuclease domains (EDMs) of *POLE* and *POLD1* have been found to be a rare cause of multiple colorectal adenomas and carcinomas. This condition is known as polymerase proofreading-associated polyposis (PPAP). The EDM of *POLE* is also somatically mutated in ~1% of colorectal cancers (CRCs) and ~8% of endometrial cancers. In this chapter we will consider the roles of these two enzymes, germline mutations that have been identified to date and their pathogenicity, the characteristics of tumours with germline or somatic mutations, clinical characteristics of patients with PPAP and the potential use of immunotherapy in patients with mutations in the EDM of *POLE*.

Keywords PPAP · Adenomatous polyposis · Exonuclease · Polymerase epsilon
Polymerase delta · DNA repair · Genetic testing · Genetic counselling
Hereditary cancer

C. Palles (✉)
Institute of Cancer and Genomic Sciences, University of Birmingham,
Birmingham B17 9JA, UK
e-mail: c.palles@bham.ac.uk

A. Latchford (✉)
The Polyposis Registry, St Mark's Hospital, Harrow, London, UK

Department of Surgery and Cancer, Imperial College London, Harrow, London, UK
e-mail: andrew.latchford@nhs.net

L. Valle (✉)
Hereditary Cancer Program, Catalan Institute of Oncology, IDIBELL and CIBERONC,
Hospitalet de Llobregat, Barcelona, Spain
e-mail: lvalle@iconcologia.net

L. Valle et al. (eds.), *Hereditary Colorectal Cancer*,
https://doi.org/10.1007/978-3-319-74259-5_8

1 Introduction

In 2013, families with colorectal polyposis and a dominant inheritance pattern were shown to carry one of two germline mutations (*POLE* p.L424V and *POLD1* p.S478N) in the exonuclease domains (EDMs) of either *POLD1* or *POLE* [1]. Both of these EDM mutations led to higher mutation rates in yeast strains constructed to carry the equivalent mutations. The exonuclease domain is responsible for proofreading replication errors made during DNA replication. Mutations in this domain effect the proofreading capabilities of polymerases ε and δ.

Since 2013 multiple groups have identified further mutations in the EDMs of *POLE* or *POLD1* [2–11]. Heterozygous mutations in *POLE* and *POLD1* account for what is now known as polymerase proofreading-associated polyposis (PPAP). *POLE* p.L424V is the most commonly observed germline EDM mutation in PPAP cases, but several additional missense mutations have been identified which impact the exonuclease function of *POLE* and *POLD1*. No additional cases of *POLD1* p.S478N have been identified that are not related to those in the initial report. Approximately 1% of patients with evidence of an inherited form of polyposis carry putative pathogenic variants in the EDM of these two genes.

The EDM of *POLE* is also somatically mutated in ~1% of colorectal cancers (CRCs) and ~8% of endometrial cancers. Interestingly somatic mutation of the EDM of *POLD1* is extremely rare. Data from TCGA (The Cancer Genome Atlas) show that as well as having a higher mutation burden, cancers where the *POLE* EDM is mutated have a particular mutation signature with a preponderance of C>A mutations flanked by Ts. This signature is signature 10 in the COSMIC Signatures of Mutational Processes in Human Cancer [12]. The most common somatic mutation, *POLE* p.P286R, has never been observed as a germline mutation, but recently another recurrent *POLE* EDM somatic mutation, *POLE* p.V411L, was seen in a patient with a phenotype resembling that of constitutional mismatch repair deficiency (CMMRD). Somatic mutation of *POLE* has also been seen as a recurrent driver event in glioblastomas of patients with CMMRD [11].

Two studies have shown that patients with somatic mutation of *POLE* have a good prognosis. This is thought to be due to the immune response elicited by these tumours as a result of the large number of neopeptides generated as a consequence of hypermutation. Clinical trials are underway to determine whether surgery alone is curative for these patients or whether immunotherapies such as anti-PD-1 are beneficial.

2 Roles of Polymerases Epsilon and Delta

Polymerases δ and ε, along with all other eukaryotic polymerases, belong to the B family of DNA-dependent DNA polymerases. Their major function is to replicate the genome. Misincorporation of nucleotides by B-family member polymerases

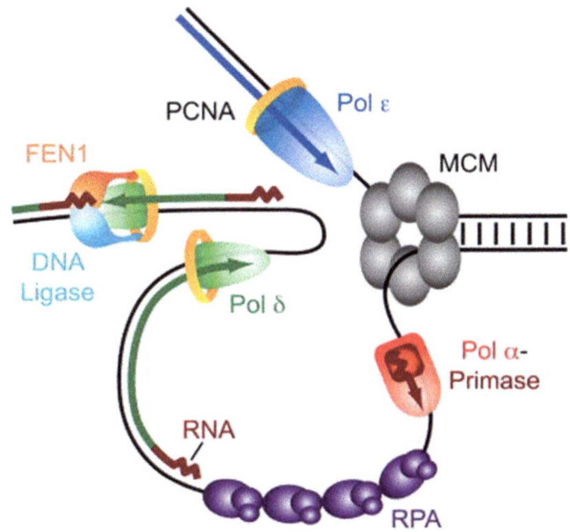

Fig. 8.1 The most recognised model of replication where polymerase ε is responsible for replication of the leading strand and polymerase δ the lagging strand (Reproduced from McElhinny et al. [15])

is low (10^{-4}–10^{-5}) [13], and fidelity of replication is enhanced further by the proofreading function of these enzymes which reduces replication errors by approximately a further 100-fold [14]. Three enzymes are responsible for eukaryotic DNA replication: polymerase *α*, polymerase *δ* and polymerase *ε*. Polymerase *α* initiates replication at origins and Okazaki fragments but carries out limited DNA synthesis. Following priming of DNA replication one or other of polymerase *δ* or polymerase *ε* takes over and extends from the primer sites. The model with the most support has polymerase *ε* synthesising the leading strand and polymerase *δ* synthesising the lagging strand under normal conditions. Data supporting this model was generated using a *Saccharomyces cerevisiae* strain *pol3-L612M msh2Δ*. The pol3-L612M allele confers an increase in mutation rate, and importantly for its utility in strand assignment, it has reduced fidelity for very specific mispairings. L612M Pol *δ* misspairs T with G with an error rate that is at least 28-fold higher than that for the complementary template A-C mispairing. Also L612M Pol δ is 11 fold more likely to delete a T base than it is to delete an A base. These biases in error rates for complementary nucleotides allowed McElhinny and authors [15] to determine which base and therefore which strand was used as a template by L612M Pol δ. By comparing the leading and lagging strand replication errors, McElhinny and authors [15] determined that over 90% of synthesis performed by L612M Pol δ use the lagging strand as template (Fig. 8.1).

3 The Exonuclease Domains of Polymerase *δ* and Polymerase *ε*

All polymerases identified to date share the same structural organisation and consist of finger, thumb and palm subdomains which collectively form the polymerase domain. The B family polymerases additionally have an EDM and an N-terminal

```
                                             Exo I
249  RGNAFPVEITRR---DDLVERPD---------PVVLAFDIETTKLPLKFPPDAETDQIMMISYMIDGQGYLITNREIVSED  316
278  KEKATQCQLEADVLWSDVVSHPPEGPWQRIAPLRVLSFDIECAGRKGIFPEPERDPVIQICSLGLRWG--------EPEP  349
                                                     Exo II
317  IEDFEFTPKPEYEG-PFCVFNEPDEAHLIQRWFEHVQETKPTIMVTYNGDFFDWPFVEARAAVHGLSMQQEIG-------  388
350  FLRLALTLRPCAPILGAKVQSYEKEEDLLQAWSTFIRIMDPDVITGYNIQNFDLPYLISRAQTLKVQTFPFLGRVAGLCS  429
                                                   Exo IV      Exo V
389  ------FQKDSQGE-----YKAPQCIHMDCLRWVKRDSYLPVGSHNLKAAAKAKLGYDPVELDPEDMCRMATEQPQT---  454
430  NIRDSSFQSKQTGRRDTKVVSMVGRVQMDMLQVLLREYKLR--SYTLNAVSFHFLGEQKEDVQHSIITDLQNGNDQTRRR  507
     Exo III
455  LATYSVSDAVATYYLY---MKYVHPFIFALCTIIPMEPDEVLRKGSGTLCEALLMVQAFHANIIFPNKQEQEFNKLTDDG  531
508  LAVYCLKDAYLPLRLLERLMVLVNAVEMARVTGVPLS--YLLSRGQQVKVVSQLLRQAMHEGLLMPVVKSEGGEDYTGAT  585
```

Fig. 8.2 Exonuclease domains of human *POLE* and *POLD1* (*POLE*: NM_006231 shown on the top line and *POLD1*:NM_002691 on the bottom line. Exo motifs of the two enzymes are highlighted in yellow and the exonuclease active site residues in the Exo 1 motif are boxed. Alignment was carried out using cobalt (https://www.ncbi.nlm.nih.gov/tools/cobalt/re_cobalt.cgi)

domain (NTD). The exonuclease domains of polymerase ε and polymerase δ are encoded by amino acids 268–471 and 304–517 of the proteins encoded by *POLE* (NM_006231) and *POLD1* (NM_002691). In humans, the exonuclease domains of both proteins contain five highly conserved EXO motifs (Fig. 8.2) [13]. Synthesis of the new DNA strand by the polymerases occurs in the 5′ to 3′ direction. The 3′ to 5′ polarity of the polymerase-associated exonuclease activities of polymerase ε and polymerase δ allows these polymerases to remove misincorporated nucleotides. During replication polymerase ε and polymerase δ switch between polymerising and editing modes. In editing mode the 3′ end of the nascent strand is in contact with the exonuclease active site, and during polymerising the 3′ end is in contact with the polymerase active site [13]. A mismatched base pair prevents the fingers of the polymerase from binding to an incoming trinucleotide phosphate, and so polymerisation stalls allowing the mismatched base to move to the exonuclease domain which can be 30 Å away.

Site-directed mutagenesis of the exonuclease domains of the Klenow fragment of *Escherichia coli* polymerase 1 and *POL2* and *POL3*, the *POLD1* and *POLE* homologues found in *Saccharomyces cerevisiae* and *Schizosaccharomyces pombe*, followed by assessment of mutator phenotypes has allowed assessment of the importance of multiple positions within the exonuclease domain [16–18]. Murphy et al. [17] performed a mutagenesis screen to identify "mutator strains". Mutated *POL3* was integrated into the chromosomal *POL3*, and clones that had acquired a mutation to revert a change in a gene involved in biosynthesis of histidine, *HIS7*, such that they can survive in media in which this amino acid is absent, were selected for. The rationale being that mutator polymerases would be more likely to revert a mutation in *HIS7* than wild-type polymerase. This rationale is also the basis of using fluctuation assays to measure the mutator phenotypes of mutations identified in patients in order to determine functional effect and likely pathogenicity of variants.

Mutation of the exonuclease active sites *POL3* p.D321 and *POL3* p.E323 (equivalent to *POLE* p.D275 and *POLE* p.E277; *POLD1* p.D316 and *POLD1* p.E318) leads to barely detectable levels of exonuclease activity in experiments assessing the degradation of labelled DNA substrates and very strong mutator phenotypes. As demonstrated by both Derbyshire and Murphy, mutation of other residues within the exonuclease domain also leads to similar phenotypes, for example, the *POL3* equivalent of the *POLE* p.L424V mutation (*POL3* p.479) was identified in the mutation screen conducted by Murphy et al. [17].

4 Germline Mutations Identified in the Exonuclease Domains of *POLD1* or *POLE*

Table 8.1 shows the characteristics of patients screened for germline mutations in the EDMs of *POLE* and *POLD1*, reports of which were published as of May 2017. As can be seen from Table 8.1, the majority of patients selected for screening have a similar phenotype to that of the patients in which *POLE*/*POLD1* EDM were first reported, namely, CRC polyposis cases or familial colorectal cancer. Some papers only describe screening for the variants reported in [1], whilst others describe results from screening all of the coding regions of *POLE* and *POLD1*. *POLE* EDMs have been picked up in exome sequencing studies of familial cases of cutaneous malignant melanoma [2] and families with a multiple tumour-type phenotype [6, 7].

Table 8.2 shows the variants mapping to the EDMs of *POLD1* and *POLE* that have been published as of May 2017. This table is an updated version of that which appears in [19]. *POLE* p.L424V accounts for 21 families with PPAP, and less frequent mutations in *POLD1* p.D316G, p.D316H, p.L474P and p.S478N account for a further 7 families. All other variants have been identified in single cases or families. Variants highlighted in grey currently lack supporting functional evidence from yeast mutation rate or biochemical assays. They are included here to highlight the challenges in determining the pathogenicity of variants mapping to a protein domain with a known function. As well as functional mutations, there seem to be rare variants mapping to the EDMs of *POLE* and *POLD1* which are less likely to be pathogenic. *POLE* p.D287E is most likely not pathogenic as it does not co-segregate with affection status. This variant and *POLD1* p.G321S were identified as germline changes in cases with suspected Lynch syndrome and microsatellite unstable cancers. Whilst it has not been possible to test the microsatellite status of all tumours from the *POLE*/*POLD1* EDM carriers identified to date, most cases with a proven pathogenic germline mutation have microsatellite stable cancers. Somatic *POLE* mutations do occasionally co-occur with microsatellite instability (see tumour characteristics section). Whilst there are examples of germline carriers of a proven pathogenic EDM mutation (5,57), these are rare and so novel germline *POLE*/*POLD1* EDM variants identified in patients with tumours displaying microsatellite instability or patients without polyposis phenotypes require particularly careful interpretation. If correct screening strategies and correct treatment stratification (see later in the chapter) are to be applied, careful classification of germline and somatic mutations in *POLE* and *POLD1* will be required.

Table 8.1 Publications that have identified or screened for germline exonuclease domain mutations in patients with colorectal adenomas or cancers

References	Types of cases screened	Discovery set	Validation set	Genotyping/sequencing method used for discovery set	Genotyping/sequencing method used for validation set
Palles et al. [1]	Familial cases with 10 or more colorectal tumours diagnosed <age 60	15 probands and 5 additional relatives	3805 cases, 6721 controls. Cases enriched for family history of colorectal tumours, multiple adenomas and early-onset disease. Majority of cases MMR proficient	Whole genome sequencing	Competitive allele-specific PCR (KASP genotyping)
Rohlin et al. [8]	Single family with multiple cases of CRC and additional cases of endometrial, ovarian, brain, pancreatic and gastric cancers	4 affected family members	NA	Exome sequencing	NA
Valle [10]	1. Familial and/or early-onset colorectal cancer and/or polyposis patients without known causal mutations in CRC predisposition genes. 2. Uncharacterised hereditary CRC and/or polyposis index patients	612 of case type 1 and 246 of case type 2	NA	Competitive allele-specific PCR (KASP genotyping) specific to *POLD1* p.S478N and *POLE* p.L424V used for cases of type 1, sanger sequencing of exons containing *POLD1* p.S478N and *POLE* p.L424V used to evaluate cases of type 2	NA
Aoude [2]	Familial cases of cutaneous malignant melanoma	34 probands and 53 additional relatives	1243 probands	Whole genome or exome sequencing	Ion torrent targeted sequencing of *POLE*

Chubb [4]	Early-onset familial CRC cases, MMR proficient or deficient	626	NA	Exome sequencing	NA
Elsayed et al. [5]	1. Polyposis cases 2. Familial CRC	485 of case type 1 and 703 of case type 2		Competitive allele-specific PCR (KASP genotyping) used to genotype *POLD1* p.S478N and *POLE* p.L424V	
Hansen et al. [6]	Single family case report. Multiple cases of CRC and additional cases of brain, bladder, pancreatic, gastric, lung and prostate cancers	14 affected or unaffected family members	95 CRC families fulfilling the Amsterdam criteria but with no pathogenic mutation in the known CRC predisposition genes	Exome sequencing	Haloplex targeted sequencing of *POLE*
Spier et al. [9]	1. Polyposis cases 2. Familial CRC	219 of case type 1 and 47 of case type 2	NA	Illumina targeted sequencing of *POLE*, *POLE2*, *POLE3*, *POLE4*, *POLD1*, *POLD2*, *POLD3*, *POLD4* or in the case of 75 polyposis cases exome sequencing	
Bellido [3]	1. Familial MMR-proficient CRC 2. Colorectal polyposis cases	456 of case type 1, 88 of type 2	NA	*POLE* exons 9–14 and *POLD1* exons 6–12 were amplified from pooled DNA samples which were sequenced on the Hiseq-2000. Sanger sequencing was used to deconvolute pools and confirm mutations	NA
Jansen [57]	Suspected lynch syndrome	62	NA	Coding regions of *MLH1*, *MSH2*, *MSH6*, *PMS2*, *POLE* and *POLD1* sequenced using Ion Torrent	NA

(continued)

Table 8.1 (continued)

References	Types of cases screened	Discovery set	Validation set	Genotyping/sequencing method used for discovery set	Genotyping/ sequencing method used for validation set
Wimmer [11]	Single case report	Suspected case of constitutional mismatch repair deficiency	NA	Sanger sequencing of exonuclease domains of *POLD1* and *POLE*	NA
Esteban-Jurado [20]	1. Polyposis cases 2. Familial CRC 3. Mismatch repair-deficient CRC	83 of type 1, 59 of type 2 and 13 of type 3	NA	Sanger sequencing of entire exonuclease domains of *POLD1* and *POLE*. Additional flanking intronic sequences were also screened (*POLE*: Complete sequencing of introns 9, 11,13, partial sequencing of introns 8, 10, 12, 14, *POLD1*: Complete sequencing of introns 7, 8, 9 and 11, partial sequencing of 10, 12 13)	NA

Table 8.2 Germline mutations that have been identified in the exonuclease domains of *POLE* and *POLD1*

Protein change (nucleotide change)	Evidence supporting pathogenicity of variant				Segregates with affection status	Number of carriers (Number of unrelated carriers)[c]	Mean age at diagnosis (range)	% of carriers with cancer type						% of carriers with		Other cancers reported in carriers	References	Missense somatic mutation reported in TCGA at same amino acid		
	Structure	PhyloP score[a]	Yeast fluctuation assays	Biochemical evidence for functional change[b]				CRC	EC	BrC	DuC	OC	GBM	Duodenal A or P	Colonic A or P			Protein change	Cancer Type (number of tumours with change)	Number of mutations in cancer
pol*ε*																				
P282S (844C→T)	Exo I motif	2.6	NR	NR	NR	1 (1)	55									Cutaneous malignant melanoma, merkel cell carcinoma	[2]	P282L	Glioma (1)	1226
D287E (861T→A)	Flanking exo I motif	0.4	NR	NR	No	5 (4)	61 (48–73)	20								Cutaneous malignant melanoma, non Hodgkins lymphoma, breast cancer, squamous cell carcinoma	[2, 57]	D287E	DLBC (1)	466
W347C (1041G→T)	Outside exo motifs	2.71	Yes [2]	NR	No[e]	11 (1)	49 (14–70)	0	0	0	0	0	0	NA	NA	Prostate, cutaneous and uveal malignant melanoma	[2]	W347G	Breast (1)	1086
N363K (1089C→A)	ExoII motif active Site	4.9a	NA	NR	Yes	12 (1)	41 (28–56)	75	17	0	0	25	0	NA	83	pancreas	[7]	N363D	CRC (1)	351
D368V (1103A→T)	Exo II motif active site	5.13	NR	Yes [58]	NR	1 (1)	47	100	0	0	0	0	0	0	0	None	[4]	NR		
V411L (1231G→C)	Flanking Exo IV	2.66	NR	Yes [18]	NA	1 (1)	14	100						100	100			V411L	CRC, EC, Stomach, Medulo-blastoma (26)	3383 (112–10498)

(continued)

Table 8.2 (continued)

Protein change (nucleotide change)	Evidence supporting pathogenicity of variant				Segregates with affection status	Number of carriers (Number of unrelated carriers)[c]	Mean age at diagnosis (range)	% of carriers with cancer type						% of carriers with		Other cancers reported in carriers	References	Missense somatic mutation reported in TCGA at same amino acid		
	Structure	PhyloP score[a]	Yeast fluctuation assays	Biochemical evidence for functional change[b]				CRC	EC	BrC	DuC	OC	GBM	Duodenal A or P	Colonic A or P			Protein change	Cancer Type (number of tumours with change)	Number of mutations in cancer
L424V (1270C→G)	Exo IV motif active site	2.66	Yes [17]	Yes [18]	Yes. 2 de novo carriers	48 (21)	39 (16–64)	61	2	2	2	2	4	19	92	Oligodendroglioma, neuro-endocrine carcinoma	[1, 4, 5, 7, 9, 10]	L424V	EC, non-small cell lung cancer, BrC (4)	1770 (49–6761)
P436S 1306C→T	Within exo V motif	3.53[a]	NA	NA	de novo	1 (1)	31	100	0	0	0	0	0	100	100	None	[9]	P436S P436R P436H	Thyroid CRC Bladder (3)	411 6541 13
R446Q (G1337→A)	Flanking exo V	2.66	NA	NA	NR	1	38									cutaneous malignant melanoma	[9]	R446Q R446W	Lung(squ) CRC (2)	274 287
Y458F 1373A→T	Exo III motif active site	4.97	NA	Yes [16]	yes	13 (2)	48 (38–63)	62	0	0	15	8		NA	62	Pancreas	[6]	Y458H	EC (1)	5502
polδ																				
D316G (947A→G)	Exo I motif, catalytic residue	1.93	Yes [17]	Yes [16, 58]	Yes	2 (1)	51 (44–57)	50	100	50	0	0	0	0	50	None	[3]	D316N	Stomach (1)	6580
D316H (946G→C)	Exo I motif catalytic residue	1.16	Yes [17]	Yes [58, 16]	Yes	2 (1)	61 (58–64)	50	0	50	0	0	0	0	100	Mesothelioma	[3]	D316N	Stomach (1)	6580

Protein change (nucleotide change)	Evidence supporting pathogenicity of variant				Segregates with affection status	Number of carriers (Number of unrelated carriers)[c]	Mean age at diagnosis (range)	% of carriers with cancer type						% of carriers with		Other cancers reported in carriers	References	Missense somatic mutation reported in TCGA at same amino acid		
	Structure	PhyloP score[a]	Yeast fluctuation assays	Biochemical evidence for functional change[b]				CRC	EC	BrC	DuC	OC	GBM	Duodenal A or P	Colonic A or P			Protein change	Cancer Type (number of tumours with change)	Number of mutations in cancer
G321S (961G→A)	Exo I motif	2.38	NA	NA	NR	1	41	100									[57]	NR		
R409W (1225C→T)	Flanking exo II motif	2.26	NA	NA	NA	1 (1)	32	100	0	0	0	0	0	0	100		[3]	R409W R409Q	Cervical (1) CRC, skin (non-melanoma) (3)	101 206 (73–435)
L474P (1421T→C)	Exo IV motif, paralogue of L424V	1.92	Yes [17]	Yes [18]	Yes	6 (2)	40 (23–52)	67	33	0	0	0	0	0	17		[3, 10]	NR		
P327L (981C→G)	Flanking exo I motif	2.16	Yes [32]	Yes [18][d]	NA	1 (1)	70	0	0	0	0	0	0	0	100		[1]	NR		
S478N (1433G→A)	Exo IV motif	1.19	Yes [1]	NA	Yes	11 (3)	35 (26–52)	45	36	0	0	0	0	0	91	Astrocytoma	[1, 4]	S478R	Oesophagogastric (1)	7

Variants shown in grey currently lack in vitro evidence of pathogenicity from either yeast mutation rate assays or biochemical assays of exonuclease function

A or P adenomas or polyps, *BrC* Breast cancer, *CRC* colorectal cancer, *DuC* Duodenal carcinoma, *EC* Endometrial cancer, *GBM* Glioblastoma, *NR* Not reported, *OC* Ovarian cancer, *ODG* Oligodendroglioma

[a]PhyloP (phylogenetic conservation) scores were calculated per nucleotide using alignment of 46 vertebrates dbNSFPv23. If a variant mapped to the third position of a codon the average PhyloP score for the codon is displayed

[b]Data from functional studies of B family polymerases

[c]Reported as of May 2017. Mean age at diagnosis in years refers to cancer or adenoma diagnosis, whichever was earliest

[d]Functional studies of the corresponding residue in Pol ε

[e]Six mutation carriers were unaffected

Mutations with functional evidence of pathogenicity are found in ~1–2% of cases enriched for colorectal polyposis or familial CRC. In certain populations PPAP may be rarer. Esteban-Jurado et al. [20] screened 155 cases with multiple polyps or early-onset colorectal cancer and did not identify any germline mutations in the EDMs of *POLE* or *POLD1*. As can be seen in Table 8.1, the majority of carriers identified to date have colonic phenotypes (polyposis or cancer), but the presence of other cancers seems to be mutation specific, and there is a higher burden of colonic adenomas and polyps in *POLE* EDM carriers compared to *POLD1* EDM carriers.

The majority of sites (8/11) of *POLD1* and *POLE* EDMs, identified in the germline setting, are also somatically mutated but are only observed in 1 to 4 cancers within TCGA (*POLE* p.V411L is seen more frequency and is discussed below). Five of the eight sites where both germline and somatic mutations arise show evidence of hypermutation in the tumours from the somatic case (defined as more than 600 mutations). As can be seen from Table 8.2, different germline and/or somatic mutations affect the same amino acid but result in different substitutions, and this may lead to markedly different mutation rates in the tumours.

The most common somatic mutation *POLE* p.P286R has never been observed as a germline mutation, but as shown in Table 8.2, *POLE* p.V411L which has been observed 26 times in TCGA tumours was recently identified in a patient with a phenotype reminiscent of constitutional mismatch repair deficiency (CMMRD). This variant was not carried by the patient's healthy mother, and it is presumed it was also not carried by the patient's healthy father whose DNA was not available for genetic testing. The most likely explanation is a de novo mutation at this site. De novo mutations resulting in *POLE* p.L424V have also been reported [10]. The phenotype of this patient, being very reminiscent of CMMRD, differs from the phenotypes of other PPAP patients reported to date but suggests that *POLE* and perhaps also *POLD1* EDMs should be screened for in other patients with similar phenotypes and no mutations in mismatch repair genes. Somatic mutation of *POLE* has also been seen as a recurrent driver event in glioblastomas of patients with CMMRD. In contrast to other tumours in these patients, the glioblastomas were ultra-mutated with no copy number changes and microsatellite stable [21].

5 Tumour Characteristics

In addition to the tumours from germline *POLE* and *POLD1* mutation carriers, somatic *POLE* proofreading domain mutations are identified in 6–12% of endometrial cancers [22–25], 1–2% of colorectal tumours [26–28] and more rarely in tumours of the stomach, pancreas, brain, breast and ovary [18, 29, 30]. In contrast to *POLE* and for reasons yet to be discovered, somatic *POLD1* proofreading mutations are extremely rare (reviewed by Rayner et al.) [19].

5.1 Molecular Characteristics

Polymerase ε and δ proofreading is essential for replication fidelity; therefore, its disruption by pathogenic heterozygous mutations, either germline or somatic, leads to a phenotype of tumour ultramutation. The mutation incidence in these tumours often exceeds 100 mutations per megabase. Moreover, the spectrum of nucleotide changes is distinct from the mutation spectrum observed in tumours with and without microsatellite instability, and it is characterised by a 100-fold increase in C→A transversions in the context TCT and a 30-fold increase in C→T transitions in the context TCG [12, 18, 22]. This translates into a strong bias for particular amino acid changes, with over-representation of serine to tyrosine or leucine, and arginine to isoleucine or glutamine, as well as increased glutamic acid to stop codon mutations [18]. In contrast to the mutation burden, proofreading-mutated tumours display very few copy number alterations [22, 23, 26, 27].

There is considerable variation in the number of mutations among tumours with polymerase proofreading mutations, and there is evidence that specific proofreading mutations have different effects on the mutation spectrum [18, 22, 31, 32]. It has been suggested that the severity of hypermutation and relative excess of G:C > T:A transversions might correlate with the degree of alteration of the residues within and close to the Exo motifs required for exonuclease activity [22].

The spectrum of mutations caused by polymerase proofreading defects causes a distinct pattern of missense and truncating mutations in oncogenes and tumour suppressors. For this reason, mutations rarely seen in tumours with microsatellite instability (MSI) or microsatellite stablity (MSS), are identified in proofreading-mutated cancers, including *PIK3CA* p.R88Q, *PTEN* p.R130Q, *TP53* p.R213X, *APC* p.R1114X, *APC* p.Q1338X, *MSH6* p.E946X, *MSH6* p.E1322X and *FBXW7* p.E369X, among others [1, 18, 22, 26, 27, 33].

Most of the tumours caused by germline *POLE* and *POLD1* proofreading domain mutations are microsatellite stable; nevertheless, microsatellite instability and/or MMR gene mutations have been detected in some cases [5, 21, 23, 26, 33, 34]. In these cases, although the cause and effect chain has not yet been experimentally established, it seems most probable that the deficient proofreading activity causes a secondary mutation in one DNA mismatch repair (MMR) gene, and therefore microsatellite instability, and not the other way around, i.e. the MMR deficiency being the cause of the polymerase proofreading mutation, as there are no microsatellites within the sequence encoding the polymerase exonuclease domain. Despite the fact that these tumours have a combination of defective proofreading and MMR deficiency, which might have resulted in a mutation rate that exceeds the maximum for tumour fitness [35, 36], the mutation rate is similar to those without the additional MMR deficiency (TCGA data, not shown). It would be of interest to know the timing and clonality of both repair defects and, as has been speculated [19], to examine the presence of "antimutator" mutations that allow continued viability, as demonstrated in yeast [37, 38].

POLE and *POLD1* are thought to be non-classic tumour suppressor genes. Second hits, such as loss of heterozygosity or mutations, are not common in the tumours, and whenever tested, expression of the proteins, assessed by immunohistochemistry, has been detected [1, 5]. From a functional point of view, heterozygous *POLE* and *POLD1* mutations, causing 50% of proofreading activity, would probably be enough to increase the mutation frequency; however, it remains uncertain whether that is sufficient to overwhelm the MMR system [31].

5.2 Prognosis, Immune Response and Therapeutic Targeting

The presence of somatic *POLE* proofreading mutations has been associated wit h a good prognosis in endometrial cancer [23–25, 34, 39, 40], glioblastomas [30] and colorectal tumours [28], even though proofreading-mutated cancers are usually high-grade tumours. Pending empirical corroboration (and reporting), this same observation is expected in tumours caused by germline polymerase proofreading mutations.

Motivated by the excellent prognosis together with the observation that *POLE*-mutated tumours show strikingly high density of tumour-infiltrating lymphocytes (TILs), often accompanied by a Crohn-like reaction, researchers hypothesised that the immune system was controlling tumour growth and therefore was the primary cause of the favourable prognosis of these tumours [22, 24, 40, 41]. Previous studies had confirmed that tumour missense mutations can lead to presentation of antigenic neo-epitopes by MHC-I molecules, resulting in activation of T-cell-mediated cytotoxicity [42–44]. In fact, *POLE*-mutated tumours are characterised by a striking CD8+ lymphocytic infiltration, a gene signature of T-cell infiltration and upregulation of cytotoxic T-cell effector markers [28, 45]. Moreover, as consequence of the high mutation burden, proofreading-mutated tumours are predicted to display more antigenic peptides than other tumours [39, 45]. Figure 8.3, taking endometrial cancer as example, shows the mechanisms linking proofreading mutations, immune response and favourable cancer prognosis [46].

Immune checkpoint inhibition is a relatively new therapeutic strategy that has shown promising efficacy in cancer treatment. In particular, significant response rates have been observed in mismatch repair (MMR)-deficient CRCs [47], which are characterised by a high mutation rate and therefore high neo-epitope load, making them more immunogenic (See Chap. 23). Based on the similar, even more accentuated, immunogenic properties of polymerase proofreading-mutated tumours, together with the presence of CD8+ lymphocytic infiltration, good response to immunotherapy was anticipated. Moreover, proofreading-mutated tumours show upregulation of genes encoding immunosuppressive checkpoints such as PD1 (programmed cell death protein 1), PDL1 (PD1 ligand 1), CTLA4 (cytotoxic T lymphocyte-associated antigen 4), LAG3 (lymphocyte activation gene 3), TIM3 (T-cell immunoglobulin mucin receptor 3) and TIGIT (T-cell immunoreceptor with immunoglobulin and ITIM domains) [28], making them

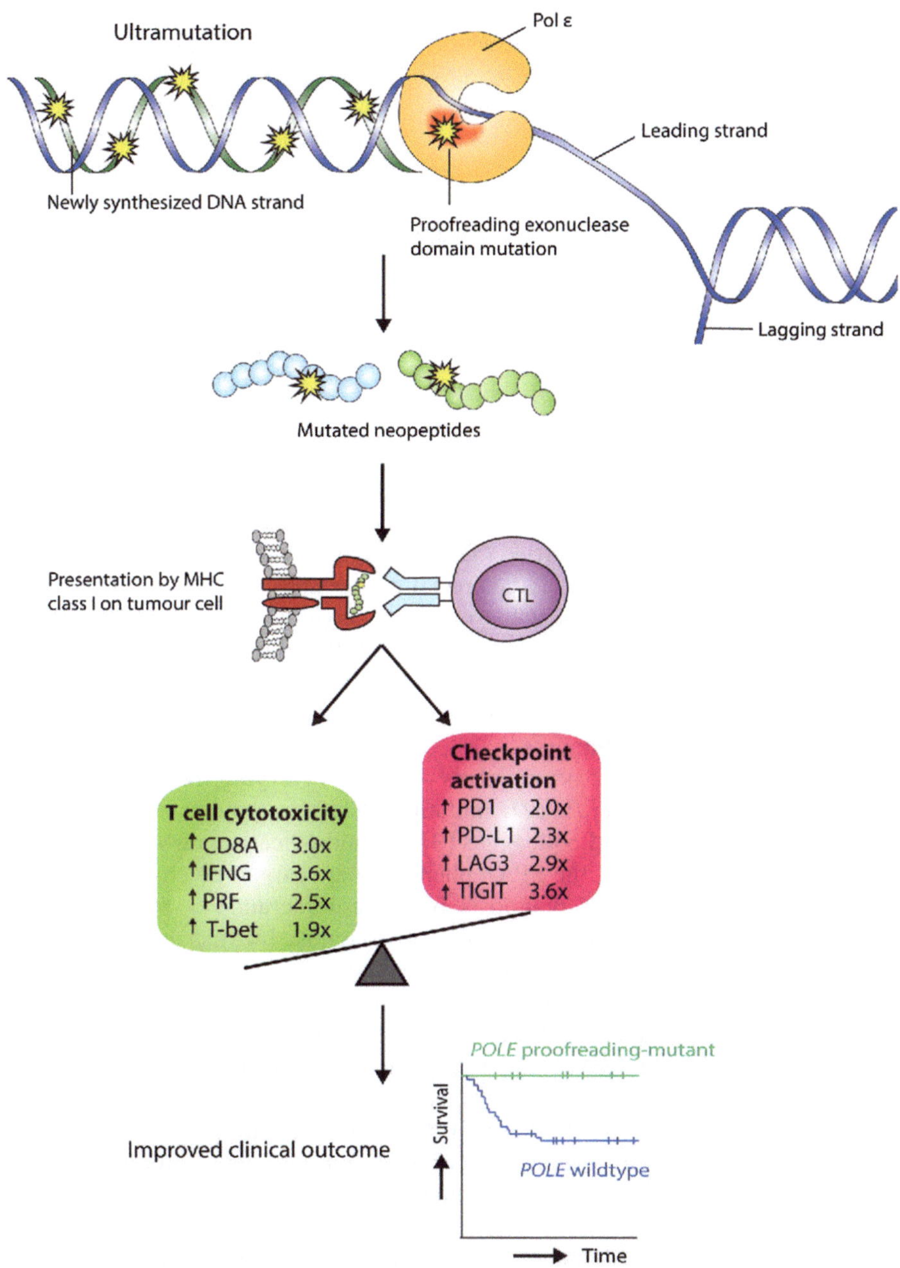

Fig. 8.3 Possible mechanism linking polymerase proofreading mutation, immune response and favourable cancer prognosis. POLE mutations in endometrial tumours are represented as an example (Reproduced from Van Gool et al. [46])

particularly sensitive to immune checkpoint inhibitors. The efficacy of checkpoint inhibitors in the context of germline and somatic polymerase proofreading-mutated tumours has been proven for several tumour types, even in the presence of metastasis [48, 49]. The progressive treatment of additional patients and/or their inclusion in clinical trials will unveil the real potential of the immune blockade therapy in the treatment of these tumours and the mechanisms of tumour resistance to these drugs [19, 50], as reported in melanoma [51]. Also, combination treatment of immune blockade therapy with radiotherapy, recently demonstrated to potentiate immune checkpoint inhibition [52, 53], may be worthwhile exploring in clinical trials.

6 Clinical Features

The first description of polymerase proofreading-associated polyposis (PPAP) was in 2013 [1]. Palles and colleagues described three pedigrees (two of which carried a *POLE* mutation and the other carried *POLD1* mutation) which included 23 affected individuals. Thirteen patients had colorectal cancer and 19 patients had multiple adenomas, with cumulative adenoma numbers ranging from 5 to 68. No extra-colonic neoplasia was observed in individuals with *POLE* mutations. In contrast, in the family with *POLD1* mutation, endometrial cancer was also a feature, diagnosed at a median age of 45 years. One subject with the *POLD1* mutation was also reported to have two primary brain tumours.

Subsequently there have been reports of cohorts carrying the same germline *POLE* mutation and further *POLD1* mutation, the phenotypic data of which was summarised by Bellido and colleagues [3]. In total 69 carriers from 29 families were included. Altogether, the PPAP phenotype appears to be characterised by an attenuated adenomatous polyposis of the colorectum (> 80% of *POLE* and > 60% of *POLD1* mutation carriers were diagnosed with ≥ 2 adenomas; on average, 16 adenomas), colorectal cancer (60–64% of carriers) and probably brain tumours (6%). Phenotypic data regarding the upper gastrointestinal tract is limited. Duodenal adenomas were detected in 57% of the 14 patients with *POLE* mutation who underwent upper GI endoscopy. In addition to an intestinal phenotype, the *POLD1* phenotypic spectrum includes endometrial (57% of female carriers) and breast tumours (14% of female carriers). All 21 *POLE/POLD1* mutation carriers without cancer were found to have colorectal adenomas which were resected, suggesting that the colorectal phenotype is strongly or completely expressed.

The phenotype of *POLE* mutation carriers has been expanded with the description of novel mutations not included in the summary by Bellido et al. [3]. Rohlin et al. (2014) identified a large family which demonstrated highly penetrant intestinal and extra-intestinal tumours, including colon, endometrium, ovaries brain and pancreas. The mutation identified in this family is also located in the proofreading exonuclease domain [8]. More recently Hansen et al. expanded the phenotypic spectrum further in a family in which in addition to the colorectum, cancers of the ovary, stomach and small intestine were observed. In addition, three cases of early-onset pancreatic cancer were observed. This novel mutation was also located in the exonuclease domain of *POLE* [6]. The finding of novel mutations with differing phenotypes has led some to postulate that a genotype-phenotype correlation may exist for *POLE*. A recent case report has also highlighted a novel *POLE* mutation within the exonuclease domain, which may predispose to a more severe phenotype. Wimmer and colleagues described a 14-year-old boy with polyposis and a rectosigmoid carcinoma; the youngest reported cancer patient with PPAP. Somewhat unusually the patient had other clinical features which are associated with constitutional mismatch repair deficiency, namely, multiple café au lait macules and a pilomatricoma [11]. Although the prospect of a *POLE* genotype-phenotype correlation is tempting, the small data set precludes any meaningful conclusions. Finally, a pathogenic germline mutation outside the exonuclease domain has been described, in an individual with young-onset CRC who also had a family history of CRC [20].

Although our understanding of genotype and phenotype is improving, the data on patients with PPAP remain sparse. It is difficult to draw meaningful conclusions regarding cancer penetrance in such a small dataset. Conclusions are further hampered by the undoubted presence of ascertainment bias in the studies. The phenotype does appear to overlap with an attenuated adenomatous polyposis syndrome, as well as Lynch syndrome. In contrast to Lynch syndrome the cancers arising in PPAP are usually microsatellite stable, arising due to chromosomal instability, with driver mutations in genes such as *APC* and *KRAS*.

7 Clinical Management

7.1 Genetic Testing

There are currently no clear recommendations to guide as to who should undergo genetic testing to look for mutations in the PPAP genes. The limited data regarding phenotype of PPAP makes any firm recommendations difficult. Bellido and colleagues have provided proposed criteria for genetic testing [3] (Table 8.3). It is likely however that with the more widespread use of next-generation sequencing and multigene panel testing for cancer and polyposis assessment, that strict criterion for testing may not be required.

For those families where a pathogenic mutation is identified, predictive genetic testing may be performed. Again there is no consensus as to what age this should be offered, but given the phenotypic data, it would seem reasonable to offer predictive testing around the age of 14–16 years.

Table 8.3 Proposed criteria for genetic testing [3]

POLE	*POLD1*
Attenuated adenomatous polyposis	Attenuated adenomatous polyposis
Amsterdam I criteria (CRC only)	Amsterdam II criteria (CRC and EC)
CRC and oligopolyposis both diagnosed under age 50 years	CRC < 50 years or EC <60 years and oligopolyposis <50 years
CRC or oligopolyposis and FDR with CRC under 50 years	CRC or EC or oligopolyposis and FDR CRC < 50 years or EC < 60 years
CRC or oligopolyposis and >/= 2 first or second degree relatives with CRC regardless of age	CRC or EC or oligopolyposis and >/= 2 first or second degree relatives with CRC or EC, regardless of age

Oligopolyposis, 5–20 adenomas; attenuated polyposis, 20–100 adenomas
CRC colorectal cancer, *EC* endometrial cancer

7.2 Surveillance

Consensus is lacking as to how patients with PPAP should be managed clinically, again reflecting the paucity of phenotypic data and lack of clarity regarding cancer penetrance. However, the manifestation of colorectal adenomas described in the second decade and the increased risk and multiplicity of CRCs from the third decade of life, colonoscopy surveillance is advised. It has been proposed that this should consist of colonoscopy every 1–2 years from the age of 18 years [3, 54], which seems a very reasonable approach, although the report from Wimmer et al. [11] may suggest that an earlier start may be required with carrying the *POLE* p.Val411Leu mutation. Whether or not prophylactic surgery is required will depend upon the individual patient's phenotype, which will also dictate the choice of prophylactic surgical intervention required. This decision-making regarding surgery can be based on the phenotype parameters that have been employed in FAP [55]; using this guidance it is likely that for most individuals with PPAP requiring prophylactic surgery, colectomy and ileo-rectal anastomosis would be appropriate. No strong recommendations can be given regarding surgical choice in those known to have PPAP who develop CRC. The choice between segmental or more extensive surgery will depend on the individuals colorectal phenotype, predicted functional outcome and possible metachronous CRC risk.

The high prevalence of duodenal adenomas and the reports of duodenal cancer suggest that upper GI tract surveillance is also recommended, as is performed in patients with FAP. This would comprise initiating upper GI endoscopy (usually with a side-viewing endoscope) from the age of 25 years, with the surveillance interval being the shortest of that as determined by the Spigelman stage and the presence or absence of ampullary pathology (Tables 8.4a and 8.4b).

Bellido and colleagues also suggested the need for extra-intestinal surveillance and proposed adding endometrial cancer screening beginning at age 40 years for *POLD1* female carriers [3], although not stated this would likely be using transvaginal ultrasound with endometrial sampling. This may seem reasonable but

Table 8.4a Suggested upper gastrointestinal tract surveillance according to Spigelman stage

	Points allocated		
	1	2	3
Number of polyps	1–4	5–20	>20
Polyp size (mm)	1–4	5–10	>10
Histological type	Tubular	Tubulovillous	Villous
Degree of dysplasia	Mild	Moderate	Severe
Total points	**Spigelman stage**	**Recommended follow-up interval**	
0	0	5 years	
1–4	I	5 years	
5–6	II	3 years	
7–8	III	1 year and consider endoscopic therapy	
9–12	IV	1 year (consider prophylactic duodenectomy)	

Table 8.4b Suggested upper gastrointestinal tract surveillance according to Ampulla classification

Ampullary classification	Endoscopic/histological features	Surveillance interval
Major	Ampullary polyp >1cm moderate/severe dysplasia villous component	1 year
Minor	Ampullary polyp <1cm mild dysplasia no villous component	3 years
Normal		5 years

one should be mindful that there is no evidence to support gynaecological screening in Lynch syndrome (although it is performed in some centres) and that many instead recommend a discussion regarding risk-reducing gynaecological surgery [56]. The reported predisposition to breast cancer means that it is unlikely to fall into the risk category that would require routine screening. However if familial clustering is observed, then individual families may meet local/national guidelines for screening on the basis of their family history alone. Certainly awareness and self-examination should be encouraged in female mutation carriers.

No doubt as our understanding of this condition evolves, more extensive clinical guidelines will be developed (Fig. 8.3).

References

1. Palles C, Cazier JB, Howarth KM, Domingo E, Jones AM, Broderick P, et al. Germline mutations affecting the proofreading domains of POLE and POLD1 predispose to colorectal adenomas and carcinomas. Nat Genet. 2013;45(2):136–44. https://doi.org/10.1038/ng.2503.
2. Aoude LG, Heitzer E, Johansson P, Gartside M, Wadt K, Pritchard AL, et al. POLE mutations in families predisposed to cutaneous melanoma. Familial Cancer. 2015;14(4):621–8. https://doi.org/10.1007/s10689-015-9826-8.

3. Bellido F, Pineda M, Aiza G, Valdes-Mas R, Navarro M, Puente DA, et al. POLE and POLD1 mutations in 529 kindred with familial colorectal cancer and/or polyposis: review of reported cases and recommendations for genetic testing and surveillance. Genet Med. 2016;18(4):325–32. https://doi.org/10.1038/gim.2015.75.
4. Chubb D, Broderick P, Frampton M, Kinnersley B, Sherborne A, Penegar S, et al. Genetic diagnosis of high-penetrance susceptibility for colorectal cancer (CRC) is achievable for a high proportion of familial CRC by exome sequencing. J Clin Oncol. 2015;33(5):426–32. https://doi.org/10.1200/JCO.2014.56.5689.
5. Elsayed FA, Kets CM, Ruano D, van den Akker B, Mensenkamp AR, Schrumpf M, et al. Germline variants in POLE are associated with early onset mismatch repair deficient colorectal cancer. Eur J Hum Genet. 2015;23(8):1080–4.
6. Hansen MF, Johansen J, Bjornevoll I, Sylvander AE, Steinsbekk KS, Saetrom P, et al. A novel POLE mutation associated with cancers of colon, pancreas, ovaries and small intestine. Familial Cancer. 2015;14(3):437–48. https://doi.org/10.1007/s10689-015-9803-2.
7. Rohlin A, Eiengard F, Lundstam U, Zagoras T, Nilsson S, Edsjo A, et al. GREM1 and POLE variants in hereditary colorectal cancer syndromes. Genes Chromosom Cancer. 2016;55(1):95–106. https://doi.org/10.1002/gcc.22314.
8. Rohlin A, Zagoras T, Nilsson S, Lundstam U, Wahlstrom J, Hulten L, et al. A mutation in POLE predisposing to a multi-tumour phenotype. Int J Oncol. 2014;45(1):77–81. https://doi.org/10.3892/ijo.2014.2410.
9. Spier I, Holzapfel S, Altmuller J, Zhao B, Horpaopan S, Vogt S, et al. Frequency and phenotypic spectrum of germline mutations in POLE and seven other polymerase genes in 266 patients with colorectal adenomas and carcinomas. Int J Cancer. 2015;137(2):320–31. https://doi.org/10.1002/ijc.29396.
10. Valle L, Hernandez-Illan E, Bellido F, Aiza G, Castillejo A, Castillejo MI, et al. New insights into POLE and POLD1 germline mutations in familial colorectal cancer and polyposis. Hum Mol Genet. 2014;23(13):3506–12. https://doi.org/10.1093/hmg/ddu058.
11. Wimmer K, Beilken A, Nustede R, Ripperger T, Lamottke B, Ure B, et al. A novel germline POLE mutation causes an early onset cancer prone syndrome mimicking constitutional mismatch repair deficiency. Familial Cancer. 2017;16(1):67–71.
12. Alexandrov LB, Nik-Zainal S, Wedge DC, Aparicio SA, Behjati S, Biankin AV, et al. Signatures of mutational processes in human cancer. Nature. 2013;500(7463):415–21. https://doi.org/10.1038/nature12477.
13. Shevelev IV, Hubscher U. The 3′ 5′ exonucleases. Nat Rev Mol Cell Biol. 2002;3(5):364–76. https://doi.org/10.1038/nrm804.
14. McCulloch SD, Kunkel TA. The fidelity of DNA synthesis by eukaryotic replicative and translesion synthesis polymerases. Cell Res. 2008;18(1):148–61. https://doi.org/10.1038/cr.2008.4.
15. Nick McElhinny SA, Gordenin DA, Stith CM, Burgers PM, Kunkel TA. Division of labor at the eukaryotic replication fork. Mol Cell. 2008;30(2):137–44. https://doi.org/10.1016/j.molcel.2008.02.022.
16. Derbyshire V, Grindley ND, Joyce CM. The 3′-5′ exonuclease of DNA polymerase I of Escherichia coli: contribution of each amino acid at the active site to the reaction. EMBO J. 1991;10(1):17–24.
17. Murphy K, Darmawan H, Schultz A, Fidalgo da Silva E, Reha-Krantz LJ. A method to select for mutator DNA polymerase deltas in Saccharomyces cerevisiae. Genome. 2006;49(4):403–10. https://doi.org/10.1139/g05-106.
18. Shinbrot E, Henninger EE, Weinhold N, Covington KR, Goksenin AY, Schultz N, et al. Exonuclease mutations in DNA polymerase epsilon reveal replication strand specific mutation patterns and human origins of replication. Genome Res. 2014;24(11):1740–50.
19. Rayner E, van Gool IC, Palles C, Kearsey SE, Bosse T, Tomlinson I, et al. A panoply of errors: polymerase proofreading domain mutations in cancer. Nature Rev. 2016;16(2):71–81.
20. Esteban-Jurado C, Gimenez-Zaragoza D, Munoz J, Franch-Exposito S, Alvarez-Barona M, Ocana T, et al. POLE and POLD1 screening in 155 patients with multiple polyps and

early-onset colorectal cancer. Oncotarget. 2017;8(16):26732–43. https://doi.org/10.18632/oncotarget.15810.
21. Shlien A, Campbell BB, de Borja R, Alexandrov LB, Merico D, Wedge D, et al. Combined hereditary and somatic mutations of replication error repair genes result in rapid onset of ultra-hypermutated cancers. Nat Genet. 2015;47(3):257–62. https://doi.org/10.1038/ng.3202.
22. Church DN, Briggs SE, Palles C, Domingo E, Kearsey SJ, Grimes JM, et al. DNA polymerase epsilon and delta exonuclease domain mutations in endometrial cancer. Hum Mol Genet. 2013;22(14):2820–8.
23. Kandoth C, Schultz N, Cherniack AD, Akbani R, Liu Y, Shen H, et al. Integrated genomic characterization of endometrial carcinoma. Nature. 2013;497(7447):67–73.
24. Church DN, Stelloo E, Nout RA, Valtcheva N, Depreeuw J, ter Haar N, et al. Prognostic significance of POLE proofreading mutations in endometrial cancer. J Natl Cancer Inst. 2015;107(1):402.
25. Talhouk A, McConechy MK, Leung S, Li-Chang HH, Kwon JS, Melnyk N, et al. A clinically applicable molecular-based classification for endometrial cancers. Br J Cancer. 2015;113(2):299–310.
26. Cancer Genome Atlas Network. Comprehensive molecular characterization of human colon and rectal cancer. Nature. 2012;487(7407):330–7.
27. Seshagiri S, Stawiski EW, Durinck S, Modrusan Z, Storm EE, Conboy CB, et al. Recurrent R-spondin fusions in colon cancer. Nature. 2012;488(7413):660–4.
28. Domingo E, Freeman-Mills L, Rayner E, Glaire M, Briggs S, Vermeulen L, et al. Somatic POLE proofreading domain mutation, immune response, and prognosis in colorectal cancer: a retrospective, pooled biomarker study. Lancet. 2016;1(3):207–16.
29. Zou Y, Liu FY, Liu H, Wang F, Li W, Huang MZ, et al. Frequent POLE1 p.S297F mutation in Chinese patients with ovarian endometrioid carcinoma. Mutat Res. 2014;761:49–52.
30. Erson-Omay EZ, Caglayan AO, Schultz N, Weinhold N, Omay SB, Ozduman K, et al. Somatic POLE mutations cause an ultramutated giant cell high-grade glioma subtype with better prognosis. Neuro-Oncology. 2015;17(10):1356–64.
31. Briggs S, Tomlinson I. Germline and somatic polymerase epsilon and delta mutations define a new class of hypermutated colorectal and endometrial cancers. J Pathol. 2013;230(2):148–53.
32. Kane DP, Shcherbakova PV. A common cancer-associated DNA polymerase epsilon mutation causes an exceptionally strong mutator phenotype, indicating fidelity defects distinct from loss of proofreading. Cancer Res. 2014;74(7):1895–901.
33. Heitzer E, Tomlinson I. Replicative DNA polymerase mutations in cancer. Curr Opin Genet Dev. 2014;24:107–13.
34. Billingsley CC, Cohn DE, Mutch DG, Stephens JA, Suarez AA, Goodfellow PJ. Polymerase varepsilon (POLE) mutations in endometrial cancer: clinical outcomes and implications for lynch syndrome testing. Cancer. 2014;121(3):386–94.
35. Sole RV, Deisboeck TS. An error catastrophe in cancer? J Theor Biol. 2004;228(1):47–54.
36. Loeb LA. Human cancers express mutator phenotypes: origin, consequences and targeting. Nature Rev. 2011;11(6):450–7.
37. Herr AJ, Ogawa M, Lawrence NA, Williams LN, Eggington JM, Singh M, et al. Mutator suppression and escape from replication error-induced extinction in yeast. PLoS Genet. 2011;7(10):e1002282.
38. Williams LN, Herr AJ, Preston BD. Emergence of DNA polymerase epsilon antimutators that escape error-induced extinction in yeast. Genetics. 2013;193(3):751–70.
39. Meng B, Hoang LN, McIntyre JB, Duggan MA, Nelson GS, Lee CH, et al. POLE exonuclease domain mutation predicts long progression-free survival in grade 3 endometrioid carcinoma of the endometrium. Gynecol Oncol. 2014;134(1):15–9.
40. Stelloo E, Bosse T, Nout RA, MacKay HJ, Church DN, Nijman HW, et al. Refining prognosis and identifying targetable pathways for high-risk endometrial cancer; a TransPORTEC initiative. Mod Pathol. 2015;28(6):836–44.

41. Hussein YR, Weigelt B, Levine DA, Schoolmeester JK, Dao LN, Balzer BL, et al. Clinicopathological analysis of endometrial carcinomas harboring somatic POLE exonuclease domain mutations. Mod Pathol. 2015;28(4):505–14.
42. Matsushita H, Vesely MD, Koboldt DC, Rickert CG, Uppaluri R, Magrini VJ, et al. Cancer exome analysis reveals a T-cell-dependent mechanism of cancer immunoediting. Nature. 2012;482(7385):400–4.
43. DuPage M, Mazumdar C, Schmidt LM, Cheung AF, Jacks T. Expression of tumour-specific antigens underlies cancer immunoediting. Nature. 2012;482(7385):405–9.
44. van Rooij N, van Buuren MM, Philips D, Velds A, Toebes M, Heemskerk B, et al. Tumor exome analysis reveals neoantigen-specific T-cell reactivity in an ipilimumab-responsive melanoma. J Clin Oncol. 2013;31(32):e439–42.
45. van Gool IC, Eggink FA, Freeman-Mills L, Stelloo E, Marchi E, de Bruyn M, et al. POLE proofreading mutations elicit an antitumor immune response in endometrial cancer. Clin Cancer Res. 2015;21(14):3347–55.
46. van Gool IC, Bosse T, Church DN. POLE proofreading mutation, immune response and prognosis in endometrial cancer. Oncoimmunology. 2016;5(3):e1072675.
47. Le DT, Uram JN, Wang H, Bartlett BR, Kemberling H, Eyring AD, et al. PD-1 blockade in tumors with mismatch-repair deficiency. N Engl J Med. 2015;372(26):2509–20.
48. Johanns TM, Miller CA, Dorward IG, Tsien C, Chang E, Perry A, et al. Immunogenomics of Hypermutated Glioblastoma: a patient with Germline POLE deficiency treated with checkpoint blockade immunotherapy. Cancer Discov. 2016;6(11):1230–6.
49. Santin AD, Bellone S, Buza N, Choi J, Schwartz PE, Schlessinger J, et al. Regression of chemotherapy-resistant polymerase epsilon (POLE) ultra-mutated and MSH6 hyper-mutated endometrial tumors with nivolumab. Clin Cancer Res. 2016;22(23):5682–7.
50. Piulats JM, Matias-Guiu X. Immunotherapy in endometrial cancer: in the Nick of time. Clin Cancer Res. 2016;22(23):5623–5.
51. Zaretsky JM, Garcia-Diaz A, Shin DS, Escuin-Ordinas H, Hugo W, Hu-Lieskovan S, et al. Mutations associated with acquired resistance to PD-1 blockade in melanoma. N Engl J Med. 2016;375(9):819–29.
52. Twyman-Saint Victor C, Rech AJ, Maity A, Rengan R, Pauken KE, Stelekati E, et al. Radiation and dual checkpoint blockade activate non-redundant immune mechanisms in cancer. Nature. 2015;520(7547):373–7.
53. Dovedi SJ, Cheadle EJ, Popple A, Poon E, Morrow M, Stewart R, et al. Fractionated radiation therapy stimulates anti-tumor immunity mediated by both resident and infiltrating polyclonal T-cell populations when combined with PD1 blockade. Clin Cancer Res. 2017;23(18):5514–26.
54. Spier I, Holzapfel S, Altmuller J, Zhao B, Horpaopan S, Vogt S, et al. Frequency and phenotypic spectrum of germline mutations in POLE and seven other polymerase genes in 266 patients with colorectal adenomas and carcinomas. Int J Cancer. 2014;137(2):320–31.
55. Sinha A, Tekkis PP, Rashid S, Phillips RK, Clark SK. Risk factors for secondary proctectomy in patients with familial adenomatous polyposis. Br J Surg. 2010;97(11):1710–5.
56. Vasen HF, Blanco I, Aktan-Collan K, Gopie JP, Alonso A, Aretz S, et al. Revised guidelines for the clinical management of Lynch syndrome (HNPCC): recommendations by a group of European experts. Gut. 2013;62(6):812–23.
57. Jansen AM, van Wezel T, van den Akker BE, Ventayol Garcia M, Ruano D, Tops CM, et al. Combined mismatch repair and POLE/POLD1 defects explain unresolved suspected Lynch syndrome cancers. Eur J Hum Genet. 2016;24(7):1089–92. https://doi.org/10.1038/ejhg.2015.252.
58. Abdus Sattar AK, Lin TC, Jones C, Konigsberg WH. Functional consequences and exonuclease kinetic parameters of point mutations in bacteriophage T4 DNA polymerase. Biochemistry. 1996;35(51):16621–9. https://doi.org/10.1021/bi961552q.

Chapter 9
Adenomatous Polyposis Syndromes: MUTYH-Associated Polyposis

Maartje Nielsen and Stephan Aretz

Abstract MUTYH-associated polyposis was first described in 2002. It is inherited recessively, and patients usually develop between tens and hundreds of adenomas throughout life. The risk of developing colon cancer when surveillance is not started in time is very high. In this chapter the clinical aspects, cancer risk, mutation spectrum, risk for heterozygotes and tumour characteristics will be described.

Keywords MUTYH- associated polyposis (MAP) · Polyposis · MUTYH

1 General

MUTYH-associated polyposis (MAP, OMIM 608456) is an autosomal recessive inherited disease caused by germline mutations in the *MUTYH* gene. DNA base excision repair (BER) plays a vital role in the cellular defence against oxidative damage. It was discovered in 2002, when, after identifying an excess of somatic G > T transversions (especially GAA > TAA) in the *APC* gene in adenomas in a Welsh family, Al-Tassan et al. suspected an underlying *MUTYH* deficiency. Next, patients from this family were indeed shown to harbour biallelic *MUTYH* germline mutations [1].

M. Nielsen (✉)
Department of Clinical Genetics, Leiden University Medical Centre, Leiden, The Netherlands
e-mail: m.nielsen@lumc.nl

S. Aretz
Institute of Human Genetics, Center for Hereditary Tumor Syndromes, University of Bonn, Bonn, Germany

L. Valle et al. (eds.), *Hereditary Colorectal Cancer*,
https://doi.org/10.1007/978-3-319-74259-5_9

2 Genetics

The *MUTYH* gene is a BER gene located on chromosome 1p34.1. There are three major *MUTYH* transcripts (α, β and γ) and at least ten isoforms of the MUTYH protein (429–549 amino acids) [2, 3]. The longest transcript variant, NM_001128425.1 (alpha 5), is being used as the coding DNA reference.

MUTYH is the only protein that recognizes an 8-oxo-7,8-dihydro-2′-deoxyguanosine (8-oxodG) incorporated opposite to a adenine (8-oxoG:A mismatch) and excises the undamaged (but misincorporated) adenine base using a base-flipping mechanism preventing the G:C > T:A transversion from occurring in the next replication round [4] (Fig. 9.1). DNA polymerases can subsequently restore an 8-oxoG:C pair that can be acted upon by another BER-glycosylase, OGG1, to replace the oxidized guanine with a guanine. Since OGG1 preferentially excises 8-oxoG opposite cytosine and not adenine, MUTYH indirectly promotes 8-oxoG repair by OGG1 [5].

Until now more than 100 different *MUTYH* variants have been described (see LOVD database, http://chromium.lovd.nl/LOVD2/colon_cancer/home.php?select_db=MUTYH). However, two European founder mutations, c.536A>G (p.Tyr179Cys) in exon 7 and c.1187G>A (p.Gly396Asp) in exon 13, predominate in the Western world and are found in 70–90% of MAP patients, depending on the geographic region [6, 7]. To date, these pathogenic variants have not been found in Japanese, Koreans or Jewish individuals of European origin [8–11]. Several other founder mutations have been reported (Table 9.1). The heterozygous frequency in normal controls is reported to be 1–2% in a UK cohort and Australian/Canadian/US cohorts [1, 12]. In the ExAC (Exome Aggregation Consortium) database though, the reported heterozygous frequency for 35 reported (likely)

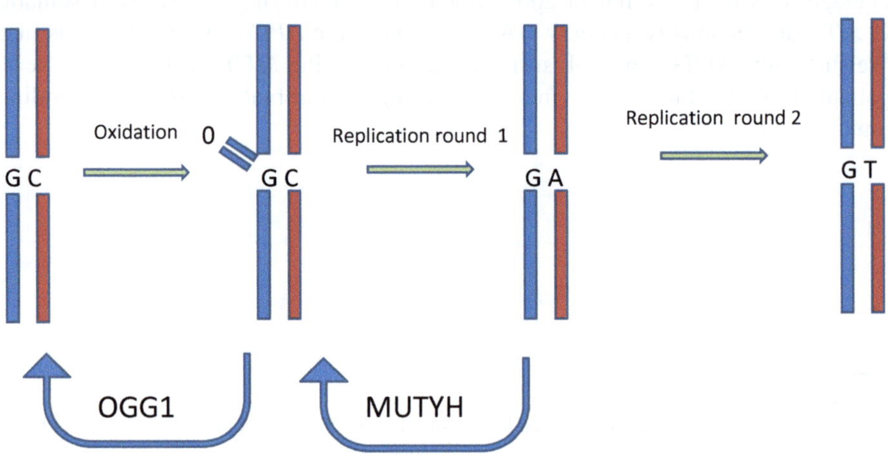

Fig. 9.1 Three-component system of 8-oxoG repair. The MUTYH protein recognizes 8-oxoG:A base pair and excises the improperly incorporated adenine during replication, after which other reparation proteins can place a cytosine opposite the 8-oxoG. OGG1 then excises the 8-oxoG from the 8-oxoG:C base-pair

Table 9.1 *MUTYH* founder mutations in patients from different ethnical backgrounds [10, 11, 13–22]

Ethnical background/country of origin	Coding DNA annotation	Protein annotation
Western countries	c.536A>G c.1187G>A	p.Gly396Asp p.Tyr179Cys
Pakistani	c.312C>A	p.Tyr104*
Northern European	c.1147delC	p.Ala385Profs*23
Dutch	c.1214C>T	p.Pro405Leu
Italian	c.1437_1439del	p.Glu480del
British Indian	c.1438G>T	p.Glu480*
Spanish, Portuguese and Tunisian	c.1227_1228dup	p.Glu410Glyfs*43
Spanish, French, Brazilian	deletion of exons 4–16	
Japanese, Korean	c.1118C>T c.857G>A	p.Ala373Val p.Gly286Glu

*indicates that the amino acid is predicted to change to a stop codon (Ter)

pathogenic *MUTYH* mutations, including the common two founder mutations, is somewhat less, about 0.8%.

Functional studies have shown that the p.Y179C mutation has a worse effect on the glycosylase function than the p.G382D mutation [1]. In fact, individuals with homozygous p.Y179C have a more severe phenotype than homozygous p.G396D, showing a younger age of onset (mean age of CRC diagnosis of 46 years compared to 58 years) [15]. A recent study in Italian patients showed an even more severe phenotype for MAP patients carrying the p.Glu480del mutation than those carrying p.Gly396Asp and/or p.Tyr179Cys, as they presented with a younger age at polyp diagnosis [17]. So far, these genotype-phenotype correlations do not support differences in surveillance.

Missense mutations are common in the *MUTYH* gene; therefore, their classification as pathogenic usually requires functional studies that assess their effect, complete or partial, on the glycosylase activity [11, 23–28].

3 Clinical Characteristics

Most reported MAP patients have between 10 and 500 polyps, although MAP patients with very few polyps in combination with CRC or very rarely with multiple hundreds of adenomas as in classical familial adenomatous polyposis (FAP) have also been described [29–34]. The diagnosis of the colorectal polyposis in MAP patients is made at an average age of 48. Colorectal carcinoma is present in about 60% of reported MAP patients at the time of diagnosis [35–37]. Estimates indicate that the risk of CRC in MAP patients is about 43% at age 60 and the lifetime risk is assumed to be close to 100% in the absence of timely colon surveillance [31, 38]. The high number of adenomas is most likely responsible for this increased cancer risk. As occurs in Lynch syndrome, MAP adenomas seem to display an accelerated progression to carcinomas [39].

Population-based studies show that MAP is responsible for 0.4% of all colon cancers and up to 1–2% of familial and early-onset (i.e. <50 years) colorectal cancers. It is noteworthy that of the MAP patients that have been discovered in population colorectal cancer studies, half had no or only a few polyps, indicating a possible role for other genetic or external modifiers in the development of adenomas [31, 32, 38, 40–44].

Besides colorectal cancer, higher risks for several other malignancies and benign tumours have been described. In a large retrospective European study of 276 MAP patients, standard incidence ratios for several tumours were calculated [45]. It was shown that the prevalence of duodenal polyposis in the MAP patient cohort was 17%, and the cumulative risk of duodenal carcinoma was 4%, comparable to that in APC-associated polyposis [45]. In a recent retrospective study (combined UK/Netherlands series) in 92 MAP patients, duodenal adenomas were detected in 31 patients (34%) at a median age of 50 years. At first diagnosis a majority of these (84%) had few small polyps, without high-grade dysplasia or villous features (Spigelman stages I or II). Subsequent evaluation showed disease progression in a minority of the cases, as only 2/18 patients reached Spiegelman stage IV in the follow-up (9.5 years) [46].

Win et al. analysed 266 probands (91% Caucasians) with an *MUTYH* mutation (41 biallelic and 225 monoallelic) from the Colon Cancer Family Registry, including Australian, US and Canadian patients. Hazard ratios (HRs) and 95% confidence intervals (CIs) were calculated for biallelic and monoallelic *MUTYH* mutation carriers. Moreover, Win et al. and Vogt et al. reported a significant increased risk for urinary bladder cancer (HR = 19; standardized incidence ratio (SIR) = 7) and ovarian cancer risk (HR = 19; SIR = 6) [47, 45] (Table 9.2).

In a European cohort, a significant increased risk for skin cancer (SIR = 2.8), including melanomas, basal cell carcinomas and squamous cell carcinomas, was also reported, as well as a significant increase in the incidence of breast cancer (SIR = 3.0; 95% CI, 1.5–5.3). This breast cancer incidence was only significant increased when the number of breast cancers was weighed instead of the number of affected women. So far, surveillance recommendations have not been modified based on these findings. Other tumours found in MAP patients include sebaceous gland tumours which are present in about 2% of patients [45]. Notably, these are also relatively often found in patients with Lynch syndrome and can be regarded as marker lesions of both syndromes [48].

A study from the USA revealed abnormal thyroid ultrasound examinations in 16 of 24 MAP individuals: a multinodular goitre in 7, and a single nodule in 6. Three of the 24 patients were diagnosed with papillary thyroid cancer (abstract Laguardia, described in [49]). Only two individuals with thyroid cancer were found in a cohort of 276 persons with MAP; a third individual with thyroid cancer was reported elsewhere [50, 45]. A high incidence of thyroid cancer was not found by others and may point to possible selection bias in the US study. More research is needed to clarify this risk.

Few MAP patients display FAP-related clinical features. Jaw-bone cysts have been reported in 3–4% (11/276) individuals with MAP [45] and congenital hypertrophy of retinal pigment epithelium (CHRPE) in 5.5%. This last figure may also include misdiagnoses since pigment anomalies of the retina are quite frequent in the general population [51].

Table 9.2 Extracolonic cancer risk reported in *MUTYH* biallelic and monoallelic mutation carriers [47, 45]

	Biallelic *MUTYH* patients (MAP)		Median age at diagnosis (range)	Cumulative risk at age 70/75	Monoallelic *MUTYH* (heterozygotes)	Cumulative risk at age 70
Study	Vogt et al. SIR, (95% CI)	Win et al. HR, (95% CI)	Vogt et al.	Vogt- Win et al. (95% CI)	Win et al.	Win et al.
Duodenal ca.	129 (15.7–465.9	NA	61 (56–65)	4% – NA	NA	NA
Bladder ca.	7.2 (2.0–18.4)	19 (3.7–97)	61 (45–67)	6% (0–12) ♂ and ♀ – 25% (5–77%) ♂ and 8% (2–33%) ♀	NA	NA
[a]Skin ca.	2.8; (1.5–4.8)	NA	58 (30–71)	17 (4–29) – NA		
Gastric ca.	4.2 (0.9–12.3)	NA	38 (17–48)	1 (0–3) – NA	9.3 (6.7–13)	5% (4–7) ♂ 2.3% (1.7–3.3%) ♀
Hepatobiliary ca.	Not increased	NA	NA	NA	4.5 (2.7–7.5)	3% (2–5%) ♂ 1% (0.8–2.3%) ♀
Pancreatic ca.	NA	NA	NA	NA	2.3 (0.2–4.1)	NA
Brain ca.	NA	NA	NA	NA	2.1 (0.9–4.9)	NA
Renal pelvis/ kidney ca.	NA	NA	NA	NA	2.3 (0.1–3.1)	NA
Ovarian ca.	5.7 (1.2–16.7)	17 (2.4–115)	51 (45–56)	14% (2–65%) – NA		NA
Endometrial ca.	4.6 (0.6–16.5)	NA	1 (47–54)	3 (0–7) – NA	2.1 (1.1–3.9)	3% (2%–6%)
Breast ca.	3.0 (1.5–5.3)	NA	53 (45–76)	25 (0–51) – NA	1.4 (1.0–2.0).	11% (8–16%)
Prostate ca.	NA	NA	NA	NA	0.5 (0.3–1.0)	NA

Abbreviations: *ca* cancer, *NA* not analysed because underpowered, ♂ male, ♀ female
[a]Including melanomas, squamous epithelial carcinomas and basal cell cancers

4 *MUTYH* Heterozygotes

As already mentioned, the frequency of monoallelic *MUTYH* mutations in the general population is about 1–2%. These individuals will not develop polyposis, but a marginally increased risk (OR = 1.1–1.2 in meta-analyses) for developing CRC has been shown in large population-based studies [49, 33, 34]. First-degree relatives of MAP patients consequently show higher risks (OR = 2–3) due to a potential clustering of risk factors in a family-based setting [52–55]. A cumulative CRC risk through age 70 of 7.2% for heterozygous males and 5.6% for heterozygous females was shown in a large family-based study consisting of 9504 relatives of MAP patients, independent of family history. For individuals with a first-degree relative diagnosed with sporadic CRC before age 50 years, the risk of CRC was 12.5% for men and 10% for women [55]. This was significantly higher in comparison with males and females from the general population (2.9% and 2.1%, respectively) in this study.

Heterozygous *MUTYH* mutation carriers in a MAP family should therefore be advised to undergo screening based on their family history. This includes taking part in population CRC screening or every-5-year colonoscopy starting from age 45, when CRC is present in non-MAP first-degree relatives.

A number of studies showed an increased risk of breast cancer for *MUTYH* heterozygotes, including large family-based studies [47, 56, 57]. A two-time higher frequency of monoallelic *MUTYH* mutations in families with both breast and colorectal cancer compared with the population has also been reported [58]. A slightly increased HR and cumulative risk for monoallelic *MUTYH* mutation carriers in gastric, hepatobiliary, endometrial and breast cancer have been reported by Win et al. (Table 9.2). Others did not find an association between *MUTYH* and

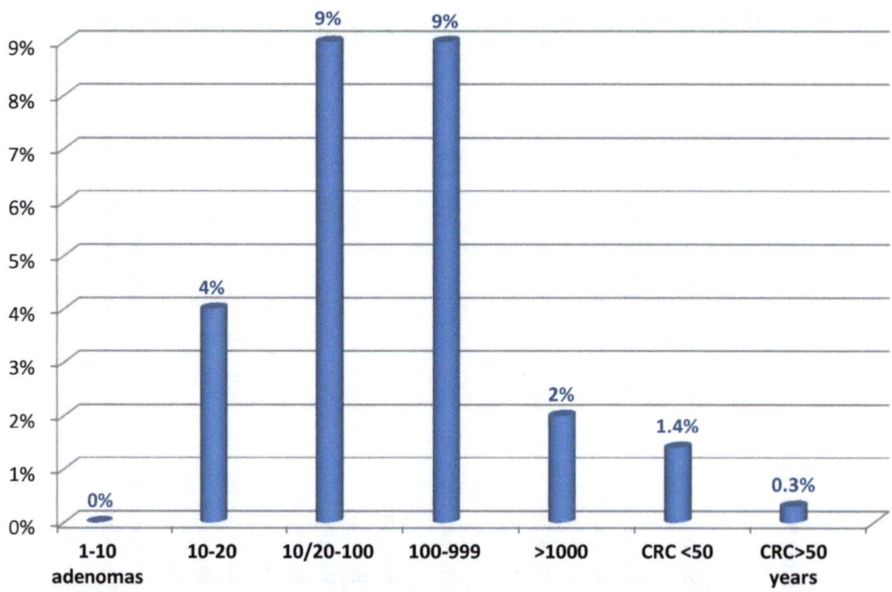

Fig. 9.2 Detection rate of biallelic *MUTYH* mutations (Adapted from meta-analysis in GeneReviews Nielsen et al.)

breast cancer or hepatocellular carcinoma which may also be due to the lack of power given the small increase and small sample size in these studies [59–61]. Furthermore, the cumulative risk for these cancers does not designate the need for surveillance advice.

Finally, recent studies of adrenocortical (ACCs) and neuroendocrine (NET) tumours of the pancreas found an unexpectedly high number of *MUTYH* heterozygotes, 2 out of 45 (4%) and 8 out of 160 (5%), respectively. In all tumours loss of heterozygosity (LOH) of the second allele was present. Moreover, these tumours showed the G > T transversion mutational profile, similar to the MUTYH-associated signature (COSMIC: signature 18), supporting the role of *MUTYH* in the tumorigenesis [62, 63]. Previously, no ACCs, pancreas carcinomas or NETs were reported in 176 biallelic *MUTYH* patients. Notably, Scarpa et al. did not identify the *MUTYH* mutational signature or pattern in 100 pancreatic ductal adenocarcinomas using the same analysis pipeline [63]. A nonsignificant hazard ratio for pancreatic cancer (HR = 2.3 95% CI = 0.2–4.1) in monoallelic mutation carriers has been reported, although histology was not mentioned in these cases [47].

Recently, an increased spontaneous mutation frequency in lymphoblastoid cell lines (LCLs) has been shown for heterozygous p.Tyr179Cys and p.Arg245His carriers compared to controls [64] supporting the notion that these patients might also have a higher risk for tumorigenesis.

5 Diagnosis of MAP

The chances of finding *MUTYH* biallelic mutations strongly depends on the number of adenomatous polyps identified in the patient (Fig. 9.2) and the pattern of inheritance. Since MAP is an autosomal recessive disease, the disease usually manifests itself in a single generation (with siblings). Exceptionally, biallelic mutations can occur in successive generations (pseudodominant pattern; see, for example, pedigree in Fig. 9.3) [36]. This option should be considered if no *APC* mutation is being found in families with 10–500 polyps in two generations or in consanguineous families.

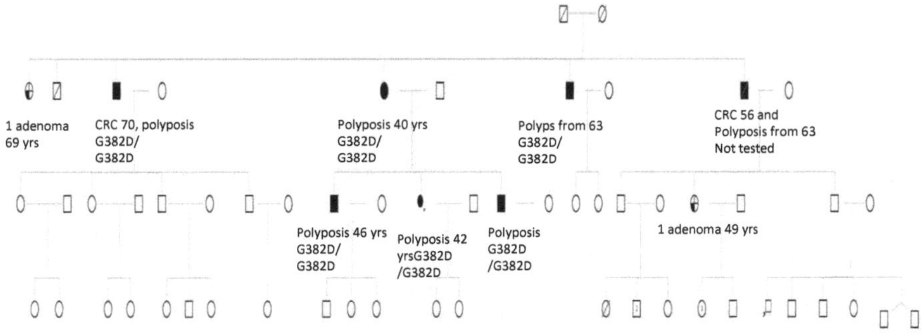

Fig. 9.3 Example of a MAP family with a pseudodominant pattern of inheritance

In most cases, MAP will be detected in isolated polyposis cases or an affected sibling. Usually, MAP patients have more than ten synchronous adenomatous colorectal polyps at time of detection. In patients with CRC and no or only a few polyps, the a priori likelihood of an underlying MAP is low; however, this increases considerably when the somatic *KRAS* hotspot mutation c.34 G > T in codon 12 (exon 1) is present in the tumour. It is important to know that adenomas as well as hyperplastic polyps can be present in MAP patients [65]. Recently, a study from Ohio reported that an important part of MAP patients under surveillance showed studding of hyperplastic polyps (10 out of 16 MAP patients) [66].

6 Tumour Characteristics

The characteristics of MAP carcinomas are somewhat comparable to Lynch and sporadic mismatch repair deficient tumours, with a frequently proximal location in the colon, secondary colon cancers, a high number of tumour-infiltrating lymphocytes and relatively often mucinous histotype [15] (Fig. 9.4).

The high number of tumour-infiltrating lymphocytes suggests an increased immune response, which might also be an explanation for the finding that MAP patients with colorectal carcinoma show a significantly better survival than sporadic cases, as has also been demonstrated in Lynch patients [67]. As in Lynch syndrome, the higher somatic mutation load in the tumours might cause modified (frameshift) peptides which might activate the immune system more early and more effective than in cancers without an early-onset DNA repair defect. Indeed, comparable to MMR-deficient colorectal tumours, loss of HLA class I expression is a frequent event in MAP carcinomas. This indicates that evasion of the activated immune system is an important step in MAP tumorigenesis because the extensive mutagenic background of these tumours most likely triggers a strong selective pressure favouring the outgrowth of tumour cell clones with an immune evasive phenotype [68].

Only few studies investigated the molecular features of MAP tumours. In two studies analysing a limited number of cancer genes, mostly *APC* (14–83%, with a

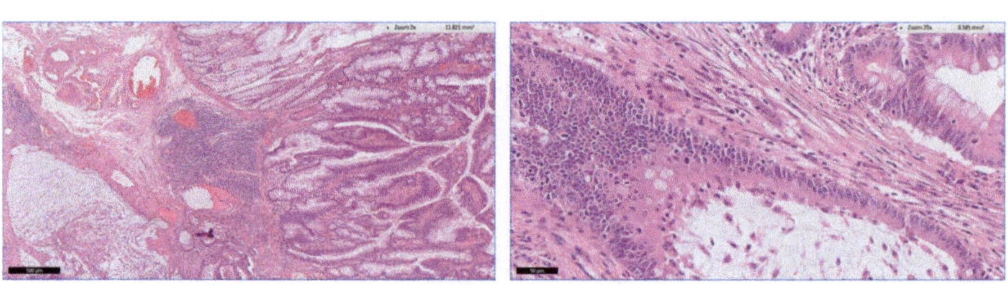

Fig. 9.4 Multiple polyps and two carcinomas in a 60-year-old female MAP patient. Picture showing adenocarcinoma of the ascending colon, marked lymphocytic infiltrate on the right (2× enlarged) and Crohn's-like infiltrate on the left (20× enlarged) (Depicted from: http://www.hereditarypathology.org, with courtesy of Prof. Dr. Hans Morreau, LUMC)

predilection for G bases in AGAA or TGAA motifs) and *KRAS* mutations were found and, to a lesser extent, *TP53* and *SMAD4* mutations (21–60% and 0–26%, respectively) [67, 69]. An important characteristic for *MUTYH* carcinomas is a *KRAS* hotspot mutation, c.34G>T in codon 12, present in about 60% of all MAP CRCs [43]. This mutation is present in only 8% of sporadic tumours [70], and a germline mutation analysis of *MUTYH* should therefore be strongly considered if this mutation is present [43].

In contrast to APC-related tumorigenesis, either sporadic or inherited, MUTYH-associated tumours are often near-diploid (52–92%) [69, 71] and frequently have chromosomal regions of copy-neutral loss of heterozygosity (LOH) (71%) [71].

MAP has been identified in 7/225 (3%) families meeting Lynch-like syndrome criteria [20]. Microsatellite instability (MSI) or DNA mismatch repair (MMR) deficiency can be present in MAP tumours, as described in two small studies (MSI-high phenotype in 1/3 and 1/6 MAP CRCs, respectively), and is usually caused by somatic (biallelic) MMR mutations due to the underlying DNA repair defect. One study also found a MAP patient when analysing 85 previously unresolved patients with MMR deficient tumors [74] MMR-deficient tumours should therefore not be an exclusion criterion for *MUTYH* genetic screening. See Fig. 9.5 for an example of a Lynch-like family that turned out to be a MAP family [75].

When analysing the mutation spectrum for 409 cancer-related genes in two CRCs from individuals with biallelic *MUTYH* germline mutations, Weren et al. showed that tumours had four and three somatic driver mutations, respectively, of which the majority (5/7) involved C:G > A:T transversions. Mutations were present in *ADAMTS20*, *PIK3CG*, *SMAD4*, *SMARCA4*, *APC*, *KRAS* and *NLRP1* [76].

Rashid et al. focused on the early evolution of adenomas from MAP (and FAP) patients. Whole-exome analysis of colorectal adenomas (eight MAP and six FAP)

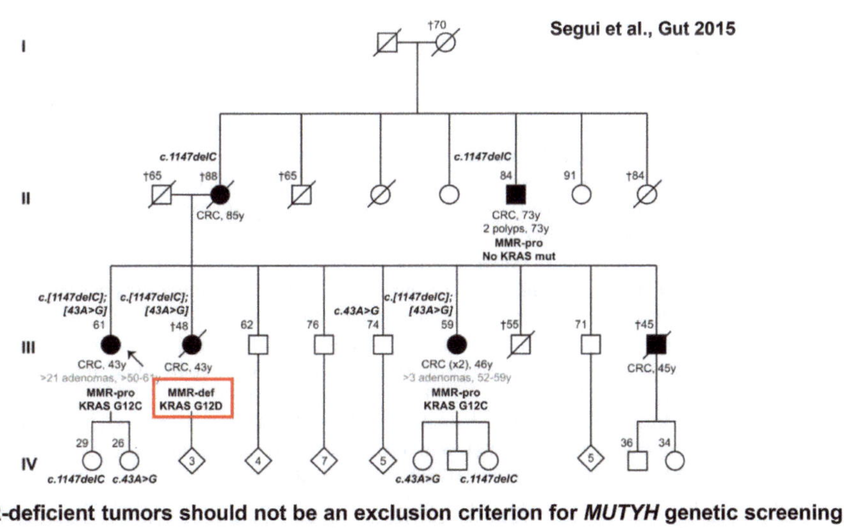

Fig. 9.5 MAP can mimic Lynch phenotype with pseudodominant pattern of inheritance [75]

and normal tissue DNA of MAP and FAP patients was done. Additionally, targeted next-generation sequencing of 20 oncogenes and direct automated sequencing of *WTX* and *KRAS* were performed in 55 adenomas (33 MAP, 22 FAP) [77]. This study showed that MAP adenomas have approximately two to four times more coding somatic mutations than FAP adenomas. The mean somatic mutational burden was 0.65 mutations per megabase (Mb) compared to 0.16 mutations per Mb in FAP adenomas ($p < 0.014$), being MUTYH-associated mutations overwhelmingly G:C > T:A changes. The most frequently mutated gene, harbouring a somatic mutation in 50% of analysed tumours, was *APC*, followed by *WTX*, mutated in 17% of MAP adenomas. Only 4 of the 33 adenomas had *KRAS* mutations and all four were the p.G12C transversion. Other genes that were mutated in MAP adenomas include, among others, *FBXW7*, *MAP3K5* and *APOB* [77]. In FAP, tumour suppressor genes undergo allelic loss as a second hit, rather than being disrupted by point mutations as occurs in MAP [78].

References

1. Al-Tassan N, Chmiel NH, Maynard J, Fleming N, Livingston AL, Williams GT, et al. Inherited variants of MYH associated with somatic G:C–>T:A mutations in colorectal tumors. Nat Genet. 2002;30(2):227–32. https://doi.org/10.1038/ng828.
2. Out AA, Tops CM, Nielsen M, Weiss MM, van Minderhout IJ, Fokkema IF, et al. Leiden open variation database of the MUTYH gene. Hum Mutat. 2010;31(11):1205–15. https://doi.org/10.1002/humu.21343.
3. Ohtsubo T, Nishioka K, Imaiso Y, Iwai S, Shimokawa H, Oda H, et al. Identification of human MutY homolog (hMYH) as a repair enzyme for 2-hydroxyadenine in DNA and detection of multiple forms of hMYH located in nuclei and mitochondria. Nucleic Acids Res. 2015;43(7):3870–1. https://doi.org/10.1093/nar/gkv264.
4. Michaels ML, Cruz C, Grollman AP, Miller JH. Evidence that MutY and MutM combine to prevent mutations by an oxidatively damaged form of guanine in DNA. Proc Natl Acad Sci U S A. 1992;89(15):7022–5.
5. Boiteux S, Coste F, Castaing B. Repair of 8-oxo-7,8-dihydroguanine in prokaryotic and eukaryotic cells: properties and biological roles of the Fpg and OGG1 DNA N-glycosylases. Free Radic Biol Med. 2016. https://doi.org/10.1016/j.freeradbiomed.2016.11.042.
6. Nielsen M, Morreau H, Vasen HF, Hes FJ. MUTYH-associated polyposis (MAP). Crit Rev Oncol Hematol. 2011;79(1):1–16. https://doi.org/10.1016/j.critrevonc.2010.05.011;S1040-8428(10)00147-2 [pii].
7. Aretz S, Tricarico R, Papi L, Spier I, Pin E, Horpaopan S, et al. MUTYH-associated polyposis (MAP): evidence for the origin of the common European mutations p.Tyr179Cys and p.Gly396Asp by founder events. Eur J Hum Genet. 2014;22(7):923–9.
8. Miyaki M, Iijima T, Yamaguchi T, Hishima T, Tamura K, Utsunomiya J, et al. Germline mutations of the MYH gene in Japanese patients with multiple colorectal adenomas. Mutat Res. 2005;578(1–2):430–3. https://doi.org/10.1016/j.mrfmmm.2005.01.017.
9. Peterlongo P, Mitra N, Sanchez de Abajo A, de la Hoya M, Bassi C, Bertario L, et al. Increased frequency of disease-causing MYH mutations in colon cancer families. Carcinogenesis. 2006;27(11):2243–9. https://doi.org/10.1093/carcin/bgl093.
10. Kim DW, Kim IJ, Kang HC, Jang SG, Kim K, Yoon HJ, et al. Germline mutations of the MYH gene in Korean patients with multiple colorectal adenomas. Int J Color Dis. 2007;22(10):1173–8. https://doi.org/10.1007/s00384-007-0289-8.

11. Yanaru-Fujisawa R, Matsumoto T, Ushijima Y, Esaki M, Hirahashi M, Gushima M, et al. Genomic and functional analyses of MUTYH in Japanese patients with adenomatous polyposis. Clin Genet. 2008;73(6):545–53. https://doi.org/10.1111/j.1399-0004.2008.00998.x.
12. Win AK, Jenkins MA, Dowty JG, Antoniou AC, Lee A, Giles GG, et al. Prevalence and penetrance of major genes and polygenes for colorectal cancer. Cancer Epidemiol Biomark Prev: Publ Am Assoc Cancer Res Cosponsored Am Soc Prev Oncol. 2016. https://doi.org/10.1158/1055-9965.EPI-16-0693.
13. Dolwani S, Williams GT, West KP, Newman J, Stock D, Griffiths AP, et al. Analysis of inherited MYH/(MutYH) mutations in British Asian patients with colorectal cancer. Gut. 2007;56(4):593. https://doi.org/10.1136/gut.2006.094532.
14. Prior TW, Bridgeman SJ. Identifying mutations for MYH-associated polyposis. Curr Protoc Hum Genet. 2010; Chapter 10:Unit 10 3. https://doi.org/10.1002/0471142905.hg1013s64.
15. Nielsen M, J-vdB MC, Jones N, Vogt S, Tops CM, Vasen HF, et al. Analysis of MUTYH genotypes and colorectal phenotypes in patients with MUTYH-associated polyposis. Gastroenterology. 2009;136(2):471–6. https://doi.org/10.1053/j.gastro.2008.10.056;S0016-5085(08)01894-5 [pii].
16. Gismondi V, Meta M, Bonelli L, Radice P, Sala P, Bertario L, et al. Prevalence of the Y165C, G382D and 1395delGGA germline mutations of the MYH gene in Italian patients with adenomatous polyposis coli and colorectal adenomas. Int J Cancer (Journal International du Cancer). 2004;109(5):680–4. https://doi.org/10.1002/ijc.20054.
17. Ricci MT, Miccoli S, Turchetti D, Bondavalli D, Viel A, Quaia M, et al. Type and frequency of MUTYH variants in Italian patients with suspected MAP: a retrospective multicenter study. J Hum Genet. 2017;62(2):309–15. https://doi.org/10.1038/jhg.2016.132.
18. Rouleau E, Zattara H, Lefol C, Noguchi T, Briaux A, Buecher B, et al. First large rearrangement in the MUTYH gene and attenuated familial adenomatous polyposis syndrome. Clin Genet. 2011;80(3):301–3. https://doi.org/10.1111/j.1399-0004.2011.01699.x.
19. Torrezan GT, da Silva FC, Krepischi AC, Santos EM, Ferreira Fde O, Rossi BM, et al. Breakpoint characterization of a novel large intragenic deletion of MUTYH detected in a MAP patient: case report. BMC Med Genet. 2011;12:128. https://doi.org/10.1186/1471-2350-12-128.
20. Castillejo A, Vargas G, Castillejo MI, Navarro M, Barbera VM, Gonzalez S, et al. Prevalence of germline MUTYH mutations among Lynch-like syndrome patients. Eur J Cancer. 2014;50(13):2241–50.
21. Gomez-Fernandez N, Castellvi-Bel S, Fernandez-Rozadilla C, Balaguer F, Munoz J, Madrigal I, et al. Molecular analysis of the APC and MUTYH genes in Galician and Catalonian FAP families: a different spectrum of mutations? BMC Med Genet. 2009;10:57. https://doi.org/10.1186/1471-2350-10-57.
22. Abdelmaksoud-Dammak R, Miladi-Abdennadher I, Amouri A, Tahri N, Ayadi L, Khabir A, et al. High prevalence of the c.1227_1228dup (p.Glu410GlyfsX43) mutation in Tunisian families affected with MUTYH-associated-polyposis. Familial Cancer. 2012;11(3):503–8. https://doi.org/10.1007/s10689-012-9543-5.
23. Shinmura K, Kato H, Goto M, Yamada H, Tao H, Nakamura S, et al. Functional evaluation of nine missense-type variants of the human DNA glycosylase enzyme MUTYH in the Japanese population. Hum Mutat. 2016;37(4):350–3. https://doi.org/10.1002/humu.22949.
24. Shinmura K, Goto M, Tao H, Matsuura S, Matsuda T, Sugimura H. Impaired suppressive activities of human MUTYH variant proteins against oxidative mutagenesis. World J Gastroenterol. 2012;18(47):6935–42. https://doi.org/10.3748/wjg.v18.i47.6935.
25. Shinmura K, Goto M, Tao H, Kato H, Suzuki R, Nakamura S, et al. Impaired 8-Hydroxyguanine repair activity of MUTYH variant p.Arg109Trp found in a Japanese patient with early-onset colorectal cancer. Oxidative Med Cell Longev. 2014. https://doi.org/10.1155/2014/617351. Artn 617351.
26. Goto M, Shinmura K, Nakabeppu Y, Tao H, Yamada H, Tsuneyoshi T, et al. Adenine DNA glycosylase activity of 14 human MutY homolog (MUTYH) variant proteins found in patients with colorectal polyposis and cancer. Hum Mutat. 2010;31(11):E1861–74. https://doi.org/10.1002/humu.21363.

27. Bai H, Grist S, Gardner J, Suthers G, Wilson TM, Lu AL. Functional characterization of human MutY homolog (hMYH) missense mutation (R231L) that is linked with hMYH-associated polyposis. Cancer Lett. 2007;250(1):74–81. https://doi.org/10.1016/j.canlet.2006.09.016.
28. Ali M, Kim H, Cleary S, Cupples C, Gallinger S, Bristow R. Characterization of mutant MUTYH proteins associated with familial colorectal cancer. Gastroenterology. 2008;135(2):499–507. https://doi.org/10.1053/j.gastro.2008.04.035.
29. Aretz S, Uhlhaas S, Goergens H, Siberg K, Vogel M, Pagenstecher C, et al. MUTYH-associated polyposis: 70 of 71 patients with biallelic mutations present with an attenuated or atypical phenotype. Int J Cancer (Journal International du Cancer). 2006;119(4):807–14. https://doi.org/10.1002/ijc.21905.
30. Isidro G, Laranjeira F, Pires A, Leite J, Regateiro F, Castro e Sousa F, et al. Germline MUTYH (MYH) mutations in Portuguese individuals with multiple colorectal adenomas. Hum Mutat. 2004;24(4):353–4. https://doi.org/10.1002/humu.9282.
31. Lubbe SJ, Di Bernardo MC, Chandler IP, Houlston RS. Clinical implications of the colorectal cancer risk associated with MUTYH mutation. J Clin Oncol: Off J Am Soc Clin Oncol. 2009;27(24):3975–80. https://doi.org/10.1200/JCO.2008.21.6853.
32. Wang L, Baudhuin LM, Boardman LA, Steenblock KJ, Petersen GM, Halling KC, et al. MYH mutations in patients with attenuated and classic polyposis and with young-onset colorectal cancer without polyps. Gastroenterology. 2004;127(1):9–16.
33. Croitoru ME, Cleary SP, Di Nicola N, Manno M, Selander T, Aronson M, et al. Association between biallelic and monoallelic germline MYH gene mutations and colorectal cancer risk. J Natl Cancer Inst. 2004;96(21):1631–4. https://doi.org/10.1093/jnci/djh288.
34. Theodoratou E, Campbell H, Tenesa A, Houlston R, Webb E, Lubbe S, et al. A large-scale meta-analysis to refine colorectal cancer risk estimates associated with MUTYH variants. Br J Cancer. 2010;103(12):1875–84. https://doi.org/10.1038/sj.bjc.6605966.
35. Sieber OM, Lipton L, Crabtree M, Heinimann K, Fidalgo P, Phillips RK, et al. Multiple colorectal adenomas, classic adenomatous polyposis, and germ-line mutations in MYH. N Engl J Med. 2003;348(9):791–9. https://doi.org/10.1056/NEJMoa025283.
36. Nielsen M, Franken PF, Reinards TH, Weiss MM, Wagner A, van der Klift H, et al. Multiplicity in polyp count and extracolonic manifestations in 40 Dutch patients with MYH associated polyposis coli (MAP). J Med Genet. 2005;42(9):e54. https://doi.org/10.1136/jmg.2005.033217.
37. Sampson JR, Dolwani S, Jones S, Eccles D, Ellis A, Evans DG, et al. Autosomal recessive colorectal adenomatous polyposis due to inherited mutations of MYH. Lancet. 2003;362(9377):39–41.
38. Farrington SM, Tenesa A, Barnetson R, Wiltshire A, Prendergast J, Porteous M, et al. Germline susceptibility to colorectal cancer due to base-excision repair gene defects. Am J Hum Genet. 2005;77(1):112–9.
39. Nieuwenhuis MH, Vogt S, Jones N, Nielsen M, Hes FJ, Sampson JR, et al. Evidence for accelerated colorectal adenoma--carcinoma progression in MUTYH-associated polyposis? Gut. 2012;61(5):734–8. https://doi.org/10.1136/gut.2010.229104.
40. Balaguer F, Castellvi-Bel S, Castells A, Andreu M, Munoz J, Gisbert JP, et al. Identification of MYH mutation carriers in colorectal cancer: a multicenter, case-control, population-based study. Clin Gastroenterol Hepatol. 2007;5(3):379–87.
41. Fleischmann C, Peto J, Cheadle J, Shah B, Sampson J, Houlston RS. Comprehensive analysis of the contribution of germline MYH variation to early-onset colorectal cancer. Int J Cancer. 2004;109(4):554–8.
42. Avezzu A, Agostini M, Pucciarelli S, Lise M, Urso ED, Mammi I, et al. The role of MYH gene in genetic predisposition to colorectal cancer: another piece of the puzzle. Cancer Lett. 2008;268(2):308–13.
43. van Puijenbroek M, Nielsen M, Tops CM, Halfwerk H, Vasen HF, Weiss MM, et al. Identification of patients with (atypical) MUTYH-associated polyposis by KRAS2 c.34G > T prescreening followed by MUTYH hotspot analysis in formalin-fixed paraffin-embedded tissue. Clin Cancer Res: Off J Am Assoc Cancer Res. 2008;14(1):139–42. https://doi.org/10.1158/1078-0432.ccr-07-1705.

44. Cleary SP, Cotterchio M, Jenkins MA, Kim H, Bristow R, Green R, et al. Germline MutY human homologue mutations and colorectal cancer: a multisite case-control study. Gastroenterology. 2009;136(4):1251–60.
45. Vogt S, Jones N, Christian D, Engel C, Nielsen M, Kaufmann A, et al. Expanded extracolonic tumor spectrum in MUTYH-associated polyposis. Gastroenterology. 2009;137(6):1976–85 e1-10. https://doi.org/10.1053/j.gastro.2009.08.052.
46. Walton SJ, Kallenberg FG, Clark SK, Dekker E, Latchford A. Frequency and features of duodenal adenomas in patients with MUTYH-associated polyposis. Clin Gastroenterol Hepatol: Off Clin Pract J Am Gastroenterol Assoc. 2016;14(7):986–92. https://doi.org/10.1016/j.cgh.2016.02.020.
47. Win AK, Reece JC, Dowty JG, Buchanan DD, Clendenning M, Rosty C, et al. Risk of extracolonic cancers for people with biallelic and monoallelic mutations in MUTYH. Int J Cancer (Journal International du Cancer). 2016;139(7):1557–63. https://doi.org/10.1002/ijc.30197.
48. Roberts ME, Riegert-Johnson DL, Thomas BC, Rumilla KM, Thomas CS, Heckman MG, et al. A clinical scoring system to identify patients with sebaceous neoplasms at risk for the Muir-Torre variant of Lynch syndrome. Genet Med: Off J Am Coll Med Genet. 2014;16(9):711–6. https://doi.org/10.1038/gim.2014.19.
49. Nielsen M, Lynch H, Infante E, Brand R. MUTYH-associated polyposis. In: Pagon RA, Adam MP, Ardinger HH, Wallace SE, Amemiya A, Bean LJH, et al., editors. GeneReviews(R). Seattle: University of Washington; 1993, All rights reserved.
50. Ponti G, Ponz DL, Maffei S, Pedroni M, Losi L, Di Gregorio C, et al. Attenuated familial adenomatous polyposis and Muir-Torre syndrome linked to compound biallelic constitutional MYH gene mutations. Clin Genet. 2005;68(5):442–7.
51. Coleman P, Barnard NA. Congenital hypertrophy of the retinal pigment epithelium: prevalence and ocular features in the optometric population. Ophthalmic Physiol Opt. 2007;27(6):547–55. https://doi.org/10.1111/j.1475-1313.2007.00513.x.
52. Jones N, Vogt S, Nielsen M, Christian D, Wark PA, Eccles D, et al. Increased colorectal cancer incidence in obligate carriers of heterozygous mutations in MUTYH. Gastroenterology. 2009;137(2):489–94, 94 e1; quiz 725-6. https://doi.org/10.1053/j.gastro.2009.04.047.
53. Jenkins MA, Croitoru ME, Monga N, Cleary SP, Cotterchio M, Hopper JL, et al. Risk of colorectal cancer in monoallelic and biallelic carriers of MYH mutations: a population-based case-family study. Cancer Epidemiol Biomark Prev: Publ Am Assoc Cancer Res Cosponsored Am Soc Prev Oncol. 2006;15(2):312–4. https://doi.org/10.1158/1055-9965.EPI-05-0793.
54. Win AK, Cleary SP, Dowty JG, Baron JA, Young JP, Buchanan DD, et al. Cancer risks for monoallelic MUTYH mutation carriers with a family history of colorectal cancer. Int J Cancer (Journal International du Cancer). 2011;129(9):2256–62. https://doi.org/10.1002/ijc.25870.
55. Win AK, Dowty JG, Cleary SP, Kim H, Buchanan DD, Young JP, et al. Risk of colorectal cancer for carriers of mutations in MUTYH, with and without a family history of cancer. Gastroenterology. 2014;146(5):1208–11.e1-5. https://doi.org/10.1053/j.gastro.2014.01.022.
56. Rennert G, Lejbkowicz F, Cohen I, Pinchev M, Rennert HS, Barnett-Griness O. MutYH mutation carriers have increased breast cancer risk. Cancer. 2012;118(8):1989–93. https://doi.org/10.1002/cncr.26506.
57. Zhu M, Chen X, Zhang H, Xiao N, Zhu C, He Q, et al. AluYb8 insertion in the MUTYH gene and risk of early-onset breast and gastric cancers in the Chinese population. Asian Pac J Cancer Prev. 2011;12(6):1451–5.
58. Wasielewski M, Out AA, Vermeulen J, Nielsen M, van den Ouweland A, Tops CM, et al. Increased MUTYH mutation frequency among Dutch families with breast cancer and colorectal cancer. Breast Cancer Res Treat. 2010;124(3):635–41. https://doi.org/10.1007/s10549-010-0801-7.
59. Beiner ME, Zhang WW, Zhang S, Gallinger S, Sun P, Narod SA. Mutations of the MYH gene do not substantially contribute to the risk of breast cancer. Breast Cancer Res Treat. 2009;114(3):575–8.
60. Out AA, Wasielewski M, Huijts PE, van Minderhout IJ, Houwing-Duistermaat JJ, Tops CM, et al. MUTYH gene variants and breast cancer in a Dutch case-control study. Breast Cancer Res Treat. 2012;134:219–27.

61. Baudhuin LM, Roberts LR, Enders FT, Swanson RL, Mettler TA, Aderca I, et al. MYH Y165C and G382D mutations in hepatocellular carcinoma and cholangiocarcinoma patients. J Cancer Res Clin Oncol. 2006;132(3):159–62.
62. Pilati C, Shinde J, Alexandrov LB, Assie G, Andre T, Helias-Rodzewicz Z, et al. Mutational signature analysis identifies MUTYH deficiency in colorectal cancers and adrenocortical carcinomas. J Pathol. 2017;242(1):10–5. https://doi.org/10.1002/path.4880.
63. Scarpa A, Chang DK, Nones K, Corbo V, Patch AM, Bailey P, et al. Whole-genome landscape of pancreatic neuroendocrine tumours. Nature. 2017;543(7643):65–71. https://doi.org/10.1038/nature21063.
64. Grasso F, Giacomini E, Sanchez M, Degan P, Gismondi V, Mazzei F, et al. Genetic instability in lymphoblastoid cell lines expressing biallelic and monoallelic variants in the human MUTYH gene. Hum Mol Genet. 2014;23(14):3843–52. https://doi.org/10.1093/hmg/ddu097.
65. Boparai KS, Dekker E, Van Eeden S, Polak MM, Bartelsman JF, Mathus-Vliegen EM, et al. Hyperplastic polyps and sessile serrated adenomas as a phenotypic expression of Myh-Associated Polyposis (Map). Gastroenterology. 2008;135:2014–8.
66. Church J, Kravochuck S. The "studded" rectum: phenotypic evidence of MYH-associated polyposis. Dis Colon Rectum. 2016;59(6):565–9. https://doi.org/10.1097/DCR.0000000000000575.
67. Nielsen M, de Miranda NF, van Puijenbroek M, Jordanova ES, Middeldorp A, van Wezel T, et al. Colorectal carcinomas in MUTYH-associated polyposis display histopathological similarities to microsatellite unstable carcinomas. BMC Cancer. 2009;9:184. https://doi.org/10.1186/1471-2407-9-184.
68. de Miranda NF, Nielsen M, Pereira D, van Puijenbroek M, Vasen HF, Hes FJ, et al. MUTYH-associated polyposis carcinomas frequently lose HLA class I expression – a common event amongst DNA-repair-deficient colorectal cancers. J Pathol. 2009;219(1):69–76. https://doi.org/10.1002/path.2569.
69. Lipton L, Halford SE, Johnson V, Novelli MR, Jones A, Cummings C, et al. Carcinogenesis in MYH-associated polyposis follows a distinct genetic pathway. Cancer Res. 2003;63(22):7595–9.
70. Andreyev HJ, Norman AR, Cunningham D, Oates J, Dix BR, Iacopetta BJ, et al. Kirsten ras mutations in patients with colorectal cancer: the 'RASCAL II' study. Br J Cancer. 2001;85(5):692–6.
71. Middeldorp A, van Puijenbroek M, Nielsen M, Corver WE, Jordanova ES, ter HN, et al. High frequency of copy-neutral LOH in MUTYH-associated polyposis carcinomas. J Pathol. 2008;216(1):25–31.
72. Lefevre JH, Rodrigue CM, Mourra N, Bennis M, Flejou JF, Parc R, et al. Implication of MYH in colorectal polyposis. Ann Surg. 2006;244(6):874–9.
73. Colebatch A, Hitchins M, Williams R, Meagher A, Hawkins NJ, Ward RL. The role of MYH and microsatellite instability in the development of sporadic colorectal cancer. Br J Cancer. 2006;95(9):1239–43.
74. Morak M, Heidenreich B, Keller G, Hampel H, Laner A, de la Chapelle A, Holinski-Feder E.Biallelic MUTYHmutations can mimic Lynch syndrome.Eur J Hum Genet. 2014 Nov;22(11):1334-7. doi: 10.1038/ejhg.2014.15. Epub 2014 Feb 12.
75. Segui N, Navarro M, Pineda M, Koger N, Bellido F, Gonzalez S, et al. Exome sequencing identifies MUTYH mutations in a family with colorectal cancer and an atypical phenotype. Gut. 2015;64(2):355–6. https://doi.org/10.1136/gutjnl-2014-307084.
76. Weren RD, Ligtenberg MJ, Kets CM, de Voer RM, Verwiel ET, Spruijt L, et al. A germline homozygous mutation in the base-excision repair gene NTHL1 causes adenomatous polyposis and colorectal cancer. Nat Genet. 2015;47(6):668–71. https://doi.org/10.1038/ng.3287.
77. Rashid M, Fischer A, Wilson CH, Tiffen J, Rust AG, Stevens P, et al. Adenoma development in familial adenomatous polyposis and MUTYH-associated polyposis: somatic landscape and driver genes. J Pathol. 2016;238(1):98–108. https://doi.org/10.1002/path.4643.
78. Cardoso J, Molenaar L, de Menezes RX, van Leerdam M, Rosenberg C, Moslein G, et al. Chromosomal instability in MYH- and APC-mutant adenomatous polyps. Cancer Res. 2006;66(5):2514–9.

Chapter 10
Adenomatous Polyposis Syndromes: NTHL1-Associated Polyposis / Tumor Syndrome

Maartje Nielsen and Stephan Aretz

Abstract In 2015 a second recessive inheritable form of polyposis was described, caused by mutations in the base excision repair gene, *NTHL1*. So far only 12 affected individuals have been described. Most had between 10 and 50 adenomas and two thirds had already developed CRC. Other cancers described include breast and endometrial cancer. In this chapter the clinical characteristics, genetics, tumor characteristics, and prevalence will be discussed.

Keywords NTHL1- associated polyposis · NAP · NTHL1 tumor syndrome · NAT Polyposis · CRC

Thirteen years after the discovery of the MUTYH-associated polyposis, a second recessive inherited form of adenomatous polyposis was discovered in 2015. Using a whole-exome sequencing approach in unsolved polyposis patients, biallelic mutations in the *NTHL1* gene were detected in three polyposis patients from unrelated Dutch families. The NTHL1 protein, similar to MUTYH, is involved in base excision repair. This syndrome was named NTHL1-associated polyposis (NAP, OMIM 616415), but since there is a wide tumor spectrum besides polyps, it can also be named NTHL1-associated tumor syndrome (NAT).

M. Nielsen (✉)
Department of Clinical Genetics, Leiden University Medical Centre, Leiden, The Netherlands
e-mail: m.nielsen@lumc.nl

S. Aretz
Institute of Human Genetics, Center for Hereditary Tumor Syndromes, University of Bonn, Bonn, Germany

L. Valle et al. (eds.), *Hereditary Colorectal Cancer*,
https://doi.org/10.1007/978-3-319-74259-5_10

1 Clinical Characteristics

At the moment, including the first clinical report, biallelic *NTHL1* mutations have been reported in 12 affected individuals from 8 different families [1–5].

Almost all patients described until now had between 10 and 50 polyps, although 1 patient only had 8 adenomatous polyps. Furthermore, one of the patients reported had 5 hyperplastic polyps next to more than 15 adenomatous polyps [2]. The age of diagnosis was between 40 and 67 years in reported cases. In 8 of 12 patients, CRC was reported (age range 40–67 years). Four patients developed a second CRC.

Furthermore, extracolonic tumors were reported in the majority of the carriers ($n = 8/12$), including duodenal cancer ($n = 1$, 52 years), endometrial cancer ($n = 2$, 57–74 years), breast cancer ($n = 3$, one bilateral, 47–58 years), bladder cancer ($n = 2$, 44–66 years), meningioma ($n = 2$, 47 and 54 years), basal cell carcinoma ($n = 3$, 52–63 years), and others which have been reported only once. Benign tumors included, among others, multiple duodenal adenomas in one patient and a parotid gland tumor in another one [1–5].

2 Surveillance

Currently the same surveillance scheme as for MAP has been advised (see Chap. 20 for MAP recommendations). Annual screening from age 40 for the breasts and endometrium might be added for females in the future, but reporting of additional carriers is required to establish more accurate risks for specific extracolonic tumors.

3 Genetics

The *NTHL1* gene is located on chromosome 16p13.3. Until now three different, all truncating, germline mutations have been reported (Table 10.1). The NTHL1 protein is a base excision repair protein involved in repairing a number of oxidized bases, although it is not clear at the moment which oxidation product is target for NTHL1. A fraction of *NTHL1* double-knockout mice develop liver (about 15%) and lung tumors (2–4%) during the second year of life, and the *KRAS* GGT to GAT transition was detected in DNA isolated from the lung tumors [6]. Similarly, C:G > T:A transitions were found when analyzing tumors of *NTHL1*-associated patients [1, 4].

Table 10.1 Biallelic *NTHL1* mutations reported in patient groups

1.5%	3/197	Polyposis patients NL [1]
2.27%	2/88	Polyposis patients ES [2]
0%	0/134	Polyposis patients UK [11]
0.12%	1/863	Early-onset familial CRC cases UK [5]
0%	0/523	Familial mismatch repair-proficient nonpolyposis CRC ES [2]
0%	0/48	Amsterdam-positive families ES [2]

It had been previously reported that the NTHL1 protein is involved in repairing a number of oxidized bases, including thymine glycol and 2,2,4-triamino-5(2H)-oxazolone (Oz), an oxidation product of 8-oxoG that causes G-to-C transversions in DNA [7, 8]. Since these mutations were not seen in *NTHL1* knockout mice, the existence of a yet unidentified oxidatively modified base was speculated, whose repair is mediated by NTHL1 and whose mutagenic properties lead to GC > TC transitions [6].

4 Tumor Characteristics

To assess the somatic mutation spectra in 3 carcinomas from NAP individuals, a cancer panel analysis of 409 cancer-related genes was performed. In total, 13 to 17 somatic mutations per tumor were found. All three carcinomas carried mutations in *APC*, *TP53*, *KRAS*, and *PIK3CA*. The number of mutations was higher than that reported in MAP carcinomas in the same study, although lower than that previously reported for hypermutated tumors. Notably, 15 of the 16 reported mutations in the driver genes were C:G > T:A transitions, significantly higher than in controls and similar to what has previously been described in mouse studies [9]. The tumors studied from another reported NAP patient were also enriched for somatic C:G > T:A transitions [4]. A causal link between NTHL1 deficiency and mutational signature 30 (COSMIC) has been recently described by clonal outgrowth of colon organoids with NTHL1 knock-out [12].

5 Prevalence

Almost all detected NAP patients were found among polyposis patient cohorts. Weren et al. analyzed 48 index polyposis patients using whole-exome sequencing, finding biallelic mutations in the index cases of 3 different families. A subsequent analysis in 149 polyposis patients did not yield any additional biallelic *NTHL1* mutation carriers [1].

Belhadj et al. found 2 biallelic carriers of c.268C>T (p.Gln90*) in 88 polyposis patients of Spanish descent. The recurrent mutation was not detected in homozygosis or as compound heterozygote in a cohort of 523 familial mismatch repair-proficient nonpolyposis CRCs, including 48 Amsterdam-positive families [2].

Broderick et al. found a biallelic *NTHL1* mutation in a 41-year-old male case with coincident polyposis among 863 early-onset familial CRC cases, with no other CRC/polyposis germline gene mutation found previously with whole-exome sequencing. No inactivating homozygotes or compound heterozygotes were found among 1604 controls [10].

Only one *NTHL1* biallelic mutation has been found in cohorts of Lynch-like, young CRC patients, or CRC families currently without a polyposis phenotype as of today (Table 10.1).

The highest prevalence of the p.Gln90* recurrent variant is encountered in subjects of European descent. Weren et al. screened for the Gln90* variant in an addi-

Table 10.2 Heterozygous *NTHL1* mutations reported in controls and polyposis/CRC patients

Nucleotide change	Protein change	Population MAF (ExAC) (*n* = 61,486 exomes)	Controls	CRC/polyposis patients
c.268C>T	p.Gln90*	0.15% (total cohort) 0.24% (European) 0.37% (Dutch) 0.37% (Finnish)	0.36% (17/2329, NL [1] 0.56% (2/359, UK) [11] 0.43%(12/2743, ES) [2]	0.7% (1/134) polyposis UK [11] 0.38% (2/523) nonpolyposis ES [2] 0.22% (3/1348) CRC cases ES [2] 0% (0/94) CRC cases UK [10]
c.709+1G>A		0.001%		
c.859C>T	p.Gln287*	0.019%		

Abbreviations: *MAF* minor allele frequency, *ExAC* Exome Aggregation Consortium (http://exac.broadinstitute.org)

tional cohort of individuals without a suspected hereditary form of cancer (*n* = 2329) and a mutation frequency of 0, finding a 0.36% of heterozygous carriers. The frequency in the ExAC database, which contains all germline variants identified in exomes derived from unrelated individuals of African, Asian, European, or Latino descent, is about 0.15% and 0.23% when only including persons from European descent. Based on this last percentage, about 1 out of 75,000 persons is expected to be homozygous for this mutation in the European population. The most prevalent mutation in *NTHL1* seems therefore to be more common in individuals of European and possible Dutch/UK origin (Table 10.2). However, the identification of the mutation in different ethnicities all around the world indicates that it may be a mutation hotspot rather than a European founder mutation.

Based on the above findings, *NTHL1* genetic testing should be performed in polyposis patients, after screening of *MUTYH* and *APC,* or simultaneously, at least for the Gln90* recurrent mutation. The prevalence of *NTHL1* mutations among (young) CRC, familial and nonfamilial, nonpolyposis cases seems to be too low to advise specific *NTHL1* mutation screening in those patient groups; however, when multigene panel testing is applied for routine genetic testing, *NTHL1* should be included.

References

1. Weren RD, Ligtenberg MJ, Kets CM, de Voer RM, Verwiel ET, Spruijt L, et al. A germline homozygous mutation in the base-excision repair gene NTHL1 causes adenomatous polyposis and colorectal cancer. Nat Genet. 2015;47(6):668–71. https://doi.org/10.1038/ng.3287;ng.3287 [pii].
2. Belhadj S, Mur P, Navarro M, Gonzalez S, Moreno V, Capella G, et al. Delineating the phenotypic spectrum of the NTHL1-associated polyposis. Clin Gastroenterol Hepatol Off Clin Pract J Am Gastroenterol Assoc. 2017;15(3):461–2. https://doi.org/10.1016/j.cgh.2016.09.153.

3. Kenwrick S, Spasic-Boskovic O, Taylor A, Brugger K, Rai H, Abbs S, Wyke J, Tischkowitz M, Maher E, Whitworth J. Compound heterozygosity for two novel mutations in NTHL1 in an individual with adenomatous polyposis and multiple tumours. Abstract joint meeting UK/ Dutch clinical genetics societies. 2016.
4. Rivera B, Castellsague E, Bah I, van Kempen LC, Foulkes WD. Biallelic NTHL1 mutations in a woman with multiple primary tumors. N Engl J Med. 2015;373(20):1985–6. https://doi.org/10.1056/NEJMc1506878.
5. Broderick P, Dobbins SE, Chubb D, Kinnersley B, Dunlop MG, Tomlinson I, et al. Validation of recently proposed colorectal cancer susceptibility gene variants in an analysis of families and patients-a systematic review. Gastroenterology. 2017;152(1):75–7 e4. https://doi.org/10.1053/j.gastro.2016.09.041.
6. Chan MK, Ocampo-Hafalla MT, Vartanian V, Jaruga P, Kirkali G, Koenig KL, et al. Targeted deletion of the genes encoding NTH1 and NEIL1 DNA N-glycosylases reveals the existence of novel carcinogenic oxidative damage to DNA. DNA Repair. 2009;8(7):786–94. https://doi.org/10.1016/j.dnarep.2009.03.001.
7. Kino K, Takao M, Miyazawa H, Hanaoka F. A DNA oligomer containing 2,2,4-triamino-5(2H)-oxazolone is incised by human NEIL1 and NTH1. Mutat Res. 2012;734(1-2):73–7. https://doi.org/10.1016/j.mrfmmm.2012.03.007.
8. Hazra TK, Das A, Das S, Choudhury S, Kow YW, Roy R. Oxidative DNA damage repair in mammalian cells: a new perspective. DNA Repair. 2007;6(4):470–80. https://doi.org/10.1016/j.dnarep.2006.10.011.
9. Chan AT, Arber N, Burn J, Chia WK, Elwood P, Hull MA, et al. Aspirin in the chemoprevention of colorectal neoplasia: an overview. Cancer Prev Res. 2012;5(2):164–78. https://doi.org/10.1158/1940-6207.CAPR-11-0391.
10. Broderick P, Bagratuni T, Vijayakrishnan J, Lubbe S, Chandler I, Houlston RS. Evaluation of NTHL1, NEIL1, NEIL2, MPG, TDG, UNG and SMUG1 genes in familial colorectal cancer predisposition. BMC Cancer. 2006;6:243. https://doi.org/10.1186/1471-2407-6-243.
11. Dallosso AR, Dolwani S, Jones N, Jones S, Colley J, Maynard J, et al. Inherited predisposition to colorectal adenomas caused by multiple rare alleles of MUTYH but not OGG1, NUDT1, NTH1 or NEIL 1, 2 or 3. Gut. 2008;57(9):1252–5. https://doi.org/10.1136/gut.2007.145748.
12. Drost J, van Boxtel R, Blokzijl F, Mizutani T, Sasaki N, Sasselli V, de Ligt J, Behjati S, Grolleman JE, van Wezel T, Nik-Zainal S, Kuiper RP, Cuppen E, Clevers H (2017) Use of CRISPR-modified human stem cell organoids to study the origin of mutational signatures in cancer. Science 358 (6360):234–8

Chapter 11
Adenomatous Polyposis Syndromes: Germline Biallelic Inactivation of Mismatch Repair Genes

Stefan Aretz and Maartje Nielsen

Abstract Early-onset multiple colorectal adenomas or a colorectal adenomatous polyposis is a common, but until recently not well-recognized, feature in the majority of patients with constitutional MMR deficiency (CMMRD), a recessively inherited condition caused by biallelic germline mutations in MMR genes, in particular in cases with *PMS2* and *MSH6* mutations. Adenomatous polyps occur in both the small intestine and large bowel, the gastrointestinal manifestations are extremely variable in numbers and age of onset, and the family history is often inconspicuous regarding LS-associated cancers. In particular the presence of high-grade dysplasia, early-onset cancer, and café-au-lait macules distinguishes this syndrome from ordinary adenomatous polyposis forms. An attenuated adenomatous colorectal and duodenal polyposis was also present in all individuals with a novel rare, autosomal recessive polyposis syndrome caused by biallelic *MSH3* germline mutations and characterized by a specific type of microsatellite instability (EMAST) in tumor tissue.

Keywords Hereditary tumor syndrome · CMMRD · MSH3 · Childhood cancer

Biallelic germline mutations in the Lynch syndrome-associated mismatch repair (MMR) genes lead to constitutional MMR deficiency (CMMRD), a recessively inherited tumor syndrome with a different phenotype characterized by multiple tumors and childhood onset [1, 2] (see Chap. 3). Interestingly, increasing evidence suggests that a number of affected individuals present with features overlapping those of colorectal adenomatous polyposis.

S. Aretz (✉)
Institute of Human Genetics, Centre for Hereditary Tumor Syndromes, University of Bonn, Bonn, Germany
e-mail: Stefan.Aretz@uni-bonn.de

M. Nielsen
Department of Clinical Genetics, Leiden University Medical Centre, Leiden, The Netherlands

L. Valle et al. (eds.), *Hereditary Colorectal Cancer*,
https://doi.org/10.1007/978-3-319-74259-5_11

1 Genetics

The majority of CMMRD cases published so far (50–60%) and around two thirds of those with gastrointestinal manifestations were carriers of a biallelic *PMS2* germline mutation [2–4]. Multiple colorectal adenomas or colorectal adenomatous polyposis is a common feature in patients with biallelic *PMS2* and *MSH6* mutations but is rarely described in biallelic *MSH2* and almost absent in biallelic *MLH1* carriers; however, this might be related to the small number of cases, lack of data and short follow-up time due to the severe phenotype of *MLH1-/MSH2*-related CMMRD rather than a specific gene-phenotype correlation.

In patients with a CMMRD-associated adenomatous polyposis, all types of loss-of-function mutations (truncating, missense, splice sites, large deletions) were reported, and all combinations of mutation types are possible. Although a truncating or splice site mutation together with a presumed missense mutation was frequently found, biallelic truncating or biallelic missense mutations were observed. The majority of mutations are private and located in a broad range across the genes. Due to the frequency of consanguineous couples, homozygous mutations are common [2, 3]. Rarely, a single heterozygous *PMS2* germline mutation has been identified despite a complete CMMRD phenotype; in other cases variants of unclear clinical significance (VUS) precluded a clear genetic diagnosis.

In the vast majority of CMMRD-associated gastrointestinal cancers and extraintestinal malignancies (glioblastomas, astrocytomas, bladder cancer, sarcomas), high MSI and an IHC result consistent with the mutated gene was found. However, there are few exceptions with a combined loss of MMR proteins in the case of *MSH6* and *PMS2* mutations or confirmed cases with MSH-L or even MSS, in particular when brain tumors were examined [2, 3].

Germline mutations of other MMR genes have neither been consistently linked to a Lynch-like phenotype nor described in cases with a gastrointestinal polyposis. Very recently, however, differing compound heterozygous truncating germline mutations in the MMR gene *MSH3* have been identified in two families with an adenomatous polyposis and extracolonic lesions, characterizing a novel rare, autosomal recessive polyposis syndrome [5]. Together with MSH2, MSH3 forms the DNA mismatch recognition heterodimer MutSß that has a strong affinity for larger base-indel loops with up to ten unpaired nucleotides. Consistently, the patients' tumor tissue demonstrated a specific type of microsatellite instability, high *microsatellite instability of di- and tetranucleotides (EMAST)*, and immunohistochemical staining a complete loss of nuclear MSH3 in normal and tumor tissue, confirming the loss-of-function effect and causal relevance of the mutations.

2 Clinical Characteristics

Typically, CMMRD is characterized by early-onset gastrointestinal tumors, brain tumors, hematological malignancies, and features suggestive of neurofibromatosis type 1, specifically café-au-lait (CAL) skin macules, and other malignancies including embryonic tumors [1, 2] (see Chap. 3). Since several of the extraintestinal manifestations occur at early age and are often fatal, data on the gastrointestinal phenotype is obtained from limited patient numbers and somehow biased [6]. However, colorectal and small bowel cancers represent a dominating tumor type in CMMRD patients which is reported in 40% of cases; in one to two thirds, gastrointestinal cancer or adenomas were even the first manifestation of the CMMRD syndrome [1, 3, 7].

The occurrence of multiple gastrointestinal polyps was not always recognized in earlier reports; nonetheless, recent data and larger cohorts showed that colorectal adenomas are a frequent finding in CMMRD. Only a small minority of patients present without any polyps; the vast majority had at least one adenoma. A polyposis-like phenotype with multiple adenomas meeting the established diagnostic criteria for adenomatous polyposis (>10–15 colorectal adenomas) was observed in about one third till 70% of patients [3, 6–8].

Adenomatous polyps have been identified in both the small intestine and large bowel. The gastrointestinal manifestations are highly dependent on age of examination and are extremely variable ranging from single or multiple early-onset adenomas (sometimes up to 100) in the first or second decade to few polyps not before the third or even fourth decade of life [8]. However, significant findings are usually not diagnosed during infancy (below the age of 6–8) [6]. The mean age at diagnosis was found to be 14 and 17 years, respectively, with a broad range (6–46 years) [3, 8].

The histology reveals tubulous, villous, or tubulovillous adenomas. Although the polyps are often asymptomatic, progression from adenoma to carcinoma can be rapid indicating an accelerated adenoma-carcinoma sequence for both adenoma formation and the adenoma-carcinoma transition due to the greatly enhanced mutation rate in neoplastic and nonneoplastic tissue [1, 8]. In agreement with this, CRC may develop within 1–2 years after a normal colonoscopy [7], and most (around 70%) of the CMMRD patients with adenomas showed high-grade dysplasia in at least one lesion or had synchronous bowel cancer at young age [8].

Duodenal adenomas are found in 5% of cases with a mean age at diagnosis of 14 years (range 10–32) [8]. Similar to the colorectum, an aggressive phenotype with frequent syn- or metachronous, early-onset duodenal, and proximal jejunal adenocarcinomas was noticed.

There is no marked gene-phenotype correlation besides the tendency of biallelic *MLH1* or *MSH2* mutation carriers to develop each tumor entity at lower age compared to *MSH6* and *PMS2* biallelics [8]. It was assumed that patients with a biallelic *PMS2* mutation had a greater incidence of LS-associated tumors or that LS-associated malignancies occurred only in the *PMS2* and *MSH6* mutation groups, respectively [2]; however, these observations might be due to other factors such as the severe phenotype of *MLH1/MSH2* biallelics resulting in missing data and short follow-up time rather than true gene-specific differences. In a recent study including 146 CMMRD patients, no significant difference in the frequency of LS-associated tumors was observed between the genes, but brain tumors occurred significantly more often in *PMS2* and hematological malignancies significantly more often in *MLH1-/MSH2*-associated CMMRD [8].

Although attention to the family history is important, pedigrees of CMMRD patients often show a paucity of LS-associated cancers or a familial history of cancer is lacking at all. Thus, most parents are unaffected, which is in particular due to the low penetrance of monoallelic *PMS2* and *MSH6* germline mutations [1, 2, 6].

As a consequence, until recently the majority of cases with multiple adenomas were misclassified as mutation-negative (attenuated) FAP or labeled as having Turcot syndrome in the case of a syn- or metachronous brain tumor. However, although the gastrointestinal findings might be very similar to simple adenomatous polyposis, there are striking differences in the majority of patients.

In particular, the phenotype of CMMRD patients is more severe with often very early onset in terms of polyp formation, high-grade dysplasia, syn- and metachronous (CRC) carcinomas, and an uncommon cancer localization (jejunum). Almost all patients display Neurofibromatosis 1 (NF1)-like skin macules and many of them extraintestinal cancers, so that awareness to extracolonic features, in particular CAL macules, is important. In addition, affected siblings and consanguineous parents indicate autosomal recessive inheritance [2]. In summary, in particular the presence of high-grade dysplasia, early-onset cancer, and CAL macules distinguishes this syndrome from ordinary adenomatous polyposis forms.

All four patients with an *MSH3*-associated polyposis from two unrelated families, which have been described recently [5], presented with an attenuated colorectal and duodenal involvement and no or late-onset cancer. This is similar to the phenotype observed in persons with other subtypes of attenuated adenomatous polyposis (MAP, NAP, PPAP, AFAP) and consistent with the findings described in *MSH3*-knockout mice. Interestingly, two of the four carriers are reported to have extraintestinal tumors including an early-onset astrocytoma. Since *MSH3*-induced EMAST occurs in different tumor types, there might be a broad clinical overlap with the tumor spectrum observed in CMMRD.

Consequently, even in the absence of cancer, a CMMRD syndrome should be considered in individuals with childhood-onset multiple colorectal adenomas and signs of NF1, if no germline mutation in the established adenomatous polyposis genes could be identified. Proposed criteria for CMMRD testing include multiple bowel adenomas at age <25 years and absence of *APC/MUTYH* mutation(s) or a single high-grade dysplasia adenoma at age <25 years [8].

References

1. Durno CA, Sherman PM, Aronson M, Malkin D, Hawkins C, Bakry D, Bouffet E, Gallinger S, Pollett A, Campbell B, Tabori U, International BMMRD Consortium. Phenotypic and genotypic characterisation of biallelic mismatch repair deficiency (BMMR-D) syndrome. Eur J Cancer. 2015;51:977–83.
2. Lavoine N, Colas C, Muleris M, Bodo S, Duval A, Entz-Werle N, Coulet F, Cabaret O, Andreiuolo F, Charpy C, et al. Constitutional mismatch repair deficiency syndrome: clinical description in a French cohort. J Med Genet. 2015;52:770–8.

3. Herkert JC, Niessen RC, Olderode-Berends MJ, Veenstra-Knol HE, Vos YJ, van der Klift HM, Scheenstra R, Tops CM, Karrenbeld A, Peters FT, et al. Paediatric intestinal cancer and polyposis due to bi-allelic PMS2 mutations: case series, review and follow-up guidelines. Eur J Cancer. 2011;47:965–82.
4. van der Klift HM, Mensenkamp AR, Drost M, Bik EC, Vos YJ, Gille HJ, Redeker BE, Tiersma Y, Zonneveld JB, García EG, Letteboer TG, Olderode-Berends MJ, van Hest LP, van Os TA, Verhoef S, Wagner A, van Asperen CJ, Ten Broeke SW, Hes FJ, de Wind N, Nielsen M, Devilee P, Ligtenberg MJ, Wijnen JT, Tops CM. Comprehensive mutation analysis of PMS2 in a large cohort of probands suspected of Lynch syndrome or constitutional mismatch repair deficiency syndrome. Hum Mutat. 2016;37:1162–79.
5. Adam R, Spier I, Zhao B, Kloth M, Marquez J, Hinrichsen I, Kirfel J, Tafazzoli A, Horpaopan S, Uhlhaas S, Stienen D, Friedrichs N, Altmüller J, Laner A, Holzapfel S, Peters S, Kayser K, Thiele H, Holinski-Feder E, Marra G, Kristiansen G, Nöthen MM, Büttner R, Möslein G, Betz RC, Brieger A, Lifton RP, Aretz S. Exome sequencing identifies biallelic MSH3 germline mutations as a recessive subtype of colorectal adenomatous polyposis. Am J Hum Genet. 2016;99:337–51.
6. Levi Z, Kariv R, Barnes-Kedar I, Goldberg Y, Half E, Morgentern S, Eli B, Baris HN, Vilkin A, Belfer RG, Niv Y, Elhasid R, Dvir R, Abu-Freha N, Cohen S. The gastrointestinal manifestation of constitutional mismatch repair deficiency syndrome: from a single adenoma to polyposis-like phenotype and early onset cancer. Clin Genet. 2015;88:474–8.
7. Vasen HF, Ghorbanoghli Z, Bourdeaut F, Cabaret O, Caron O, Duval A, Entz-Werle N, Goldberg Y, Ilencikova D, Kratz CP, Lavoine N, Loeffen J, Menko FH, Muleris M, Sebille G, Colas C, Burkhardt B, Brugieres L, Wimmer K, EU-Consortium Care for CMMR-D (C4CMMR-D). Guidelines for surveillance of individuals with constitutional mismatch repair-deficiency proposed by the European consortium "care for CMMR-D" (C4CMMR-D). J Med Genet. 2014;51:283–93.
8. Wimmer K, Kratz CP, Vasen HF, Caron O, Colas C, Entz-Werle N, Gerdes AM, Goldberg Y, Ilencikova D, Muleris M, Duval A, Lavoine N, Ruiz-Ponte C, Slavc I, Burkhardt B, Brugieres L, EU-Consortium Care for CMMRD (C4CMMRD). Diagnostic criteria for constitutional mismatch repair deficiency syndrome: suggestions of the European consortium 'care for CMMRD' (C4CMMRD). J Med Genet. 2014;51:355–65.

Chapter 12
Adenomatous Polyposis Syndromes: Unexplained Colorectal Adenomatous Polyposis

Stefan Aretz and Maartje Nielsen

Abstract In a considerable number of patients with clinically confirmed colorectal adenomatous polyposis, no germline mutation in known genes can be identified, although a genetic etiology is likely. The phenotype of these cases is characterized by a more attenuated course, no evident extracolonic manifestations, and an unsuspicious or unclear family history in at least half of the patients. Diagnostic and technical difficulties to identify mutations in established genes might be relevant, in particular low-level APC mutational mosaicism seems to be the underlying cause in a large fraction of unexplained cases. During the last decades, several efforts had been made to uncover further genetic causes. Using different approaches including exome sequencing, however, only few and very rare novel genetic subtypes could be delineated pointing to extreme genetic heterogeneity. Consequently, large cohorts provided by international collaborations and novel analytic strategies are required to uncover the genetic basis in those patients.

Keywords Etiology · Mutation negative polyposis · Colorectal cancer Classification · Multiple adenomas

Gastrointestinal polyposes are genetically heterogeneous conditions. The likelihood to detect a pathogenic disease-causing germline mutation in one of the established genes strongly depends on the colorectal phenotype and family history.

In up to 30–50% of patients with a clinically confirmed colorectal adenomatosis (>10–15 synchronous adenomas), no germline mutation in known genes can be identified. However, the syn- or metachronous occurrence of dozens to hundreds of polyps strongly argues for an underlying genetic basis, although it remains unclear so far whether the predisposing genetic factors mainly act in a monogenic fashion

S. Aretz (✉)
Institute of Human Genetics, Center for Hereditary Tumor Syndromes, University of Bonn, Bonn, Germany
e-mail: Stefan.Aretz@uni-bonn.de

M. Nielsen
Department of Clinical Genetics, Leiden University Medical Centre, Leiden, The Netherlands

L. Valle et al. (eds.), *Hereditary Colorectal Cancer*,
https://doi.org/10.1007/978-3-319-74259-5_12

or contribute as low or moderately penetrant variants to a more complex, oligo/polygenic trait.

The phenotype of unexplained patients is characterized by a more attenuated course, no evident extracolonic manifestations, and an unsuspicious or unclear family history in at least half of the patients. However, the detailed presentation strongly depends on the inclusion and selection criteria and the extent of clinical examinations and shows marked differences between published cohorts. In general, the majority of cases exhibit 10–50 adenomas, and the mean age of diagnosis (44–60 years) is correlated with the polyp number. A personal history of CRC was reported in 4–49%, duodenal adenomas in 0–35%, extraintestinal lesions in 0–14%, and a positive family history regarding polyposis of CRC in up to 59% of unexplained polyposis patients [1–4].

Reasons for missing a molecular delineation might be diagnostic difficulties. An incomplete histologic work-up where an insufficient number of polyps were examined prevents the evaluation of the dominating polyp histology. Patients with mixed polyp types or conditions with a phenotypic overlap such as Lynch syndrome, CMMRD, or Peutz-Jeghers syndrome, where multiple adenomas might occur, can result in misclassification. In around 8% of patients with more than five colorectal adenomas, germline mutations in hamartomatous polyposis-associated genes were found [5]. Further reasons are the identification of rare missense variants of unknown significance (VUS) [6] or cryptic mutations not discovered by routine methods, such as deep intronic mutations [7, 8] or promoter alterations. A considerable fraction of cases might be explained by low-level *APC* mutational mosaicism [9, 10] (see Fig. 6.1 in Chap. 6). Up to one third of unexplained adenomatous polyposis showed a decreased allele-specific APC expression pointing to undiscovered *APC* alterations which may include epigenetic changes [11]. There are also speculations about environmental factors, in particular late effects of irradiation, that might explain few cases [12].

During the last decades, several efforts had been made to uncover further genetic causes. Classical approaches to gene identification such as linkage analysis are feasible in a few families only, since most of the cases are sporadic or characterized by an uncertain family history and an attenuated course of the disease where parents are already deceased [1, 2, 13]. Over the past two decades, a number of candidate gene studies have been performed including genes from the Wnt, TGFb, or BER pathways without convincing results [3, 6, 14–17]. Neither loss-of-heterozygosity (LOH) analyses nor specific somatic mutational profiles could contribute to the identification of promising novel genetic causes. Germline mutations in the *BUB* gene family (*BUB1B*, *BUB1*, *BUB3*) were found in patients with gastrointestinal tumors and early-onset CRC [18, 19]. Rare germline copy number variants (CNVs) and low-penetrant single-nucleotide variants might contribute to the genetic predisposition for the formation of adenomas [1, 20].

Currently, exome sequencing is considered the most powerful tool for the identification of new causative genes in Mendelian disorders of unknown etiology [21]. The underlying strategies include screening for recurrently mutated genes (overlap strategy), the biallelic hit strategy for a suspected recessive inheritance, and the tumor suppressor model in cancer predisposition syndromes (selection of genes which harbor both a heterozygous truncating germline mutation and a somatic mutation). Those studies were successful in delineating few genetic subtypes, so far [4, 22, 23]. However, the data also consistently show that mutations in newly identified causative genes associated with adenomatous polyposis are very rare indicating extreme genetic heterogeneity. As a consequence, identifying further recurrently mutated genes and a more complex genetic architecture will require large cohorts which can be provided only by international collaborations and consortia such as the European Reference Network (ERN) GENTURIS (www.genturis.eu). In light of the abovementioned studies, it might be reasonable to carefully exclude *APC* mutational mosaicism and clearly reduced allele-specific APC expression prior to admittance of these patients in studies that aim to identify new causative, highly penetrant genes.

References

1. Hes FJ, Ruano D, Nieuwenhuis M, et al. Colorectal cancer risk variants on 11q23 and 15q13 are associated with unexplained adenomatous polyposis. J Med Genet. 2014;51:55–60.
2. Thirlwell C, Howarth KM, Segditsas S, et al. Investigation of pathogenic mechanisms in multiple colorectal adenoma patients without germline APC or MYH/MUTYH mutations. Br J Cancer. 2007;96:1729–34.
3. Mongin C, Coulet F, Lefevre JH, et al. Unexplained polyposis: a challenge for geneticists, pathologists and gastroenterologists. Clin Genet. 2012;81:38–46.
4. Adam R, Spier I, Zhao B, Kloth M, Marquez J, Hinrichsen I, Kirfel J, Tafazzoli A, Horpaopan S, Uhlhaas S, Stienen D, Friedrichs N, Altmüller J, Laner A, Holzapfel S, Peters S, Kayser K, Thiele H, Holinski-Feder E, Marra G, Kristiansen G, Nöthen MM, Büttner R, Möslein G, Betz RC, Brieger A, Lifton RP, Aretz S. Exome sequencing identifies biallelic MSH3 germline mutations as a recessive subtype of colorectal adenomatous polyposis. Am J Hum Genet. 2016;99:337–51.
5. Ngeow J, Heald B, Rybicki LA, Orloff MS, Chen JL, Liu X, Yerian L, Willis J, Lehtonen HJ, Lehtonen R, Mester JL, Moline J, Burke CA, Church J, Aaltonen LA, Eng C. Prevalence of germline PTEN, BMPR1A, SMAD4, STK11, and ENG mutations in patients with moderate-load colorectal polyps. Gastroenterology. 2013;144:1402–9.
6. Azzopardi D, Dallosso AR, Eliason K, Hendrickson BC, Jones N, Rawstorne E, Colley J, Moskvina V, Frye C, Sampson JR, Wenstrup R, Scholl T, Cheadle JP. Multiple rare nonsynonymous variants in the adenomatous polyposis coli gene predispose to colorectal adenomas. Cancer Res. 2008;68:358–63.
7. Spier I, Horpaopan S, Vogt S, Uhlhaas S, Morak M, Stienen D, Draaken M, Ludwig M, Holinski-Feder E, Nöthen MM, Hoffmann P, Aretz S. Deep intronic APC mutations explain a substantial proportion of patients with familial or early-onset adenomatous polyposis. Hum Mutat. 2012;33:1045–50.
8. Nieminen TT, Pavicic W, Porkka N, Kankainen M, Järvinen HJ, Lepistö A, Peltomäki P. Pseudoexons provide a mechanism for allele-specific expression of APC in familial adenomatous polyposis. Oncotarget. 2016;7(43):70685–98.
9. Spier I, Drichel D, Kerick M, Kirfel J, Horpaopan S, Laner A, Holzapfel S, Peters S, Adam R, Zhao B, Becker T, Lifton RP, Perner S, Hoffmann P, Kristiansen G, Timmermann B, Nöthen MM, Holinski-Feder E, Schweiger MR, Aretz S. Low-level APC mutational mosaicism is the underlying cause in a substantial fraction of unexplained colorectal adenomatous polyposis cases. J Med Genet. 2016;53:172–9.

10. Jansen AM, Crobach S, Geurts-Giele WR, van den Akker BE, Garcia MV, Ruano D, Nielsen M, Tops CM, Wijnen JT, Hes FJ, van Wezel T, Dinjens WN, Morreau H. Distinct patterns of somatic mosaicism in the APC gene in neoplasms from patients with unexplained adenomatous polyposis. Gastroenterology. 2017;152:546–9.
11. Aceto GM, Fantini F, De Iure S, Di Nicola M, Palka G, Valanzano R, Di Gregorio P, Stigliano V, Genuardi M, Battista P, Cama A, Curia MC. Correlation between mutations and mRNA expression of APC and MUTYH genes: new insight into hereditary colorectal polyposis predisposition. J Exp Clin Cancer Res. 2015;34:131.
12. Rigter LS, Kallenberg FG, Bastiaansen B, van Os TA, van Leeuwen FE, van Leerdam ME, Dekker E. A case series of intestinal adenomatous polyposis of unidentified etiology; a late effect of irradiation? BMC Cancer. 2016;16:862.
13. Knudsen AL, Bisgaard ML, Bülow S. Attenuated familial adenomatous polyposis (AFAP). A review of the literature. Familial Cancer. 2003;2:43–55.
14. Fearnhead NS, Wilding JL, Winney B, et al. Multiple rare variants in different genes account for multifactorial inherited susceptibility to colorectal adenomas. Proc Natl Acad Sci USA. 2004;101:15992–7.
15. Lefevre JH, Bonilla C, Colas C, et al. Role of rare variants in undetermined multiple adenomatous polyposis and early-onset colorectal cancer. J Hum Genet. 2012;57:709–16.
16. Dallosso AR, Dolwani S, Jones N, et al. Inherited predisposition to colorectal adenomas caused by multiple rare alleles of MUTYH but not OGG1, NUDT1, NTH1 or NEIL 1, 2 or 3. Gut. 2008;57:1252–5.
17. Will O, Carvajal-Carmona LG, Gorman P, Howarth KM, Jones AM, Polanco-Echeverry GM, Chinaleong JA, Gunther T, Silver A, Clark SK, Tomlinson I. Homozygous PMS2 deletion causes a severe colorectal cancer and multiple adenoma phenotype without extraintestinal cancer. Gastroenterology. 2007;132:527–30.
18. Rio Frio T, Lavoie J, Hamel N, et al. Homozygous BUB1B mutation and susceptibility to gastrointestinal neoplasia. N Engl J Med. 2010;363:2628–37.
19. de Voer RM, Geurts van Kessel A, Weren RD, Ligtenberg MJ, Smeets D, Fu L, Vreede L, Kamping EJ, Verwiel ET, Hahn MM, Ariaans M, Spruijt L, van Essen T, Houge G, Schackert HK, Sheng JQ, Venselaar H, van Ravenswaaij-Arts CM, van Krieken JH, Hoogerbrugge N, Kuiper RP. Germline mutations in the spindle assembly checkpoint genes BUB1 and BUB3 are risk factors for colorectal cancer. Gastroenterology. 2013;145:544–7.
20. Horpaopan S, Spier I, Zink AM, Altmüller J, Holzapfel S, Laner A, Vogt S, Uhlhaas S, Heilmann S, Stienen D, Pasternack SM, Keppler K, Adam R, Kayser K, Moebus S, Draaken M, Degenhardt F, Engels H, Hofmann A, Nöthen MM, Steinke V, Perez-Bouza A, Herms S, Holinski-Feder E, Fröhlich H, Thiele H, Hoffmann P, Aretz S. Genome-wide CNV analysis in 221 unrelated patients and targeted high-throughput sequencing reveal novel causative candidate genes for colorectal adenomatous polyposis. Int J Cancer. 2015;136:E578–89.
21. Gilissen C, Hoischen A, Brunner HG, Veltman JA. Disease gene identification strategies for exome sequencing. Eur J Hum Genet. 2012;20:490–7.
22. Palles C, et al. Germline mutations affecting the proofreading domains of POLE and POLD1 predispose to colorectal adenomas and carcinomas. Nat Genet. 2013;45(2):136–44.
23. Weren RD, Ligtenberg MJ, Kets CM, de Voer RM, Verwiel ET, Spruijt L, van Zelst-Stams WA, Jongmans MC, Gilissen C, Hehir-Kwa JY, Hoischen A, Shendure J, Boyle EA, Kamping EJ, Nagtegaal ID, Tops BB, Nagengast FM, Geurts van Kessel A, van Krieken JH, Kuiper RP, Hoogerbrugge N. A germline homozygous mutation in the base-excision repair gene NTHL1 causes adenomatous polyposis and colorectal cancer. Nat Genet. 2015;47(6):668–71.

Chapter 13
Hamartomatous Polyposis Syndromes

Joanne Ngeow, Eliza Courtney, Kiat Hon Lim, and Charis Eng

Abstract The hamartomatous polyposis syndromes (HPS) include a small but appreciable number of the gastrointestinal hereditary cancer syndromes and are characterized by the presence of gastrointestinal (GI) hamartomatous polyps. Hamartomatous polyps account for a very small percentage of all GI polyps. They arise from excessive proliferation of the epithelial and stromal cells native to the tissue of origin and contain components from any of the three germ layers forming the intestines. The process underlying the progression of hamartomatous polyps to cancer is not fully understood. HPS occur at approximately one tenth of the frequency of adenomatous polyposis syndromes and account for less than 1% of colorectal cancer cases, although their prevalence may be higher than originally

J. Ngeow
Division of Medical Oncology, National Cancer Centre, Singapore, Singapore

Oncology Academic Clinical Program, Duke-NUS Graduate Medical School, Singapore, Singapore

Genomic Medicine Institute, Cleveland Clinic, Cleveland, OH, USA

E. Courtney
Division of Medical Oncology, National Cancer Centre, Singapore, Singapore

K. H. Lim
Division of Pathology, Singapore General Hospital, Singapore, Singapore

C. Eng (✉)
Genomic Medicine Institute, Cleveland Clinic, Cleveland, OH, USA

Lerner Research Institute, Cleveland Clinic, Cleveland, OH, USA

Taussig Cancer Institute, Cleveland Clinic, Cleveland, OH, USA

Department of Genetics and Genome Sciences, Case Western Reserve University School of Medicine, Cleveland, OH, USA

Germline High Risk Focus Group, Case Comprehensive Cancer Center, Case Western Reserve University, Cleveland, OH, USA
e-mail: engc@ccf.org

L. Valle et al. (eds.), *Hereditary Colorectal Cancer*,
https://doi.org/10.1007/978-3-319-74259-5_13

thought. It is now well recognized that these syndromes confer a substantial risk of colonic and extracolonic malignancies, therefore making it important to identify individuals with HPS for further risk management.

Keywords Cowden syndrome · Juvenile polyposis · Peutz-Jeghers syndrome · PTEN · Hamartomas · Colorectal cancers · Extra-colonic cancer risk

The hamartomatous polyposis syndromes (HPS) include a small but appreciable number of the gastrointestinal hereditary cancer syndromes and are characterized by the presence of gastrointestinal (GI) hamartomatous polyps. Hamartomatous polyps account for a very small percentage of all GI polyps. They arise from excessive proliferation of the epithelial and stromal cells native to the tissue of origin and contain components from any of the three germ layers forming the intestines. Figure 13.1a–c compares the histological features of hamartomatous polyps, juvenile polyps (hamartomatous polyp subtype), and adenomatous polyps. The process

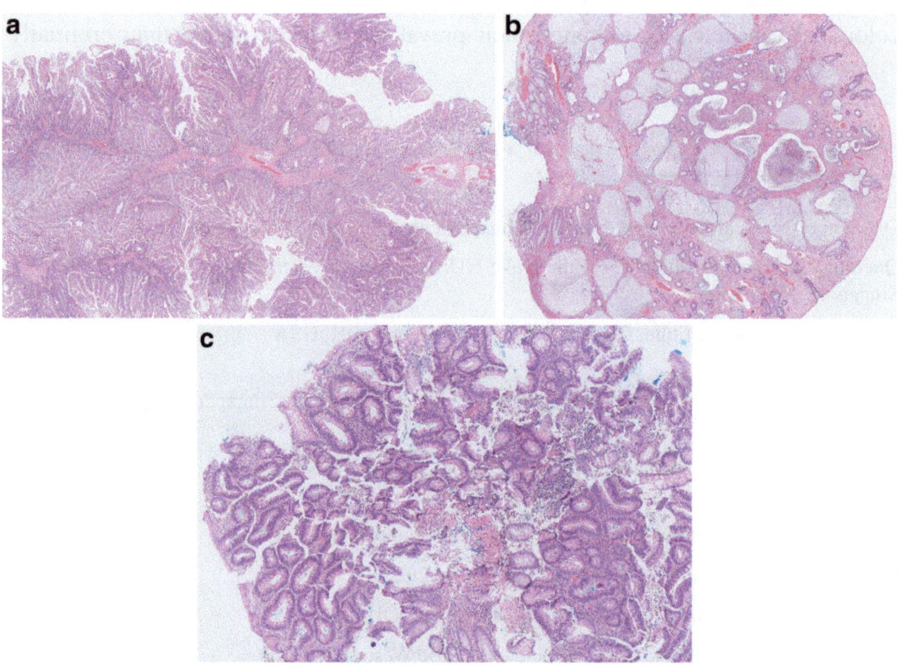

Fig. 13.1 (**a**) Hamartomatous polyp. HE X20. Elongated and proliferative glands with branching "arborizing" smooth muscle bands. (**b**) Juvenile polyp. HE X50. Cystic and dilated glands with edematous and markedly inflamed lamina propria. (**c**) Adenomatous polyp. HE X20. Round and tubular glands with columnar cells displaying nuclear stratification amounting to low-grade dysplasia

underlying the progression of hamartomatous polyps to cancer is not fully understood. HPS occur at approximately one tenth of the frequency of adenomatous polyposis syndromes and account for less than 1% of colorectal cancer cases [1], although their prevalence may be higher than originally thought [2]. It is now well recognized that these syndromes confer a substantial risk of colonic and extracolonic malignancies, therefore making it important to identify individuals with HPS for further risk management.

HPS predominantly include Peutz-Jeghers syndrome (PJS), juvenile polyposis syndrome (JPS), and the PTEN-hamartoma tumor syndromes (PHTS), although hamartomatous polyps have also been reported in other syndromes [3]. They are autosomal dominant conditions, and although there are clinical criteria available for most HPS [4], there are a number of confounding factors that result in atypical presentations that do not fulfill criteria. These include reduced penetrance, vast inter- and intrafamilial variation in expression, and significant de novo rates, where individuals have no relevant family history. Furthermore, there are phenotypic features shared among HPS, making the ability to differentiate among them sometimes difficult. Genetic testing has helped resolve some of these diagnostic complications; however, gene mutations cannot be identified in all individuals with HPS and so are not used to exclude a diagnosis [3]. It is important for clinicians to be aware of the phenotypic features (particularly extracolonic; see Table 13.1) associated with HPS, as well as the confounding factors that make diagnostics difficult, so they can offer genetic counseling to their patients where appropriate.

In this chapter, we will describe the clinical characteristics and genetics for the three aforementioned HPS, as well as the current risk management recommendations for each.

1 Peutz-Jeghers Syndrome

1.1 Clinical Characteristics

PJS (OMIM 175200) is characterized by the presence of the so-called Peutz-Jeghers-type hamartomatous polyps in the GI tract and mucocutaneous pigmentation. The incidence of PJS is approximately 1 in 8300 to 1 in 230,000 live births [5], although a more recent report estimates the lower limit at 1 in 50,000 [6].

Peutz-Jeghers polyps have a distinctive frond-like structure, appropriate epithelium for each area of the GI tract, and associated smooth muscle proliferation. Histologically, Peutz-Jeghers polyps have convoluted, stretched glands and an arborizing branching pattern of smooth muscle growth [7]. Rarely focal dysplastic glands can be observed [8, 9]. Polyp numbers can vary from one to hundreds and occur most commonly in the small bowel, but also frequently in the colon and stomach [10]. They are occasionally found in the gall bladder, the bronchi, the urinary bladder, and the ureter [11]. More than half of individuals with PJS will experience polyp-related symptoms before the age of 20, with the median age of onset being

Table 13.1 Extra-gastrointestinal features in hamartomatous polyposis syndromes

Syndrome	Dermatologic	Head/Neck	Musculoskeletal	Endocrine	Neurologic	Gonadal	Pulmonary	Others
PJS	Mucocutaneous hyperpigmentation			Thyroid cancer		Sex cord and Sertoli tumors of the testes Gynecomastia Ovarian cysts Sex cord tumor with annular tubules of the ovary	Bronchial polyps Lung cancer	Ureteral polyps Bladder polyps Pancreatic cancer Breast cancer
JPS		Cleft lip and palate Macrocephaly Hypertelorism	Digital clubbing Polydactyly				Pulmonary arteriovenous malformation	Malrotation of the gut Other congenital abnormalities
CS	Papillomatous papules Acral/plantar keratosis Trichilemommas	Brain tumors (Lhermitte-Duclos disease) Macrocephaly Dolichocephaly		Thyroid cancer		Endometrial cancer Uterine leiomyomas	Bronchial polyps Lung cancer	Fibrocystic breast disease Thyroid goiters Breast cancer Renal cell carcinoma
BRRS[a]	Lipomas Pigmented macules of the glans penis	Macrocephaly	Myopathy in proximal muscles Joint Hyperextensibility Pectus excavatum Scoliosis		Developmental delay Mental deficiency			Large birth weight

[a]Individuals with BRRS who have a germline *PTEN* mutation are also thought to have a similar cancer risk to CS.
Abbreviations: *PJS* Peutz-Jeghers syndrome, *JPS* juvenile polyposis syndrome, *CS* Cowden syndrome, *BRRS* Bannayan-Riley-Ruvalcaba syndrome

13 years [3, 12]. The most common symptoms are small bowel intussusception and obstruction, abdominal pain, rectal bleeding, and anemia.

Mucocutaneous pigmentation is present in approximately 95% of individuals with PJS and is found on the vermillion border of the lips, buccal mucosa, and the perianal region [10]. Typically these lesions present as small, brown macules in infancy and often fade after puberty, but sometimes persist in the buccal mucosa [3].

The clinical diagnostic criteria are based on a consensus of European experts [10] and include (i) two or more histologically confirmed PJS polyps; (ii) any number of PJS polyps detected in one individual, who has family history of PJS in a close relative(s); (iii) characteristic mucocutaneous pigmentation in an individual who has a family history of PJS in a close relative(s); or (iv) any number of PJS-type polyps in an individual who also had characteristic mucocutaneous pigmentations.

There have been a number of large-scale publications evaluating cancer risk in PJS [5, 13–17]. Using a retrospective cohort study design, Resta et al. [17] estimated that the cumulative lifetime risk for any cancer was 89%. This is consistent with previous findings including 85% [14], 81% [16], and 93% [13]. The most common cancers identified in individuals with PJS were those located in the GI tract including the esophagus, stomach, small bowel, colon, and pancreas. Breast cancer in women is also commonly reported in these studies, although some argue the degree of risk may not as high as routinely quoted [18]. Other PJS-associated cancers are those of the reproductive organs. Females are at increased risk for developing sex-cord tumors with annular tubules of the ovary and adenoma malignum of the cervix, which can cause irregular menstruation and precocious puberty. Males are at increased risk for developing testicular tumors of the sex-cord and Sertoli-cell types, often resulting in sexual precocity and gynecomastia [5, 14]. It is important to note that the cancer risk figures given in these studies may be overestimated, due to difficulties with ascertainment bias.

Cancer risks and relevant risk management recommendations are described in Table 13.2. Although there is little evidence documenting the efficacy of surveillance in individuals with PJS, recommendations have been established based on expert opinion [5, 7, 10, 15, 19]. Surveillance of the GI tract is crucial for individuals with PJS because of the risk of complications from polyps, such as intussusception [20, 21]. Given that the cumulative risk of intussusception increases in childhood (15% by age 10), it is reasonable to begin surveillance for polyps around this age [21], with some evidence suggesting to commence even younger at age 4–5 [22]. Screening of the small bowel has traditionally been difficult, as the vast majority of its mucosa is not easily viewed or accessible by endoscopy. Other techniques such as video capsule endoscopy (VCE), barium follow through (BaFT), double-balloon enteroscopy, or magnetic resonance endoscopy (MRE) have been suggested. Studies have illustrated favorable characteristics for VCE, including reduced radiation and greater sensitivity to detecting small polyps (<1 cm), and are generally better tolerated [19, 23]. However, larger polyps (>15 mm) may be missed with VCE, and studies so far have shown MRE and enteroscopy to be effective in these cases [23, 24]. Polyps greater than 1 cm in size should be removed endoscopically, and often a combined approach with laparoscopy or laparotomy is required to reach the region

Table 13.2 Cancer risk and suggested management for hamartomatous polyposis syndromes

Phenotype	Cancer risk (%)	Age to commence	Interval	Intervention
Peutz-Jeghers syndrome				
Colon cancer	39	25	2–3 years	Colonoscopy
Proximal GI tract/ small bowel cancer	11–29	10	2–3 years	GI endoscopy, VCE, BaFT or MRE (annual hemoglobin in childhood)
Pancreatic cancer	11–26	30	1–2 years	Endoscopic ultrasound Transabdominal ultrasound
Breast cancer	45	25	2 years	Mammogram
			1 year	Self-exam
Gynecological cancer/tumors	18	20	1 year	Transvaginal ultrasound Endometrial biopsy
		18–20	1 year	Exo-cervix pap smear Pelvic examination
Testicular tumor	9	10	1 year	Physical exam Ultrasound if clinically indicated
Juvenile polyposis syndrome				
Colon cancer	38	15	2 years	Colonoscopy
			1 year	Colonoscopy (if polyps detected)
			–	Consider colectomy if polyp burden too high
Proximal GI tract cancer	21 (if multiple polyps)	15	2 years	GI endoscopy
			1 year	GI endoscopy (if polyps detected)
HHT management for *SMAD4* carriers only				
AVM		<6 months or at diagnosis	–	MRI (unenhanced for children)
PAVM		At diagnosis	5–10 years (additional after puberty, pre/post pregnancy)	TTCE
GI bleeding	*SMAD4* carriers	35	1 year	Hemoglobin or hematocrit levels
Cowden syndrome				
Breast cancer	85	25	6–12 months	Clinical breast exam
		30–35	1 year	Mammogram, MRI
Endometrial cancer	28	30–35	Annual	Transvaginal ultrasound Endometrial biopsy

(continued)

Table 13.2 (continued)

Phenotype	Cancer risk (%)	Age to commence	Interval	Intervention
Thyroid cancer (mainly follicular)	35	At diagnosis	1 Year	Clinical exam plus baseline ultrasound
Colon cancer	9	35	5 years	Colonoscopy
Melanoma	6	15	1 year	Consider annual dermatologic exam
Renal cancer	34	40	1–2 years	Consider renal ultrasound

of interest. Women are recommended to undergo breast and gynecological surveillance, although there is little evidence to support this recommendation in the PJS context specifically.

1.2 Genetics

PJS is caused by the presence of germline mutations in the tumor suppressor gene *STK11* (*LKB1*) located at 19p13.3. It is 23 kb in size, is composed of ten exons (nine of which are coding), and encodes a 433 amino acid STK (serine-threonine kinase) protein [7]. The mutation detection rate in individuals fulfilling the diagnostic criteria for PJS is 94% when using sequencing and multiplex ligation-dependent probe amplification (MLPA) [25]. Approximately 38–50% of individuals with a germline *STK11* gene have no family history of PJS [25, 26]. The majority of mutations associated with disease are truncating or missense which eliminate the kinase function of the protein. Importantly, up to 30% of mutations may be large deletions which are often not detected by sequencing alone [25], and so caution should be taken regarding testing methodologies in certain circumstances. There are conflicting reports regarding genotype-phenotype correlations. One group reported a higher mutation detection rate for those who present more classically than those with isolated features [25], and another have reported a relationship between the mutation type and age of onset [12]. Other studies have not found the same relationships [14, 27].

Once an *STK11* mutation has been identified in the proband, at-risk blood relatives can then undergo predictive testing. Parents of apparently de novo cases should be carefully evaluated for PJS features. Testing can be considered for the proband's siblings regardless of the parents' results due to the small possibility of gonadal mosaicism (although this has not been reported in PJS previously). Offspring of the proband are at 50% risk of inheriting the *STK11* mutation and should be offered testing.

2 Juvenile Polyposis Syndrome

2.1 Clinical Characteristics

JPS (OMIM 174900) is characterized by the presence of multiple juvenile-type hamartomatous polyps throughout the GI tract, although they occur most commonly in the colon and rectum [28]. The estimated incidence is 1 in 100,000 live births [29, 30].

Juvenile polyps are lobulated and spherical in shape and are histologically characterized by overgrowth of an edematous lamina propria with inflammatory cells and dilated cystic glands (Fig. 13.1b; [31]). Moderate to marked inflammatory infiltrate is commonly seen. No smooth muscle proliferation or normal glands are present. They can vary in size from a few millimeters to several centimeters. Although juvenile polyps are well described, they are sometimes difficult to distinguish from inflammatory polyps. Singular juvenile polyps are detected in approximately 2% of all children, and the risk of cancer in these sporadic cases is not thought to be high [28, 32, 33], therefore highlighting the importance of distinguishing those with JPS. Diagnosis is made between 16 and 18 years of age on average, although there is variability in age of onset and 50% will have family history [34]. The clinical presentation of JPS has been distinguished into three forms: (i) juvenile polyposis of infancy, (ii) juvenile polyposis coli, and (iii) generalized JPS [35, 36].

Juvenile polyposis of infancy occurs very early on in life (usually by 2 years of age) and is the rarer form of JPS. Individuals in this group generally have poor prognosis. They typically present with recurrent GI bleeding, diarrhea, hypoproteinemia, and malnutrition and usually have larger, recurrent polyps that cause rectal prolapse and intussusception. In addition, many suffer from congenital abnormalities, including macrocephaly and generalized hypotonia [31]. It is believed that this severe phenotype is the result of a contiguous gene deletion of *BMPR1A* (JPS associated gene) and *PTEN* (PHTS associated gene) [37, 38], although this has been somewhat disputed by others reporting variable phenotypes in individuals with large deletions [39]. Juvenile polyposis coli and generalized JPS are associated with varied expression and penetrance, with polyps in the former typically occurring in the colon. Symptoms in these forms tend to present in the second decade of life, and polyp numbers can vary over their lifetime. The typical presentation for these JPS forms includes chronic or acute GI bleeding, anemia, prolapsed rectal polyps, abdominal pain, and diarrhea [28, 30, 40]. Approximately 20% of JPS patients have manifestations other than hamartomatous polyposis including congenital abnormalities of the heart, cranium, and urinary-sexual systems, cleft lip and palate, finger clubbing, polydactyly, macrocephaly, hypertelorism, and malrotation of the gut [28, 41]. However, the diagnoses of the reported JPS cases in these studies have been made based solely on clinical criteria, and there is a possibility their phenotypes are due to a different genetic syndrome entirely. When JPS is the result of a germline *SMAD4* mutation, individuals are at higher risk of large gastric polyps and upper GI malignancy than when due to a

BMPR1A mutation [42, 43]. Additionally, hereditary hemorrhagic telangiectasia (HHT) occurs in approximately 15–22% of individuals carrying a germline *SMAD4* mutation and is characterized by skin and mucosal telangiectasia; cerebral, pulmonary, and hepatic arteriovenous malformations; and an increased risk of associated hemorrhage [44, 45].

A clinical diagnosis of JPS is made based on the following criteria [46]: (i) more than five juvenile polyps of the colon or rectum, (ii) juvenile polyps in other parts of the GI tract, or (iii) any number of juvenile polyps together with family history of JPS.

Cancer risks and relevant risk management recommendations are described in Table 13.2. The lifetime risk for individuals with JPS of developing colorectal and upper GI (predominantly gastric) cancers is estimated to be 38% and 21%, respectively [47–49]. The median age of diagnosis is reported at 42 years. Cancers of the colon and stomach are the most commonly observed in JPS, although there are small numbers of individuals with JPS presenting with cancers of the pancreas, small bowel, duodenum, and jejunum [48, 50]. Cancers typically occur in the third or fourth decade of life. A recent publication has suggested that those harboring *SMAD4* germline mutations are associated with a more aggressive upper GI malignancy risk than those with *BMPR1A* [42], although these results should be interpreted with some caution given the small number of included subjects.

The rationale for surveillance is to reduce morbidity related to polyposis [3], and approaches can vary depending on the clinical presentation of the individual. Guidelines have been published from both the UK [51] and USA [52]. Colonoscopy is generally recommended from age 12 to 15 (or earlier if symptomatic) and repeated every 2–3 years if no polyps are detected. If polyps are present, they should be sent for histological examination and colonoscopies repeated annually thereafter. The frequency can be reduced if subsequent scopes are clear. In cases where the polyp burden is too high, colectomy can be considered. Upper GI surveillance with endoscopy is recommended to commence between age 15 and 25 (or earlier if symptomatic), with the frequency dependent on polyp findings (as described above). Additionally, surveillance and treatment for HHT complications is necessary for all *SMAD4* carriers, and international guidelines have been published [53]. Recommendations for HHT described in Table 13.2 are for asymptomatic individuals only.

2.2 Genetics

Two genes are currently known to cause JPS: *BMPR1A,* a type 1 receptor of the transforming growth factor beta (TGF-β) super family, located on 10q22.3, and *SMAD4*, a tumor suppressor gene, located on 18q21.2. Approximately 40–60% of individuals with JPS will carry a germline mutation in either the *SMAD4* or *BMPR1A* genes [44, 54]. Large deletions account for 14% of detected mutations, and a further 10% are found in the promoter region of *BMPR1A*. As mentioned previously, there is a reported genotype-phenotype correlation where mutations in the *SMAD4* gene are associated with a higher risk of large gastric polyps and a higher risk of upper GI malignancy than those in *BMPR1A* [42, 43]. Additionally, unlike *SMAD4* germline mutation carriers, those harboring *BMPR1A* germline mutations are not at risk of HHT. Both proteins encoded by *SMAD4* and *BMPR1A* work in the TGF-β pathway, which is involved in a number of cellular processes including cell growth, differentiation, apoptosis, and cellular homeostasis [3].

As is the case for PJS, once a causative mutation has been identified in the proband, at-risk blood relatives can then undergo predictive testing. Approximately 75% of JPS individuals will have an affected parent. Testing can be considered for the proband's siblings regardless of the parents' results due to the small possibility of gonadal mosaicism (although this has not been reported in PJS previously). Offspring of the proband are at 50% risk of inheriting the causative mutation and should be offered testing.

3 PTEN-Hamartoma Tumor Syndromes

3.1 Clinical Characteristics

PHTS (OMIM 601728) encompasses a number of related syndromes all caused by germline mutations in the *PTEN* gene including (i) Cowden syndrome (OMIM 158350), (ii) Bannayan-Riley-Ruvalcaba syndrome (OMIM 153480), (iii) *PTEN*-related Proteus syndrome, and (iv) Proteus-like syndrome. *PTEN*-related Proteus syndrome and Proteus-like syndrome are particularly rare overgrowth syndromes and are still not thoroughly understood and thus won't be discussed here. The phenotypic spectrum of PHTS is wide and variable, with Cowden syndrome (CS) and Bannayan-Riley-Ruvalcaba syndrome (BRRS) sharing the most overlap [3]. CS was first described in 1963 and was named after the first patient reported with the condition, Rachel Cowden [55]. It wasn't until a decade later that Bannayan described the first patient with the condition later named BRRS [56].

3.1.1 Cowden Syndrome

CS is characterized by the presence of multiple hamartomas of the skin and mucous membranes, mucocutaneous lesions, macrocephaly, and an increased risk of benign and malignant lesions of the breast, thyroid, and endometrium [57, 58]. The incidence is estimated to be 1 in 200,000 live births [59, 60], although this figure is believed to be an underestimate due to underdiagnosis. It is believed that more than 90% of individuals with germline *PTEN* mutations will be symptomatic by age 20 and 100% by age 30 [58]. The mucocutaneous lesions are pathognomonic for CS and include trichilemmomas, papillomatous papules, and acral keratosis. GI polyps are commonly reported in CS and histologically can include hamartomatous, hyperplastic, or adenomatous polyps and rarely ganglioneuromas [2, 61–64]. Upper GI involvement includes esophageal glycogenic acanthosis. Fibrocystic breast disease, uterine leiomyoma, thyroid nodules, and goiters are part of the CS spectrum.

In 1995, the International Cowden Consortium established diagnostic criteria for CS, which at the time facilitated Nelen et al. in their search for the CS candidate gene [59]. It has since been revised [57], and it is now reviewed annually by the US National Comprehensive Cancer Network (Table 13.3). Later in 2011, using phenotype and genotype data from more than 3000 CS or CSL probands, Tan et al. developed a scoring system that calculates the *PTEN* mutation likelihood for a given individual based on their age and clinical presentation [65]. This was demonstrated to have greater sensitivity and positive predictive value for germline *PTEN* mutations relative to the diagnostic criteria (described in Table 13.3). This web-based

Table 13.3 The International Cowden Consortium diagnostic criteria

Pathognomonic criteria	Major criteria	Minor criteria
Adult Lhermitte-Duclos disease (LDD)	Breast cancer	Other thyroid lesions (e.g., adenoma, multinodular goiter)
Facial trichilemmomas	Epithelial thyroid carcinoma (non-medullary, especially follicular)	Cognitive impairment
Acral keratoses	Macrocephaly	Hamartomatous intestinal polyps
Papillomatous papules	Endometrial cancer	Fibrocystic breast disease
Mucosal lesions		Lipomas
		Fibromas
		Genitourinary tumors (especially renal)
		Genitourinary malformations
		Uterine leiomyoma

An operational diagnosis of CS is made by meeting one of the following:

Pathognomonic mucocutaneous lesions combined with one of the following:

- Six or more facial papules, of which three or more must be trichilemmoma
- Cutaneous facial papules and oral mucosal papillomatosis
- Oral mucosal papillomatosis and acral keratosis
- Six or more palmoplantar keratoses

Two or more major criteria

One major and three or more minor criteria

Four or more minor criteria

In a family in which one individual meets the diagnostic criteria above, other relatives are diagnosed with CS if they meet any one of the following:

The pathognomonic criteria

Any one major criterion with or without minor criteria

Two minor criteria

History of Bannayan-Riley-Ruvalcaba syndrome

tool enables clinicians to identify those most appropriate for genetics referral and *PTEN* genetic testing.

Cancer risks and relevant risk management recommendations are described in Table 13.2. Studies evaluating malignancy in CS report high cancer risks [66–69]. Tan et al. [69] reported a lifetime risk of breast cancer to be 85.2%, thyroid cancer (tend to be follicular histology) 35.2%, endometrial cancer 28%, colorectal cancer 9%, renal carcinoma 33.6%, and melanoma 6%. Two independent studies report similarly high lifetime risks of these cancers [66, 68]. A recent study reported a family with a novel germline frameshift *PTEN* mutation and a history of esophageal cancer, suggesting variability in the PHTS-related cancer spectrum [70]. Surveillance for cancers other than breast is controversial; however, many follow the guidelines published by the National Comprehensive Cancer Network [71]. These recommend individuals with *PTEN* mutations to undergo surveillance for breast, endometrial, and thyroid cancer and colonoscopy for polyp surveillance [72, 73]. They also suggest consideration of dermatological and renal surveillance.

3.1.2 Bannayan-Riley-Ruvalcaba Syndrome

BRRS is characterized by macrocephaly, developmental delay, lipomatosis, GI hamartomatous polyps, hemangiomatosis, and pigmented macules on the glans penis in males [3, 56]. Hamartomatous polyps have been reported in approximately 45% of individuals with BRRS, particularly in the ileum and colon [74]. These polyps can increase the risk of intussusceptions and rectal bleeding; however, they are not believed to increase the risk of GI cancer. Originally it was thought that BRRS was not associated with risk of malignancy; however, it is now believed that those who carry a germline *PTEN* mutation (approximately 60%) are at a similar level of risk as those with CS and should therefore follow risk management guidelines discussed previously for PHTS [72].

3.2 Genetics

PHTS is usually caused by the presence of germline mutations in the *PTEN* tumor suppressor gene located on 10q23.3. *PTEN* [57, 75]. Depending on the inclusion criteria, the mutation detection rate is reported to be between 25% and 80% [58, 75]. A recent study estimated the de novo mutation rate to be between 10.7% and 47.6% [76]. Additionally, this study illustrated that often family history was not obvious in cases where the *PTEN* mutation was proven to be inherited, particularly in cases where the proband was a child. It is therefore important that all parents of *PTEN* mutation-positive individuals be offered predictive testing. It is also appropriate in certain cases to offer predictive testing to children relatives, given PHTS features can occur in childhood. Testing can be considered for the proband's siblings regardless of the parents' results due to the small possibility of gonadal mosaicism.

Offspring of the proband are at 50% risk of inheriting the causative mutation and should be offered testing.

There are a number of individuals who have CS or CS-like (CSL) features who do not have a detectable germline mutation in *PTEN*. There have now been a number of other possible candidate genes identified. Germline mutations in the *SDH* genes [67, 77, 78] and *KLLN* epimutations have been detected in CS/CSL individuals [67, 79]. Nizialek et al. [79] demonstrated significant levels of *KLLN* promoter methylation in CS/CSL individuals when compared with controls and that methylation load correlated with stronger CS phenotypes. The *KLLN* epimutation was also identified in *PTEN* mutation-positive individuals, thus suggesting its presence as a potential modifier of *PTEN*-related presentations. While paragangliomas and pheochromocytomas typically associated with *SDH* germline mutations are not commonly observed in CS/CSL, there is some overlap in terms of thyroid and renal cancer risk. Ni et al. [78] reported a higher frequency of breast, thyroid, and renal malignancies in those CS/CSL individuals with *SDH* germline mutations. More recently, it has been shown that *PTEN* mutations and *SDH* variants are not necessarily mutually exclusive in CS/CSL individuals and the risk of breast cancer appears to be higher when both are present as opposed to *PTEN* mutations alone [77]. This suggests that the *SDH* genes have roles both in the predisposition and risk modification for CS/CSL-related malignancies. A recent case study reported the identification of a germline gain-of-function *EGFR* mutation in an individual with Lhermitte-Duclos disease, a pathognomonic feature of CS [80]. Additionally, *SEC23B* [81] and *USF3* [82] gene mutations may be involved in the predisposition of thyroid cancer in CS/CSL individuals.

4 Other Hamartomatous Polyposis Conditions

There have been a number of other conditions where hamartomatous polyps have been reported including Gorlin syndrome (basal cell nevus syndrome), hereditary mixed polyposis syndrome, multiple endocrine neoplasia 2B (MEN2B), and neurofibromatosis type 1 (NF1). Clinicians should be aware of these differential diagnoses in the context of hamartomatous polyposis, albeit rarely the cause.

Gorlin syndrome (OMIM 109400) is characterized by multiple basal cell carcinomas, odontogenic keratocysts, childhood medulloblastoma, frontal bossing, ovarian tumors, and palmar and plantar pits. It is an autosomal dominant condition, caused by germline mutations in *PTCH1* and SUFU and rarely *PTCH2* [3]. A 1970s case report described a 54-year-old male with Gorlin syndrome who was found to have multiple gastric hamartomatous polyps and a benign mesenteric cyst [83]. However, hamartomatous polyps are not commonly seen, and so GI surveillance is not routinely recommended in Gorlin syndrome.

Hereditary mixed polyposis syndrome (OMIM 601299) is a relatively recently described condition where individuals typically present with a mixed pattern of polyps in the colon, including adenomas, hyperplastic polyps, and hamartomatous polyps. A more recent case review of 10 patients with this condition found adenomatous polyps and mixed hyperplastic and inflammatory type polyps to be the predominant finding, with no hamartomatous polyps identified in these individuals [84]. Individuals with this condition have been shown to have higher colorectal cancer risk [85]. Mapping studies have identified chromosomal regions 6q [86] and 10q23, which also encompasses *BMPR1A*, and later studies have implicated this gene in some families presenting with this condition [87, 88]. More recently, a duplication including the *SCGS* gene just upstream of the *GREM1* gene was identified in a family with hereditary mixed polyposis syndrome [85].

Ganglioneuromatosis in the GI tract has been reported in both NF1 (OMIM 162200) and MEN2B (OMIM 162300), which are among the types of polyps described in PHTS [89, 90]. The incidence of NF1 is 1 in 5000 live births and is caused by germline mutations in the *NF1* gene. It is characterized by multiple neurofibromas, café au lait macules, iris Lisch nodules, and axillary and inguinal freckling. Whilst there is associated cancer risk with NF1, GI cancer does not seem to be part of the spectrum [91, 92]. MEN2B is a specific subtype of MEN2 caused by germline mutations in the *RET* gene, typically M918 T, and is associated with medullary thyroid cancer, pheochromocytoma and distinctive facies with enlarged lips, marfanoid body habitus, ocular features, and musculoskeletal manifestations. In addition to the GI tract, the mucosal ganglioneuromas in MEN2B individuals can occur on the lips, tongue, conjunctiva, and urinary system [93]

Disclosure of Potential Conflict of Interest No author had any relevant financial or personal relationships that could inappropriately influence or bias this work.

References

1. Schreibman IR, Baker M, Amos C, McGarrity TJ. The Hamartomatous polyposis syndromes - a clinical and molecular review. Am J Gastroenterol. 2005;100:476–90.
2. Ngeow J, Heald B, Rybicki LA, et al. Prevalence of germline PTEN, BMPR1A, SMAD4, STK11, and ENG mutations in patients with moderate-load colorectal polyps. Gastroenterology. 2013;144:1402–9. https://doi.org/10.1053/j.gastro.2013.02.001.
3. Jelsig AM. Hamartomatous polyps – a clinical and molecular genetic study. Dan Med J. 2016. https://doi.org/10.1111/cge.12693.
4. Aretz S. The differential diagnosis and surveillance of hereditary gastrointestinal polyposis syndromes. Dtsch Arztebl Int. 2010;107:163–73. https://doi.org/10.3238/arztebl.2010.0163.
5. van Lier M, Wagner A, Mathus-Vliegen E, et al. High cancer risk in Peutz–Jeghers syndrome: a systematic review and surveillance recommendations. Am J Gastroenterol. 2010;105:1258–64. https://doi.org/10.1038/ajg.2009.725.
6. Latchford A, Phillips R. Gastrointestinal polyps and cancer in Peutz-Jeghers syndrome: clinical aspects. Familial Cancer. 2011;10:455–61. https://doi.org/10.1007/s10689-011-9442-1.
7. Giardiello F, Trimbath J. Peutz-Jeghers syndrome and management recommendations. Clin Gastroenterol Hepatol. 2006;4:408–15. https://doi.org/10.1016/j.cgh.2005.11.005.
8. Entius MM, Westerman AM, Giardiello FM, et al. Peutz-Jeghers polyps, dysplasia, and K-ras codon 12 mutations. Gut. 1997;41:320–2.

9. Yaguchi T, Wen-Ying L, Hasegawa K, et al. Peutz-Jeghers polyp with several foci of glandular dysplasia: report of a case. Dis Colon Rectum. 1982;25:592–6.
10. Beggs A, Latchford A, Vasen H, et al. Peutz-Jeghers syndrome: a systematic review and recommendations for management. Gut. 2010;59:975–86. https://doi.org/10.1136/gut.2009.198499.
11. Vogel T, Schumacher V, Saleh A, et al. Extraintestinal polyps in Peutz-Jeghers syndrome: presentation of four cases and review of the literature. Deutsche Peutz-Jeghers-Studiengruppe. Int J Color Dis. 2000;15:118–23.
12. Amos CI, Keitheri-Cheteri MB, Sabripour M, et al. Genotype-phenotype correlations in Peutz-Jeghers syndrome. J Med Genet. 2004;41:327–33. https://doi.org/10.1136/jmg.2003.010900.
13. Giardiello FM, Brensinger JD, Tersmette AC, et al. Very high risk of cancer in familial Peutz–Jeghers syndrome. Gastroenterology. 2000;119:1447–53. https://doi.org/10.1053/gast.2000.20228.
14. Hearle N, Schumacher V, Menko FH, et al. Frequency and Spectrum of cancers in the Peutz-Jeghers syndrome. Clin Cancer Res. 2006;12:3209–15. https://doi.org/10.1158/1078-0432.CCR-06-0083.
15. Korsse SE, Harinck F, van Lier MGF, et al. Pancreatic cancer risk in Peutz-Jeghers syndrome patients: a large cohort study and implications for surveillance. J Med Genet. 2013;50:59–64. https://doi.org/10.1136/jmedgenet-2012-101277.
16. Lim W, Olschwang S, Keller JJ, et al. Relative frequency and morphology of cancers in STK11 mutation carriers1 ☆. Gastroenterology. 2004;126:1788–94. https://doi.org/10.1053/j.gastro.2004.03.014.
17. Resta N, Pierannunzio D, Lenato GM, et al. Cancer risk associated with STK11/LKB1 germline mutations in Peutz–Jeghers syndrome patients: results of an Italian multicenter study. Dig Liver Dis. 2013;45:606–11. https://doi.org/10.1016/j.dld.2012.12.018.
18. Mehenni H, Resta N, Park J-G, et al. Cancer risks in LKB1 germline mutation carriers. Gut. 2006;55:984–90. https://doi.org/10.1136/gut.2005.082990.
19. Korsse SE, Dewint P, Kuipers EJ, van Leerdam ME. Small bowel endoscopy and Peutz-Jeghers syndrome. Best Pract Res Clin Gastroenterol. 2012;26:263–78. https://doi.org/10.1016/j.bpg.2012.03.009.
20. Jelsig AM, Qvist N, Brusgaard K, et al. Hamartomatous polyposis syndromes: a review. Orphanet J Rare Dis. 2014;9:101. https://doi.org/10.1186/1750-1172-9-101.
21. van Lier M, Mathus-Vliegen E, Wagner A, et al. High cumulative risk of intussusception in patients with Peutz–Jeghers syndrome: time to update surveillance guidelines? Am J Gastroenterol. 2011;106:940–5. https://doi.org/10.1038/ajg.2010.473.
22. Goldstein SA, Hoffenberg EJ. Peutz-Jegher syndrome in childhood. J Pediatr Gastroenterol Nutr. 2013;56:191–5. https://doi.org/10.1097/MPG.0b013e318271643c.
23. Brown G, Fraser C, Schofield G, et al. Video capsule endoscopy in Peutz-Jeghers syndrome: a blinded comparison with barium follow-through for detection of small-bowel polyps. Endoscopy. 2006;38:385–90. https://doi.org/10.1055/s-2006-925028.
24. Gupta A, Postgate AJ, Burling D, et al. A prospective study of MR Enterography versus capsule endoscopy for the surveillance of adult patients with Peutz-Jeghers syndrome. Am J Roentgenol. 2010;195:108–16. https://doi.org/10.2214/AJR.09.3174.
25. Aretz S, Stienen D, Uhlhaas S, et al. High proportion of large genomic STK11 deletions in Peutz-Jeghers syndrome. Hum Mutat. 2005;26:513–9. https://doi.org/10.1002/humu.20253.
26. Papp J, Kovacs ME, Solyom S, et al. High prevalence of germline STK11 mutations in Hungarian Peutz-Jeghers syndrome patients. BMC Med Genet. 2010;11:169. https://doi.org/10.1186/1471-2350-11-169.
27. Mehenni H, Resta N, Guanti G, et al. Molecular and clinical characteristics in 46 families affected with Peutz–Jeghers syndrome. Dig Dis Sci. 2007;52:1924–33. https://doi.org/10.1007/s10620-006-9435-3.
28. Plawski A, Cichy W, Klincewicz B. Juvenile polyposis syndrome. Arch Med Sci. 2014;10:570–7. https://doi.org/10.5114/aoms.2014.43750.

29. Chen H-M, Fang J-Y. Genetics of the hamartomatous polyposis syndromes: a molecular review. Int J Color Dis. 2009;24:865–74. https://doi.org/10.1007/s00384-009-0714-2.
30. Latchford A, Neale K, Phillips R, Clark S. Juvenile polyposis syndrome: a study of genotype, phenotype, and long-term outcome. Dis Colon Rectum. 2012;55:1038–43. https://doi.org/10.1097/DCR.0b013e31826278b3.
31. Brosens LA, Langeveld D, Arnout W, et al. Juvenile polyposis syndrome. World J Gastroenterol. 2011;17:4839–44. https://doi.org/10.3748/wjg.v17.i44.4839.
32. Kapetanakis A, Vini D, Plitsis G. Solitary juvenile polyps in children and colon cancer. Hepato-Gastroenterology. 1996;43:1530–1.
33. Nugent KP, Talbot IC, Hodgson SV, Phillips RK. Solitary juvenile polyps: not a marker for subsequent malignancy. Gastroenterology. 1993;105:698–700.
34. Coburn M, Pricolo V, DeLuca F, Bland K. Malignant potential in intestinal juvenile polyposis syndromes. Ann Surg Oncol. 1995;2:386–91.
35. Sachatello CR, Griffen WO. Hereditary polypoid diseases of the gastrointestinal tract: a working classification. Am J Surg. 1975;129:198–203.
36. Sachatello CR, Hahn IS, Carrington CB. Juvenile gastrointestinal polyposis in a female infant: report of a case and review of the literature of a recently recognized syndrome. Surgery. 1974;75:107–14.
37. Alimi A, Weeth-Feinstein LA, Stettner A, et al. Overlap of juvenile polyposis syndrome and cowden syndrome due to de novo chromosome 10 deletion involving BMPR1A and PTEN: implications for treatment and surveillance. Am J Med Genet. 2015;167:1305–8. https://doi.org/10.1002/ajmg.a.36876.
38. Delnatte C, Sanlaville D, Mougenot J-F, et al. Contiguous gene deletion within chromosome arm 10q is associated with juvenile polyposis of infancy, reflecting cooperation between the BMPR1A and PTEN tumor-suppressor genes. Am J Hum Genet. 2006;78:1066–74. https://doi.org/10.1086/504301.
39. Menko F, Kneepkens C, De Leeuw N, et al. Variable phenotypes associated with 10q23 microdeletions involving the PTEN and BMPR1A genes. Clin Genet. 2008;74:145–54. https://doi.org/10.1111/j.1399-0004.2008.01026.x.
40. Merg A, Howe JR. Genetic conditions associated with intestinal juvenile polyps. Am J Med Genet. 2004;129:44–55. https://doi.org/10.1002/ajmg.c.30020.
41. Desai D, Murday V, Phillips R, et al. A survey of phenotypic features in juvenile polyposis. J Med Genet. 1998;35:476–81.
42. Aytac E, Sulu B, Heald B, et al. Genotype-defined cancer risk in juvenile polyposis syndrome. Br J Surg. 2015;102:114–8. https://doi.org/10.1002/bjs.9693.
43. Friedl W, Uhlhaas S, Schulmann K, et al. Juvenile polyposis: massive gastric polyposis is more common in MADH4 mutation carriers than in BMPR1A mutation carriers. Hum Genet. 2002;111:108–11. https://doi.org/10.1007/s00439-002-0748-9.
44. Aretz S, Stienen D, Uhlhaas S, et al. High proportion of large genomic deletions and a genotype phenotype update in 80 unrelated families with juvenile polyposis syndrome. J Med Genet. 2007;44:702–9. https://doi.org/10.1136/jmg.2007.052506.
45. O'Malley M, LaGuardia L, Kalady MF, et al. The prevalence of hereditary hemorrhagic telangiectasia in juvenile polyposis syndrome. Dis Colon Rectum. 2012;55:886–92. https://doi.org/10.1097/DCR.0b013e31825aad32.
46. Jass J, Williams C, Bussey H, Morson B. Juvenile polyposis--a precancerous condition. Histopathology. 1988;13:619–30.
47. Brosens LA, van Hattem A, Hylind LM, et al. Risk of colorectal cancer in juvenile polyposis. Gut. 2007;56:965–7. https://doi.org/10.1136/gut.2006.116913.
48. Howe J, Mitros F, Summers R. The risk of gastrointestinal carcinoma in familial juvenile polyposis. Ann Surg Oncol. 1998;5:751–6.
49. Ma C, Giardiello FM, Montgomery EA. Upper tract juvenile polyps in juvenile polyposis patients: dysplasia and malignancy are associated with foveolar, intestinal, and pyloric differentiation. Am J Surg Pathol. 2014;38:1618–26. https://doi.org/10.1097/PAS.0000000000000283.

50. Walpole IR, Cullity G, Opitz JM, Reynolds JF. Juvenile polyposis: a case with early presentation and death attributable to adenocarcinoma of the pancreas. Am J Med Genet. 1989;32:1–8. https://doi.org/10.1002/ajmg.1320320102.
51. Cairns SR, Scholefield JH, Steele RJ, et al. Guidelines for colorectal cancer screening and surveillance in moderate and high risk groups (update from 2002). Gut. 2010;59:666–89. https://doi.org/10.1136/gut.2009.179804.
52. Syngal S, Brand RE, Church JM, et al. ACG clinical guideline: genetic testing and management of hereditary gastrointestinal cancer syndromes. Am J Gastroenterol. 2015;110:223–62. https://doi.org/10.1038/ajg.2014.435.
53. Faughnan M, Palda V, Garcia-Tsao G, et al. International guidelines for the diagnosis and management of hereditary haemorrhagic telangiectasia. J Med Genet. 2011;48:73–87. https://doi.org/10.1136/jmg.2009.069013.
54. Howe J, Sayed M, Ahmed A, et al. The prevalence of MADH4 and BMPR1A mutations in juvenile polyposis and absence of BMPR2, BMPR1B, and ACVR1 mutations. J Med Genet. 2004;41:484–91. https://doi.org/10.1136/jmg.2004.018598.
55. Daly MB, Pilarski R, Axilbund J, et al. NCCN Guidelines Insights: Genetic/Familial High-Risk Assessment:Breast and Ovarian, Version 2.2017 J Natl Compr Canc Netw 2017;15:9–20 doi:10.6004/jnccn.2017.0003.
56. Bannayan G. Lipomatosis, angiomatosis, and macrencephalia. A previously undescribed congenital syndrome. Arch Pathol. 1971;92:1–5.
57. Eng C. Will the real Cowden syndrome please stand up: revised diagnostic criteria. J Med Genet. 2000;37:828–30. https://doi.org/10.1136/jmg.37.11.828.
58. Ngeow J, Eng C. PTEN hamartoma tumor syndrome: clinical risk assessment and management protocol. Methods. 2015;77–78:11–9. https://doi.org/10.1016/j.ymeth.2014.10.011.
59. Nelen MR, Padberg GW, Peeters EAJ, et al. Localization of the gene for Cowden disease to chromosome 10q22–23. Nat Genet. 1996;13:114–6. https://doi.org/10.1038/ng0596-114.
60. Uppal S, Mistry D, Coatesworth A. Cowden disease: a review. Int J Clin Pract. 2007;61:645–52. https://doi.org/10.1111/j.1742-1241.2006.00896.x.
61. Coriat R, Mozer M, Caux E, et al. Endoscopic findings in Cowden syndrome. Endoscopy. 2011;43:723–6. https://doi.org/10.1055/s-0030-1256342.
62. Heald B, Mester J, Rybicki L, et al. Frequent gastrointestinal polyps and colorectal adenocarcinomas in a prospective series of PTEN mutation carriers. Gastroenterology. 2010;139:1927–33. https://doi.org/10.1053/j.gastro.2010.06.061.
63. Levi Z, Baris HN, Kedar I, et al. Upper and lower gastrointestinal findings in PTEN mutation-positive Cowden syndrome patients participating in an active surveillance program. Clin Transl Gastroenterol. 2011;2:e5. https://doi.org/10.1038/ctg.2011.4.
64. Stanich PP, Owens VL, Sweetser S, et al. Colonic polyposis and neoplasia in Cowden syndrome. Mayo Clin Proc. 2011;86:489–92. https://doi.org/10.4065/mcp.2010.0816.
65. Tan M-H, Mester J, Peterson C, et al. A clinical scoring system for selection of patients for PTEN mutation testing is proposed on the basis of a prospective study of 3042 probands. Am J Hum Genet. 2011;88:42–56. https://doi.org/10.1016/j.ajhg.2010.11.013.
66. Bubien V, Bonnet F, Brouste V, et al. High cumulative risks of cancer in patients with PTEN hamartoma tumour syndrome. J Med Genet. 2013;50:255–63. https://doi.org/10.1136/jmedgenet-2012-101339.
67. Ngeow J, Mester J, Rybicki LA, et al. Incidence and clinical characteristics of thyroid cancer in prospective series of individuals with Cowden and Cowden-like syndrome characterized by germline PTEN, SDH, or KLLN alterations. J Clin Endocrinol Metab. 2011;96:E2063–71. https://doi.org/10.1210/jc.2011-1616.
68. Nieuwenhuis MH, Kets CM, Murphy-Ryan M, et al. Cancer risk and genotype–phenotype correlations in PTEN hamartoma tumor syndrome. Familial Cancer. 2014;13:57–63. https://doi.org/10.1007/s10689-013-9674-3.
69. Tan M, Mester J, Ngeow J, et al. Lifetime cancer risks in individuals with germline PTEN mutations. Clin Cancer Res. 2012;18:400–7. https://doi.org/10.1158/1078-0432.CCR-11-2283.

70. Sherman SK, Maxwell JE, Qian Q, et al. Esophageal cancer in a family with hamartomatous tumors and germline PTEN frameshift and SMAD7 missense mutations. Cancer Genet. 2015;208:41–6. https://doi.org/10.1016/j.cancergen.2014.11.002.
71. NCCN. Genetic/familial high-risk assessment: breast and ovarian. Natl Compr Cancer Netw. 2016.
72. Ngeow J, Liu C, Zhou K, et al. Detecting germline PTEN mutations among at-risk patients with cancer: an age- and sex-specific cost-effectiveness analysis. J Clin Oncol. 2015;33:2537–44. https://doi.org/10.1200/JCO.2014.60.3456.
73. Ngeow J, Stanuch K, Mester JL, et al. Second malignant neoplasms in patients with Cowden syndrome with underlying germline PTEN mutations. J Clin Oncol. 2014;32:1818–24. https://doi.org/10.1200/JCO.2013.53.6656.
74. Gorlin RJ, Cohen MM, Condon LM, Burke BA. Bannayan-Riley-Ruvalcaba syndrome. Am J Med Genet. 1992;44:307–14. https://doi.org/10.1002/ajmg.1320440309.
75. Marsh D, Kum J, Lunetta K, et al. PTEN mutation spectrum and genotype-phenotype correlations in Bannayan-Riley-Ruvalcaba syndrome suggest a single entity with Cowden syndrome. Hum Mol Genet. 1999;8:1461–72.
76. Mester J, Eng C. Estimate of de novo mutation frequency in probands with PTEN hamartoma tumor syndrome. Genet Med. 2012;14:819–22. https://doi.org/10.1038/gim.2012.51.
77. Ni Y, He X, Chen J, et al. Germline SDHx variants modify breast and thyroid cancer risks in Cowden and Cowden-like syndrome via FAD/NAD-dependant destabilization of p53. Hum Mol Genet. 2012;21:300–10. https://doi.org/10.1093/hmg/ddr459.
78. Ni Y, Zbuk KM, Sadler T, et al. Germline mutations and variants in the succinate dehydrogenase genes in Cowden and Cowden-like syndromes. Am J Hum Genet. 2008;83:261–8. https://doi.org/10.1016/j.ajhg.2008.07.011.
79. Nizialek EA, Mester JL, Dhiman VK, et al. KLLN epigenotype-phenotype associations in Cowden syndrome. Eur J Hum Genet. 2015;23:1538–43. https://doi.org/10.1038/ejhg.2015.8.
80. Colby S, Yehia L, Niazi F, et al. Exome sequencing reveals germline gain-of-function EGFR mutation in an adult with Lhermitte-Duclos disease. Cold Spring Harb Mol Case Stud. 2016;2:a001230. https://doi.org/10.1101/mcs.a001230.
81. Yehia L, Niazi F, Ni Y, et al. Germline heterozygous variants in SEC23B are associated with Cowden syndrome and enriched in apparently sporadic thyroid cancer. Am J Hum Genet. 2015;97:661–76. https://doi.org/10.1016/j.ajhg.2015.10.001.
82. Ni Y, Seballos S, Fletcher B, et al. Germline compound heterozygous poly-glutamine deletion in USF3 may be involved in predisposition to heritable and sporadic epithelial thyroid carcinoma. Hum Mol Genet. ddw382. 2016. https://doi.org/10.1093/hmg/ddw382.
83. Schwartz R. Basal-cell-nevus syndrome and gastrointestinal polyposis. N Engl J Med. 1978;299:49. https://doi.org/10.1056/NEJM197807062990118.
84. Plesec T, Brown K, Allen C, et al. Clinicopathological features of a kindred with SCG5-GREM1–associated hereditary mixed polyposis syndrome. Hum Pathol. 2017;60:75–81. https://doi.org/10.1016/j.humpath.2016.10.002.
85. Jaeger E, Leedham S, Lewis A, et al. Hereditary mixed polyposis syndrome is caused by a 40-kb upstream duplication that leads to increased and ectopic expression of the BMP antagonist GREM1. Nat Genet. 2012;44:699–703. https://doi.org/10.1038/ng.2263.
86. Thomas HJ, Whitelaw SC, Cottrell SE, et al. Genetic mapping of hereditary mixed polyposis syndrome to chromosome 6q. Am J Hum Genet. 1996;58:770–6.
87. Cao X, Eu KW, Kumarasinghe MP, et al. Mapping of hereditary mixed polyposis syndrome (HMPS) to chromosome 10q23 by genomewide high-density single nucleotide polymorphism (SNP) scan and identification of BMPR1A loss of function. J Med Genet. 2006;43:e13. https://doi.org/10.1136/jmg.2005.034827.
88. O'Riordan JM, O'Donoghue D, Green A, et al. Hereditary mixed polyposis syndrome due to a BMPR1A mutation. Color Dis. 2009;12:570–3. https://doi.org/10.1111/j.1463-1318.2009.01931.x.
89. Agaimy A, Vassos N, Croner RS. Gastrointestinal manifestations of neurofibromatosis type 1 (Recklinghausen's disease): clinicopathological spectrum with pathogenetic considerations. Int J Clin Exp Pathol. 2012;5:852–62.

90. Moline J, Eng C. Multiple endocrine neoplasia type 2: an overview. Genet Med. 2011;13:755–64. https://doi.org/10.1097/GIM.0b013e318216cc6d.
91. Uusitalo E, Rantanen M, Kallionpää RA, et al. Distinctive cancer associations in patients with Neurofibromatosis type 1. J Clin Oncol. 2016;34:1978–86. https://doi.org/10.1200/JCO.2015.65.3576.
92. Walker L, Thompson D, Easton D, et al. A prospective study of neurofibromatosis type 1 cancer incidence in the UK. Br J Cancer. 2006;95:233–8. https://doi.org/10.1038/sj.bjc.6603227.
93. Wells SA, Asa SL, Dralle H, et al. Revised American Thyroid Association guidelines for the Management of Medullary Thyroid Carcinoma. Thyroid. 2015;25:567–610. https://doi.org/10.1089/thy.2014.0335.

Chapter 14
Hereditary Mixed Polyposis Syndrome

Huw Thomas and Ian Tomlinson

Abstract Hereditary mixed polyposis syndrome (HMPS) is an autosomal dominant inherited condition in which affected individuals develop colorectal polyps of multiple and mixed histological type including serrated lesions, Peutz-Jeghers polyps, juvenile polyps, conventional adenomas and colorectal carcinomas in the absence of any extra-colonic features. Most of the families described to date are Ashkenazi Jewish and have an ancestral founder mutation with a duplication of 40 kb upstream of the *GREM1* gene. This leads to increased and ectopic expression of *GREM1* in the colonic crypt. A smaller duplication of about 16 kb also upstream of *GREM1* has been reported in a Swedish HMPS family. Presymptomatic genetic testing is now available in these families, and affected individuals require careful colonoscopic surveillance from an early age, with polypectomy to prevent the development of colorectal cancer.

Keywords Hereditary mixed polyposis syndrome · HMPS · GREM1 · Colorectal cancer

1 Introduction

Other chapters in this book have described inherited polyposis syndromes associated with adenomatous, serrated, Peutz-Jeghers and juvenile colonic polyps, in which there is a clearly defined phenotype. Hereditary mixed polyposis syndrome (HMPS) is an unusual inherited condition in that the clinical phenotype includes multiple polyps of mixed histological types and, indeed, individual polyps that may

H. Thomas (✉)
St Mark's Hospital, Imperial College London, Harrow, UK
e-mail: huw.thomas@imperial.ac.uk

I. Tomlinson
Institute of Cancer and Genomic Studies, University of Birmingham, Birmingham B15 2TT, UK
e-mail: i.tomlinson@bham.ac.uk

L. Valle et al. (eds.), *Hereditary Colorectal Cancer*,
https://doi.org/10.1007/978-3-319-74259-5_14

contain mixed histology. There is a great phenotypic variation between individual gene carriers with some having serrated and adenomatous polyps and others also having juvenile or even Peutz-Jeghers-type polyps. Extra-colonic cancers have not been a consistent feature of HMPS families.

The condition was originally described in a large Ashkenazi Jewish kindred. Genetic studies showed linkage to chromosome 15q13-q31. Genetic linkage studies in other Ashkenazi Jewish families who had multiple colorectal adenomas had previously showed linkage to this region. The HMPS and multiple adenoma families were shown to have the same disease-associated haplotype on chromosome 15 indicating a founder mutation.

The genetic event causing HMPS in the Ashkenazi Jewish families has been shown to be a duplication that results in increased expression of the Gremlin-1 (*GREM1*) gene in the colonic crypt. A Swedish kindred with HMPS has been reported with a smaller duplication in the same region that also affects *GREM1* expression.

The chapter will review the clinical phenotype of HMPS and the overlap with other conditions such as attenuated polyposis, serrated polyposis and juvenile polyposis, the genetic alteration of *GREM1* and how this is thought to result in the development of mixed polyps, the role of presymptomatic diagnosis in families and the role of colonoscopic surveillance to prevent the development of colorectal cancer.

2 Clinical Phenotype

Hereditary mixed polyposis syndrome was first described in a large Ashkenazi Jewish kindred. The proband presented to St Mark's Hospital in London in 1956 at the age of 38 with rectal bleeding. Rigid sigmoidoscopy revealed polyps in his rectum. He was a member of a large family of Lithuanian origin (St Mark's Family 96) with a history of colonic polyps and colorectal cancer that appeared to be inherited in an autosomal dominant fashion. A provisional diagnosis of familial polyposis coli was made. He was regularly reviewed with barium enema and rigid sigmoidoscopy. He developed a large colonic polyp and underwent a colectomy and ileo-rectal anastomosis in 1962. In the colectomy specimen, there were six polyps, five of which were tubular adenomas and one of which was a juvenile-type polyp with overlapping histological features (Fig. 14.1). He did not have the multiple adenomas and microadenomas characteristic of familial adenomatous polyposis. The case was classified as a polyposis of unspecified type by Basil Morson.

Other family members were contacted and asked for their clinical history and a pedigree constructed. In 1995 Whitelaw et al. published a description of the phenotype of St Mark's Family 96 and called the condition hereditary mixed polyposis syndrome [1]. At that time there were 20 second-generation, 64 third-generation, 102 fourth-generation and 42 fifth-generation family members (Fig. 14.2).

Affected family members of St Mark's Family 96 had presented with bowel symptoms at a median age of 42. One hundred fifty-four colorectal polyps from family members underwent histopathological review. These included 101 tubular

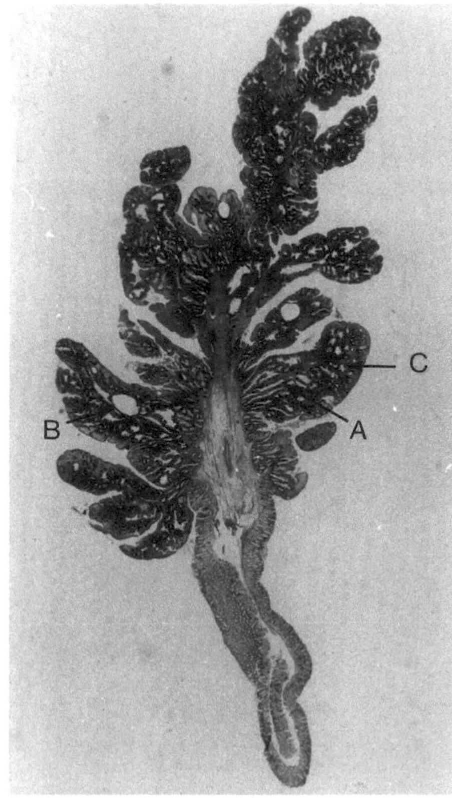

Fig. 14.1 A mixed hyperplastic/juvenile/adenomatous polyp with a hyperplastic area (**a**), juvenile area (**b**) and adenomatous area (**c**) (Fig. 2 reproduced from Whitelaw et al. [1]. Page 329)

adenomas, 7 villous adenomas, 25 hyperplastic polyps and 25 atypical or mixed juvenile polyps. Typically, fewer than 15 polyps were found at colonoscopy, and polyps had been detected at an age as young as 18 years. Eleven family members had had a colectomy. Thirteen family members had developed colorectal cancer at a median age of 47 with a range of 32 to 74. The cancers were evenly distributed through the colon and rectum. Upper gastrointestinal polyps were not reported.

In 2003 Rosen et al. reviewed 17 affected members of St Mark's Family 96 who lived in Israel [2]. They had had 10 juvenile polyps, 21 mixed juvenile and adenomatous polyps, 18 hyperplastic polyps, 1 mixed hyperplastic and adenomatous polyps, 12 serrated adenomas and 2 tubular adenomas. There were cases of pancreatic, renal and breast cancer, although these cancers were not definitively linked to HMPS.

The phenotype of other Ashkenazi Jewish families from St Mark's with the same founder mutation has been described. Affected individuals had multiple adenomatous polyps with large adenomas occurring at an age as young as 22 and 24 and serrated polyps and colorectal cancers presenting between the ages of 31 and 67 [3]. The spectrum of histological types of polyps reported in HMPS has changed over the years as sessile serrated polyps have been recognised in addition to adenomatous, hyperplastic and juvenile polyps.

A Swedish HMPS family has recently been described with a similar but smaller duplication in the *GREM1* regulatory region on chromosome 15. Affected individuals

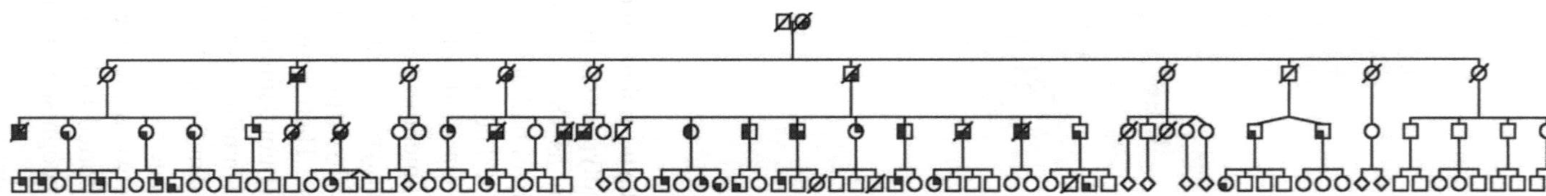

Fig. 14.2 Pedigree of St Mark's Family 96. Generations 1 (pedigree founders) to 4. Individuals affected by colorectal cancer are denoted by an obscure symbol in the lower, right-hand quadrant. An obscure upper left-hand quadrant shows the presence of atypical juvenile polyps, and an obscure lower left-hand quadrant shows the presence of adenomatous polyps. An obscure upper right-hand quadrant denotes that an individual is affected by a benign, non-hyperplastic polyp but that the pathology report did not distinguish between adenomas and juvenile-like polyps (Modified from Ballester-Vargas and Tomlinson [15])

also have polyps of mixed histological type that include adenomatous, hyperplastic and juvenile polyps. One individual was diagnosed with a colorectal cancer at the age of 33. There were two cases of gastric cancer, one of breast and one of lymphosarcoma reported in the family [4].

A patient who developed colorectal cancer at the age of 35 has been reported who had a large duplication encompassing the entire *GREM1* gene, but no further details of colonic polyps or family history are available [5].

In summary, the phenotype of HMPS is varied with polyps of diverse histological types presenting at an age as young as 18 years. In some individuals there are multiple adenomatous polyps and in others serrated, adenomatous and juvenile polyps. Cases of colorectal cancer have been diagnosed as early as 31 years of age. There are no reports of upper gastrointestinal polyps as are found in familial adenomatous polyposis.

There has been discussion about the definition of HMPS due to the overlap of the clinical phenotype with that of juvenile polyposis [6]. Inherited conditions are now defined by molecular genetics as there is a considerable phenotypic overlap between several different types of polyposis. In some cases the overlap may be due to different genes in the same pathway being altered, as is the case for juvenile polyposis and HMPS, which both involve defective bone morphogenetic protein (BMP) signalling.

3 Molecular Genetics

When the phenotype of Family 96 was originally described, it was not clear whether this was an atypical form of a recognised polyposis syndrome or a distinct disorder. Initial genetic linkage studies in Family 96 excluded linkage to the then known colorectal cancer genes *APC*, *MSH2* and *MLH1* [1].

In 1996 a genome-wide genetic linkage study mapped the gene to chromosome 6q16-q21 [7]. However, subsequently an individual (4.30) from Family 96 without the putative disease-associated haplotype on chromosome 6 developed a large colonic villous adenoma at the age of 42. This suggested that the reported location of the HMPS gene on chromosome 6 was incorrect.

Further linkage studies were undertaken with updated clinical information and a more stringent definition of affected status [8]. With these new criteria, linkage to chromosome 6 was not replicated, but linkage was found to chromosome 15q13-q21. It was noted that in colorectal cancers from family members, loss of heterozygosity at the locus on chromosome 15 was not detected suggesting that it may not be the site of a typical tumour suppressor gene.

Linkage to the same region of chromosome 15 had previously been demonstrated in another Ashkenazi Jewish family at St Mark's (Family 1311) with a dominantly inherited predisposition to multiple colorectal adenomas and colorectal cancer [3]. When the disease-associated haplotypes of the two families were compared, they were identical. Three further Ashkenazi Jewish families with multiple colorectal adenomas were also shown to have the same disease-associated haplotype.

Analysis of candidate genes in the region on chromosome 15 did not detect any significant alterations. This suggested that there might be an unusual genetic event associated with a single founder mutation [9].

Oligonucleotide arrays showed a heterozygous single copy duplication of 40Kb on chromosome 15q from intron 2 of the *SCG5* gene to a site just upstream of the *GREM1* CpG island. No difference in the expression of *SCG5* was detected in affected individuals. The duplication included enhancer elements of the *GREM1* gene, and increased expression of *GREM1* was demonstrated not only in intestinal subepithelial myofibroblasts but also at very high levels in crypt epithelial cells [10]. Increased expression was also seen in HMPS polyps [9].

GREM1 is a secreted antagonist of BMP signalling, binding to BMP ligands and preventing them from activating the pathway. Increased expression of GREM1 would be expected to reduce BMP ligand levels and promote a stem cell phenotype. It is of note that a reduction of BMP signalling is the likely cause of juvenile polyposis syndrome in which either the type 1A BMP receptor (*BMPR1A*) or the downstream effector *SMAD4* is mutated and functionally defective.

Subsequent studies in a mouse model have demonstrated that aberrant epithelial expression of GREM1 disrupts the intestinal morphogen gradients in the intestinal crypt, altering daughter cell fate and leading to the persistence of stem cell properties in cells that have exited the stem cell niche. These cells form ectopic crypts, proliferate, accumulate somatic mutations and can initiate intestinal neoplasia. Aberrant expression of *GREM1* has also been demonstrated in sporadic colonic traditional serrated adenomas that are rare, premalignant polyps [11].

GREM1 is thought to act as a landscaper gene affecting the maturation of colon crypt cells. This would explain why loss of heterozygosity on chromosome 15 is not seen in HMPS tumours as would be expected if it had been acting as a tumour suppressor gene. It may also explain the development of polyps of mixed histological type, since *GREM1* does not direct a tumour down any particular molecular pathway.

4 Presymptomatic Genetic Testing

The ancestral Ashkenazi HMPS duplication has a unique DNA sequence at the breakpoint, and this has been used to develop a simple PCR diagnostic test to determine carriage of the duplication in Ashkenazi Jewish individuals. Carriage of the duplication has been shown to be rare in the Ashkenazi Jewish population. A similar test has not yet been developed for the Swedish duplication.

5 Management of Affected and At-Risk Individuals

In HMPS significant colorectal polyps have been diagnosed at an age as young as 18 years and cases of colorectal cancer have been diagnosed as young as 31 years of age. Colonoscopic surveillance should start by 18 years of age. There is a great variation in the number and types of polyps that develop in affected individuals.

It has been suggested that initially colonoscopy should be two yearly and the frequency adjusted depending on the number and type of polyps found.

In other intestinal polyposis syndromes, upper gastrointestinal polyps have been reported, and there is an increased incidence of upper gastrointestinal cancer. Lieberman et al. have recently reported an HMPS family with the Ashkenazi duplication in which the proband's father, who carried the duplication, had a phenotype similar to that of familial adenomatous polyposis with >50 colonic adenomas, a desmoid tumour and a duodenal carcinoma [12]. There are also two cases of gastric cancer in earlier generations of the Swedish family with a duplication affecting *GREM 1* expression [4]. Upper gastrointestinal neoplasia has been recently reported in a *GREM1* duplication carrier [12]. This may need review when the genotypes of these individuals have been further analysed. Various extraintestinal cancers have been reported in HMPS families, but it is not clear whether the frequency is greater than that expected in the Ashkenazi Jewish population.

Increased COX2 expression in polyps from individuals with HMPS has been reported [13]. Aspirin has been shown to reduce the incidence of colorectal cancer in individuals at high familial risk of colorectal cancer and in those at population risk although the precise mechanism is not certain [14]. There may be a role for aspirin chemoprevention in HMPS, but it would currently not be possible to undertake an adequately powered study to investigate this.

6 Conclusion

HMPS is a rare condition in which colorectal polyps of mixed histological type develop as a consequence of mutations that affect the expression of the *GREM1* gene and alter bone morphogenetic protein signalling. There is an increased incidence of colorectal cancer. There is uncertainty as to whether it may also be associated with an increased incidence of upper gastrointestinal cancers. Affected individuals require colonoscopic surveillance and possibly upper gastrointestinal surveillance.

References

1. Whitelaw SC, Murday VA, Tomlinson IPM, Thomas HJW, Cottrell S, Ginsberg A, Bukofzer S, Hodgson SV, Skudowitz RB, Jass JR, Talbot IC, Northover JMA, Bodmer WF, Solomon E. Clinical and molecular features of hereditary mixed polyposis syndrome. Gastroenterology. 1997;112:327–34.
2. Rosen P, Samual Z, Brazowski E. A prospective study of the clinical, genetic screening and pathologic features of a family with hereditary mixed polyposis syndrome. Am J Gastroenterol. 2003;98:2317–20.
3. Tomlinson I, Rahman N, Frayling I, Mangion J, Barfoot R, Hamoudi R, Seal S, Northover J, Thomas HJ, Neale K, Hodgson S, Talbot I, Houlston R, Stratton MR. Inherited susceptibility

to colorectal adenomas and carcinomas: evidence for a new predisposition gene on 15q14-q22. Gastroenterology. 1999;116:789–95.

4. Rohlin A, Eiengard F, Lundstam U, Zagoras T, Nilsson S, Edsjo A, Pedersen J, Svensson J, Skullman S, Goran Karlsson B, Bjork J, Nordling M. GREM1 and POLE variants in hereditary colorectal cancer syndromes. Genes Chromosomes Cancer. 2016;55:95–106.
5. Venkatachalam R, Verwiel ETP, Kamping EJ, Hoenselaar E, Gorgens H, Schackert HK, van Krieken HJM, Ligtenberg MJL, Hoorerbrugge N, van Kessel AG, Kuiper RP. Identification of candidate predisposing copy number variants in familial and early-onset colorectal cancer patients. Int J Cancer. 2011;129:1635–42.
6. Tomlinson I, Jaeger E, Leedham S, Thomas H. The classification of intestinal polyposis. Nat Genet. 2013;45:2–3.
7. Thomas HJW, Whitelaw SC, Cottrell SC, Murday VA, Tomlinson IPA, Markie D, Jones T, Bishop DT, Hodgson SV, Sheer D, Northover JMA, Talbot IC, Solomon E, Bodmer WF. Genetic mapping of the hereditary mixed polyposis syndrome to chromosome 6q. Am J Hum Genet. 1996;58:770–6.
8. Jaegers EEM, Woodford-Richens KL, Lockett M, Rowan AJ, Sawyer EJ, Heinimann K, Rozen P, Murday VA, Whitelaw SC, Ginsberg A, Atkin WS, Lynch HT, Southey MC, Eng C, Bodmer WF, Talbot IC, Hodgson SV, Thomas HJW, Tomlinson IPM. An ancestral Ashkenazi haplotype at the HMPS/CRAC1 locus is associated with hereditary mixed polyposis syndrome. Am J Hum Genet. 2003;72:1261–7.
9. Jaeger E, Leedham S, Lewis A, Segditsas S, Becker M, Cuadrado PR, Davis H, Kaur K, Heinimann K, Howarth K, East J, Taylor J, Thomas H, Tomlinson I. Hereditary mixed polyposis syndrome is caused by a 40-kb upstream duplication that leads to increased and ectopic expression of the BMP antagonist GREM1. Nat Genet. 2012;44:699–703.
10. Lewis A, Freeman-Mills L, de la Calle-Mustienes E, Giráldez-Pérez RM, Davis H, Jaeger E, Becker M, Hubner NC, Nguyen LN, Zeron-Medina J, Bond G, Stunnenberg HG, Carvajal JJ, Gomez-Skarmeta JL, Leedham S, Tomlinson I. A polymorphic enhancer near GREM1 influences bowel cancer risk through differential CDX2 and TCF7L2 binding. Cell Rep. 2014;8:983–90.
11. Davis H, Irshad S, Bansal M, Rafferty H, Boitsova T, Bardella C, Jaeger E, Lewis A, Freeman-Mills L, Castro Giner F, Rodenas-Cuadrado P, Mallappa S, Clark S, Thomas H, Jeffrey R, Poulsom R, Rodriguez-Justo M, Novelli M, Chetty R, Silver A, Sansom O, Greten F, Wang LM, East J, Tomlinson I, Needham S. Subtypes of inherited and sporadic colorectal cancer result from GREM-1 induced acquisition of progenitor-like features by differentiated intestinal epithelial cells. Nat Med. 2015;21:62–70.
12. Lieberman S, Walsh T, Schechter M, Adar T, Goldin E, Beeri R, Sharon N, Baris H, Ben Avi L, Half E, Lerer I, Shirts B, Pritcahrd C, Tomlinson I, King M, Levy-Lahad E, Peretz T, Goldberg Y. Features of patients with hereditary mixed polyposis syndrome caused by duplication of GREM1 and implications for screening and surveillance. Gastroenterology. 2017;156: 1876–80.
13. Brazowski E, Misonzhnick-Bedny F, Rosen P. Immunohistochemical expression of COX-2 in polyps of hereditary mixed polyposis syndrome suggests the possibility of chemoprevention. Dig Dis Sci. 2004;49:1906–11.
14. Burn J, Gerdes A-M, McCrea F, Mecklin J-P, Moeslein G, Olschwang S, Eccles D, Evans DG, Maher ER, Bertario L, Bisgaard M-L, Dunlop M, JWC H, Hodgson SV, Lindblom A, Lubinski J, Morrison PJ, Murday V, Ramesar R, Side L, Scott RJ, Thomas HJW, Vasen HF, Barker G, Crawford G, Elliott F, Movahedi M, Pylvanainen K, Wijnen JT, Fodde R, Lynch HT, Mathers JC, Bishop DT on behalf of the CAPP2 Investigators. Long-term effect of aspirin on cancer risk in carriers of hereditary colorectal cancer: an analysis from the CAPP2 randomised controlled trial. Lancet. 2011;378:2081–7.
15. Ballester-Vargas V, Tomlinson I. Hereditary mixed polyposis syndrome. In: Boardman LA, editor. Intestinal Polyposis Syndromes: Springer. ISBN 987-3-319-28101-8.

Chapter 15
Serrated Polyposis Syndrome

Sabela Carballal, Francesc Balaguer, and Antoni Castells

Abstract Serrated polyps (SPs) are considered the precursor lesions of up to 15–30% of all colorectal carcinomas through the "serrated neoplasia pathway." Serrated polyposis syndrome (SPS), characterized by the presence large and/or numerous serrated lesions spreading throughout the colorectum, is emerging as one of the most common colorectal cancer polyp syndromes. This condition is associated with an increased personal and familial colorectal cancer risk. Clinical management includes yearly surveillance colonoscopy and surgery. Although the majority of cases occur in patients older than 50 years old with no family history of CRC, several lines of evidence support that a proportion of SPS could be the phenotypic expression of an inherited genetic syndrome, but the genetic basis for SPS remains elusive. Recent studies provided proof of the pathogenicity of *RNF43* germline mutation in a small subset of patients. Future research in SPS should be focused on understanding the phenotype and clinical management and on unraveling the pathogenesis of the syndrome.

Keywords Serrated polyp · Hyperplastic polyp · Polyposis · Colorectal carcinogenesis · Serrated pathway

1 Clinical Features

1.1 Definition and Cancer Risk

Colorectal cancer (CRC) arises through precursor lesions, called polyps, and the timely detection and removal of these polyps is essential in CRC prevention [1]. Traditionally, conventional adenomas were considered the only precursor lesions

S. Carballal · F. Balaguer · A. Castells (✉)
Gastroenterology Department, Hospital Clínic de Barcelona, Centro de Investigación, Biomédica en Red de Enfermedades Hepáticas y Digestivas (CIBERehd), Institut d'Investigacions Biomediques August Pi i Sunyer (IDIBAPS), Universitat de Barcelona, Barcelona, Spain
e-mail: castells@clinic.cat

L. Valle et al. (eds.), *Hereditary Colorectal Cancer*,
https://doi.org/10.1007/978-3-319-74259-5_15

Table 15.1 Serrated polyp subtypes: endoscopic, histological, and molecular features

Serrated polyp subtype	Endoscopic description	Pathological features	Molecular marker
Hyperplastic polyp (HP)			
Microvesicular hyperplastic polyp (MVHP)	Distal colon. Flat Multiplicity in the rectum	Small droplet ("microvesicular") mucin within the cytoplasm of most cells	*BRAF* (30–80%) *KRAS* (10%)
Goblet cell hyperplastic Polyp (GCHP)	Left colon (≈90%) Typically very small (< 0.5 cm)	Nearly exclusive presence of goblet cells, few or no luminal serrations (compared to MVHPs)	*BRAF* (20%) *KRAS* (50%)
Sessile serrated adenoma/polyp (SSA/P)	Proximal colon, flat Usually >0.5 cm Covered by mucus cap Cloud-like surface	Distorted crypt growth pattern Dilated, mucus-filled, L-shaped ("boot") and T-shaped ("anchor") crypts Serration at the basis of the crypt	*BRAF* (80–90%) *KRAS* (3–8%)
Traditional serrated adenoma (TSA)	Distal colon Sessile or pedunculated Size often >0.5 cm	Complex and distorted tubulovillous or villous ("filiform") configuration, eosinophilic cytoplasm, ectopic crypts	*BRAF* (20–60%) *KRAS* (20–25%)

that would develop into CRC through the "adenoma-carcinoma" pathway [2]. In contrast, hyperplastic polyps, typically observed in the rectum, were thought to be benign. Over the last 30 years, growing evidence has given rise to an alternative pathway, called "serrated pathway," characterized morphologically by the presence of serrated lesions and molecularly by somatic mutations in the *BRAF* proto-oncogene, hypermethylation of the promoter regions of tumor suppressor genes, and microsatellite instability. This pathway is currently considered the responsible of up to 15–30% of all CRC [3, 4].

Serrated polyps (SPs) are defined as heterogeneous group of lesions morphologically characterized by serrated ("saw-tooth") architecture of the epithelium that lines the colonic crypts [5]. The World Health Organization (WHO) classifies SPs into three subgroups: hyperplastic polyps (HPs), sessile serrated adenomas/polyps (SSA/Ps) with or without dysplasia, and traditional serrated adenomas/polyps (TSA/Ps). The main features defining each serrated polyp subtype are reported in Table 15.1.

Hyperplastic polyps (HPs) are common, accounting for 70–90% of all SP. They are characterized by the presence of straight crypts, which extend symmetrically from the surface of the polyp to the muscularis mucosae without significant distortion. Distinct subtypes of HPs have been recognized; basically HPs are subdivided into microvesicular (MVHP) and goblet cell (GCHP) types, based on the characteristics of lining epithelium. MVHPs and GCHPs are well characterized and display considerable differences in molecular and histological features as well as anatomic

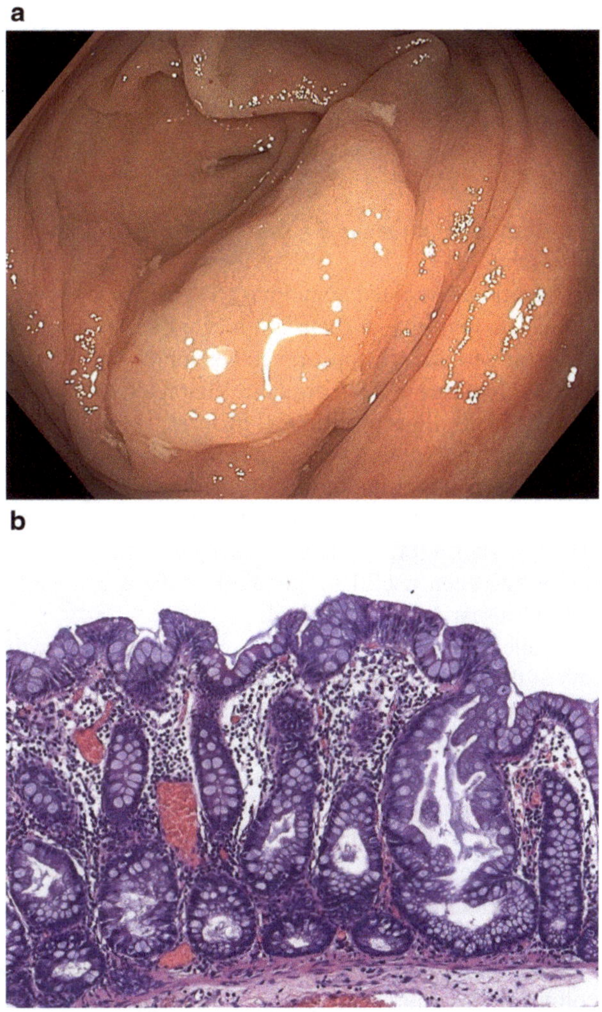

Fig. 15.1 Endoscopic and histological appearance of sessile serrated adenoma/polyps. (**a**) A slightly elevated lesion located at cecum was detected during endoscopic examination in patient with serrated polyposis syndrome. After washing the adherent mucus over the polyp surface its indistinct edges, "cloud-like" surface and color similar to surrounding mucosa could be appreciated. Polyp was removed by endoscopic mucosal resection. (**b**) Microscopically, the polyp showed a marked serration and dilated, mucus-filled T-shaped ('anchor') crypts, corresponding to a sessile serrated adenoma/polyp

distribution within the colon. HPs are considered of less clinical importance, especially if they are diminutive and located in the rectosigmoid. It is unclear whether some MVHP can progress to SSA/Ps. The significance of GCHP is poorly understood; some authors have suggested that it may represent the precursor lesion of TSA.

Sessile serrated adenomas (SSAs) are often subtle, appear flat or slightly elevated, and can be covered by yellow mucus. They are typically found in the proximal colon and they are usually larger than 0.5 mm. Histologically, the serrations are more prominent than those of hyperplastic polyps and involve the entire length of the crypt (Fig. 15.1). SSA/Ps, especially when cytological dysplasia is present, are considered the main precursors of serrated colorectal carcinomas [6, 7]. They

Table 15.2 Revised World Health Organization (WHO) criteria for SPS

Criterion I. 5 or more serrated polyps proximal to the sigmoid colon, 2 of them larger than 10 mm.
Criterion II. Any number of serrated polyps proximal to the sigmoid in an individual who has any first-degree relative with SPS
Criterion III. More than 20 serrated polyps distributed throughout the colon

represent approximately 5–25% of all SPs and are found in 3.3% of average risk population [8].

Traditional serrated adenomas (TSAs) are less common than other types of SPs (1%). The majority of them are located at the distal colon, they are often >5 mm, and their endoscopic appearance resembles conventional adenomas. The histopathological features of TSA are quite characteristic, often showing a complex and distorted tubulovillous or villous ("filiform") configuration.

Serrated polyposis syndrome (SPS) is a condition characterized by the combination of large and/or numerous serrated lesions spreading throughout the colorectum with an increased life-time risk of CRC [9–14]. Revised World Health Organization (WHO) criteria for SPS are represented in Table 15.2. Although arbitrary, this definition has been useful to standardize the diagnosis and treatment, as well as to prompt research in such a field.

While the prevalence of SPS remains unknown, this syndrome is emerging as one of the most common colorectal cancer polyp syndromes. Endoscopic detection and histopathological characterization is a challenge in clinical practice. Increased awareness of serrated polyps has likely improved the diagnosis of SPS, suggesting that the prevalence is greater than initially reported. Indeed, prevalence of SPS in primary colonoscopy or sigmoidoscopy screening programs was reported to be <0.1%, while recent data suggest a four-time higher prevalence [8]. The prevalence of SPS in preselected screening populations based on a positive fecal immunochemical test (FIT) has been reported to be considerably higher (0.34–0.66%) [15, 16]. Moreover, SPS is often missed during a first screening colonoscopy. The rate of SPS after follow-up, as reported in the FIT-based screening cohort (0.8%) and in primary colonoscopy cohort (0.4%), seems to be more accurate estimates of the true prevalence of SPS.

Initial small series of patients with SPS reported up to 70% rates of CRC [14], a figure that probably traduced an important selection bias, overestimating the perception of CRC in SPS. The prevalence of CRC reported in subsequent studies, with a larger number of patients, showed a lower risk between 7% and 35% [11, 17–21]. Few studies have tried to stratify the CRC risk based on clinical risk factors [20, 22, 23]. Indeed, patients who fulfill both WHO criteria I and III, the presence of advanced adenomas or dysplasia within serrated polyps, and the number of SSA/P are factors that have been associated with an increased risk of CRC in SPS patients. However, cancer risk in patients fulfilling criterion II remains controversial. Since proximal SPs are detected in 4.7–12.2% of the screening population [8], this criterion is probably leading to an overdiagnosis of SPS and should be revised in the near future.

This high prevalence of CRC is far from the rate of incident CRC observed in the two largest and most recent cohorts of patients with SPS. Current observations suggest that once patients with SPS undergo endoscopic surveillance with polyp removal (at least those >3 mm), the CRC risk is very low (5-year-cumulative incidence of CRC around 2%) [22, 23].

1.2 Clinical Characteristics

Characteristics of patients with SPS have been defined mainly based on the publication of series of cases, with significant heterogeneity in the description of the clinical, endoscopic, and histological features. There is no apparent sex predominance and the mean age at diagnosis is between 50 and 60 years. Cigarette smoking history and overweight/obesity have been associated with an increased risk of developing serrated polyps [24], suggesting that environmental factors are involved in the pathogenesis. In this sense, current smoking has been strongly associated with the presence of advanced SP [25]. However, recent studies suggest that the pathogenesis of SPS might be different in smokers and non-smokers [24]. History of smoking (current and former smokers) is significantly associated to fulfillment of WHO criterion III only, compared with non-smokers [23]. Additionally, the CRC risk seems to be smaller in the smokers than in the non-smokers [23]. Future research needs to clarify the role of smoking in SPS and might influence the options for therapy and surveillance for smokers in the near future.

Some authors have suggested the existence of various phenotypes within the SPS definition. Some patients display a right-sided phenotype with large SSA/P (i.e., criterion I), some present with a left-sided phenotype with a greater amount of small polyps (i.e., criterion III), and others show a mixed phenotype with shared features of the previous phenotypes [20]. As mentioned, patients who fulfill both WHO criteria I and III seem to be at increased risk to be diagnosed with CRC, compared with patients who fulfill WHO criterion I or WHO criterion III only [23]. Conventional adenomas frequently coexist with serrated polyps in patients with SPS. There is no clear evidence of an increased risk of extracolonic neoplasms in patients with SPS and their relatives [12].

Between 10 and 50% of SPS patients report a family history of CRC [14, 18–21, 26, 27], and first-degree relatives of SPS patients have an increased risk for both CRC and SPS compared with the general population. In the largest series, the standardized incidence ratio of CRC in first-degree relatives of patients with SPS was approximately five times that of the general population [20].

1.3 Clinical Management

Due to the high risk of CRC in patients with SPS, scientific societies recommend 1-year endoscopic surveillance in all patients with SPS diagnosis [28]. Patients undergoing annual colonoscopy surveillance in experienced centers, with removal of polyps >3 mm, show a low risk of developing CRC (<2% in 5 years) [12, 22]. Ongoing follow-up studies are evaluating whether endoscopic surveillance can be performed at longer time intervals in a subset of patients that do not display CRC risk factors.

Surgical management should be restricted to cases with severe polyposis that is unmanageable endoscopically, unresectable large lesions, or the presence of CRC. The decision for an extended (total colectomy with ileo-rectal anastomosis if the rectum is spared) vs. segmental colectomy needs to be individualized for each patient. After surgery, it is advisable to conduct surveillance of the remaining colorectum every 6–12 months for the risk of metachronous lesions.

First-degree relatives of patients with SPS should undergo CRC screening starting at the age of 35–40 years or 10 years before the age of diagnosis of the youngest affected family member [29, 30].

2 Molecular Features and Pathogenesis

2.1 Serrated Pathway of Carcinogenesis

The serrated pathway has recently emerged as an alternative pathway leading to sporadic CRC. The well-characterized molecular changes associated with serrated pathway are (1) mutations in *BRAF* and *KRAS* oncogenes, (2) microsatellite instability (MSI), and (3) CpG island methylator phenotype (CIMP) (Fig. 15.2).

The mitogen-activated protein kinase (MAPK) pathway activation through mutation of the *BRAF* and *KRAS* oncogenes leads to uncontrolled cell proliferation. The most distinct molecular alteration associated with the serrated neoplasia pathway is a mutation in the *BRAF* proto-oncogene [31]. Moreover, aberrant hypermethylation of CpG islands in the promoter region of a gene can result in its silencing. In practice, the CIMP status of a given lesion is determined by the assessment of the promoter methylation status of a panel 1 of five genes, in which hypermethylation of at least three genes is considered to be CIMP high and methylation of one or two genes is considered CIMP low. CIMP-high tumors have been strongly associated with the serrated neoplasia pathway [32, 33]. An example of a tumor suppressor gene that is usually silenced in CIMP tumors is the mismatch repair gene *MLH1*. The silencing of this gene results in sporadic microsatellite instability, comparable to hereditary microsatellite instability in patients with Lynch syndrome. For this reason, the serrated neoplasia pathway is often referred to as the sporadic microsatellite instability pathway. However, not all CIMP tumors develop microsatellite instability. The

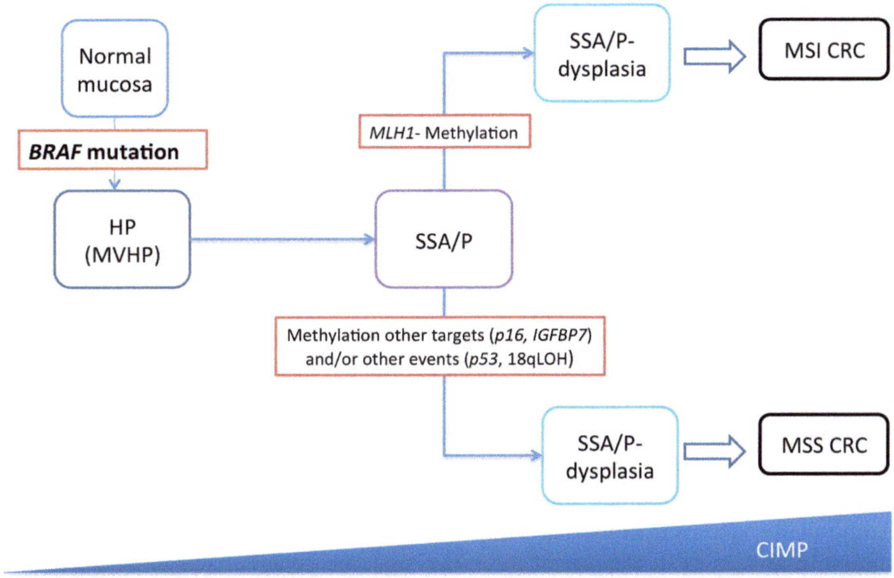

Fig. 15.2 Serrated pathway of colorectal carcinogenesis. Oncogenic *BRAF* mutation is detected in the earliest serrated lesions, especially in MVHP. *MLH1* methylation leads to MSI tumors. In contrast, methylation in other targets (i.e., *p16INK4a*, *IGFBP7*, and *MGMT*) is associated with MSS CRCs. Abbreviations: *MSI-H* high microsatellite instability, *MSS* microsatellite stability, *CIMP* CpG island methylator phenotype

silencing of other tumor suppressor genes, such as *p16INK4a*, *IGFBP7*, and *MGMT*, might also have a prominent role in the development of CIMP-high microsatellite stable tumors.

Serrated pathway of colorectal carcinogenesis is represented in Fig. 15.2. Oncogenic *BRAF* (V600E) mutation seems to be the earliest event in the "classical serrated pathway" that proposes a progression from MVHP → SSA/P → SSA/P with cytological dysplasia → CRC. This sequence occurs most commonly in the proximal colon, leading to tumors that show CIMP high.

An alternative serrated pathway has been described, characterized by *KRAS* instead of *BRAF* mutation as earliest event, CIMP low, and progression to TSA from GCHP. However, this alternate pathway remains poorly understood [34].

Despite the association between SSA/Ps and serrated adenocarcinomas, up to 50% of patients with SPS develop CRC at the rectosigmoid or left colon, and *BRAF* mutation is observed only in 33% of CRC [35]. These data suggest that, in the setting of SPS, a considerable proportion of CRCs may arise from an adenoma rather than serrated polyps. Further prospective studies are needed to clarify the relationship between histopathology and CRC development in SPS [22, 23].

2.2 Pathogenesis

Given that most patients with SPS are diagnosed in the 50s, with no family history of polyposis, and a strong association with environmental factors (i.e., smoking) [21, 23], it has been suggested that, overall, SPS is not an inherited genetic syndrome and rather behaves as a complex disorder where disease appears as a consequence of the interaction of genetic susceptibility and environment.

Nevertheless, several lines of evidence support that a small proportion of SPS could be the phenotypic expression of an inherited genetic syndrome: first-degree relatives of patients with SPS appear to have an increased risk for both CRC and SPS [26, 36]. Also, the multiplicity of lesions and the unrelenting and sometimes rapid development of colorectal neoplasia in affected individuals suggest that, for a minority of cases, a genetic basis is yet to be discovered. Both autosomal and recessive patterns of inheritance have been described. Biallelic *MUTYH* mutations have been reported in some patients fulfilling the WHO criteria of SPS usually in the context of a concomitant attenuated form of adenomatous polyposis [37]. Additionally, studies in individual families have reported linkage to loci on chromosomes 1p and 2q [37]. Despite of these findings, the genetic basis of SPS remains largely unknown.

3 RNF43-Associated Serrated Polyposis

BRAF or *KRAS* mutations that are associated with serrated polyps are alone insufficient to induce intestinal tumorigenesis. After a short period of hyperproliferation, crypt cells undergo growth arrest due to metabolic and replicative stress, a process termed oncogene-induced senescence. Recently, a whole-exome sequencing study of 20 unrelated subjects with multiple SSA/Ps identified mutations in several putative genes (*ATM, PIF1, TELO2, XAF1, RBL1,* and *RNF43*) functionally related to oncogene-induced senescence [37].

RNF43 is an E3 ubiquitin ligase expressed in colon stem cells that acts as a Wnt inhibitor by targeting Wnt receptors for degradation. It regulates Wnt signal strength through the R-spondin/LGR5/RNF43 module, with its effect antagonized by the Wnt amplifier R-spondin [38, 39]. In the mentioned study, two patients shared the same germline nonsense mutation in *RNF43* (p.R113X), indicating that it is also associated with multiple serrated polyps (odds ratio, 460; 95% confidence interval, 23.1–16.384; $p = 6.8 \times 10^{-5}$).

Another study reported a family with two siblings carrying germline nonsense *RNF43* mutation (p.R132X) and numerous serrated polyps at a young age, one of whom developed a CRC with microsatellite instability (MSI) [40].

More recently, Yan et al. [41] reported the results from a combination of whole-exome sequencing and target gene Sanger sequencing to study SPS families, sporadic SPs, and CRCs. In one out four SPS families, exome sequencing identified a germline likely pathogenic mutation in *RNF43* (c.953-1G > A; c.953_954delAG; p.E318fs). This mutation was detected in two siblings who fulfilled WHO criteria I and/or III for SPS and also in a third sibling with one SP proximal to the sigmoid (criterion II of WHO) and a rectal cancer diagnosed at 49 years old. Several SPs at right colon were also detected during screening colonoscopy in the two children of this last case (both confirmed gene carriers). One gene carrier could not be screened, and the other four family members that did not carry the germline mutation had normal colonoscopies. In addition, *RNF43* second hit by loss of heterozygosity or somatic mutation was observed in all serrated polyps (n = 16), adenomas (n = 5), and CRCs (n = 1) arising from germline *RNF43* mutation carriers. Concurrently, somatic *RNF43* mutations were identified in 34% of sporadic SSAs/TSAs, but 0% of HPs. Another recent study also reported frequent *RNF43* somatic mutations in SPs [42].

The results reported by Yan et al. suggest that germline *RNF43* mutations are responsible for a subgroup of SPS patients, and that should become part of the routine germline testing in SPS patients.

4 Unexplained Serrated Polyposis

After Yan et al. publication, the results of two genetic screens of a large cohort of individuals with SPS have been published [43]. The 295 individuals of these cohorts were recruited from the Genetics of Colorectal Polyposis Study. The first screen comprised 74 individuals with SPS selected based on early age at diagnosis, high numbers of SPs throughout the colon, and having a first-degree relative with SPS or CRC. By performing whole-exome or whole-genome sequencing, no pathogenic variants were identified; however, two uncommon non-synonymous variants predicted to be damaging were detected in a single carrier each (*RNF43* NM_017763; exon6, c.C640G; p.L214 V and exon4, c.C443G; p.A148G). A second targeted genetic screen was performed specifically testing for the *RNF43* p.R113X and p.R132X variants to determine their prevalence in individuals with SPS (n = 221). None of the tested individuals with SPS were carriers of either of these two *RNF43* germline pathogenic variants.

The scarcity of *RNF43* germline pathogenic variants in these 295 patients with SPS indicates that mutations in *RNF43* may account for only a small proportion of SPS suggesting that additional genetic risk factors for SPS are yet to be identified. Given these results, it is likely that the underlying genetic cause of SPS is genetically complex and heterogeneous.

4.1 Future Directions

Serrated polyposis syndrome is an emerging disease associated with an increased CRC risk. Although a great body of evidence has emerged in the last decade, many challenges remain ahead:

- Reassessment of the WHO definition criteria. Based on current knowledge, some aspects of the current WHO guidelines for the diagnosis of SPS could be challenged. Current diagnostic criteria exclude lesions based on their location in the rectosigmoid. This seems mainly due to the fact that diminutive HPs in the rectosigmoid should probably not be taken into account for the diagnosis of SPS. However, up to 50% of CRC in SPS occur in this location. Accordingly, it would seem reasonable to reassess the WHO criteria and not exclude lesions purely on their location without taking into account their size and histopathology. Also, as mentioned above, WHO criterion II should be probably removed from the definition of SPS. These adjustments to the current WHO guidelines could help in defining those patients who are at risk of developing CRC.
- CRC risk stratification. Which patients benefit most from surveillance colonoscopy or prophylactic surgery? Future studies should mainly focus on the safety and feasibility of personalized treatment and surveillance for patients with SPS according to CRC risk factors in order to decrease the colonoscopy burden as well as the incidence of colonoscopy interval CRCs.
- Improving colonoscopy diagnosis. The detection rate of serrated polyps is widely variable among endoscopists [44].The role of ancillary techniques (narrow band imaging, chromoendoscopy) needs to be defined in SPS.
- Unraveling the genetic cause of SPS. Although it is likely that the majority of the highly penetrant familial CRC genes have been already discovered, it is likely that SPS displays genetic heterogeneity and new candidate genes wait to be discovered. Moreover, the role of low- or moderate-penetrance genes that interact with other genetic variants and/or environmental factors (i.e., smoking) will need to be clarified.

References

1. Winawer SJ, Zauber AG, Ho MN, O'Brien MJ, Gottlieb LS, Sternberg SS, et al. Prevention of colorectal cancer by colonoscopic polypectomy. The National Polyp Study Workgroup. N Engl J Med. 1993;329(27):1977–81. https://doi.org/10.1056/NEJM199312303292701.
2. Muto T, Bussey HJ, Morson BC. The evolution of cancer of the colon and rectum. Cancer. 1975;36(6):2251–70.
3. Leggett B, Whitehall V. Role of the serrated pathway in colorectal cancer pathogenesis. Gastroenterology. 2010;138(6):2088–100. S0016-5085(10)00172-1 [pii]. https://doi.org/10.1053/j.gastro.2009.12.066.
4. Snover DC. Update on the serrated pathway to colorectal carcinoma. Hum Pathol. 2011;42(1):1–10. S0046-8177(10)00206-6 [pii]. https://doi.org/10.1016/j.humpath.2010.06.002.

5. Rex DK, Ahnen DJ, Baron JA, Batts KP, Burke CA, Burt RW, et al. Serrated lesions of the colorectum: review and recommendations from an expert panel. Am J Gastroenterol. 2012;107(9):1315–29; quiz 4, 30. doi:ajg2012161 [pii]. https://doi.org/10.1038/ajg.2012.161.
6. Oono Y, Fu K, Nakamura H, Iriguchi Y, Yamamura A, Tomino Y, et al. Progression of a sessile serrated adenoma to an early invasive cancer within 8 months. Dig Dis Sci. 2009;54(4):906–9. https://doi.org/10.1007/s10620-008-0407-7.
7. Lash RH, Genta RM, Schuler CM. Sessile serrated adenomas: prevalence of dysplasia and carcinoma in 2139 patients. J Clin Pathol. 2010;63(8):681–6. jcp.2010.075507 [pii]. https://doi.org/10.1136/jcp.2010.075507.
8. IJspeert J, Bevan R, Senore C, Kaminski MF, Kuipers EJ, Mroz A, et al. Detection rate of serrated polyps and serrated polyposis syndrome in colorectal cancer screening cohorts: a European overview. Gut. 2016. gutjnl-2015-310784 [pii]. https://doi.org/10.1136/gutjnl-2015-310784.
9. Lockett MJ, Atkin WS. Hyperplastic polyposis: prevalence and cancer risk. Gut. 2001;48(Supl 1):A4.
10. Hyman NH, Anderson P, Blasyk H. Hyperplastic polyposis and the risk of colorectal cancer. Dis Colon Rectum. 2004;47(12):2101–4. https://doi.org/10.1007/s10350-004-0709-6.
11. Boparai KS, Mathus-Vliegen EM, Koornstra JJ, Nagengast FM, van Leerdam M, van Noesel CJ, et al. Increased colorectal cancer risk during follow-up in patients with hyperplastic polyposis syndrome: a multicentre cohort study. Gut. 2010;59(8):1094–100. gut.2009.185884 [pii]. https://doi.org/10.1136/gut.2009.185884.
12. Hazewinkel Y, Tytgat KM, van Eeden S, Bastiaansen B, Tanis PJ, Boparai KS, et al. Incidence of colonic neoplasia in patients with serrated polyposis syndrome who undergo annual endoscopic surveillance. Gastroenterology. 2014;147(1):88–95. S0016-5085(14)00364-3 [pii]. https://doi.org/10.1053/j.gastro.2014.03.015.
13. Orlowska J. Hyperplastic polyposis syndrome and the risk of colorectal cancer. Gut. 2012;61(3):470–1.; author reply 1–2. gutjnl-2011-300141 [pii]. https://doi.org/10.1136/gutjnl-2011-300141.
14. Rubio CA, Stemme S, Jaramillo E, Lindblom A. Hyperplastic polyposis coli syndrome and colorectal carcinoma. Endoscopy. 2006;38(3):266–70. https://doi.org/10.1055/s-2006-925026.
15. Moreira L, Pellise M, Carballal S, Bessa X, Ocana T, Serradesanferm A, et al. High prevalence of serrated polyposis syndrome in FIT-based colorectal cancer screening programmes. Gut. 2013;62(3):476–7. gutjnl-2012-303496 [pii]. https://doi.org/10.1136/gutjnl-2012-303496.
16. Biswas S, Ellis AJ, Guy R, Savage H, Madronal K, East JE. High prevalence of hyperplastic polyposis syndrome (serrated polyposis) in the NHS bowel cancer screening programme. Gut. 2013;62(3):475. gutjnl-2012-303233 [pii]. https://doi.org/10.1136/gutjnl-2012-303233.
17. Ferrandez A, Samowitz W, DiSario JA, Burt RW. Phenotypic characteristics and risk of cancer development in hyperplastic polyposis: case series and literature review. Am J Gastroenterol. 2004;99(10):2012–8. https://doi.org/10.1111/j.1572-0241.2004.30021.x. AJG30021 [pii]
18. Lage P, Cravo M, Sousa R, Chaves P, Salazar M, Fonseca R, et al. Management of Portuguese patients with hyperplastic polyposis and screening of at-risk first-degree relatives: a contribution for future guidelines based on a clinical study. Am J Gastroenterol. 2004;99(9):1779–84. https://doi.org/10.1111/j.1572-0241.2004.30178.x. AJG30178 [pii]
19. Chow E, Lipton L, Lynch E, D'Souza R, Aragona C, Hodgkin L, et al. Hyperplastic polyposis syndrome: phenotypic presentations and the role of MBD4 and MYH. Gastroenterology. 2006;131(1):30–9. S0016-5085(06)00713-X [pii]. https://doi.org/10.1053/j.gastro.2006.03.046.
20. Kalady MF, Jarrar A, Leach B, LaGuardia L, O'Malley M, Eng C, et al. Defining phenotypes and cancer risk in hyperplastic polyposis syndrome. Dis Colon Rectum. 2011;54(2):164–70. https://doi.org/10.1007/DCR.0b013e3181fd4c15. 00003453-201102000-00007 [pii]
21. Navarro M, Gonzalez S, Iglesias S, Capella G, Rodriguez-Moranta F, Blanco I. Hyperplastic polyposis syndrome: phenotypic diversity and association to colorectal cancer. Med Clin (Barc). 2013;141(2):62–6. S0025-7753(12)00512-X [pii]. https://doi.org/10.1016/j.medcli.2012.04.024.

22. Carballal S, Rodriguez-Alcalde D, Moreira L, Hernandez L, Rodriguez L, Rodriguez-Moranta F, et al. Colorectal cancer risk factors in patients with serrated polyposis syndrome: a large multicentre study. Gut. 2015. gutjnl-2015-309647 [pii]. https://doi.org/10.1136/gutjnl-2015-309647.
23. Ijspeert J, Rana SA, Atkinson NS, van Herwaarden YJ, Bastiaansen BA, van Leerdam ME, et al. Clinical risk factors of colorectal cancer in patients with serrated polyposis syndrome: a multicentre cohort analysis. Gut. 2015. gutjnl-2015-310630 [pii]. https://doi.org/10.1136/gutjnl-2015-310630.
24. Buchanan DD, Sweet K, Drini M, Jenkins MA, Win AK, Gattas M, et al. Phenotypic diversity in patients with multiple serrated polyps: a genetics clinic study. Int J Color Dis. 2010;25(6):703–12. https://doi.org/10.1007/s00384-010-0907-8.
25. IJspeert J, Bossuyt PM, Kuipers EJ, Stegeman I, de Wijkerslooth TR, Stoop EM, et al. Smoking status informs about the risk of advanced serrated polyps in a screening population. Endosc Int Open. 2016;4(1):E73–8. https://doi.org/10.1055/s-0034-1393361.
26. Boparai KS, Reitsma JB, Lemmens V, van Os TA, Mathus-Vliegen EM, Koornstra JJ, et al. Increased colorectal cancer risk in first-degree relatives of patients with hyperplastic polyposis syndrome. Gut. 2010;59(9):1222–5. gut.2009.200741 [pii]. https://doi.org/10.1136/gut.2009.200741.
27. Oquinena S, Guerra A, Pueyo A, Eguaras J, Montes M, Razquin S, et al. Serrated polyposis: prospective study of first-degree relatives. Eur J Gastroenterol Hepatol. 2013;25(1):28–32. https://doi.org/10.1097/MEG.0b013e3283598506.
28. Lieberman DA, Rex DK, Winawer SJ, Giardiello FM, Johnson DA, Levin TR. Guidelines for colonoscopy surveillance after screening and polypectomy: a consensus update by the US Multi-Society Task Force on Colorectal Cancer. Gastroenterology. 2012;143(3):844–57. S0016-5085(12)00812-8 [pii]. https://doi.org/10.1053/j.gastro.2012.06.001.
29. Syngal S, Brand RE, Church JM, Giardiello FM, Hampel HL, Burt RW. ACG clinical guideline: genetic testing and management of hereditary gastrointestinal cancer syndromes. Am J Gastroenterol. 2015;110(2):223–62.; quiz 63. ajg2014435 [pii]. https://doi.org/10.1038/ajg.2014.435.
30. Stefanius K, Ylitalo L, Tuomisto A, Kuivila R, Kantola T, Sirnio P, et al. Frequent mutations of KRAS in addition to BRAF in colorectal serrated adenocarcinoma. Histopathology. 2011;58(5):679–92. https://doi.org/10.1111/j.1365-2559.2011.03821.x.
31. Sebolt-Leopold JS, Herrera R. Targeting the mitogen-activated protein kinase cascade to treat cancer. Nat Rev Cancer. 2004;4(12):937–47. nrc1503 [pii]. https://doi.org/10.1038/nrc1503.
32. Kim KM, Lee EJ, Ha S, Kang SY, Jang KT, Park CK, et al. Molecular features of colorectal hyperplastic polyps and sessile serrated adenoma/polyps from Korea. Am J Surg Pathol. 2011;35(9):1274–86. https://doi.org/10.1097/PAS.0b013e318224cd2e.
33. Moran A, Ortega P, de Juan C, Fernandez-Marcelo T, Frias C, Sanchez-Pernaute A, et al. Differential colorectal carcinogenesis: molecular basis and clinical relevance. World J Gastrointest Oncol. 2010;2(3):151–8. https://doi.org/10.4251/wjgo.v2.i3.151.
34. Yamane L, Scapulatempo-Neto C, Reis RM, Guimaraes DP. Serrated pathway in colorectal carcinogenesis. World J Gastroenterol. 2014;20(10):2634–40. https://doi.org/10.3748/wjg.v20.i10.2634.
35. Rosty C, Parry S, Young JP. Serrated polyposis: an enigmatic model of colorectal cancer predisposition. Pathol Res Int. 2011;2011:157073. https://doi.org/10.4061/2011/157073.
36. Win AK, Walters RJ, Buchanan DD, Jenkins MA, Sweet K, Frankel WL, et al. Cancer risks for relatives of patients with serrated polyposis. Am J Gastroenterol. 2012;107(5):770–8. ajg201252 [pii]. https://doi.org/10.1038/ajg.2012.52.
37. Gala MK, Mizukami Y, Le LP, Moriichi K, Austin T, Yamamoto M, et al. Germline mutations in oncogene-induced senescence pathways are associated with multiple sessile serrated adenomas. Gastroenterology. 2014;146(2):520–9. S0016-5085(13)01519-9 [pii]. https://doi.org/10.1053/j.gastro.2013.10.045.

38. de Lau W, Peng WC, Gros P, Clevers H. The R-spondin/Lgr5/Rnf43 module: regulator of Wnt signal strength. Genes Dev. 2014;28(4):305–16. 28/4/305 [pii]. https://doi.org/10.1101/gad.235473.113.
39. Koo BK, Spit M, Jordens I, Low TY, Stange DE, van de Wetering M, et al. Tumour suppressor RNF43 is a stem-cell E3 ligase that induces endocytosis of Wnt receptors. Nature. 2012;488(7413):665–9. nature11308 [pii]. https://doi.org/10.1038/nature11308.
40. Taupin D, Lam W, Rangiah D, McCallum L, Whittle B, Zhang Y, et al. A deleterious RNF43 germline mutation in a severely affected serrated polyposis kindred. Hum Genome Var. 2015;2:15013. https://doi.org/10.1038/hgv.2015.13.
41. Yan HH, Lai JC, Ho SL, Leung WK, Law WL, Lee JF, et al. RNF43 germline and somatic mutation in serrated neoplasia pathway and its association with BRAF mutation. Gut. 2016. gutjnl-2016-311849 [pii]. https://doi.org/10.1136/gutjnl-2016-311849.
42. Sekine S, Yamashita S, Tanabe T, Hashimoto T, Yoshida H, Taniguchi H, et al. Frequent PTPRK-RSPO3 fusions and RNF43 mutations in colorectal traditional serrated adenoma. J Pathol. 2016;239(2):133–8. https://doi.org/10.1002/path.4709.
43. Buchanan DD, Clendenning M, Zhuoer L, Stewart JR, Joseland S, Woodall S, et al. Lack of evidence for germline RNF43 mutations in patients with serrated polyposis syndrome from a large multinational study. Gut. 2016. gutjnl-2016-312773 [pii]. https://doi.org/10.1136/gutjnl-2016-312773.
44. IJspeert J, van Doorn SC, van der Brug YM, Bastiaansen BA, Fockens P, Dekker E. The proximal serrated polyp detection rate is an easy-to-measure proxy for the detection rate of clinically relevant serrated polyps. Gastrointest Endosc. 2015;82(5):870–7. S0016-5107(15)00216-3 [pii]. https://doi.org/10.1016/j.gie.2015.02.044.

Part III
Genetic Diagnostics and Clinical Management

Chapter 16
Genetic Testing in Hereditary Colorectal Cancer

Conxi Lázaro, Lidia Feliubadaló, and Jesús del Valle

Abstract Genetic testing for hereditary disorders has suffered a dramatic change in the last decade with the incorporation of next-generation sequencing (NGS) technologies in the clinical diagnostics routine. Consequently, mutation detection yield in hereditary cancer in general, and in colorectal cancer in particular, has increased due to the fact that more genes are screened at the same time with a similar cost and turnaround time. This chapter summarizes previous methodologies used to address genetic causes of hereditary colorectal cancer and tackles important issues regarding NGS implementation for clinical testing. Analytical validity and clinical validity and utility together with ELSI aspects are briefly addressed. Somatic versus germline testing is also discussed due to its relevance in new clinical scenarios where novel target therapies are introduced for particular genetic conditions. Altogether, we highlight the importance of creating multidisciplinary committees to interpret genetic and genomic results and translate them into good laboratory practice and clinical guidelines.

Keywords Genetic testing · Mutation detection · Next generation sequencing · Gene panels · Germline mutations · Somatic mutations · Lynch syndrome · Familial adenomatous polyposis · Microsatellite instability (MSI) · Variants of unknown significance (VUS) · Multilocus inherited neoplasia alleles syndrome (MINAS) · Moderate risk genes

1 Conventional Approaches for Molecular Analysis of Hereditary Colorectal Cancer Patients

1.1 Hereditary Colorectal Cancer-Associated Genes

Traditional algorithms for molecular testing in hereditary colorectal cancer (CRC) are based on patient- and tumor-specific evidence together with family history and are basically designed to distinguish hereditary nonpolyposis CRC from polyposis

C. Lázaro (✉) · L. Feliubadaló · J. del Valle
Hereditary Cancer Program, Genetic Diagnostics Unit, Catalan Institute of Oncology (ICO-IDIBELL), CIBERONC, Hospitalet de Llobregat, Barcelona, Spain
e-mail: clazaro@iconcologia.net

L. Valle et al. (eds.), *Hereditary Colorectal Cancer*,
https://doi.org/10.1007/978-3-319-74259-5_16

syndromes and sporadic cases, although other rare CRC phenotypes have been associated with hereditary forms (a revised list of genes is presented in Table 16.1).

Starting with the main clinical suspicion of CRC, a genetic testing algorithm is followed (Fig. 16.1). In the case of LS suspicion, simultaneous or sequential tests

Table 16.1 Hereditary colorectal cancer genes, associated syndromes and mode of inheritance. Shading denotes genes recently proposed to increase CCR risk but not fully validated

Gene	Syndrome	Inheritance
MLH1	Lynch syndrome	Dominant
MSH2	Lynch syndrome	Dominant
MSH6	Lynch syndrome	Dominant
PMS2	Lynch syndrome	Dominant
EPCAM[a]	Lynch syndrome	Dominant
APC	Familial adenomatous polyposis	Dominant
MUTYH	*MUTYH*-associated polyposis	Recessive
POLE	Polymerase proofreading-associated polyposis	Dominant
POLD1	Polymerase proofreading-associated polyposis	Dominant
NTHL1	Colorectal adenomatous polyposis	Recessive
MSH3	Colorectal adenomatous polyposis	Recessive
MMR[b]	Constitutional MMR deficiency	Recessive
GREM1[c]	Hereditary mixed polyposis	Dominant
SMAD4	Juvenile polyposis	Dominant
BMPR1A	Juvenile polyposis	Dominant
STK11	Peutz-Jeghers	Dominant
BUB1	Hereditary CRC	Dominant
BUB3	Hereditary CRC	Dominant
PTPN12	Hereditary CRC	Dominant
LRP6	Hereditary CRC	Dominant
RPS20	Hereditary CRC	Dominant
FAN1	Hereditary CRC	Dominant
FANCM	Hereditary CRC	Dominant
TREX2	Hereditary CRC	Dominant
TP53	Early-onset hereditary CRC	Dominant
POT1	Hereditary CRC	Dominant
POLE2	Hereditary CRC	Dominant
MRE11	Hereditary CRC	Dominant
RPS20	Hereditary CRC	Dominant

[a]Only large deletions affecting the 3′ end

[b]Biallelic mutations of MMR genes (in the same or different MMR genes, including *MLH1*, *MSH2*, *MSH6*, and *PMS2*)

[c]Only a large duplication upstream *GREM1* gene

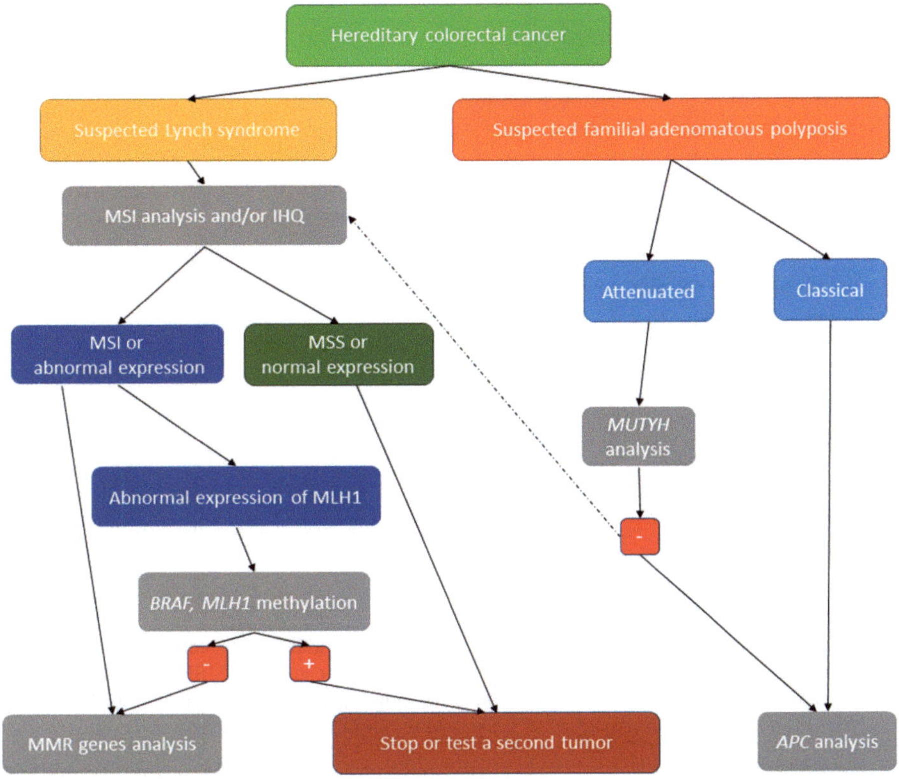

Fig. 16.1 *Hereditary CCR algorithm.* A common strategy to identify patients with hereditary colorectal cancer (Adapted from Pineda et al. [9])

are performed on the tumor sample as a prescreening tool to determine if germline genetic analysis of mismatch repair (MMR) genes is suitable. This type of algorithm was (and still is) used by many diagnostic laboratories because the cascade workflow dramatically decreased costs and turnaround times, while complete analysis of several genes with traditional methodologies is expensive and time-consuming.

1.2 *Prescreening Tests on Tumor Samples*

Since the 1990s, many different approaches have been used to analyze the possibility of hereditary CRC. The first marker used to identify hereditary CRC was microsatellite instability (MSI), described by Ionov et al. [1] and Aaltonen et al. [2] Microsatellites, or single sequence repeats, are a subcategory of tandem repeats; they consist of short nucleotide motifs (ranging in length from 1 to 10 nucleotides) that are repeated several times (from 5 to 50 times). They are spread through the

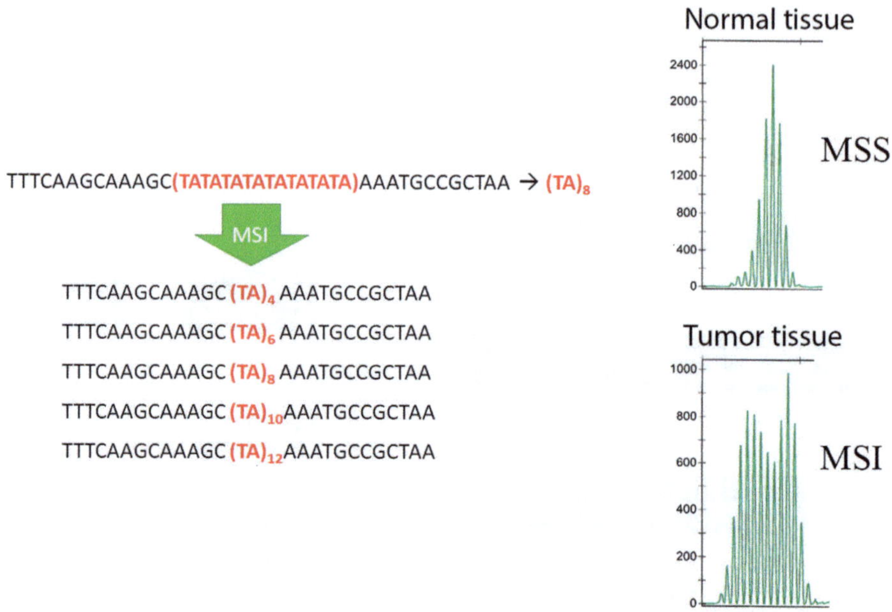

Fig. 16.2 *Microsatellite instability schemes*. Left, a dinucleotide microsatellite of thymine and adenine, illustrating the length variation of this microsatellite caused by MSI. Right, two electropherograms analyzing one microsatellite in the same individual: at the top normal tissue DNA with no MSI (MSS), at the bottom analysis of the paired tumor DNA, which clearly shows MSI

whole genome, though most often found in noncoding regions. Microsatellites mutate up to ten times faster than other regions [3], meaning that they are usually highly polymorphic, varying in length from one individual to another. Cancer MSI consists of the accumulation of errors (deletions and duplications) in microsatellite sequences during DNA replication, leading to differences in microsatellite lengths between tumor cells (Fig. 16.2).

By analyzing the length of several selected microsatellites in DNA from colon and endometrial cancer tissues, these tumors can be classified in two groups: microsatellite stable (MSS) and microsatellite instable (MSI or MSI-high). MSI is defined by instability of at least 30% of the studied microsatellite markers [4]. For this classification, the US National Cancer Institute (NCI) originally recommended the Bethesda panel of five markers (three dinucleotide and two mononucleotide repeats) [5]. However, it was subsequently demonstrated that dinucleotide microsatellites provide lower sensitivity and specificity than mononucleotide microsatellites, so a panel of five quasi-monomorphic mononucleotide microsatellites was proposed [6] and is now widely used.

MSI is originated by defects in the mismatch repair (MMR) system. Germline mutations in MMR genes lead to the accumulation of errors during DNA replication, which can be easily detected in the analysis of microsatellite markers. The presence of MSI is a hallmark of Lynch syndrome (LS), although approximately 10% of sporadic CRC show MSI [7].

Loss of MMR protein expression by immunohistochemical (IHC) analysis is a potential alternative for the identification of LS tumors. It consists of the immunohistochemical staining of the 4 LS-associated MMR proteins, MLH1, MSH2, MSH6, and PMS2, on tumor samples, mostly formalin-fixed paraffin-embedded (FFPE), to test for possible loss of expression. In addition to providing evidence indicative of LS, loss of expression of one or two MMR proteins in the tumor is very useful for selecting the specific MMR gene for germline testing, because the pattern of staining is suggestive of the underlying molecular alteration.

MSI analysis and IHC analysis provide almost equal sensitivity, although IHC may give false positive results when the antibody hybridizes to a fragment of a truncated protein [8], and not all pathogenic mutations result in loss of protein expression [9]. So, the two approaches can be complementary and are both widely used in LS screening.

Most sporadic MSI tumors (without germline alterations) also present loss of expression of MLH1/PMS2 proteins, often due to abnormal hypermethylation of the *MLH1* promoter. This methylation represses *MLH1* gene transcription and leads to the absence of normal MLH1 protein. Consequently, the analysis of *MLH1* promoter hypermethylation is a good prescreening method to avoid the study of MMR genes in sporadic cases, lowering the cost associated with gene analysis. Screening of the *BRAF* V600E mutation in tumor samples is also a valid method for identifying sporadic cases with MSI because it is strongly associated with *MLH1* promoter hypermethylation, although this mutation has occasionally been detected in LS tumors [10–12]. *MLH1* methylation is more specific than *BRAF* mutation screening and is therefore more cost-effective. However, different ranges of specificity have been reported depending on the technique and criteria used for case selection [13, 14]. Importantly, the presence of constitutional *MLH1* promoter hypermethylation, although rare, should also be considered as a possible cause of LS.

In summary, after tumor screening, genetic testing of the candidate MMR gene should be performed in selected cases (Fig. 16.1). Nevertheless, it is advisable to evaluate unusual clinical cases that do not meet the molecular criteria set for the algorithm by a multidisciplinary team before ruling out germline MMR genetic testing.

Mutations in the *POLE* and *POLD1* genes have recently been described as a cause of hereditary CRC with high penetrance [89]. Although more evidence is needed, it seems that mutations in *POLE* and *POLD1* produce a phenotype of oligo-adenomatous colorectal polyposis, CRC, and other extra-colonic tumors (mainly endometrial) [15]. The majority of pathogenic mutations are located in the exonuclease (proofreading) domains (*POLE* exons 9–14, *POLD1* exons 6–12), affecting the exonuclease activity and resulting in a reduction of the DNA replication fidelity [16]. *POLE* alterations are also associated with ultramutated sporadic colon and endometrial tumors [17]. For this reason, hypermutation assessment in MMR-proficient tumors could be a good prescreening marker for sporadic or germline cases caused by *POLE* mutations.

1.3 Germline Mutational Analysis Before the Introduction of Next-Generation Sequencing Approaches

In general, mutational analysis of the genes described above involves analysis of the whole coding region and intron-exon boundaries. For point mutations and small deletions and insertions, there are two screening approaches: (1) traditional Sanger sequencing, which is the gold standard for mutation screening, and (2) other screening methods, most based on heteroduplex conformation, such as single-strand conformation polymorphism (SSCP), denaturing high-performance liquid chromatography (dHPLC), conformation-sensitive capillary electrophoresis (CSCE) and the high-resolution melting (HRM) approach which detect point mutations with a lower sensitivity than Sanger sequencing.

None of the above methods can detect large genomic rearrangements like exonic deletions/duplications. To achieve this, several semiquantitative methods were developed in the early 2000s, the most widely used being multiplex ligation-dependent probe amplification (MLPA). The frequency of large rearrangements varies from one gene to another and between different populations but is generally around 10% of overall mutations.

1.3.1 Germline Mutations in Lynch Syndrome

LS is defined by the presence of germline mono-allelic mutations affecting the *MLH1*, *MSH2* (or the 3′ end of *EPCAM*), *MSH6*, or *PMS2* genes.

IHC analysis of MMR proteins is a powerful tool, since loss of expression is not only a hallmark of LS: in samples with loss of expression of only one of the proteins (mostly MSH6 or PMS2), the gene that codifies this protein is also the best candidate to test for deleterious mutations. When two proteins are not expressed, normally corresponding to the heterodimers MLH1/PMS2 or MSH2/MSH6, then *MLH1* or *MSH2*, respectively, is the best candidate to test first; if negative, mutation screening of the other gene is recommended [18].

It should be noted that molecular analysis of *PMS2* gene is more complex due to the presence of various pseudogenes in the genome. The presence of genomic regions with high sequence homology to *PMS2* hampers conventional analysis. The best strategy to overcome this problem is to perform long-range PCR and/or cDNA sequencing [19–21].

When testing *MSH2*, it is important to also look for large rearrangements in the *EPCAM* (*TACSTD1*) gene, which is located 5′ from to the *MSH2* promoter region, because deletions of the last exons of *EPCAM* originate hypermethylation of *MSH2* promoter, resulting in a similar clinical effect to that of pathogenic *MSH2* mutations [22, 23].

1.3.2 Germline Mutations in Familial Adenomatous Polyposis

In general, when CRC is originated in a polyposis (multiple polyps) context, it is related not to LS but to familial adenomatous polyposis (FAP). When there are 100 or more polyps in the colon and rectum (the classical form of FAP), analysis of the *APC* gene is mandatory, since more than 80% of patients with classical FAP have an *APC* mutation [9]. When the number of polyps is lower (the attenuated form of FAP), screening should be performed for biallelic mutations in *MUTYH*, a recessive form of polyposis. Some recurrent mutations in *MUTYH* account for a high proportion of the total mutations, although they differ among populations [24, 25]. To improve cost-effectiveness, some laboratories first screen for recurrent mutations. However, if even one mutation is found in the first screening, analysis of the rest of *MUTYH* should be completed. In CRC patients with a non-informative *MUTYH* test and a low number of polyps, MSI analysis should be considered in order to rule out the possibility of LS. Nevertheless, the presence of MSI-positive tumors, although rare, has also been reported in biallelic carriers of *MUTYH* mutations [26–28].

Unlike hereditary nonpolyposis CCR, in FAP prescreening of tumor samples is not effective, so it is advisable to proceed straight to gene analysis. Interestingly, the tumors of *MUTYH* biallelic germline mutants frequently carry the *KRAS* mutation G12C (c.34G > T) [26]. It has therefore been proposed that the study of cases with the attenuated form of polyposis should begin with tumor screening of the *KRAS* G12C mutation [29, 30].

2 Mutation Analysis Using Next-Generation Sequencing-Based Approaches

2.1 *Brief Introduction to Next-Generation or Massively Parallel Sequencing*

Next-generation sequencing (NGS), also known as massively parallel or high-throughput sequencing, describes a group of sequencing technologies developed in the first decade of this century to reduce the cost and increase the yield of sequencing. It analyzes many DNA molecules clonally and in parallel through different approaches and can be used for molecular diagnostics following an essentially common workflow, shown in Fig.16.3. First, a library of DNA fragments from the regions of interest, surrounded by universal priming sequences, must be prepared. If various samples need to be sequenced together, short barcoding sequences are added. This targeted library can be produced in one or two steps by simplex or multiplex PCR amplification. Other common approaches involve DNA fragmentation, oligomer ligation, and enrichment by some kind of hybridization or primer extension. The most important quality control steps in the laboratory workflow are quantification of dsDNA from the starting sample and assessment of the library quantity and quality at critical points and before pooling libraries from different samples.

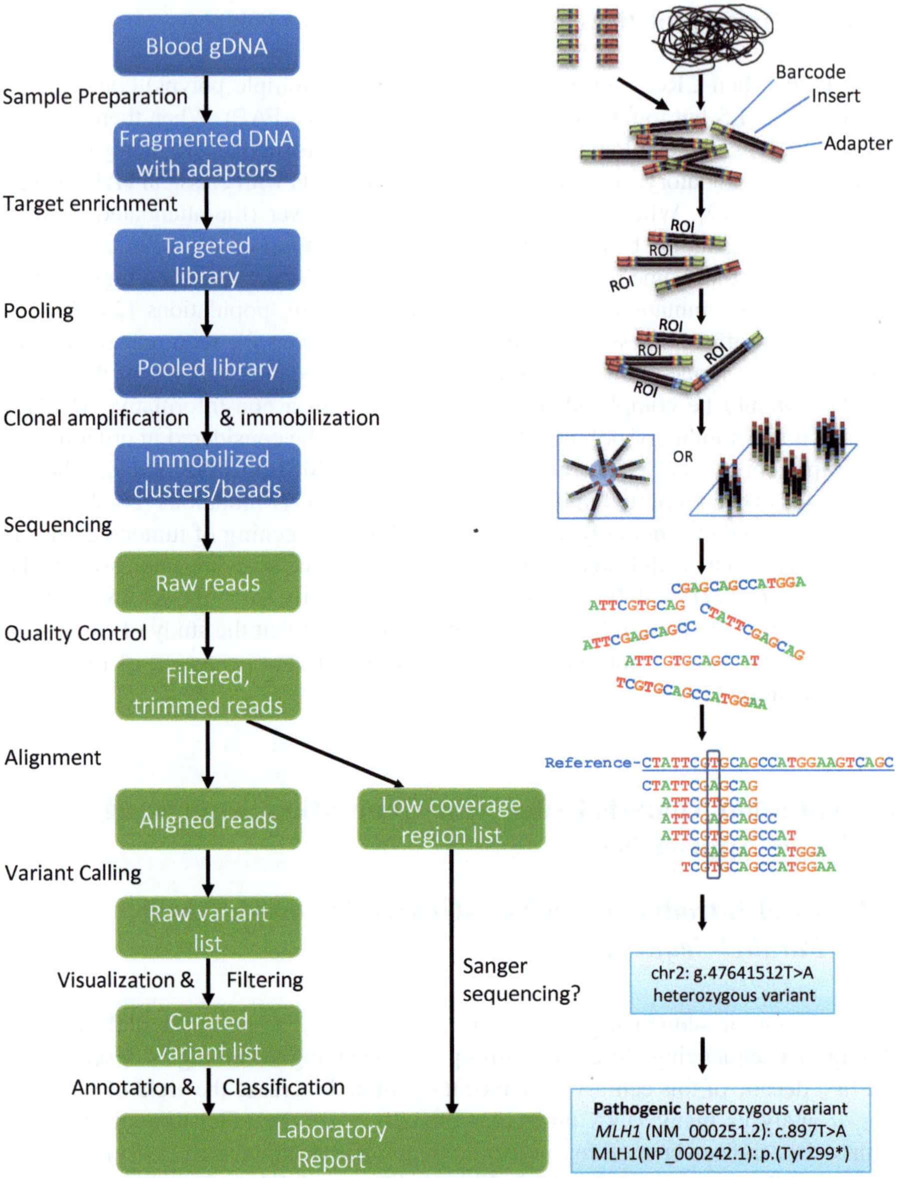

Fig. 16.3 *Basic NGS diagnostic workflow*. Left, the main steps needed to go from the sample to the laboratory report and their intermediate products (blue for the laboratory workflow, green for the bioinformatic pipeline). Right, images depicting sample and products

The main NGS technologies currently used for diagnostics are reversible termination sequencing by synthesis, provided by Illumina, and ion semiconductor sequencing, developed by Ion Torrent. Both technologies require prior clonal DNA amplification to ensure accurate detection. Reversible termination sequencing by synthesis uses bridge PCR on a surface to generate the high-density array of template DNA where sequencing takes place. Ion semiconductor sequencing employs an emulsion PCR on primer-coated beads, which are subsequently deposited in individual wells for the sequencing reaction. Illumina sequencing is based on cycles of DNA synthesis where fluorescent reversible terminator dideoxyribonucleotides are incorporated. After an image has been taken, the fluorophore is detached and the hydroxyl group regenerated for a subsequent synthesis cycle [31]. In ion semiconductor sequencing, the four natural nucleotides are supplied sequentially to the DNA polymerase. When a nucleotide is incorporated into the growing strand, the proton released is detected as an electric signal proportional to the number of nucleotides incorporated [32]. Table 16.2 lists the main characteristics of the sequencing technologies

Table 16.2 Main sequencing technologies used in molecular diagnostics

Sequencing technology	Read length (bp)	Throughput (Mb/run)/run time	Main characteristics
Sanger (chain termination)	600–900	0.002–0.1/0.3–2.3 h	Main company: Thermo fisher-applied biosystems Different alleles are read together; detection based on fluorescence imaging It has the lowest error rate (0.001–0.1%) but also the lowest throughput and is by far the most expensive Gold standard in diagnostics for several decades
Ion semiconductor	200–400	30–15,000/2–7.3 h	Company: Thermo fisher-ion torrent After clonal amplification, sequentially released natural nucleotides are incorporated. Released protons are detected as an electric signal proportional to the incorporated bases 1% error rate, prone to indel errors, especially in homopolymeric sequences Highly scalable platforms, with an intermediate price per base
Reversible termination	50–300	1.2–1,800,000/4 h–11 d	Company: Illumina After clonal amplification, sequencing consists of cycles of incorporation of fluorescently labeled reversible terminators, imaging, and fluorescence cleavage to allow addition of the next base 0.1% error rate, mainly substitution errors It reaches the highest throughput and is the cheapest

Data collected mainly from company websites; error rates extracted from Glenn's NGS Field Guide [47]

most commonly used for diagnostics. A newer generation of sequencers can sequence long single molecules without any amplification step. The most commonly used platforms of this type are developed by Pacific Biosciences, which classifies its technology as single molecule real-time (SMRT) sequencing, although it is not included in the table because as of February 2018 it has not reached the throughput, reliability, price, and ease of use that would make them suitable for application in the routine setting. Given the constant evolution of sequencing technologies, however, SMRT or another similar platform, or another technology based on a completely different approach, could become widely adopted in the near time.

NGS technologies generate a large number of sequencing reads, each derived from a clonally amplified DNA fragment. Consequently, each allele of a locus is read separately. Unfortunately, these reads are usually less accurate than Sanger sequences. To increase sequence accuracy and ensure the detection of both alleles for heterozygous variants, each locus is read several times. The number of reads supporting the base calling of a DNA position is called read depth or coverage, and, rather confusingly, a position or region is considered covered if it is represented by at least one read. Some regions may be systematically underrepresented due to biases in library preparation or sequencing.

2.2 *Next-Generation Sequencing Analysis*

The analysis workflow begins with a quality control step to detect possible problems in the data, discard low-quality reads, and trim low-quality portions of good reads. If different samples have been pooled, barcodes allow the reads from each one to be separated. An alignment algorithm maps reads to the corresponding sequences to the human reference genome. Then, a variant caller detects differences between those reads and the reference genome, generating a variant list that can be filtered to reduce false positives. Next, an annotator retrieves information from databases to help determine the possible effects of the variant. More filtering usually discards variants classified as neutral and sometimes discards variants of unknown significance (VUS). Selected variants are reported, and in parallel, a list of regions with coverage below a set threshold value can be produced. Variant detection largely depends on coverage. Poorly covered regions do not guarantee the sensitivity required for diagnostics and must be analyzed by a gap-filling technique like Sanger sequencing or at least disclosed in the diagnostics report.

There has been much debate about whether Sanger sequencing should be used to confirm variants detected by NGS [33–36]. In a recent study, Mu et al. [37] Sanger-sequenced the 7845 non-polymorphic variants found in 20,000 hereditary cancer panels comprising 47 genes and found only 98.7% concordance. Setting the variant-calling quality score to increase specificity to 100% caused 176 true variants to be missed, reducing the sensitivity to 97.8%. Based on these data, Sanger-sequencing confirmation is highly recommended.

2.3 Limitations of Next-Generation Sequencing

NGS can detect point mutations and small insertions and deletions with high accuracy in most regions. Some regions, particularly those with high GC content, often corresponding to promoters and first exons (e.g., *MSH6* first exon), are difficult to capture and can be poorly covered. This decreases the sensitivity if the problem is not addressed by improving the targeting design or complementing with Sanger sequencing [38].

Unlike Sanger sequencing, NGS can detect copy number alterations (CNAs, also called large rearrangements) from sequence data, identified as changes in the expected read depth of a region, after internal normalization, relative to the depth observed in other samples. Many factors can influence depth and reduce homogeneity within and between samples, reducing the specificity or the sensitivity of the approach [39, 40]. When the breakpoint is sequenced, sensitivity increases because single reads or read pairs can be detected partially aligning to distant positions. This also allows for the detection of copy-neutral structural variants but seldom happens in targeted sequencing, since only a small portion of the genome is sequenced [41–43].

NGS usually provides short reads, which are more difficult to align to repetitive regions. These include microsatellites (short tandem repeats, SRTs), long interspersed repeats (e.g., *Alu* repeat elements), and segmental duplications (e.g., pseudogenes). All of these are common in the human genome and can affect gene function. The most challenging example for hereditary colorectal cancer diagnostics is the existence of the multiple highly homologous *PMS2* pseudogenes, although a strategy has been described to address this [44].

NGS can also be used to analyze microsatellite instability in tumor samples, using the unstable microsatellites detected in genome data or incidentally targeted by the exome or even large or mid-size gene panels [45, 46].

2.4 Use of Gene Panels for Genetic Testing of Hereditary CRC Syndromes

With the development of the first benchtop NGS platforms, a plethora of papers were published addressing the use of NGS to tackle genetic testing for different hereditary disorders. Academic laboratories and commercial companies designed the first NGS assays to analyze single or small numbers of genes according to clinical phenotypes. The main aim was to improve on the cost-effectiveness of Sanger sequencing without losing quality control over the process [48]. Rapid advances in the development of these technologies made it possible to investigate dozens of genes simultaneously, at a similar price and turnaround time. Consequently the era for larger gene panels for genetic testing opened. Table 16.3 summarizes recent publications using different commercial or ad hoc panels for molecular diagnostics in CRC patients.

Table 16.3 Main results of gene panels used for CRC patients

First author citation no.	Patients #	Clinical selection	Panel description	Main results
Susswein [49]	10,000	Hereditary cancer patients	GeneDx, 29 genes, multigene panels	9% PAT; highest yield LS/CRC 14.8%; 34.7% VUS
LaDuca [50]	2079	Hereditary cancer patients	Ambry (14–22 genes)	8.3% global PAT, 9.2% ColoNext
Yurgelun [51]	1260	Lynch syndrome- patients	Myriad myRisk (25 genes)	9% LS genes PAT, 5.6% other HC genes, 38% VUS
Yurgelun [52]	1058	Consecutive CRC patients	Myriad myRisk (25 genes)	9.9% PAT, 31.2% VUS
Chubb [53]	626	Early-onset CRC	Exome sequencing, analysis 9 CRC genes	14.2% PAT (10.9% MMR), 10% VUS
Cragun [54]	586	CRC patients	ColoNext ambry (14 genes)	10.4% PAT, 20.1% VSD
Ricker [55]	475	Hereditary cancer patients	Different multigene panels	15.6% PAT, 43.2% VUS
Pearlman [56]	450	CRC patients <50 years	Myriad myRisk (25 genes)	16% PAT; 32.2% VUS
Slavin [57]	348	Hereditary cancer patients	Different multigene panels	17% PAT, 42% VUS
Hermel [58]	227	Hereditary cancer patients	Different multigene panels	12.3% PAT; 19.4% VUS
Howarth [59]	92	HBOC + HNPCC	Myriad myRisk/ ambry BRCAplus	10% PAT, 43% VUS
Rohlin [60]	91	6 CRC overlapping phenotypes	19 CRC genes	17.6% PAT/PPAT; 33% VUS

All of the above panels are theoretically valid, provided that quality control is maintained and meets the minimum requirements described in the previous section, although it is crucial for clinicians and molecular geneticists to reach a consensus regarding the most suitable test for their particular clinical setting. There is no single correct solution, and several factors must be taken into consideration: the number of samples to be analyzed/year, the number of different clinical conditions studied in both the clinical and laboratory settings, the desired turnaround time, the laboratory's NGS infrastructure, the availability of bioinformatic support, etc. It is particularly important for the laboratory and clinicians to fully understand and disclose the range and limitations of the tests they offer.

For the sake of concision and balance, the main conclusions of four different publications analyzing more than one thousand patients each are discussed in this section [49–52], which encompass most of the knowledge derived from the use of NGS panels for the molecular diagnosis of hereditary colorectal cancer. In addition, the main contributions of other studies are briefly summarized in Table 16.3.

2.4.1 Gene Composition of Panels

Academic laboratories and commercial firms have developed a variety of hereditary cancer panels that can be categorized as follows: (1) panels by clinical *phenotype* (Ambry [50], GeneDx [49], etc.); (2) panels by *risk*, which tend to include high- and moderate-risk genes (for instance, the 25 genes included in the myRisk panel by Myriad [51] or the 29 genes included by GeneDx [49]); and (3) comprehensive panels with a *broad unbiased* list of genes mutated in hereditary cancer syndromes (TruSight Cancer [61, 62], I2HCP [63], Table 16.4). These three types of panels provide complementary genetic information, and it is important for a comprehensive committee of clinic and academic staff to agree upon the specific panel to be used in a given institution. This agreement is especially essential in public health systems where a balance between clinical utility and translation of scientific evidence should be achieved.

2.4.2 Frequency of Pathogenic Mutations and Detection Yield by Cancer Type

The number of pathogenic mutations identified varies according to the clinical selection of patients and the gene content of the panel used. For instance, Yurgelun et al. [51], using a 25-gene panel, identified 14.4% of pathogenic mutations in a

Table 16.4 Genes targeted by some panels used for hereditary cancer diagnostics

ColoNext Ambry	MyRisk Myriad	CRC GeneDx	CRC Invitae	TruSight Cancer Illumina[59]			I2HCP Castellanos et al.[60]			
APC	*APC*	*APC*	*APC*	*AIP*	*FANCC*	*RAD51C*	*A2ML1*^{a}	*ERCC8*	*MSH2*	*RB1*
BMPR1	*ATM*	*ATM*	*AXIN2*	*ALK*	*FANCD2*	*RAD51D*	*AIP*	*EXO1*	*MSH3*	*RET*
CDH1	*BARD1*	*AXIN2*	*BMPR1*	*APC*	*FANCE*	*RB1*	*ALK*	*EXT1*	*MSH6*	*RIT1*^{a}
CHEK2	*BMPR1*	*BMPR1*	*CDH1*	*ATM*	*FANCF*	*RECQL4*	*APC*	*EXT2*	*MUTYH*	*RNASEL*
EPCAM	*BRCA1*	*CDH1*	*CHEK2*	*BAP1*	*FANCG*	*RET*	*ARAF*	*FAN1*^{a}	*NBN*	*RRAS*^{a}
GREM1	*BRCA2*	*CHEK2*	*EPCAM*	*BLM*	*FANCI*	*RHBDF2*	*ATM*	*FANCA*	*NF1*	*SBDS*
MLH1	*BRIP1*	*EPCAM*	*GREM1*	*BMPR1*	*FANCL*	*RUNX1*	*BAP1*	*FANCB*	*NF2*	*SDHAF2*
MSH2	*CDH1*	*GREM1*	*MLH1*	*BRCA1*	*FANCM*	*SBDS*	*BARD1*	*FANCC*	*NRAS*	*SDHB*
MSH6	*CDK4*	*MLH1*	*MSH2*	*BRCA2*	*FH*	*SDHAF2*	*BLM*	*FANCD*	*NTHL1*^{a}	*SDHC*
MUTYH	*CDKN2*	*MSH2*	*MSH6*	*BRIP1*	*FLCN*	*SDHB*	*BMPR1*	*FANCE*	*PALB2*	*SDHD*
PMS2	*CHEK2*	*MSH6*	*MUTYH*	*BUB1B*	*GATA2*	*SDHC*	*BRAF*	*FANCF*	*PDGFB*	*SHOC2*
POLD1	*EPCAM*	*MUTYH*	*PMS2*	*CDC73*	*GPC3*	*SDHD*	*BRCA1*	*FANCG*	*PDGFRA*	*SLX4*
POLE	*GREM1*	*PMS2*	*POLD1*	*CDH1*	*HNF1A*	*SLX4*	*BRCA2*	*FANCI*	*PHOX2B*	*SMAD4*
PTEN	*MLH1*	*POLD1*	*POLE*	*CDK4*	*HRAS*	*SMAD4*	*BRIP1*	*FANCL*	*PIK3CA*^{a}	*SMARCA4*
SMAD4	*MSH2*	*POLE*	*PTEN*	*CDKN1*	*KIT*	*SMARCB*	*BUB1B*	*FANCM*	*PMS1*	*SMARCB1*
STK11	*MSH6*	*PTEN*	*SMAD4*	*CDKN2*	*MAX*	*STK11*	*CBL*	*FH*	*PMS2*	*SMARCE1*
TP53	*MUTYH*	*SMAD4*	*STK11*	*CEBPA*	*MEN1*	*SUFU*	*CDC73*	*FLCN*	*POLD1*	*SOS1*
	NBN	*STK11*	*TP53*	*CEP57*	*MET*	*TMEM12*	*CDH1*	*GPC3*	*POLE*	*SOS2*^{a}
	PALB2	*TP53*		*CHEK2*	*MLH1*	*TP53*	*CDK4*	*GRB2*^{a}	*POLH*	*SPRED1*
	PMS2			*CYLD*	*MSH2*	*TSC1*	*CDKN1*	*HNF1A*	*POT1*^{a}	*STK11*
	POLD1			*DDB2*	*MSH6*	*TSC2*	*CDKN2*	*HRAS*	*PPM1D*	*SUFU*
	POLE			*DICER1*	*MUTYH*	*VHL*	*CDKN2*	*KIT*	*PRKAR1*	*TGFBR2*
	PTEN			*DIS3L2*	*NBN*	*WRN*	*CHEK2*	*KLLN*	*PRSS1*	*TMEM127*
	RAD51C			*EGFR*	*NF1*	*WT1*	*CYLD*	*KRAS*	*PTCH1*	*TP53*
	RAD51D			*EPCAM*	*NF2*	*XPA*	*DDB1*	*LZTR1*^{a}	*PTEN*	*TSC1*
	SMAD4			*ERCC2*	*NSD1*	*XPC*	*DDB2*	*MAP2K1*	*PTPN11*	*TSC2*
	STK11			*ERCC3*	*PALB2*		*DICER1*	*MAP2K2*	*RAD50*	*TSHR*
	TP53			*ERCC4*	*PHOX2B*		*ELAC2*	*MAX*	*RAD51*	*VHL*
				ERCC5	*PMS1*		*EPCAM*	*MEN1*	*RAD51B*^{a}	*WRN*
				EXT1	*PMS2*		*ERCC2*	*MET*	*RAD51C*	*WT1*
				EXT2	*PRF1*		*ERCC3*	*MLH1*	*RAD51D*	*XPA*
				EZH2	*PRKAR1*		*ERCC4*	*MLH3*	*RAF1*	*XPC*
				FANCA	*PTCH1*		*ERCC5*	*MN1*	*RASA1*	*XRCC2*
				FANCB	*PTEN*		*ERCC6*	*MRE11A*	*RASA2*^{a}	

Genes present in more than one panel are denoted by bold text, with darker shading indicating presence in more panels. Genes present in all six panels are denoted by white text

[a]Genes not present in the published panel version; they correspond to I2HCP v2.2

cohort of patients with clinical suspicion of Lynch syndrome. Interestingly, around 9% of the patients had a LS mutation but 5.6% carried non-LS mutations. These mutations would have been lost if only LS genes were screened. The largest study published to date includes the analyses of more than 10,000 samples with clinical suspicion of hereditary cancer using a 29-gene panel [49] in which the global mutation rate is 9.0%, although individuals with colon/stomach cancer had the highest yield of positive results (14.8%). While the majority of mutations were in well-established colon cancer genes, 28.2% were in genes considered nonclassical for gastrointestinal cancer, a third of them in *BRCA1* and *BRCA2*, and the remainder in *CHEK2*, *ATM*, *PALB2*, *BRIP1*, and *RAD51D*. Notably, in this comprehensive study, pathogenic mutations in the whole hereditary cancer cohort were divided almost evenly between well-established genes such as LS genes, *BRCA1/2* and other high-risk genes (51.8%), and recently described genes with moderate or unknown risk (48.2%). For endometrial cancer, the mutation detection yield was 11.9%, with mutations in LS genes—predominantly in *MSH6*—present in 61.1% of the carrier patients. *CHEK2* and *BRCA1/2* were also equally mutated in more than 10% of patients.

2.4.3 Frequency of Variants of Unknown Significance

The number of VUS identified differs in the literature and is associated not with patient phenotype but with the number of genes in the panel. The highest VUS frequency is observed on the largest panels due to the larger DNA sequence analyzed. Moreover, the larger panels contain fewer well-studied genes or newly characterized genes for which few missense variants have been functionally analyzed or studied in families, as well as including genes of moderate or low penetrance in which cosegregation analysis or case-control studies have less statistic power. Additionally, VUS frequency has been related to ancestry; in the study by Susswein, patients of Hispanic and Caucasian ancestry have the lowest rate of VUS across panels (around 20%), compared to those of Asian or African-American ancestry (around 37%). There is discussion between molecular geneticists and clinical specialists as to whether VUS should be reported, since they can be misinterpreted by patients and by doctors without specific expertise [64]. Conflicting interpretations of variants have also been described [65]. As such, the potential stress to patients caused by the identification of a VUS should be carefully considered when performing cost analyses of panels.

2.4.4 Identification of Multiple Mutations (MINAS)

Of 901 mutated patients in the Susswein study, 28 had more than one pathogenic mutation (3.1%), representing 0.3% of the total patients analyzed (28/10030). Six of these patients reported multiple primary cancers [49]. The presence of inherited pathogenic mutations in multiple cancer genes has recently been suggested as a clinical entity, for which the acronym MINAS (multilocus inherited neoplasia alleles syndrome) has been proposed [66]. Whitworth and colleagues described five new cases and collected data on 82 cases identified by a systematic literature review. Their main conclusion seems to be that deleterious variants appeared to act independently in many cases but not consistent effect was discernable. Several of the papers shown in Table 16.3 reported a similar proportion of patients with more than one pathogenic mutation (around 2–3%), but no clear genotype-phenotype association has been described to date. In order to increase knowledge in this field, Whitworth and colleagues proposed to create a public MINAS database using the Leiden Open Variation Database (LOVD) platform.

Although it cannot be considered a multilocus syndrome, it is worth mentioning a clinical entity fully described in the hereditary CRC field: constitutional mismatch repair-deficiency (CMMR-D) syndrome, in which biallelic mismatch repair gene mutations result in a more pronounced phenotype characterized by a broad spectrum of early-onset malignancies and a phenotype resembling that of neurofibromatosis type 1 (reviewed by Wimmer et al.) [67].

2.4.5 Unexpected Findings

The analysis of broad gene panels comprises the identification of mutations in genes where they are not expected, on the basis of the patient/family clinical characteristics. Of clinical relevance is the identification of mutations in highly penetrant genes, especially genes such as *TP53* and *CDH1* that are associated with high risk of cancer, whose management options include prophylactic surgery and/or extensive surveillance measures that do not always offer the required precision (NCCN Guidelines). In the Susswein study, 6 out of 18 patients with pathogenic *TP53* mutations did not meet any Li-Fraumeni or Li-Fraumeni-like criteria, and 2 out of 4 patients with pathogenic *CDH1* mutations did not meet international gastric cancer criteria either. Although de novo mutations may account for some of these cases, more knowledge is needed and caution should be exercised in the surveillance of these unexpected molecular results.

2.4.6 Moderate-Risk Genes

As described above, most panel studies detect almost half of the pathogenic mutations in genes of moderate or unknown risk. This represents a clinical dilemma, since uncertain risk impedes the use of established guidelines for the medical surveillance of patients and because it is difficult to determine if these mutations are the sole cause of cancer in the patient/family in question. The clinical utility of mutations in these genes remains a matter of debate, so clinicians should plan how these putative results should be given to patients in pre-genetic testing consultations and offer clear recommendations in posttesting consultations about how patients should proceed in the event of positive results.

2.4.7 Use of Gene Panels in Nonselected Consecutive CRC Patients

A recent paper presented the analysis of a panel of 25 genes associated with inherited cancer risk in 1058 CRC cases without preselection for age at diagnosis, personal/family history, or MSI/MMR results [52]. One or more mutations were identified in 9.9% (105/1058) of patients; 33 harbored LS mutations and 74 had non-LS mutations. In the non-LS group, 23 patients presented mutations in high-penetrance genes, and 15 did not have clinical histories suggestive of their underlying mutation; 38 patients had moderate-penetrance CRC risk gene mutations. These results demonstrate that multigene panel analysis without clinical preselection can identify pathogenic mutations in genes where primary or secondary cancer prevention is recommended. Interestingly, *APC* and biallelic *MUTYH* mutations were present in 0.8% of patients, and half of these probands lacked diffuse colorectal polyposis, indicating that polyp number is an imperfect indicator of germline mutations in these genes. Interestingly, *BRCA* mutations were present in 1% of all patients, making them more common than FAP and MAP combined. The main conclusion of this study is that neither proband age at CRC diagnosis nor family or personal history of CRC or other cancers significantly predicts the presence of germline mutations in non-LS genes. In addition, Pearlman and colleagues analyzed a cohort of 450 CRC patients younger than 50 years of age and found that one-third of mutation-positive patients did not meet established criteria for the affected gene(s) [56]. These results opened discussion about the efficacy of multigene germline testing for CRC, irrespective of phenotype, due to the fact that the cost of panels is falling and the cancer risks for most of these genes are being more accurately defined. A recent study concluded that multigene panel testing was cost-effective as a first-line test for patients with suspicion of hereditary CRC syndrome [68].

2.5 *Whole Exome Sequencing*

The exome is the collection of all protein-coding regions (exons) and constitutes about 1% (30 Mb) of the human genome [69]. However, it is thought to contain 85% of disease-causing mutations [70], which makes it a cost-effective sequencing option in many clinical situations [71]. Whole exome sequencing (WES) seeks to sequence all protein-coding exons but also their intron-exon boundaries and, in many cases, functional non-protein-coding elements such as microRNA, long intergenic noncoding RNA, and untranslated regions (UTRs). The main NGS companies produce exome capture kits, with different designs and characteristics, which are reviewed in Warr et al. [72] and whose performance has been thoroughly assessed by Chilamakuri et al. [73] and Meienberg et al. [74]

WES has been successfully used to identify the gene responsible for several diseases in which the candidate-gene approach was unfeasible or had proved unsuccessful [70, 75–77]. The diagnostic yield of exome sequencing largely depends on the type of disease; two large successive-case series [78, 79] suggest that it ranges from 9% to 41%, with an average frequency of 1 in 4. WES has been also used to associate *PALB2* with familial pancreatic cancer [80] and, with the help of linkage analysis, tumor analysis and functional studies, to identify the new hereditary colorectal cancer predisposition gene *RPS20* [81]. The usefulness of WES for hereditary CRC diagnostics was demonstrated in a study by Chubb et al. of 626 early-onset familial CRC cases from the UK national registry, where sequence data were filtered for the candidate genes *MLH1*, *MSH2*, *MSH6*, *PMS2*, *APC*, *MUTYH*, *SMAD4*, *BMPR1A*, *POLD1*, and *POLE*. A pathogenic or likely pathogenic variant was found in 14.2% of cases [53]. The main question, then, regarding the use of WES for hereditary cancer diagnostics is not whether it is possible but if it is cost-effective. If the WES platform will be used in the same way as a gene panel, it is probable not worth it, since the cost is higher and the coverage and, consequently, the sensitivity are usually lower [38, 50]. However, WES should be considered if the approach envisages the analysis of other genes after a negative result, whenever a new gene reaches clinical utility for the disease, and in a research setting.

2.6 *Whole Genome Sequencing*

The most comprehensive approach to identify potentially disease-causing variants is to resequence the two times 3 billion base pairs that compose the diploid human genome. Although Sanger sequencing of the first human genome took about 11 years and cost $2.7 billion, since 2014 NGS technology has made it possible to resequence the genome at 30x coverage in 3-and-a-half days at a cost of approximately $1000. Whole genome sequencing (WGS) has identified many disease alleles [82–84] and cancer risk genes, such as *MITF* for familial melanoma [85], *ATM* for pancreatic cancer [86], *MAX* for familial pheochromocytoma [87], *BRIP1* for ovarian cancer [88], and *POLE* and *POLD1* for colorectal cancer [89]. These studies often involved several rounds of variant filtering to reduce the list from the 4,000,000 variants typically found in a WGS[28] (compared to 20,000 in WES) [69] to a small number that can be functionally validated.

Whole genome sequencing does not require the enrichment step, which simplifies library preparation and ensures more homogeneous coverage and more accurate variant calling at equal or slightly lower mean coverages [90–92]. Although exome targeting kits are improving, sequencing costs are decreasing, and WGS may eventually cost no more than WES for the same sensitivity in coding regions. The additional information provided for noncoding regions and structural variants is advantageous, but the higher data volume and computing time and a lack of information on the clinical significance of most noncoding variants make WGS less appealing for routine laboratory analysis.

2.7 *Pros and Cons of Next-Generation Sequencing Approaches*

This chapter reviews the evolution of molecular diagnostics for hereditary CRC. Table 16.5 summarizes the main pros and cons of each approach.

Table 16.5 highlights the importance of knowing the limitations of the different technologies used for genetic testing, in order to be fully aware of the possible results, costs, time frames, and additional findings. Good communication between laboratory suppliers and clinicians is essential, as are professional pretest and post-test visits. Patients must be given clear and unbiased information, and this should be reflected in the consent form.

Table 16.5 Pros and cons of different genetic testing approaches

	Sanger-specific genes	CRC gene panels	HC panels	Exomes	Genomes
Number of VUS found	+	++	+++	+++++	+++++++
Detection of mosaicism	Difficult if it is less than 5–10%	Possible, depending on coverage	Possible, depending on coverage	Difficult to be cost-effective	Difficult to be cost-effective
CNV detection	MLPA or similar	Array-CGH or NGS algorithms[a]	Array-CGH or NGS algorithms[a]	NGS algorithms[a]	NGS algorithms[a]
Turnaround time	+ (only one gene), ++++ (many genes)	+	++	+++	++++
Bioinformatic data volume	+	++	+++	++++	++++++
Noncoding mutations	No	No	No	No	Yes
Unexpected mutations	No	No	Yes, but related to cancer	Yes, related or not to cancer	Yes, related or not to cancer
Incorporation of new risk genes	After technical setup	If custom panel, after technical setup If commercial, depending on the company	If custom panel, after technical setup If commercial, depending on the company	Immediate, even retrospective	Immediate, even retrospective
Clinical management of positive results	Clear guidelines	Clear guidelines for most genes	Clear guidelines for most genes	Not clear guidelines for a large set of genes	Not clear guidelines for a large set of genes
Relative cost	+	+	++	+++	++++

[a]Not fully validated

3 Final Considerations

As can be seen, many technical and analytical challenges remain in the use of NGS for hereditary cancer diagnostics. Moreover, the introduction of new target therapies for particular genetic status is changing genetic testing scenarios. Several clinical laboratories currently offer genetic tumor testing for treatment purposes. In these cases it is very important to sequence matching germline and tumor DNA for proper identification of somatic and germline mutations. Patients should be carefully informed of the possibility of identifying germline variants prior to testing [93]. The incorporation of new technologies has improved our understanding of several CRC cases, as well as highlighting the limits of our current knowledge.

Future studies of whole genomes in larger cohorts of patients will make it possible to establish more accurate genotype-phenotype correlations and will ultimately lead to precise and personalized management of CRC patients and their relatives. In the meantime, scientists and clinicians should build bridges of communication and create multidisciplinary committees to interpret genetic and genomic results and translate them into good laboratory practice and clinical guidelines.

Acknowledgments We thank all patients who contributed to our studies and have helped us to better understand the molecular basis underlying colorectal cancer and other hereditary cancer syndromes. The authors would also like to thank all current and former members of the Hereditary Cancer Program at the Catalan Institute of Oncology (ICO). The authors would like to particularly acknowledge the support of the Asociación Española Contra el Cáncer (AECC), the Instituto de Salud Carlos III (organismo adscrito al Ministerio de Economía y Competitividad) and "Fondo Europeo de Desarrollo Regional (FEDER), una manera de hacer Europa" (PI10/01422, PI13/00285, PIE13/00022, PI16/00563, and CIBERONC), and the Institut Català de la Salut and Autonomous Government of Catalonia (2017SGR1282, 2017SGR496 and PERIS Project MedPerCan).

References

1. Ionov Y, Peinado MA, Malkhosyan S, Shibata D, Perucho M. Ubiquitous somatic mutations in simple repeated sequences reveal a new mechanism for colonic carcinogenesis. Nature. 1993;363(6429):558–61.
2. Aaltonen LA, Peltomaki P, Leach FS, Sistonen P, Pylkkanen L, Mecklin JP, et al. Clues to the pathogenesis of familial colorectal cancer. Science (New York, NY). 1993;260(5109):812–6.
3. Verstrepen KJ, Jansen A, Lewitter F, Fink GR. Intragenic tandem repeats generate functional variability. Nat Genet. 2005;37(9):986–90.
4. Cicek MS, Lindor NM, Gallinger S, Bapat B, Hopper JL, Jenkins MA, et al. Quality assessment and correlation of microsatellite instability and immunohistochemical markers among population- and clinic-based colorectal tumors results from the colon cancer family registry. J Mol Diagn: JMD. 2011;13(3):271–81.
5. Boland CR, Thibodeau SN, Hamilton SR, Sidransky D, Eshleman JR, Burt RW, et al. A National Cancer Institute Workshop on Microsatellite Instability for cancer detection and familial predisposition: development of international criteria for the determination of microsatellite instability in colorectal cancer. Cancer Res. 1998;58(22):5248–57.

6. Suraweera N, Duval A, Reperant M, Vaury C, Furlan D, Leroy K, et al. Evaluation of tumor microsatellite instability using five quasimonomorphic mononucleotide repeats and pentaplex PCR. Gastroenterology. 2002;123(6):1804–11.
7. Yamamoto H, Imai K. Microsatellite instability: an update. Arch Toxicol. 2015;89(6):899–921.
8. Vasen HF, Moslein G, Alonso A, Bernstein I, Bertario L, Blanco I, et al. Guidelines for the clinical management of Lynch syndrome (hereditary non-polyposis cancer). J Med Genet. 2007;44(6):353–62.
9. Pineda M, Gonzalez S, Lazaro C, Blanco I, Capella G. Detection of genetic alterations in hereditary colorectal cancer screening. Mutat Res. 2010;693(1–2):19–31.
10. Deng G, Bell I, Crawley S, Gum J, Terdiman JP, Allen BA, et al. BRAF mutation is frequently present in sporadic colorectal cancer with methylated hMLH1, but not in hereditary nonpolyposis colorectal cancer. Clin Cancer Res: Off J Am Assoc Cancer Res. 2004;10(1 Pt 1):191–5.
11. Gausachs M, Mur P, Corral J, Pineda M, Gonzalez S, Benito L, et al. MLH1 promoter hypermethylation in the analytical algorithm of Lynch syndrome: a cost-effectiveness study. Eur J Hum Genet: EJHG. 2012;20(7):762–8.
12. Parsons MT, Buchanan DD, Thompson B, Young JP, Spurdle AB. Correlation of tumour BRAF mutations and MLH1 methylation with germline mismatch repair (MMR) gene mutation status: a literature review assessing utility of tumour features for MMR variant classification. J Med Genet. 2012;49(3):151–7.
13. Moreira L, Munoz J, Cuatrecasas M, Quintanilla I, Leoz ML, Carballal S, et al. Prevalence of somatic mutl homolog 1 promoter hypermethylation in Lynch syndrome colorectal cancer. Cancer. 2015;121(9):1395–404.
14. Newton K, Jorgensen NM, Wallace AJ, Buchanan DD, Lalloo F, McMahon RF, et al. Tumour MLH1 promoter region methylation testing is an effective prescreen for Lynch syndrome (HNPCC). J Med Genet. 2014;51(12):789–96.
15. Bellido F, Pineda M, Aiza G, Valdes-Mas R, Navarro M, Puente DA, et al. POLE and POLD1 mutations in 529 kindred with familial colorectal cancer and/or polyposis: review of reported cases and recommendations for genetic testing and surveillance. Genetics in medicine : Off J Am Coll Med Genet. 2016;18(4):325–32.
16. Shinbrot E, Henninger EE, Weinhold N, Covington KR, Goksenin AY, Schultz N, et al. Exonuclease mutations in DNA polymerase epsilon reveal replication strand specific mutation patterns and human origins of replication. Genome research. 2014;24(11):1740–50.
17. Mertz TM, Baranovskiy AG, Wang J, Tahirov TH, Shcherbakova PV. Nucleotide selectivity defect and mutator phenotype conferred by a colon cancerassociated DNA polymerase delta mutation in human cells. Oncogene. 2017;36(31):4427–33.
18. Bellizzi AM, Frankel WL. Colorectal cancer due to deficiency in DNA mismatch repair function: a review. Adv Anat Pathol. 2009;16(6):405–17.
19. Etzler J, Peyrl A, Zatkova A, Schildhaus HU, Ficek A, Merkelbach-Bruse S, et al. RNA-based mutation analysis identifies an unusual MSH6 splicing defect and circumvents PMS2 pseudogene interference. Hum Mutat. 2008;29(2):299–305.
20. van der Klift HM, Tops CM, Bik EC, Boogaard MW, Borgstein AM, Hansson KB, et al. Quantification of sequence exchange events between PMS2 and PMS2CL provides a basis for improved mutation scanning of Lynch syndrome patients. Hum Mutat. 2010;31(5):578–87.
21. Vaughn CP, Robles J, Swensen JJ, Miller CE, Lyon E, Mao R, et al. Clinical analysis of PMS2: mutation detection and avoidance of pseudogenes. Hum Mutat. 2010;31(5):588–93.
22. Kovacs ME, Papp J, Szentirmay Z, Otto S, Olah E. Deletions removing the last exon of TACSTD1 constitute a distinct class of mutations predisposing to lynch syndrome. Hum Mutat. 2009;30(2):197–203.
23. Ligtenberg MJ, Kuiper RP, Chan TL, Goossens M, Hebeda KM, Voorendt M, et al. Heritable somatic methylation and inactivation of MSH2 in families with Lynch syndrome due to deletion of the 3′ exons of TACSTD1. Nat Genet. 2009;41(1):112–7.
24. Nielsen M, Morreau H, Vasen HF, Hes FJ. MUTYH-associated polyposis (MAP). Crit Rev Oncol Hematol. 2011;79(1):1–16.

25. Grover S, Kastrinos F, Steyerberg EW, Cook EF, Dewanwala A, Burbidge LA, et al. Prevalence and phenotypes of APC and MUTYH mutations in patients with multiple colorectal adenomas. JAMA. 2012;308(5):485–92.
26. Castillejo A, Vargas G, Castillejo MI, Navarro M, Barbera VM, Gonzalez S, et al. Prevalence of germline MUTYH mutations among lynch-like syndrome patients. Eur J Cancer. 2014;50(13):2241–50.
27. Morak M, Heidenreich B, Keller G, Hampel H, Laner A, de la Chapelle A, et al. Biallelic MUTYH mutations can mimic lynch syndrome. Eur J Hum Genet : EJHG. 2014;22(11):1334–7.
28. Segui N, Navarro M, Pineda M, Koger N, Bellido F, Gonzalez S, et al. Exome sequencing identifies MUTYH mutations in a family with colorectal cancer and an atypical phenotype. Gut. 2015;64(2):355–6.
29. van Puijenbroek M, Nielsen M, Tops CM, Halfwerk H, Vasen HF, Weiss MM, et al. Identification of patients with (atypical) MUTYH-associated polyposis by KRAS2 c.34G > T prescreening followed by MUTYH hotspot analysis in formalin-fixed paraffin-embedded tissue. Clin Cancer Res : Off J Am Assoc Cancer Res. 2008;14(1):139–42.
30. Knopperts AP, Nielsen M, Niessen RC, Tops CM, Jorritsma B, Varkevisser J, et al. Contribution of bi-allelic germline MUTYH mutations to early-onset and familial colorectal cancer and to low number of adenomatous polyps: case-series and literature review. Familial Cancer. 2013;12(1):43–50.
31. Bentley DR, Balasubramanian S, Swerdlow HP, Smith GP, Milton J, Brown CG, et al. Accurate whole human genome sequencing using reversible terminator chemistry. Nature. 2008;456(7218):53–9.
32. Rothberg JM, Hinz W, Rearick TM, Schultz J, Mileski W, Davey M, et al. An integrated semiconductor device enabling non-optical genome sequencing. Nature. 2011;475(7356):348–52.
33. Aziz N, Zhao Q, Bry L, Driscoll DK, Funke B, Gibson JS, et al. College of American Pathologists' laboratory standards for next-generation sequencing clinical tests. Arch Pathol Lab Med. 2015;139(4):481–93.
34. Rehm HL, Bale SJ, Bayrak-Toydemir P, Berg JS, Brown KK, Deignan JL, et al. ACMG clinical laboratory standards for next-generation sequencing. Genet Med : Off J Am Coll Med Genet. 2013;15(9):733–47.
35. Strom SP, Lee H, Das K, Vilain E, Nelson SF, Grody WW, et al. Assessing the necessity of confirmatory testing for exome-sequencing results in a clinical molecular diagnostic laboratory. Genet Med : Off J Am Coll Med Genet. 2014;16(7):510–5.
36. Baudhuin LM, Lagerstedt SA, Klee EW, Fadra N, Oglesbee D, Ferber MJ. Confirming variants in next-generation sequencing panel testing by Sanger sequencing. J Mol Diagn : JMD. 2015;17(4):456–61.
37. Mu W, Lu HM, Chen J, Li S, Elliott AM. Sanger confirmation is required to achieve optimal sensitivity and specificity in next-generation sequencing panel testing. J Mol Diagn : JMD. 2016;18(6):923–32.
38. Feliubadaló L, Tonda R, Gausachs M, Trotta JR, Castellanos E, Lopez-Doriga A, et al. Benchmarking of whole exome sequencing and ad hoc designed panels for genetic testing of hereditary cancer. Sci Rep. 2017;7:37984.
39. Campbell PJ, Stephens PJ, Pleasance ED, O'Meara S, Li H, Santarius T, et al. Identification of somatically acquired rearrangements in cancer using genome-wide massively parallel paired-end sequencing. Nat Genet. 2008;40(6):722–9.
40. Yoon S, Xuan Z, Makarov V, Ye K, Sebat J. Sensitive and accurate detection of copy number variants using read depth of coverage. Genome Res. 2009;19(9):1586–92.
41. Ye K, Schulz MH, Long Q, Apweiler R, Ning Z. Pindel: a pattern growth approach to detect break points of large deletions and medium sized insertions from paired-end short reads. Bioinformatics. 2009;25(21):2865–71.
42. Chen K, Wallis JW, McLellan MD, Larson DE, Kalicki JM, Pohl CS, et al. BreakDancer: an algorithm for high-resolution mapping of genomic structural variation. Nat Methods. 2009;6(9):677–81.

43. Bartenhagen C, Dugas M. Robust and exact structural variation detection with paired-end and soft-clipped alignments: SoftSV compared with eight algorithms. Brief Bioinform. 2016;17(1):51–62.
44. Li J, Dai H, Feng Y, Tang J, Chen S, Tian X, et al. A comprehensive strategy for accurate mutation detection of the highly homologous PMS2. J Mol Diagn : JMD. 2015;17(5):545–53.
45. Kim TM, Laird PW, Park PJ. The landscape of microsatellite instability in colorectal and endometrial cancer genomes. Cell. 2013;155(4):858–68.
46. Salipante SJ, Scroggins SM, Hampel HL, Turner EH, Pritchard CC. Microsatellite instability detection by next generation sequencing. Clin Chem. 2014;60(9):1192–9.
47. Glen T. 2016 NGS field guide. 2016. The Molecular Ecologist. 2017, March. Available from: http://www.molecularecologist.com/next-gen-fieldguide-2016/.
48. Feliubadaló L, Lopez-Doriga A, Castellsague E, del Valle J, Menendez M, Tornero E, et al. Next-generation sequencing meets genetic diagnostics: development of a comprehensive workflow for the analysis of BRCA1 and BRCA2 genes. Eur J Hum Genet : EJHG. 2013;21(8):864–70.
49. Susswein LR, Marshall ML, Nusbaum R, Vogel Postula KJ, Weissman SM, Yackowski L, et al. Pathogenic and likely pathogenic variant prevalence among the first 10,000 patients referred for next-generation cancer panel testing. Genet Med : Off J Am Coll Med Genet. 2016;18(8):823–32.
50. LaDuca H, Farwell KD, Vuong H, Lu HM, Mu W, Shahmirzadi L, et al. Exome sequencing covers >98% of mutations identified on targeted next generation sequencing panels. PLoS One. 2017;12(2):e0170843.
51. Yurgelun MB, Allen B, Kaldate RR, Bowles KR, Judkins T, Kaushik P, et al. Identification of a variety of mutations in cancer predisposition genes in patients with suspected lynch syndrome. Gastroenterology. 2015;149(3):604–13 e20.
52. Yurgelun MB, Kulke MH, Fuchs CS, Allen BA, Uno H, Hornick JL, et al. Cancer susceptibility gene mutations in individuals with colorectal cancer. J Clin Oncol. 2017;35(10):1086–95.
53. Chubb D, Broderick P, Frampton M, Kinnersley B, Sherborne A, Penegar S, et al. Genetic diagnosis of high-penetrance susceptibility for colorectal cancer (CRC) is achievable for a high proportion of familial CRC by exome sequencing. J Clin Oncol. 2015;33(5):426–32.
54. Cragun D, Radford C, Dolinsky JS, Caldwell M, Chao E, Pal T. Panel-based testing for inherited colorectal cancer: a descriptive study of clinical testing performed by a US laboratory. Clin Genet. 2014;86(6):510–20.
55. Ricker C, Culver JO, Lowstuter K, Sturgeon D, Sturgeon JD, Chanock CR, et al. Increased yield of actionable mutations using multi-gene panels to assess hereditary cancer susceptibility in an ethnically diverse clinical cohort. Cancer Genet. 2016;209(4):130–7.
56. Pearlman R, Frankel WL, Swanson B, Zhao W, Yilmaz A, Miller K, et al. Prevalence and spectrum of germline cancer susceptibility gene mutations among patients with early-onset colorectal cancer. JAMA Oncol. 2017;3(4):464–471. doi:10.1001/jamaoncol.2016.5194.
57. Slavin TP, Niell-Swiller M, Solomon I, Nehoray B, Rybak C, Blazer KR, et al. Clinical application of multigene panels: challenges of next-generation counseling and cancer risk management. Front Oncol. 2015;5:208.
58. Hermel DJ, McKinnon WC, Wood ME, Greenblatt MS. Multi-gene panel testing for hereditary cancer susceptibility in a rural Familial Cancer Program. Familial Cancer. 2017;16(1):159–66.
59. Howarth DR, Lum SS, Esquivel P, Garberoglio CA, Senthil M, Solomon NL. Initial results of multigene panel testing for hereditary breast and ovarian cancer and lynch syndrome. Am Surg. 2015;81(10):941–4.
60. Rohlin A, Rambech E, Kvist A, Torngren T, Eiengard F, Lundstam U, et al. Expanding the genotype-phenotype spectrum in hereditary colorectal cancer by gene panel testing. Familial Cancer. 2017;16(2):195–203.
61. Illumina. TruSight Cancer Gene List (.xls). 2017. Available from: https://www.google.es/url?sa=t&rct=j&q=&esrc=s&source=web&cd=3&cad=rja&uact=8&ved=0ahUKEwiJ24PerKTTAhUKthoKHSAdALsQFgg4MAI&url=https%3A%2F%2Fwww.illumina.

com%2Fcontent%2Fdam%2Fillumina-marketing%2Fdocuments%2Fproducts%2Fgene_lists%2Fgene_list_trusight_cancer.xlsx&usg=AFQjCNEJE1drO3kJvcytgOlazl2GfLIvGw&sig2=QnYf4jA2e2gvW8YGrd2RTA&bvm=bv.152479541,d.d2s.
62. Illumina. TruSight Cancer. 2017. Available from: https://www.illumina.com/products/by-type/clinical-research-products/trusight-cancer.html.
63. Castellanos E, Gel B, Rosas I, Tornero E, Santin S, Pluvinet R, et al. A comprehensive custom panel design for routine hereditary cancer testing: preserving control, improving diagnostics and revealing a complex variation landscape. Sci Rep. 2017;7:39348.
64. Eccles DM, Mitchell G, Monteiro AN, Schmutzler R, Couch FJ, Spurdle AB, et al. BRCA1 and BRCA2 genetic testing-pitfalls and recommendations for managing variants of uncertain clinical significance. Ann oncol : Off J Eur Soc Med Oncol. 2015;26(10):2057–65.
65. Balmana J, Digiovanni L, Gaddam P, Walsh MF, Joseph V, Stadler ZK, et al. Conflicting interpretation of genetic variants and cancer risk by commercial laboratories as assessed by the prospective registry of multiplex testing. J Clin Oncol. 2016;34(34):4071–8.
66. Whitworth J, Skytte AB, Sunde L, Lim DH, Arends MJ, Happerfield L, et al. Multilocus inherited Neoplasia alleles syndrome: a case series and review. JAMA Oncol. 2016;2(3):373–9.
67. Wimmer K, Kratz CP. Constitutional mismatch repair-deficiency syndrome. Haematologica. 2010;95(5):699–701.
68. Gallego CJ, Shirts BH, Bennette CS, Guzauskas G, Amendola LM, Horike-Pyne M, et al. Next-generation sequencing panels for the diagnosis of colorectal cancer and polyposis syndromes: a cost-effectiveness analysis. J Clin Oncol. 2015;33(18):2084–91.
69. Ng SB, Turner EH, Robertson PD, Flygare SD, Bigham AW, Lee C, et al. Targeted capture and massively parallel sequencing of 12 human exomes. Nature. 2009;461(7261):272–6.
70. Choi M, Scholl UI, Ji W, Liu T, Tikhonova IR, Zumbo P, et al. Genetic diagnosis by whole exome capture and massively parallel DNA sequencing. Proc Natl Acad Sci U S A. 2009;106(45):19096–101.
71. Harding KE, Robertson NP. Applications of next-generation whole exome sequencing. J Neurol. 2014;261(6):1244–6.
72. Warr A, Robert C, Hume D, Archibald A, Deeb N, Watson M. Exome sequencing: current and future perspectives. G3 (Bethesda). MD. 2015;5(8):1543–50.
73. Chilamakuri CS, Lorenz S, Madoui MA, Vodak D, Sun J, Hovig E, et al. Performance comparison of four exome capture systems for deep sequencing. BMC Genomics. 2014;15:449.
74. Meienberg J, Zerjavic K, Keller I, Okoniewski M, Patrignani A, Ludin K, et al. New insights into the performance of human whole-exome capture platforms. Nucleic Acids Res. 2015;43(11):e76.
75. Wang JL, Yang X, Xia K, Hu ZM, Weng L, Jin X, et al. TGM6 identified as a novel causative gene of spinocerebellar ataxias using exome sequencing. Brain. 2010;133(Pt 12):3510–8.
76. Vissers LE, de Ligt J, Gilissen C, Janssen I, Steehouwer M, de Vries P, et al. A de novo paradigm for mental retardation. Nat Genet. 2010;42(12):1109–12.
77. Ng SB, Buckingham KJ, Lee C, Bigham AW, Tabor HK, Dent KM, et al. Exome sequencing identifies the cause of a mendelian disorder. Nat Genet. 2010;42(1):30–5.
78. Lee H, Deignan JL, Dorrani N, Strom SP, Kantarci S, Quintero-Rivera F, et al. Clinical exome sequencing for genetic identification of rare Mendelian disorders. JAMA. 2014;312(18):1880–7.
79. Yang Y, Muzny DM, Xia F, Niu Z, Person R, Ding Y, et al. Molecular findings among patients referred for clinical whole-exome sequencing. JAMA. 2014;312(18):1870–9.
80. Jones S, Hruban RH, Kamiyama M, Borges M, Zhang X, Parsons DW, et al. Exomic sequencing identifies PALB2 as a pancreatic cancer susceptibility gene. Science (New York, NY). 2009;324(5924):217.
81. Nieminen TT, O'Donohue MF, Wu Y, Lohi H, Scherer SW, Paterson AD, et al. Germline mutation of RPS20, encoding a ribosomal protein, causes predisposition to hereditary nonpolyposis colorectal carcinoma without DNA mismatch repair deficiency. Gastroenterology. 2014;147(3):595–8 e5.

82. Lupski JR, Reid JG, Gonzaga-Jauregui C, Rio Deiros D, Chen DC, Nazareth L, et al. Whole-genome sequencing in a patient with Charcot-Marie-tooth neuropathy. N Engl J Med. 2010;362(13):1181–91.
83. Sobreira NL, Cirulli ET, Avramopoulos D, Wohler E, Oswald GL, Stevens EL, et al. Whole-genome sequencing of a single proband together with linkage analysis identifies a Mendelian disease gene. PLoS Genet. 2010;6(6):e1000991.
84. Rios J, Stein E, Shendure J, Hobbs HH, Cohen JC. Identification by whole-genome resequencing of gene defect responsible for severe hypercholesterolemia. Hum Mol Genet. 2010;19(22):4313–8.
85. Yokoyama S, Woods SL, Boyle GM, Aoude LG, MacGregor S, Zismann V, et al. A novel recurrent mutation in MITF predisposes to familial and sporadic melanoma. Nature. 2011;480(7375):99–103.
86. Roberts NJ, Jiao Y, Yu J, Kopelovich L, Petersen GM, Bondy ML, et al. ATM mutations in patients with hereditary pancreatic cancer. Cancer Discov. 2012;2(1):41–6.
87. Comino-Mendez I, Gracia-Aznarez FJ, Schiavi F, Landa I, Leandro-Garcia LJ, Leton R, et al. Exome sequencing identifies MAX mutations as a cause of hereditary pheochromocytoma. Nat Genet. 2011;43(7):663–7.
88. Rafnar T, Gudbjartsson DF, Sulem P, Jonasdottir A, Sigurdsson A, Jonasdottir A, et al. Mutations in BRIP1 confer high risk of ovarian cancer. Nat Genet. 2011;43(11):1104–7.
89. Palles C, Cazier JB, Howarth KM, Domingo E, Jones AM, Broderick P, et al. Germline mutations affecting the proofreading domains of POLE and POLD1 predispose to colorectal adenomas and carcinomas. Nat Genet. 2013;45(2):136–44.
90. Belkadi A, Bolze A, Itan Y, Cobat A, Vincent QB, Antipenko A, et al. Whole-genome sequencing is more powerful than whole-exome sequencing for detecting exome variants. Proc Natl Acad Sci U S A. 2015;112(17):5473–8.
91. Lelieveld SH, Spielmann M, Mundlos S, Veltman JA, Gilissen C. Comparison of exome and genome sequencing Technologies for the Complete Capture of protein-coding regions. Hum Mutat. 2015;36(8):815–22.
92. Meynert AM, Ansari M, FitzPatrick DR, Taylor MS. Variant detection sensitivity and biases in whole genome and exome sequencing. BMC bioinformatics. 2014;15:247.
93. Abdel-Rahman MH, Rai K, Pilarski R, Davidorf FH, Cebulla CM. Germline BAP1 mutations misreported as somatic based on tumor-only testing. Familial Cancer. 2016;15(2):327–30.

Chapter 17
Universal Tumor Screening for Lynch Syndrome

Heather Hampel, Rachel Pearlman, and Deborah Cragun

Abstract Lynch syndrome is estimated to affect 1 out of every 279 individuals worldwide. However, 95% of individuals with Lynch syndrome are not aware of their diagnosis. Therefore, it is important that we maximize all possible efforts to diagnose individuals with Lynch syndrome. Universal tumor screening is one approach that has been successful in helping to identify patients who might not have been referred for a genetics assessment otherwise. Universal tumor screening consists of testing the paraffin-embedded tumor from individuals with colorectal or endometrial cancer for features of deficient mismatch repair including microsatellite instability and/or absence of any of the four mismatch repair proteins (MLH1, MSH2, MSH6, and PMS2) using immunohistochemical (IHC) staining. Several professional organizations have recommended universal tumor screening of all newly diagnosed colorectal cancer patients at the time of diagnosis. Reasons for this recommendation are that patients whose tumors exhibit microsatellite instability (whether proven by MSI testing or extrapolated from abnormal IHC testing) have a better prognosis may need different treatment from those without microsatellite instability, and are more likely to have Lynch syndrome. Patients whose tumors exhibit MSI or have abnormal IHC without *MLH1* methylation are suspicious for having Lynch syndrome and are candidates for genetic counseling and germline genetic testing. Best practices for implementing universal tumor screening have been explored.

H. Hampel (✉) · R. Pearlman
Division of Human Genetics, Department of Internal Medicine, The Ohio State University Comprehensive Cancer Center, Columbus, OH, USA
e-mail: Heather.Hampel@osumc.edu

D. Cragun
Department of Global Health, College of Public Health, University of South Florida, Tampa, FL, USA

L. Valle et al. (eds.), *Hereditary Colorectal Cancer*,
https://doi.org/10.1007/978-3-319-74259-5_17

Keywords Hereditary · Colorectal cancer · Universal tumor screening · Microsatellite instability · Immunohistochemical staining · Mismatch repair proteins

1 Introduction

Lynch syndrome is estimated to affect 1 out of every 279 individuals worldwide [1]. In the United States alone, the American Cancer Society predicts that there will be 135,430 new cases of colorectal cancer diagnosed in 2017 [2]. It is projected that 4063 of these patients (3%) have Lynch syndrome and another 12,189 of their family members also have Lynch syndrome [3, 4]. However, it is estimated that 95% of individuals with Lynch syndrome are not aware of their diagnosis [5]. Therefore, it is important that we maximize all possible efforts to diagnose individuals with Lynch syndrome. Universal tumor screening is one approach that has been successful in helping to identify patients who might not have been referred for a genetics assessment otherwise. Universal tumor screening consists of testing the paraffin-embedded tumor from individuals with colorectal or endometrial cancer for features of deficient mismatch repair (MMR) including microsatellite instability (MSI: a characteristic found in 77–89% of tumors from individuals with Lynch syndrome) and/or absence of any of the four mismatch repair proteins (MLH1, MSH2, MSH6, and PMS2) using immunohistochemical (IHC) staining (one or more of these proteins are absent in 83% of tumors from individuals with Lynch syndrome) [6]. Reasons for this recommendation are that patients whose tumors exhibit MSI (whether proven by MSI testing or extrapolated from abnormal IHC testing) (1) have a better prognosis [7], (2) may need different treatment from those without microsatellite instability [8, 9], and (3) are more likely to have Lynch syndrome [3, 4] (Table 17.1). For cases with MSI-high tumors or tumors that are missing the MLH1 and PMS2 proteins, additional testing to determine if this was caused by acquired *MLH1* promoter methylation follows. This can be done directly by assessing the methylation level of the *MLH1* promoter or indirectly by testing for the somatic *BRAF* V600E mutation. If *MLH1* promoter methylation or the *BRAF* V600E mutation is found, the patient generally does not need additional follow-up. The remaining patients whose tumors exhibit MSI or have abnormal IHC without *MLH1* promoter methylation are suspicious for having Lynch syndrome and are candidates for genetic counseling and germline genetic testing. Several professional organizations have recommended universal tumor screening of all newly diagnosed colorectal cancer patients at the time of diagnosis [10–13]. Best practices for implementing universal tumor screening have been explored. There are many possible barriers to the implementation of universal tumor screening for all newly diagnosed CRC patients, but one of the most significant is that many cancer centers do not have cancer genetics professionals on staff to provide genetic counseling and follow-up genetic testing to the patients whose tumors have defective mismatch repair.

Table 17.1 The case for routine tumor screening for Lynch syndrome

• Lynch syndrome is common: ~3% of colorectal patients
• Reduce morbidity and mortality
• Recommended by several professional organizations
• Cost-effective
• Meets public health screening program criteria
• Becoming standard of care
• Identifies substantially more patients with Lynch syndrome [37–40]. Routine tumor screening identifies over 95% of patients with Lynch syndrome. In contrast, clinical criteria (Bethesda or Amsterdam) fail to identify a substantial proportion of individuals with Lynch syndrome, and these criteria are inconsistently applied
• Referral of patients with abnormal screen results for genetic counseling and molecular testing for germline MMR mutations allows for diagnostic confirmation for the patient and accurate testing for family members
• Identification of a colorectal cancer patient with Lynch syndrome affects future screening for colorectal cancer and other Lynch syndrome-associated malignancies
• Evidence suggests a diagnosis of Lynch syndrome may affect surgical and chemotherapeutic management decisions

This chapter will address all of the issues surrounding universal tumor screening for Lynch syndrome.

2 Universal Tumor Screening for Lynch Syndrome

2.1 Tumor Screening Methods

There are many algorithms available for tumor screening for Lynch syndrome. All involve the testing of tumor tissue.

MSI Approximately 77–89% of colon tumors from individuals with Lynch syndrome demonstrate microsatellite instability (MSI), whereas only approximately 15% of sporadic colon tumors exhibit this molecular feature. Thus, MSI testing is useful in identifying patients who are more or less likely to have Lynch syndrome.

IHC Tumors from individuals with Lynch syndrome are likely to demonstrate loss of mismatch repair protein expression. The pattern of observed protein loss can provide information about which gene is not functioning properly. As a result, immunohistochemistry (IHC) testing can be helpful both in providing information about the likelihood of Lynch syndrome and in directing germline genetic testing to a specific gene.

***MLH1* Promoter Methylation** The majority of tumors that are MSI-high or are missing the MLH1 and PMS2 proteins on IHC are caused by acquired methylation of the *MLH1* promoter. This can be assessed directly by studying CpG islands in the

MLH1 promoter. This is very important to universal tumor screening programs because it limits the number of individuals who need follow-up genetic counseling and testing. Those with acquired *MLH1* promoter methylation generally do not need germline genetic testing.

***BRAF* V600E Somatic Testing** The somatic *BRAF* V600E mutation can be used as a surrogate for *MLH1* promoter methylation testing in colorectal tumors, but not in endometrial tumors. This mutation is found in 68% of colorectal tumors with *MLH1* methylation, so it can identify the majority of cases with methylation, but not all. It is important to note that cases without the *BRAF* V600E mutation may still have *MLH1* methylation [6]. This mutation is studied for treatment purposes in many cancers, so it is generally easier for hospitals to add this multipurpose test than to develop an *MLH1* methylation test which would be used solely for universal tumor screening.

There is no consensus on whether MSI, IHC, or both are the ideal screening tool for Lynch syndrome. Immunohistochemistry was originally shown to be more cost-effective because it could reduce the number of genes that needed to be sequenced by identifying the 1–2 genes most likely to be mutated. However, with the advent of next-generation sequencing panels, the cost of genetic testing is now generally the same regardless of the number of genes included, which should make the cost-effectiveness of MSI and IHC more equivalent. There are limitations to both tests. For example, MSI alone may not detect all patients with *MSH6* mutations since not all *MSH6*-related tumors have MSI. On the other hand, IHC alone may not detect all patients with Lynch syndrome because some mutations will still result in a full-length protein, so the protein will be present on IHC even though it is dysfunctional (e.g., pathogenic missense mutations). Some centers perform both tests simultaneously or sequentially to provide as much information as possible, but this is not the most cost-effective approach. The majority of centers use IHC as the screening test out of convenience since it does not require a molecular laboratory and *BRAF* as the follow-up test to rule out *MLH1*-methylated cases for tumors with the absence of MLH1 and PMS2 on IHC (Fig. 17.1).

3 Applications of Universal Tumor Screening for Lynch Syndrome: Screening All Tumors Versus a Subset of Tumors

When universal tumor screening was first proposed, multiple groups considered how to limit the screening test to the smallest number of patients possible by proposing age cutoffs or scoring systems based on histologic features. However, it became clear that restricting tumor screening to a subset of cases would result in patients with Lynch syndrome being missed, so the lack of sensitivity had to be weighed against the decrease in cost. The largest meta-analysis of universal tumor

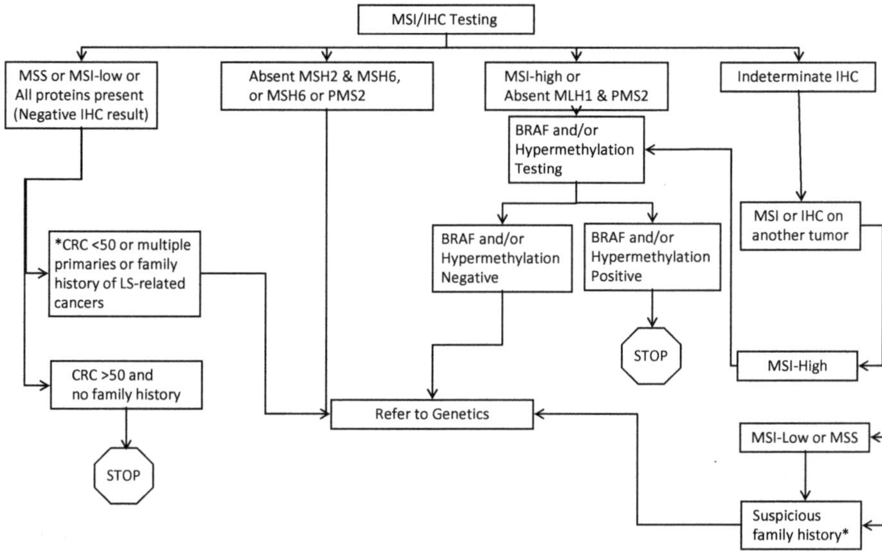

Fig. 17.1 Flowchart for universal tumor screening for Lynch syndrome

screening for Lynch syndrome among colorectal cancers recommended one of two possible approaches to the screening population. First, centers could elect to screen all cases of colorectal cancer regardless of age at diagnosis. This is the most sensitive approach but does cost the most, and the ratio of positive cases to all cases screened becomes quite low in the oldest age groups. As a cost-saving measure, they also recommended that centers could elect to screen all cases of colorectal cancer diagnosed under age 70 and only the cases diagnosed at or after age 70 who met Bethesda criteria. While this might save money, it would likely lead to no testing in patients age 70 and older because pathology departments are unlikely to know the patient's prior cancer history or family history and therefore are unable to determine who does and does not meet the Bethesda guidelines. In addition, most pathologists agree that it is much easier to adopt a policy of screening all cases of colorectal cancer since this makes it less likely that cases will fall through the cracks due to high volume.

4 Cost-Effectiveness

Most articles demonstrate positive cost-effectiveness data for universal tumor screening programs [14–24], including one from an integrated healthcare organization's perspective [18]. For universal tumor screening among colorectal cancers, all studies agree screening age ≤ 70 is cost-effective (US healthcare) [5, 6], and many support true universal tumor screening with no age restrictions [16, 17, 19]. Results and conclusions vary due to differences in screening protocols (and associated costs), societal value judgment ($50,000 per life year saved), number of at-risk relatives tested, and other assumptions that must be made. Prior to widespread use of panel-based gene testing, the most cost-effective strategy involved IHC testing first, followed by testing for the *BRAF* mutation among those with absent MLH1 staining, and subsequent targeted MMR gene sequencing and deletion analysis among those with absent staining for other proteins and those without the *BRAF* mutation, with an incremental cost-effectiveness ratio of less than $40,000 per life year saved compared with age-targeted testing [16, 17, 19]. Cascade testing among at-risk relatives is one of the key factors influencing the cost-effectiveness of universal tumor screening for Lynch syndrome, with screening becoming more cost-effective as increasing numbers of relatives undergo genetic counseling and testing [16, 17, 19]. In addition, as noted previously, IHC was found to be more cost-effective prior to the advent of next-generation sequencing panels when genetic testing required Sanger sequencing of one gene at a time. As a result, IHC was more cost-effective since it predicted in which gene the mutation likely occurred. Now that all of the Lynch syndrome genes can be tested simultaneously using next-generation sequencing for the same cost as testing one gene using Sanger sequencing, the cost-effectiveness of MSI is likely more similar to that of IHC (with the exception of requiring *BRAF* testing or *MLH1* methylation testing on all MSI-high cases instead of just those with the absence of MLH1 and PMS2 in the case of IHC).

5 Professional Organizations Endorsing Universal Tumor Screening

Screening for Lynch syndrome on all newly diagnosed colorectal cancers is recommended by several organizations (Table 17.2), and it is a Healthy People 2020 objective. It is already performed in more than 100 hospitals nationwide and numerous hospitals around the world (www.lynchscreening.net). The first organization to recommend universal tumor screening for Lynch syndrome was the Evaluation of Genomic Applications in Practice and Prevention (EGAPP) group out of the Centers for Disease Control (CDC). In 2009, the EGAPP Working Group found sufficient evidence to recommend offering testing for Lynch syndrome to patients with newly diagnosed colorectal cancer, citing its ability to reduce morbidity and mortality in relatives. They did not specify which screening test to use, finding that both were nearly equally effective. Due to the poor performance of the Amsterdam and Bethesda criterion, the EGAPP Working Group did not recommend use of family history to exclude individuals from screening. In 2013, the National Comprehensive Cancer Network guidelines recommended tumor screening for Lynch syndrome for all colorectal cancer patients or colorectal cancer patients diagnosed before age 70 and those 70 years and above who met Bethesda guidelines and all endometrial cancer patients up to age 50. The guidelines also address diagnostic criteria and management for Lynch syndrome and include a helpful algorithm for following up on tumor testing results. The US Multi-Society Task Force on Colorectal Cancer

Table 17.2 Professional organizations that have recommended universal tumor screening for Lynch syndrome among colorectal cancer patients

Tumor to Screen	Professional organization	Year recommendation released
Colorectal cancer	Evaluation of Genetic Applications in Practice and Prevention [10] (CDC)	2009
	Healthy People 2020	2010
	National Comprehensive Cancer Network	2013
	European Society of Medical Oncology [29]	2013
	US Multi-society Task Force on Colorectal Cancer [11]	2014
	American College of Gastroenterology [13]	2015
	American Society of Clinical Oncology [27]	2015
	National Institute for Health and Care Excellence [28] (UK)	2017

released a consensus statement guideline on genetic evaluation and management of Lynch syndrome in 2014 [11]. The National Society for Genetic Counselors (NSGC) and Collaborative Group of the Americas on Inherited Colorectal Cancer (CGA-ICC) guideline [25] does not specifically recommend universal screening for Lynch syndrome; however, it did endorse IHC as the preferred method of screening when universal screening for Lynch syndrome is being implemented based on cost considerations at the time. No recommendation was made about the use of *MLH1* promoter methylation and/or *BRAF* testing after abnormal MLH1 and PMS2 results from IHC. This guideline also provides a review of the literature on Lynch syndrome with emphasis on tumor analysis and testing.

Universal tumor screening for Lynch syndrome is also recommended by the American Society of Clinical Oncology [26], the National Institute for Health and Care Excellence in the United Kingdom [27], the European Society for Medical Oncology [28], and the American College of Gastroenterology [13].

6 Adoption of Universal Tumor Screening for Lynch Syndrome

Universal tumor screening for Lynch syndrome is increasingly being adopted. When adoption was assessed in 2012 [29], 71% of NCI-Comprehensive Cancer Centers were performing universal tumor screening for Lynch syndrome. However, only 36% of College of Surgeons-accredited community hospital comprehensive cancer programs and 15% of community hospital cancer programs were performing universal tumor screening at that time.

7 Impact of Immunotherapy for Microsatellite Unstable Tumors

Patients with MSI-high tumors appear to respond well to immunotherapy [30]. A phase II clinical trial has shown that patients with MSI-high metastatic colorectal cancer may benefit from pembrolizumab, an anti-programmed death 1 immune checkpoint inhibitor [30]. The immune-related objective response rate was 40% (4/10) in patients with mismatch repair-deficient colorectal cancer, with an immune-related progression-free survival rate of 78% (7/9) in patients whose disease had progressed on prior standard chemotherapies [30]. Thus, the benefits of identifying patients with tumors that are MSI-high, or that have lost MMR protein expression, extend beyond screening for Lynch syndrome. See Chaps. 16, 23 and 24 in the Genetic Diagnostics, Clinical Management section of this book for more information.

8 Implementing Tumor Screening for Lynch Syndrome

Tumor screening programs can be challenging to implement due to the many different stakeholders (e.g., healthcare providers from various specialties, patients, administrators) who need to be involved in the process, variety of approaches that can be considered, and multiple steps that need to be well coordinated to ensure that patients and their family members truly benefit from tumor screening programs. A guide, summarized in Table 17.3, was developed by the authors to help institutions through the complex process of developing an implementation plan while considering issues of quality. This guide is based on our own research [31, 32] as well as the Consolidated Framework for Implementation Research (CFIR) process domain, which includes concepts from various implementation theories and/or research demonstrating how they relate to rates of adoption or implementation effectiveness of evidence-based recommendations [33].

Regardless of the type of systematic screening or testing approach selected, there are many different factors that can influence implementation success and the likelihood of desired outcomes. We have used data from our own implementation research and practical experiences to identify several recommendations that may increase the likelihood of successful implementation and high uptake of genetic counseling and germline genetic testing by patients [31, 32]. These recommendations are summarized according to CFIR constructs within Table 17.4 below.

Once implemented, the most significant barrier is getting patients with abnormal tumor screening to undergo genetic counseling with consideration of genetic testing. These patients are different from those seen in the traditional genetic counseling model because they did not seek out genetics due to concerns about their personal or family history, range in age from 18 to 89+, may have little to no knowledge about Lynch syndrome or hereditary cancers, and are dealing with their own new

Table 17.3 Considerations for planning routine Lynch syndrome tumor screening based on the process domain of the Consolidated Framework for Implementation Research (CFIR)

Engaging stakeholders	
Who are the stakeholders?	Centers that have successfully implemented tumor screening tend to include representatives from several key stakeholder groups early on in the planning stage. These stakeholders may include: • Surgery • Pathology • Oncology • Gastroenterology • Genetics • Gynecology • Patients • Families • Hospital administrators
How can we engage stakeholders?	Starting and maintaining successful screening programs is easier and more likely to be successful with upfront support and input from all key stakeholders. Some ways to engage stakeholders include: • Find champions from each stakeholder group because healthcare providers and others are often more likely to listen to someone from their own specialty or group • Evaluate stakeholders' interests and motivations • Hold a conference or meeting (tumor board) • Make the case (provide supporting evidence and cost-effectiveness data, list institutions that have already adopted the approach, show the impact on patients and families, provide supporting guidelines from various professional organizations) • Elicit and address barriers
Planning: Tumor screening approach	
Which patients to screen?	As described previously, we favor tumor screening for *all* newly diagnosed colorectal cancer patients. Limiting based on various criteria will miss an estimated 25–75% of patients, depending on the screening criteria used. Additional time and resources must be expended to gather and review data when complex screening criteria are used, and it is harder to automate or routinize the process. Pathologists do not usually have access to complete family histories to implement Bethesda criteria, and patients meeting the criteria are likely to be missed.
Which specimens to screen (biopsies versus tumor resections)?	• Screening biopsies allow for surgical decision-making (subtotal vs. segmental resection) • Rectal tumors have not been exposed to neoadjuvant chemotherapy and radiation yet, so IHC on these biopsies is more reliable than after neoadjuvant chemotherapy • Biopsies often do not have enough tumor or normal tissue to do MSI. • Screening could be done twice (once on biopsy and once on surgical resection), thereby decreasing cost-effectiveness. • Patient may be lost to follow-up if they don't have surgery or if they have surgery elsewhere.

(continued)

Table 17.3 (continued)

What about informed consent?	Issues of consent slowed implementation at several centers that were among the early adopters of tumor screening. Consider using arguments from these institutions to circumvent concerns about informed consent for tumor screening early on: • Ethics committees have determined that explicit informed consent for screening is *not* necessary and that patients can consent for germline testing if the tumor screen is suggestive of Lynch syndrome. • Most centers do *not* obtain consent for screening. • Some centers provide patient information about screening and/or include a general statement in the pre-op consent form.
Who orders the screen?	Requiring a separate order for each patient or leaving it up to each healthcare provider to order the screening increases the chance that cases will be missed and patients will receive inadequate care. For these reasons, we believe the best approach is to have a standing order or an automated procedure allowing pathologists to automatically screen all tumors.
What method should be used to screen tumors (i.e., MSI versus IHC versus both)? Alternatively, should institutions go straight to germline panel-based testing?	• Using IHC *or* MSI as a first screen can be cost-effective, but doing both simultaneously is *not* a cost-effective approach. • The sensitivity and specificity are comparable between IHC and MSI (assuming that pathologists are experienced with IHC). • Most institutions have implemented IHC, probably because it was initially more cost-effective. However, with the advent of next-generation sequencing and panel-based testing of multiple genes simultaneously at relatively low cost, IHC may not necessarily be more cost-effective than MSI. • Germline panel-based testing as a first-line test has *not* been implemented at most centers presumably due to logistical concerns related to the need to obtain informed consent for this diagnostic test. However, given the additional opportunity to identify hereditary cancer syndromes other than lynch syndrome, it may be prudent to offer such testing (at least to a subset of those diagnosed at a young age, who should be referred for genetic counseling even if tumor screening finds no evidence of mismatch repair deficiency) [41] • Once costs fall, tumor sequencing may become the preferred approach because it will simplify the screening protocol, reduce the need for reflex testing (described below), and may provide additional prognostic or treatment information. Furthermore, tumor testing can be done without explicit informed consent because patients subsequently consent for germline testing if the tumor testing is suggestive of Lynch syndrome.

(continued)

Table 17.3 (continued)

Should we perform automatic reflex testing to help determine patients with mismatch repair deficiency that is unlikely due to Lynch syndrome?	Approximately 15% of sporadic tumors will demonstrate mismatch repair deficiency, usually as a result of *MLH1* promoter hypermethylation. Determining which cases are likely sporadic is possible with additional testing on either all tumors with microsatellite instability if MSI is used or on tumors with absence of *MLH1* and *PMS2* if IHC is used. Reflex testing (using *MLH1* hypermethylation or *BRAF* mutation testing) may streamline your protocol and reduce the added time, cost, and patient anxiety that can be associated with the need to be evaluated by genetics. Furthermore, we have hypothesized that reducing the number seen by genetics who do not end up having Lynch syndrome makes it less likely that providers or patients will just assume that the positive screen was due to *MLH1* promoter hypermethylation and can create more of an urgency to follow through with germline testing for those cases without evidence of hypermethylation.
What method should we use for reflex testing (i.e., *MLH1* hypermethylation versus *BRAF* V600E mutation testing)?	*BRAF* testing only detects ~2/3 of colorectal tumors with hypermethylation [6]. However, hypermethylation could erroneously eliminate patients with Lynch syndrome who have a germline *PMS2* mutation or *MLH1* mutation with hypermethylation as their second hit (at this point it is not known how common this is though). The type of reflex testing selected appears to depend largely on what is available at certain institutions. Many centers have *BRAF* available in house and do not want to send out samples for hypermethylation testing [note: *BRAF* testing does not work for endometrial tumors because very few of these tumors have hypermethylation that is caused by *BRAF* mutations].
Planning: Results follow-up	
Where and to whom will positive screening results go (i.e., those demonstrating MSI-high or absent proteins on IHC staining)?	Screen-positive results should be entered into the pathology report and flagged in the electronic medical record so that the surgeon and other physicians working with the patient are aware of this result. This is important because patients with evidence of mismatch repair deficiency (i.e., MSI-high tumors or absent proteins on IHC) have a better prognosis than other colorectal cancer patients and may have different treatment options

(continued)

Table 17.3 (continued)

Who will be responsible for disclosing the positive results to patients?	• All individuals involved in screening need to understand the importance of patient follow-up with genetic counseling and germline genetic testing. Without follow-up, patients and their family members are unlikely to benefit from tumor screening programs, and the programs will *not* be cost-effective. • Roles and responsibilities should be well defined including designating who is responsible to follow up on all screen-positive results. Without follow-up and tracking mechanisms in place, several centers reported that tumor screening results were getting lost in medical records. There was often *no record* that patients were offered genetic counseling and germline genetic testing, raising concerns about legal liability. • Several institutions have found it helpful to have a single person (with a backup person) who is responsible for all results disclosure or follow-up. • Having a genetic counselor follow-up has been helpful for several institutions because they already have the knowledge about Lynch syndrome and deal with this routinely. Plus, this takes the burden off physicians who have many other competing demands and may be unable to prioritize spending time discussing genetic implications. • A few institutions where tumor screening has been successful have indicated that when genetic counselors disclose screening results, they indicate they are working with Dr. _______ (the patient's treating physician). • Unfortunately these strategies are not feasible options at some institutions, making patient follow-through with counseling/germline testing more challenging. Nonetheless, some centers have been relatively successful when the treating physicians are in routine communication with genetic counselors who remind them which patients need follow-up and the physicians subsequently stress to the patient the importance of follow-up.
How will the patients be informed of a screen-positive result?	Several institutions report difficulty contacting patients and overcame this by meeting them at a post-op appointment for a brief pretest counseling session to facilitate germline testing. The experiences at OSU and Cleveland Clinic provide data to support the value of this approach. [42, 43] Regardless of whether patients are informed by phone or at a post-op appointment, it is important to identify and implement ways to help ensure patients receive appropriate counseling and follow-up (see below). Follow-up with a letter may be useful, especially in cases when there is difficulty contacting the patients. Sample letters for screen-positive and screen-negative patients are included in the implementation section of the Lynch Syndrome Screening Network (LSSN) website (www.lynchscreening.net) and are tailored according to whether IHC or MSI is used. Other useful information such as sample reports are also included in the website.

(continued)

Table 17.3 (continued)

How will patients with screen-positive results receive appropriate counseling?	Patients with a positive screen will need information about germline testing in order to make an informed decision and benefit from the information. Patients can either receive a full pretest genetic counseling session or a shorter informed consent session with plans for a full genetic counseling session once results of germline testing are available.
What steps can you put into place to facilitate patient follow-through with genetic counseling and reduce patient barriers?	• Eliminate the need for the patient to be referred to genetics, or automate the referral and scheduling process. • Schedule genetic counseling follow-up to coincide with another follow-up visit. • Have a genetic service provider meet the patient at a follow-up appointment. • Have all healthcare providers involved in patient care stress the importance of follow-up. • Make patients aware of available funds for germline testing of uninsured patients who meet certain qualifications or any other funding that may be available to ensure patients can access germline testing. • Follow up again with patients if they have not followed through because they may have fewer competing demands or feel a bit less overwhelmed after treatment is complete. • Send a letter to the patient if they have not followed up after a certain period of time. • Send a letter to the treating physician to remind them to follow up with the patient and/or to send a referral (included in the implementation section of the LSSN website). • Communicate during tumor boards to remind treating physicians when patients still need to follow up with genetics. • Put an electronic reminder system in place.
Where and to whom will negative screening results go?	Results should be documented in the chart. Additionally, having an active tracking mechanism or someone review basic information about the patients with negative results can be helpful in identifying others for whom a genetics referral is appropriate if your center has time and resources available to do this. This improves quality of care and has resulted in the diagnosis of other hereditary cancer syndromes.
How and by whom will the patients be informed of negative results?	Some centers generate a standardized letter which informs the patient that their tumor was screened. This is useful in case they are asked about this in the future, and it also provides an opportunity to explain that there may be other causes of hereditary cancer, and encourage the patient to talk with their physician, and/or make an appointment if they have "red flags" that would suggest genetic counseling is indicated. Other centers may have physicians mention the results to the patient, and review whether a genetics appointment is warranted for other reasons (e.g., polyposis, strong family history, multiple primaries, early age at diagnosis). Simply putting results in the chart means that the opportunity to catch patients at high risk for other hereditary cancer syndromes may be lost.

(continued)

Table 17.3 (continued)

Executing the plan	
Will you document how the plan is executed?	Ways in which screening is executed can positively or negatively influence patient follow-up (e.g., who discloses and tracks results, whether processes are automated, timeliness of results disclosure and follow-up). Documenting whether the plan was executed as intended is important as deviations can make tumor screening more or less successful. Maintaining records on changes that are made (and on what dates) is critical when evaluating outcomes. Regardless of how much you plan, it is unlikely that you can anticipate everything. Straying from your original plan may be necessary to improve patient follow-up. Most institutions we have talked to have altered their plans.
Reflecting and evaluating	
How and who will record and track whether patients followed through after a positive screen?	Keeping track and verifying that patient tumors are being screened as intended are critical for quality assurance. Several centers have found that as providers and personnel change, the processes can break down even if they are routinized or automated. Develop a tracking system to monitor outcomes regularly, and make changes to the protocol as necessary. Most successful screening programs have made changes over time.
Will someone be monitoring and tracking for any negative outcomes?	Although few negative outcomes have been reported thus far, tracking of any perceived negative outcomes is critical to making improvements or averting issues in the future. For example, some sites have run into challenges with following up on tumor screening results of prison inmates.
Under what circumstances and at what intervals will stakeholders reflect on the implementation process?	• By talking about the tumor screening process and discussing what seems to work and what does not, several centers have developed ways to streamline or improve their process. • This should be done periodically and whenever there are any changes in key personnel, challenges with patient follow-through, or any perceived negative outcomes.
How will you know if you are successful?	• In addition to patient follow-through with genetic counseling and germline testing, other implementation outcomes have been measured at several different institutions, and this data is relatively easy to collect and compare with expected outcomes based on data from large centers that have been doing screening for years. • An excel spreadsheet available on the LSSN website has been created where you can track the number of screen-positive patients you can expect, the number who will require counseling and germline testing (depending on your screening protocol), and the number of patients with Lynch syndrome who are expected to be identified. This can be used for quality control if the numbers are substantially different than expected (though if volumes are low, numbers could differ from what is expected simply due to chance) [note: This excel spreadsheet can also be a useful tool to anticipate counseling volumes when preparing to start a screening program].

diagnosis of cancer. It has been shown that institutions with a high level of patient follow-through with genetic counseling and testing following a screen-positive result all utilize genetic counselors to disclose the screen-positive results to the patients, and genetic counselors either facilitate physician referrals to genetics or eliminated the need for referrals through an agreement with the treating surgeons and oncologist [31]. It is also important to include tests (somatic *BRAF* mutation testing or *MLH1* promoter methylation testing) to identify patients with acquired *MLH1* promoter methylation who do not need follow-up genetic counseling and testing.

Tumor screening for Lynch syndrome may change with time as newer technologies are adopted. However, many of the challenges and lessons we have learned through implementing routine tumor screening are likely to be applicable in the context of other genomic technologies. Consequently, it can be valuable for stakeholders involved in the identification of hereditary cancer syndromes to be familiar with concepts related to implementation science and apply these in a similar fashion as we have done here.

9 Cascade Testing

In controlled research settings, it has been shown that six at-risk relatives can be tested for every colorectal cancer patient identified with Lynch syndrome, with three of those relatives testing positive [3, 4]. Because this testing occurred in a research setting, the genetic counseling and testing were free, and the counselor provided services locally in the families' homes, churches, or doctor's offices. However, outside the research setting, it appears that 3.6 relatives or fewer are tested for every individual diagnosed with Lynch syndrome [34]. Demographic factors (age < 50, female sex, parenthood, level of education, employment, participation in medical studies), psychological factors (lack of depressive symptoms), and possible family history (greater number of relatives with cancer) were positively associated with uptake of genetic testing. Another study found that individuals with Lynch syndrome share their results with first-degree relatives (parents, children, and siblings) but they are significantly less likely to share their results with more distant relatives [35]. It is very important that rates of cascade testing within known Lynch syndrome families improve. In fact, this is the key factor influencing the cost-effectiveness of universal tumor screening for Lynch syndrome, with screening becoming more cost-effective as increasing numbers of relatives under genetic counseling and testing [16, 17, 19].

Efforts to improve uptake of cascade testing of at-risk relatives once a diagnosis of Lynch syndrome is made in a family will be applicable for all adult-onset genetic conditions (e.g., hereditary breast-ovarian cancer syndrome, familial hypercholesterolemia), so the potential benefits are enormous. Researchers are beginning to explore ways to improve cascade testing through the use of secure website for sharing results (Kintalk.org), videos that can be sent to relatives explaining the impor-

Table 17.4 Recommendations when implementing tumor screening for Lynch syndrome organized according to four additional domains from the Consolidated Framework for Implementation Research (CFIR)

Domain	CFIR constructs	Relevant experiences and recommendations
Intervention characteristics	Intervention source Perception of stakeholders about whether tumor screening is internally or externally developed and the legitimacy of the source	Tumor screening should be developed by multiple different stakeholders to improve acceptance and legitimacy.
	Evidence strength and quality Stakeholder perceptions of the quality and validity of evidence that tumor screening will have on the desired outcomes	Effectiveness of tumor screening has been established (assuming it is well implemented). Recognize that evidence is not always the most important factor in decision-making among some stakeholders.
	Relative advantage Belief about the benefits of routine tumor screening compared to no routine screening or other methods of identifying Lynch syndrome	Family history alone is insufficient and difficult to collect routinely, whereas routine tumor screening can improve the ability to diagnose Lynch syndrome. When planning there are many advantages and disadvantages to the different approaches that should be considered (see Table 17.3).
	Adaptability Ease of tailoring tumor screening to meet the institution's needs	The initial protocol doesn't always work. Programs have changed their protocol over time to improve efficiency or effectiveness. Each tumor screening program looks different given their own structure or limitations. Know your patient populations, and find the best screening protocol based on other institutions' experiences, but recognize adaptations may be needed to fit your institution and available resources.
	Trialability Ability to test tumor screening on a small scale before it is fully adopted	Some centers that faced resistance have had success by starting with a subset of tumors (e.g., all under age 50) before advancing to routine screening of all tumors. Several centers started with either screening of endometrial or colorectal tumors first before screening the other tumor type.

(continued)

Table 17.4 (continued)

Domain	CFIR constructs	Relevant experiences and recommendations
	Complexity Degree of difficulty in developing a tumor screening program	Program complexity reduces successful implementation. Simplify the protocol and automate or routinize steps as much as possible. Screening all tumors is easier than screening based on complex criteria that requires elicitation and review of tumor pathology and/or detailed clinical and family history. Reducing the number of steps that patients and providers must take to follow up on positive screens is critical for success.
	Cost Cost of implementing and running a tumor screening program	Providers at most institutions we have talked with lack information about tumor screening reimbursement. Confusion exists about billing strategies. Clinicians are generally not aware of problems with reimbursement for screening. When performed on surgical resections, Medicare patients are not billed for tumor screening because reimbursement occurs as part of the diagnosis-related group (DRG). Screening can be billed separately if performed on biopsies. There are several reported cases we are aware of where Medicare would not pay for follow-up germline genetic testing or hypermethylation testing unless certain clinical and/or family history criteria are met (some of these involved endometrial tumor screening, but at least one was colorectal cancer screening).
Outer setting	Patient needs and resources Degree to which the needs of cancer patients are accurately assessed and continually addressed	Facilitate patient follow-up by scheduling it when it is convenient for patients (i.e., meet patients at post-op visits if possible). *MLH1* hypermethylation or *BRAF* testing is important in the screening protocol to rule out patients who do not likely have lynch syndrome. Adding *BRAF* testing or *MLH1* hypermethylation to the protocol may prevent patient harm because it eliminates the need for several patients who likely do not have Lynch syndrome from having genetic counseling or worrying about the possibility of Lynch syndrome or follow-up testing

(continued)

Table 17.4 (continued)

Domain	CFIR constructs	Relevant experiences and recommendations
	Cosmopolitanism Degree to which the organization is networked with external organizations (from which they can attain knowledge/ resources)	Lynch Syndrome Screening Network (LSSN) resources and information on starting a screening program may be helpful www.lynchscreening.net. Joining the LSSN listserv allows people to connect with and seek advice from others who work at centers that have been conducting lynch syndrome screening and testing for many years.
	Peer pressure Pressure to implement tumor screening from other organizations with established tumor screening	Drawing attention to other institutions currently performing tumor screening (particularly competing hospitals in your area) can be a great motivation for implementation. The LSSN maintains a list of member institutions doing routine tumor screening who have agreed to be listed.
	External policies and incentives Strategies or policies and recommendations from outside organizations that influence the adoption of tumor screening	Present guidelines from EGAPP, the National Comprehensive Cancer Center (NCCN), and other professional organizations to support implementation (as previously described).
Inner setting	Structural characteristics Effect of social architecture and size of an institution on tumor screening	Large institutions with multiple healthcare providers can present challenges, highlighting the importance of ensuring everyone is well informed. Sometimes centralizing follow-up responsibilities with a small number of individuals can help to overcome this structural challenge.
	Networks and communication Quality and extent of communication among those involved in tumor screening and results follow-up	Communication with key stakeholders is critical to successful implementation. Successful programs have communication that occurs regularly between physicians, genetics, and pathology. Tumor board is a great way to keep lines of communication open. Assigning one or two genetic counselors to communicate screening results to patients and promote patient follow-up has been helpful at some institutions. Sending letters to physicians and reminders for follow-up counseling has worked relatively well at one center, but can be time-consuming.

(continued)

Table 17.4 (continued)

Domain	CFIR constructs	Relevant experiences and recommendations
	Implementation climate Capacity for change and support for tumor screening within the organization • Tension for change • Compatibility • Relative priority • Organizational incentives/rewards • Goals and feedback • Learning climate	Having a team of motivated key stakeholders who value tumor screening as well as some key individuals who make it a priority is critical for success. Set goals and keep track of patient outcomes. Share outcomes at your center with physicians, so they can see the patients and family members who are not being diagnosed through the methods in current practice. Once implemented, share information about those patients who were identified, but may have been missed if screening had not been done or if the patient did not follow through with germline testing.
	Readiness for implementation • Leadership Engagement • Available resources • Access to information and knowledge	Increase readiness by accessing the LSSN website at www.lynchscreening.net for useful information about screening. Make a list of available resources. Determine if you have a follow-up plan because there is no point in starting to screen tumors if patients and family members are not actually being identified by undergoing germline testing.
Characteristics of individuals	Knowledge and beliefs, self-efficacy, individual identification with organization	Physicians' level of knowledge and attitudes can influence whether patients follow through with genetic counseling and testing. Knowledge and attitudes among physicians is even more critical if they are disclosing the results and if they are going to encourage patient follow-through with genetic counseling and testing. Providing information about Lynch syndrome screening through tumor boards or an educational fact sheet about the screening protocol may increase physician awareness.

tance of genetic counseling and testing for Lynch syndrome, and direct contact of at-risk relatives by the clinician helping to take this burden off the original family member with a diagnosis of Lynch syndrome who may be dealing with their own cancer diagnosis. The results of two nationwide cascade testing programs for familial hypercholesterolemia have been published. The program in the Netherlands was very successful and resulted in testing 25.7 relatives per proband compared to 4.5 relatives tested per proband in Norway [36]. The Netherlands program involved direct contact of the at-risk family members by a genetic field worker who arranged to take a blood sample from the family members at their homes for testing with treatment for those found to have familial hypercholesterolemia then coordinated by local specialist clinics. The program in Norway relied on the proband and the genetic counselor to contact the relatives and request follow-up testing coordinated by the primary care physician, which required an appointment. In the future, public policy may play a role if the United States was to consider some type of coordinated effort at a nationwide cascade testing program for adult-onset conditions where early detection has been shown to improve outcomes and testing has been proven to be cost-effective.

10 Conclusions

With the growing importance of immunotherapy in the treatment of MSI-high cancers, we are confident that universal tumor screening for Lynch syndrome will truly become "universal" in the next few years. Testing improves as technology changes, so it may be done using different technology, but the need to identify all colorectal (and other) cancers with MSI for treatment purposes will help drive the continued adoption of this approach. As a result, we must now focus on ways to optimize universal tumor screening so that all cases with abnormal screening have access to genetic counseling and follow-up genetic testing. Moreover, we must work to improve cascade testing efforts within families once a diagnosis of Lynch syndrome has been made. To truly reap the benefits of universal tumor screening, we must ensure the identification of as many unaffected at-risk relatives as possible. One can imagine a day when we will not need to do universal tumor screening for the detection of Lynch syndrome anymore (even though it will always be needed to identify MSI-high patients for treatment purposes) because the majority of families and individuals with Lynch syndrome will have been diagnosed.

References

1. Win AK, Jenkins MA, Dowty JG, Antoniou AC, Lee A, Giles GG, et al. Prevalence and penetrance of major genes and polygenes for colorectal cancer. Cancer Epidemiol Biomark Prev. 2017;26(3):404–12. https://doi.org/10.1158/1055-9965.EPI-16-0693.
2. American Cancer Society. Key statistics for colorectal cancer. 2016. http://www.cancer.org/cancer/colonandrectumcancer/detailedguide/colorectal-cancer-key-statistics. Accessed 2 May 2016.
3. Hampel H, Frankel WL, Martin E, Arnold M, Khanduja K, Kuebler P, et al. Feasibility of screening for Lynch syndrome among patients with colorectal cancer. J Clin Oncol. 2008;26(35):5783–8. https://doi.org/10.1200/JCO.2008.17.5950.
4. Hampel H, Frankel WL, Martin E, Arnold M, Khanduja K, Kuebler P, et al. Screening for the Lynch syndrome (hereditary nonpolyposis colorectal cancer). N Engl J Med. 2005;352(18):1851–60. https://doi.org/10.1056/NEJMoa043146.
5. Cross D, Rahm A, Le A, Webster J, Potosky A, Feigelson H, et al. PS1-08: Lynch syndrome screening pattering in colorectal cancer patients in a large multi-institutional cohort. Clin Med Res. 2012;10(3):146.
6. Palomaki GE, McClain MR, Melillo S, Hampel HL, Thibodeau SN. EGAPP supplementary evidence review: DNA testing strategies aimed at reducing morbidity and mortality from Lynch syndrome. Genet Med. 2009;11(1):42–65.
7. Popat S, Hubner R, Houlston RS. Systematic review of microsatellite instability and colorectal cancer prognosis. J Clin Oncol. 2005;23(3):609–18.

8. Des Guetz G, Schischmanoff O, Nicolas P, Perret GY, Morere JF, Uzzan B. Does microsatellite instability predict the efficacy of adjuvant chemotherapy in colorectal cancer? A systematic review with meta-analysis. Eur J Cancer. 2009;45(10):1890–6.
9. Diaz LA Jr, Le DT. PD-1 blockade in tumors with mismatch-repair deficiency. N Engl J Med. 2015;373(20):1979. https://doi.org/10.1056/NEJMc1510353.
10. Recommendations from the EGAPP Working Group. Genetic testing strategies in newly diagnosed individuals with colorectal cancer aimed at reducing morbidity and mortality from Lynch syndrome in relatives. Genet Med. 2009;11(1):35–41.
11. Giardiello FM, Allen JI, Axilbund JE, Boland CR, Burke CA, Burt RW, et al. Guidelines on genetic evaluation and management of Lynch syndrome: a consensus statement by the US Multi-society Task Force on Colorectal Cancer. Am J Gastroenterol. 2014;109(8):1159–79. https://doi.org/10.1038/ajg.2014.186.
12. Referenced with permission from the NCCN Guidelines® for Genetic/Familial High-Risk Assessment: Colorectal V.1.2016 © National Comprehensive Cancer Network IArrAJ, https://www.nccn.org/store/login/login.aspx?
13. Syngal S, Brand RE, Church JM, Giardiello FM, Hampel HL, Burt RW. ACG clinical guideline: genetic testing and management of hereditary gastrointestinal cancer syndromes. Am J Gastroenterol. 2015;110(2):223–62.; ; quiz 63. https://doi.org/10.1038/ajg.2014.435.
14. Bessa X, Balleste B, Andreu M, Castells A, Bellosillo B, Balaguer F, et al. A prospective, multicenter, population-based study of BRAF mutational analysis for Lynch syndrome screening. Clin Gastroenterol Hepatol. 2008;6(2):206–14. https://doi.org/10.1016/j.cgh.2007.10.011.
15. Gausachs M, Mur P, Corral J, Pineda M, Gonzalez S, Benito L, et al. MLH1 promoter hypermethylation in the analytical algorithm of Lynch syndrome: a cost-effectiveness study. Eur J Hum Genet. 2012;20(7):762–8. https://doi.org/10.1038/ejhg.2011.277.
16. Grosse SD. When is genomic testing cost-effective? Testing for Lynch syndrome in patients with newly-diagnosed colorectal cancer and their relatives. Health. 2015;3(4):860–78.
17. Grosse SD, Palomaki GE, Mvundura M, Hampel H. The cost-effectiveness of routine testing for Lynch syndrome in newly diagnosed patients with colorectal cancer in the United States: corrected estimates. Genet Med. 2015;17(6):510–1. https://doi.org/10.1038/gim.2015.53.
18. Gudgeon JM, Williams JL, Burt RW, Samowitz WS, Snow GL, Williams MS. Lynch syndrome screening implementation: business analysis by a healthcare system. Am J Manag Care. 2011;17(8):e288–300. doi:50524 [pii]
19. Mvundura M, Grosse SD, Hampel H, Palomaki GE. The cost-effectiveness of genetic testing strategies for Lynch syndrome among newly diagnosed patients with colorectal cancer. Genet Med. 2010;12(2):93–104.
20. Snowsill T, Huxley N, Hoyle M, Jones-Hughes T, Coelho H, Cooper C, et al. A systematic review and economic evaluation of diagnostic strategies for Lynch syndrome. Health Technol Assess. 2014;18(58):1–406. https://doi.org/10.3310/hta18580.
21. Ladabaum U, Wang G, Terdiman J, Blanco A, Kuppermann M, Boland CR, et al. Strategies to identify the lynch syndrome among patients with colorectal cancer: a cost-effectiveness analysis. Ann Intern Med. 2011;155(2):69–79. https://doi.org/10.1059/0003-4819-155-2-201107190-00002. 155/2/69 [pii]
22. Severin F, Stollenwerk B, Holinski-Feder E, Meyer E, Heinemann V, Giessen-Jung C, et al. Economic evaluation of genetic screening for Lynch syndrome in Germany. Genet Med. 2015;17(10):765–73. https://doi.org/10.1038/gim.2014.190.
23. Wang G, Kuppermann M, Kim B, Phillips KA, Ladabaum U. Influence of patient preferences on the cost-effectiveness of screening for Lynch syndrome. Am J Manag Care. 2012;18(5):e179–85.
24. Gould-Suarez M, El-Serag HB, Musher B, Franco LM, Chen GJ. Cost-effectiveness and diagnostic effectiveness analyses of multiple algorithms for the diagnosis of Lynch syndrome. Dig Dis Sci. 2014;59(12):2913–26. https://doi.org/10.1007/s10620-014-3248-6.
25. Weissman SM, Burt R, Church J, Erdman S, Hampel H, Holter S, et al. Identification of individuals at risk for lynch syndrome using targeted evaluations and genetic testing: National

Society of Genetic Counselors and the Collaborative Group of the Americas on Inherited Colorectal Cancer joint practice guideline. J Genet Couns. 2012;21(4):484–93. https://doi.org/10.1007/s10897-011-9465-7.
26. Stoffel EM, Mangu PB, Gruber SB, Hamilton SR, Kalady MF, Lau MW, et al. Hereditary colorectal cancer syndromes: American Society of Clinical Oncology Clinical Practice Guideline endorsement of the familial risk-colorectal cancer: European Society for Medical Oncology Clinical Practice Guidelines. J Clin Oncol. 2015;33(2):209–17. https://doi.org/10.1200/JCO.2014.58.1322.
27. Monahan KJ, Alsina D, Bach S, Buchanan J, Burn J, Clark S, et al. Urgent improvements needed to diagnose and manage Lynch syndrome. BMJ. 2017;356:j1388. https://doi.org/10.1136/bmj.j1388.
28. Balmana J, Balaguer F, Cervantes A, Arnold D. Familial risk-colorectal cancer: ESMO Clinical Practice Guidelines. AnnOncol: Off J EurSocMed Oncol/ESMO. 2013;24(Suppl 6):vi73–80. https://doi.org/10.1093/annonc/mdt209.
29. Beamer LC, Grant ML, Espenschied CR, Blazer KR, Hampel HL, Weitzel JN, et al. Reflex immunohistochemistry and microsatellite instability testing of colorectal tumors for lLynch syndrome among US cancer programs and follow-up of abnormal results. J Clin Oncol. 2012;30(10):1058–63. JCO.2011.38.4719 [pii] 31.1200/JCO.2011.38.4719
30. Le DT, Uram JN, Wang H, Bartlett BR, Kemberling H, Eyring AD, et al. PD-1 blockade in tumors with mismatch-repair deficiency. N Engl J Med. 2015;372(26):2509–20. https://doi.org/10.1056/NEJMoa1500596.
31. Cragun D, DeBate RD, Vadaparampil ST, Baldwin J, Hampel H, Pal T. Comparing universal Lynch syndrome tumor-screening programs to evaluate associations between implementation strategies and patient follow-through. Genet Med. 2014;16(10):773–82. https://doi.org/10.1038/gim.2014.31.
32. Cragun D, Pal T, Vadaparampil ST, Baldwin J, Hampel H, DeBate RD. Qualitative comparative analysis: a hybrid method for identifying factors associated with program effectiveness. J Mixed Methods Res. 2016;10(3):251–72. https://doi.org/10.1177/1558689815572023.
33. Damschroder LJ, Aron DC, Keith RE, Kirsh SR, Alexander JA, Lowery JC. Fostering implementation of health services research findings into practice: a consolidated framework for advancing implementation science. Implement Sci: IS. 2009;4:50. https://doi.org/10.1186/1748-5908-4-50.
34. Sharaf RN, Myer P, Stave CD, Diamond LC, Ladabaum U. Uptake of genetic testing by relatives of Lynch syndrome probands: a systematic review. Clin Gastroenterol Hepatol. 2013;11(9):1093–100. https://doi.org/10.1016/j.cgh.2013.04.044.
35. Stoffel EM, Ford B, Mercado RC, Punglia D, Kohlmann W, Conrad P, et al. Sharing genetic test results in Lynch syndrome: communication with close and distant relatives. Clin Gastroenterol Hepatol. 2008;6(3):333–8. https://doi.org/10.1016/j.cgh.2007.12.014.
36. Hadfield SG, Humphries SE. Implementation of cascade testing for the detection of familial hypercholesterolaemia. Curr Opin Lipidol. 2005;16(4):428–33.
37. Mills AM, Liou S, Ford JM, Berek JS, Pai RK, Longacre TA. Lynch syndrome screening should be considered for all patients with newly diagnosed endometrial cancer. Am J Surg Pathol. 2014;38(11):1501–9. https://doi.org/10.1097/PAS.0000000000000321.
38. Morrison J, Bronner M, Leach BH, Downs-Kelly E, Goldblum JR, Liu X. Lynch syndrome screening in newly diagnosed colorectal cancer in general pathology practice: from the revised Bethesda guidelines to a universal approach. Scand J Gastroenterol. 2011;46(11):1340–8. https://doi.org/10.3109/00365521.2011.610003.
39. Ryan P, Mulligan AM, Aronson M, Ferguson SE, Bapat B, Semotiuk K, et al. Comparison of clinical schemas and morphologic features in predicting Lynch syndrome in mutation-positive patients with endometrial cancer encountered in the context of familial gastrointestinal cancer registries. Cancer. 2012;118(3):681–8. https://doi.org/10.1002/cncr.26323.
40. Trano G, Sjursen W, Wasmuth HH, Hofsli E, Vatten LJ. Performance of clinical guidelines compared with molecular tumour screening methods in identifying possible Lynch syndrome among colorectal cancer patients: a Norwegian population-based study. Br J Cancer. 2010;102(3):482–8. https://doi.org/10.1038/sj.bjc.6605509.

41. Pearlman R, Frankel WL, Swanson B, Zhao W, Yilmaz A, Miller K, et al. Prevalence and spectrum of germline cancer susceptibility gene mutations among patients with early-onset colorectal cancer. JAMA Oncol. 2016;3(4):464–71. https://doi.org/10.1001/jamaoncol.2016.5194.
42. Heald B, Plesec T, Liu X, Pai R, Patil D, Moline J, et al. Implementation of universal microsatellite instability and immunohistochemistry screening for diagnosing lynch syndrome in a large academic medical center. J Clin Oncol. 2013;31(10):1336–40. https://doi.org/10.1200/JCO.2012.45.1674.
43. Hampel H, Lattimer I, Frankel W. Universal Lynch syndrome screening result notification: efficacy affected by method. J Genet Couns. 2012;21(6):888–9.

Chapter 18
Classification of Genetic Variants

Maurizio Genuardi, Elke Holinski-Feder, Andreas Laner, and Alexandra Martins

Abstract Widespread resequencing for research and diagnostic purposes has disclosed a huge amount of genetic variability in the human genome, including the genes associated with inherited predisposition to colorectal cancer. The functional and clinical consequences of the gene variants identified are often difficult to predict. Therefore, it has becoming increasingly evident that standardized approaches for the clinical interpretation of gene variants are needed in order to maximize the clinical utility of molecular testing. In this chapter, we discuss strategies for variant classification, with special reference to hereditary colorectal cancer genes and to the functional and clinical points of evidence that are available for their interpretation.

Keywords mRNA functional studies · Alternative splicing · Nonsense- mediated mRNA decay · In vitro protein assays · In silico prediction tools · Multifactorial Bayesian analysis · Variants of uncertain significance (VUS)

M. Genuardi (✉)
Institute of Genomic Medicine, Catholic University of the Sacred Heart, Rome, Italy

Fondazione Policlinico Universitario "A. Gemelli", Rome, Italy
e-mail: maurizio.genuardi@unicatt.it

E. Holinski-Feder
Medizinische Klinik und Poliklinik IV, Campus Innenstadt, Klinikum der Universität München, Munich, Germany

MGZ – Medizinisch Genetisches Zentrum, Munich, Germany

A. Laner
MGZ - Medizinisch Genetisches Zentrum, Munich, Germany

A. Martins
Inserm-U1245-IRIB, Normandy Centre for Genomic and Personalized Medicine, University of Rouen, Rouen, France

L. Valle et al. (eds.), *Hereditary Colorectal Cancer*,
https://doi.org/10.1007/978-3-319-74259-5_18

1 General Principles

High-throughput genetic technologies have revealed the extent of DNA sequence variation in humans. While two individuals differ on average by 1 nucleotide per kilobase in their coding sequences, the differences may involve a fraction as high as 0.5% of the whole genome [1].

The functional significance of such a vast genetic variability is largely unknown. Consequently, sequencing entire genomes, exomes or large gene panels yields a huge amount of data on variants of unknown consequences. In current medical practice, specific multigene molecular diagnostic tests are often preferred over exome or full genome sequencing. The former are typically focused on functionally relevant regions of specific genes, (mostly exons and exon-intron boundaries, occasionally regulatory 5′ and 3′ sequences, or other regions, depending on the underlying molecular mechanisms known for the condition tested). While more is known about the organization and function of these specific sequences (as compared to the entire genome), the effects of DNA changes identified must still be determined very carefully, given the implications for the genetic counseling of the tested individuals and their families. Therefore, clinical interpretation of DNA variants must be performed by adopting well-defined procedures that take into account multiple lines of evidence in favor or against pathogenicity.

In the case of hereditary colorectal cancer genetic screens, the data useful for variant interpretation pertain to three different domains (Table 18.1): (1) characteristics inherent to the DNA sequence; (2) clinical information on the patients and their families, including pathology and molecular tumor studies; and (3) functional data derived from studies assessing the consequences on either RNA synthesis/processing or the protein(s) encoded by the variant allele.

Table 18.1 Types of evidence used for DNA variant classification

Categories of evidence		
DNA sequence	Clinical	Functional
Variant location (i.e., coding, noncoding, mutation hotspot, functional domain)	Phenotype (type of cancer, tumor features, age of onset)	mRNA splicing level, allelic-specific expression and splicing pattern (in vitro and in vivo assays)
Predicted effects (i.e., truncating, splicing, missense, synonymous, intronic)	Co-segregation with the phenotype	Quantitative mRNA expression
For missense changes: Involvement of a codon previously affected by pathogenic amino acid substitutions	Type of inheritance (for semidominant and recessive conditions: correlation with phenotype if co-occurrence in trans with a known pathogenic variant)	Protein expression level, localisation and function (in vitro and in vivo assays)
	Population frequency De novo variant with negative family history Tumor molecular studies (i.e., microsatellite instability (MSI), specific mutational signatures)	In silico predictions (RNA, protein)

2 Characteristics of the DNA Sequence

The type and location of the sequence change are the first important elements to consider. Importantly, these information are known for most variants, notable exceptions being some large rearrangements (inversions, amplifications) while clinical and/or functional data may not be available.

Some types of variants have a very high a priori likelihood of pathogenicity. For tumor suppressor or "mutator" genes, such as those involved in colorectal cancer (CRC) predisposition, these include the overwhelming majority of variants leading to the introduction of premature stop codons (i.e., nonsense, frameshift, and some splice site variants). Notable exceptions are changes that are not predicted to disrupt important protein functional domains, e.g. those that introduce stop codons in the most 3′ portion of a gene or small in-frame alterations.

Other variants, such as deep intronic and synonymous changes, have a lower likelihood of disrupting gene function. However, since they can occasionally have consequences on RNA processing, their clinical effects cannot be established in the absence of other types of evidence.

Nucleotide substitutions that cause potential missense changes are often the most problematic variants for clinical assessment. Their effects depend on a number of factors: (1) functional relevance of the affected amino acid. This can be also assessed indirectly by comparing the amino acids present in the equivalent position in orthologous sequences from other species. Also, previous involvement of the same codon in a pathogenic missense change suggests a relevant role for the wild-type amino acid, although it does not automatically imply that any substitution in that position is deleterious. (2) Type of amino acid substitution (i.e., conservative vs. non-conservative change, based on chemical and physical characteristics of the wild type and of the variant amino acid). (3) Lastly, but importantly, potential consequences on RNA, namely, splicing alterations induced by the nucleotide change; in the latter case, the amino acid change does not occur at all in the mRNA or is associated only with a fraction of the transcripts produced by the variant allele. The impact of nucleotide variants on RNA and protein integrity/function can be assessed by in vitro and/or in vivo assays (see below).

Changes in 5′ and 3′ regulatory regions can theoretically have effects on RNA processing and stability, which can be determined by RNA studies (see below).

3 Clinical Evidence: Phenotype Information

Information on the phenotype of the patient/family should be provided by referring physicians. For genes with (nearly) complete penetrance that are usually associated with highly characteristic phenotypes, such as *APC*, the detection of a variant in an individual who is healthy or who does not show the typical manifestations (i.e., late-onset CRC in the absence of multiple adenomas) is a clue in favor of non-pathogenicity. On the other hand, the consistent association of an *APC* variant with classical adenomatous polyposis in multiple unrelated families is suggestive of its pathogenicity.

The same applies to hereditary CRC syndromes associated with less specific phenotypes, such as Lynch syndrome (LS). However, in this case, the value of clinical information is lower and must be weighed against reduced penetrance and variable phenotypic expression.

The principles of traditional Bayesian linkage analysis can be very useful to assess the pathogenicity of a variant. If multiple family members are available for analysis, co-segregation of the variant with gene-specific phenotypic manifestations can be investigated, and odds ratios in favor of causality can be determined [2]. Gene-specific penetrance values must be considered, since *MSH6* and *PMS2* are associated with significantly lower disease risks compared to *MLH1* and *MSH2* [3, 4]. For diseases with reduced penetrance, it is particularly important to obtain information on cancer-affected family members, since unaffected individuals have a relatively high chance of being carriers and are therefore less informative.

Segregation analysis is also important to verify the phase when the variant of interest is found in an individual who also has a bona fide pathogenic variant, if the associated condition is autosomal recessive or autosomal dominant and shows semi-dominance (i.e., a more severe phenotype in individuals who are compound heterozygotes or homozygotes for pathogenic variants compared to simple heterozygotes). Among hereditary CRC conditions, the latter phenomenon is well documented for LS, where biallelic constitutional inactivation of a mismatch repair (MMR) locus is associated with a condition characterized by early-onset pediatric cancers and manifestations of type 1 neurofibromatosis [5]. Co-occurrence in trans of two pathogenic variants in the same MMR gene is expected to lead to this phenotype, named constitutional mismatch repair deficiency (CMMRD), which is more severe than LS. On the other hand, if the two variants are in cis, no inference on the sequence change under scrutiny can be made, since the phenotype could be caused by the associated pathogenic change alone. Therefore, if two variants, one pathogenic and one of unknown significance, are detected in a CMMRD patient, and segregation studies show that each one is inherited from a different parent, this is considered evidence in favor of pathogenicity. On the contrary, their detection in trans in an individual with a diagnosis of LS, for whom CMMRD can be excluded, provides evidence against pathogenicity [6]. The same principle underlies the use of co-occurrence analysis for the interpretation of variants identified in genes causing autosomal recessive conditions [7], such as *MUTYH*-associated polyposis (MAP): in a patient with attenuated or classical colorectal polyposis, the finding of a pathogenic variant and an unclassified *MUTYH* variant in trans supports pathogenicity for the latter.

Although not strictly pertaining to the clinical setting, allele population frequencies, derived from the analyses of biological samples of control subjects or stored in public genetic databases, such as gnomAD [8], are an important source of information for variant interpretation. In principle, the higher the frequency of a variant allele, the lower the likelihood of pathogenicity. However, some pathogenic alleles may attain polymorphic or nearly polymorphic frequencies in specific ethnic groups due to a founder effect. In addition, alleles causing autosomal recessive conditions, such as MAP, tend to be more frequent than dominant disease alleles. Hence when using allele frequency data as evidence for variant interpretation, one should take into account both the type of inheritance and disease prevalence, and disease-specific thresholds should be set [7].

4 Clinical Evidence: Tumor Pathology

Tumors associated with hereditary cancer syndromes often have characteristics that are unusual in the nonhereditary counterparts. For instance, medullary or triple-negative ductal breast carcinoma is significantly more frequent in carriers of *BRCA1* pathogenic variants [9, 10]. In hereditary polyposis syndromes, the histology of intestinal polyps is a very important diagnostic clue: hamartomatous polyps of the juvenile or Peutz-Jeghers types are characteristic of juvenile polyposis and Peutz-Jeghers syndrome, respectively [11]. In LS patients, CRCs tend to develop in the right colon and are often mucinous with a prominent lymphocytic infiltration.

The most useful type of information for LS is derived from molecular studies. The molecular tests commonly used to identify markers of LS, microsatellite instability (MSI) and immunohistochemistry (IHC) of MMR proteins, can be equated to a sort of in vivo functional test [12]. A high degree of instability (MSI-H) or the absence of one or more MMR proteins in a tumor is indicative of MMR deficiency. Therefore, the consistent association of a MMR gene variant with MSI-H and/or with loss of the protein encoded by the variant allele is evidence for its pathogenicity. Conversely, if the tumor is microsatellite stable (MSS) or shows normal expression of the protein encoded by the variant gene and by its heterodimeric partner, the likelihood of pathogenicity is lower.

Tumors arising in subjects with other types of hereditary CRC predisposition, especially those caused by impairment of DNA repair genes, are often associated with specific molecular alterations. The base excision repair (BER) protein MUTYH is involved in the repair of oxidative damage that leads to the production of 8-oxoguanine, which mispairs with adenine. Hence, somatic G > T transversions in driver genes, such as *KRAS* and *APC*, are more frequent in MAP-associated tumors compared to non-MAP CRCs [13]. Likewise, the most common type of mutations in tumors from biallelic carriers of pathogenic variants in *NTHL1*, another BER gene with different repair specificity, are C > T transitions [14]. Finally, CRCs from patients with PPAP (polymerase proofreading-associated polyposis) tend to have an ultramutated phenotype, often associated with inactivation of the MMR system [15–17]. In principle, these molecular signatures could be useful for the clinical interpretation of sequence variants identified in *MUTYH*, *NTHL1*, *POLD1*, and *POLE*, and further studies on larger number of samples are needed to establish how they can be incorporated in the classification algorithms.

In principle, clinically useful information could also derive from molecular tumor studies for the search of second hits in tumor suppressor or genome integrity maintenance genes, such as *APC* and the MMR genes. While it has been shown that loss of heterozygosity is not a useful marker of pathogenicity for MMR genes [18], the value of somatic MMR gene mutations ascertained by sequencing of tumor DNA has yet to be determined.

5 The Role of RNA Studies

It is now widely accepted that every nucleotide variant can potentially affect RNA expression by directly altering either the level of transcription of a gene of interest (e.g. modifications of promoter or enhancer sequences), mRNA maturation (e.g. disruption of splicing or polyadenylation signals) or mRNA stability.

Mutations affecting pre-mRNA splicing are a major cause of genetic disease, including hereditary CRC [19]. The biological and clinical interpretation of sequence variations should therefore always take into consideration a potential impact on RNA splicing. Nucleotide variants may alter the splicing pattern of the genes to which they map to, either partially (leaky variants) or totally (complete loss of the reference full-length transcript). These alterations may be due to simple events resulting in a single aberrant transcript or, less frequently, to complex anomalies yielding multiple abnormal RNAs [20–22]. As illustrated in Fig. 18.1, simple events include (i) exon skipping, (ii) deletion of a portion of an exon, (iii) retention of a contiguous intronic fragment, (iv) retention of an entire intron (no splicing),

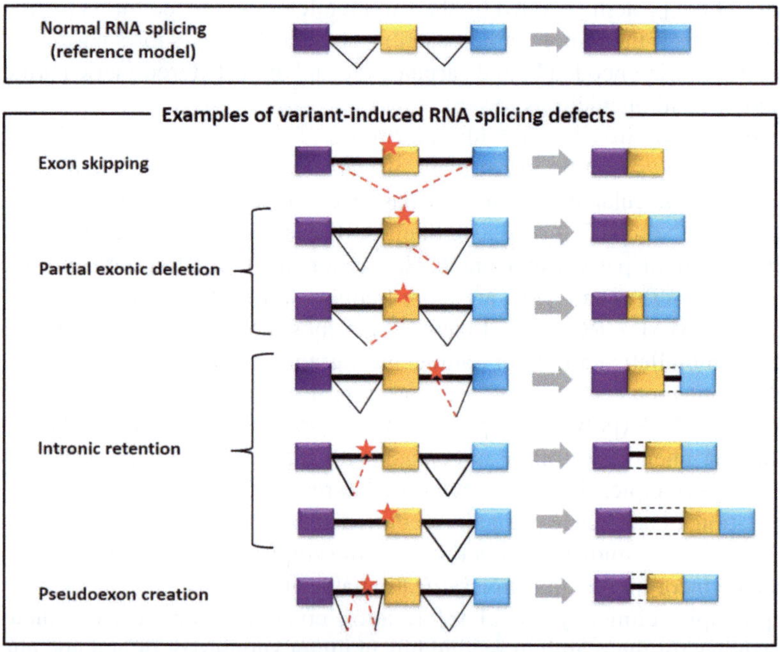

Fig. 18.1 Examples of variant-induced RNA splicing defects

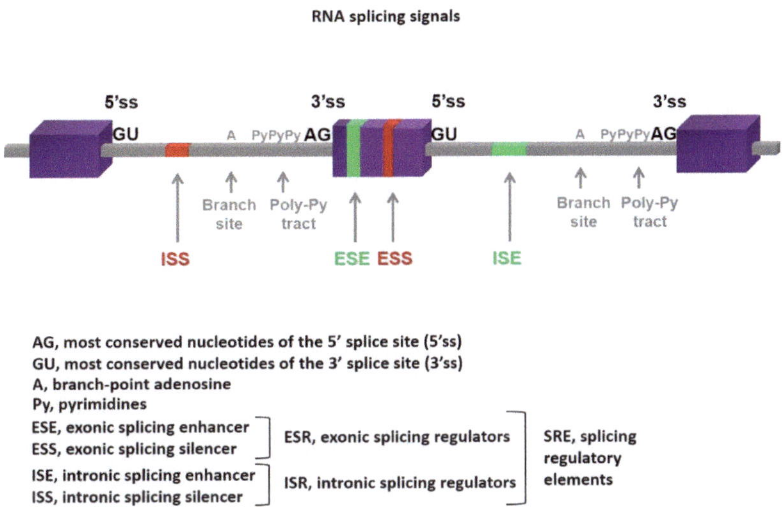

Fig. 18.2 RNA splicing signals

and (v) exonization of an intronic fragment located in a region noncontiguous to reference exons (e.g., inclusion of a so-called pseudoexon). Complex anomalies are often due to a combination of different simple events arising simultaneously. Moreover, some RNA splicing alterations do not necessarily result in aberrant RNA species but in changes in the ratio of normal alternative transcripts [23, 24].

In most cases, variant-induced splicing defects are due to modifications of cis-acting signals that are crucial for proper RNA splicing (Fig. 18.2). The best known signals include the sequences that directly define the splice sites, i.e., the splice sites themselves (donor sites and acceptor sites) and the branch sites, as well as sequences that contribute to the recognition of the splice sites and help regulating the splicing pattern of constitutive and alternative exons [21]. The latter are generally referred to as splicing regulatory elements (SRE), can be exonic or intronic (ESR or ISR for exonic or intronic splicing regulators), and either have an enhancer or silencer role in exon inclusion (ESE and ISR, or ESS and ISS, respectively). Whereas variant-induced alterations of splice sites are relatively easy to foretell by using computational tools, those affecting potential SRE are still difficult to predict, though recent studies highlighted the promising value of new ESR-dedicated in silico tools [25–30]. Besides the abovementioned major splicing signals, other sequence features can influence RNA splicing patterns, such as chromatin conformation, promoter strength, and RNA secondary structure. Importantly, it is currently estimated that splicing alterations may account for at least 15% up to 50–70% of all described pathogenic variants [19, 30–33].

Several cases of splicing alterations caused by nucleotide variants mapping to genes implicated in hereditary colorectal cancer (CRC) have been reported to date, including variants in *APC*, *MLH1*, *MSH2*, *MSH3*, *MSH6*, *MUTYH*, *PMS2*, *POLE*, *PTEN*, and *STK11*. A few examples are described in Table 18.2, among which one

Table 18.2 Examples of RNA splicing anomalies caused by variants identified in genes implicated in hereditary colorectal cancer

RNA splicing anomalies			
Gene	Variant	RNA data	References
Exon skipping			
APC	c.423G>T	Skipping of exon 4	[34]
MLH1	c.793C>T	Skipping of exon 10	[30]
MSH2	c.942+3A>T	Skipping of exon 5	[35]
MSH3	c.2319-1G>A	Skipping of exon 17	[36]
MSH6	c.3991C>T	Skipping of exon 9	[37]
MUTYH	c.690G>A	Skipping of exon 8	[38]
MUTYH	c.933+3A>C	Skipping of exon 10	[39]
PMS2	c.989-2A>G	Skipping of exon 10	[40]
POLE	c.4444+3A>G	Skipping of exon 34	[41]
PTEN	c.209+5G>A	Skipping of exon 3	[42]
PTEN	c.511C>T	Skipping of exon 6	[43]
STK11	c.597+1G>A	Skipping of exon 4	[44]
Partial deletion of an exon			
APC	c.1409-1G>A	Deletion of first nt of exon 11	[34]
APC	c.1959-2A>G	Deletion of first 12 nt of exon 15	[34]
MLH1	c.589-2A>G	Deletion of first 4 nt of exon 8	[45]
MSH2	c.1915C>T	Deletion of last 92 nt of exon 12	[35]
PMS2	c.164-2A>G	Deletion of first 8 nt of exon 3	[40]
PMS2	c.825A>G	Deletion of first 22 nt of exon 8	[45]
PTEN	c.164+1G>A	Deletion of last 5 nt of exon 2	[46]
PTEN	c.334C>G	Deletion of last 159 nt of exon 5	[47]
Retention of a contiguous intronic fragment			
APC	c.532-8G>A	Retention of 6 last nt of intron 4	[48]
MLH1	c.1667G>T	Retention of first 88 nt of intron 14	[49]
MSH2	c.646-3T>G	Retention of last 24 nt of intron 3	[50]
MSH2	c.1387-9T>A	Retention of last 7 nt of intron 3	[51]
PTEN	c.801+1G>A	Retention of first 75 nt of intron 7	[52]
Retention of an entire intron			
MUTYH	c.934-2A>G	Retention of full intron 10	[53]
STK11	c.597+31_598-32	Retention of full intron 4	[54]
Pseudoexon inclusion			
APC	c.[532-941G>A(;) c.532-845A>G]	167 nt pEx (intron 4)	[55]
APC	c.646-1806T>G	127 nt pEx (intron 5)	[56]
APC	c.1408+729A>G	83 nt pEx (intron 10)	[56]
APC	c.1408+735A>T	83 nt pEx (intron 10)	[55]
MSH2	c.212-478T>G	75 nt pseudoexon (intron 1)	[57]
Complex splicing anomalies			
PMS2	c.538-3C>G	Skipping of exon 6 and partial deletion of the first 49 nt of exon 8	[36]
PMS2	c.989-1G>T	Skipping of exon 10 and partial deletion of first 27 nt of exon 10	[58]

APC (NM_001127510.2), *MLH1* (NM_000249.2), *MSH2* (NM_000251.2), *MSH3* (NM_002439.4), *MSH6* (NM_000179.1), *MUTYH* (NM_001128425.1), *PMS2* (NM_000535.5), *POLE* (NM_006231.2), *PTEN* (NM_000314.4), *STK11* (NM_00455)
nt nucleotides, *pEx* pseudoexon

can find nucleotide variants mapping at exon-intron junctions, within the body of the exons, or deep in the introns. As shown, splicing defects may include noncoding variants and also variants otherwise considered as missense, nonsense, or even translationally silent (synonymous). These examples illustrate why any nucleotide variant, independently of their position or coding potential, should be investigated for their eventual impact on RNA splicing, CRC-associated variants being no exception.

Contrary to RNA splicing mutations, knowledge on variants susceptible of affecting the transcription level of CRC-implicated genes is currently scarce. Most variants identified within the minimal promoters of the MMR genes remain unstudied, only a few having been classified as non-pathogenic (Class 1), likely non-pathogenic (Class 2) or of unknown significance (Class 3). The exception is *MSH2* c.-78_-77del, a promoter variant that is now considered as probably pathogenic (Class 4) in the context of Lynch syndrome [59, 60]. Another example of a genomic deletion in a promoter region which leads to a clinically relevant reduction of the expression level of the corresponding gene is the deletion of promoter 1B in the *APC* gene, which has been detected in several families with familial polyposis [61, 62]. Further studies are needed to assess the functional impact of variants mapping to the promoter regions of CRC-genes, for instance by measuring endogenous allele-specific expression, performing luciferase reporter assays, and determining alterations in transcription factor binding [59]. Moreover, one has to keep in mind that promoter function can also be affected by distant changes. An example of such situation can be found in Lynch syndrome patients carrying germline deletions in the 3' portion of the *EPCAM* gene. These deletions lead to *EPCAM* transcription readthrough, causing silencing of the downstream *MSH2* promoter [63].

Finally, variants which alter the stability and the turnover of mRNA have been demonstrated to modulate expression levels of cancer genes and are implicated in tumorigenesis. These variants may affect the secondary structure of 5′ or 3′ untranslated regions, miRNA binding sites, or the polyadenylation site [64]. Interestingly, even if DNA or RNA analyses do not identify a causative variant, the confirmation of a functional impact, such as dramatically reduced expression of a MMR gene, may nevertheless warrant specific clinical recommendations.

6 Strategies for RNA Analyses

Variant-induced splicing anomalies are usually detected upon performing experimental work that is in many cases motivated by preceding bioinformatic analyses. For obvious reasons, most molecular diagnostic laboratories rely on the availability of patients' RNA samples and on conventional gene-specific RT-PCR approaches to conduct RNA splicing analyses. This type of strategy, which allowed the identification of a large number of splicing mutations in genes implicated in hereditary CRC, such as most of those described in Table 18.1, implies a deep knowledge of the normal/alternative splicing pattern of the genes of interest, and the analysis of patients' RNA in parallel to those of several control individuals [65, 66]. Moreover, patients' RNA studies need to take into consideration that, in the absence of a co-occuring exonic variant, it is difficult to trace intronic splicing mutations especially if abnormal frameshift transcripts are produced and degraded by nonsense-mediated decay (NMD). Treatment of cellular cultures with NMD inhibitors such as puromycin or cycloheximide can be used to outwit this limitation [30, 35, 66]. Complementary strategies include: (i) functional in cellulo assays based on the use of minigenes and (ii) massively parallel high throughput RNA sequencing (RNA-seq), each method having its advantages and limitations [18–20, 30, 35, 45, 56, 66–68]. For instance, minigene-based assays allow to both circumvent the need for patients RNA samples and to establish a direct causality effect, but depending on the type of construct, may miss complex splicing anomalies involving multiple exons. RNA-seq analyses have the advantage of interrogating multiple transcripts in parallel and at high resolution, but remain expensive for routine diagnostic applications [68, 69].

RT-PCR analyses of RNA samples from patients suspected of hereditary CRC have thus far been very useful for the identification of: (i) deleterious splicing mutations (for examples please see Table 18.1 and [6]), (ii) genetic inversions [70], (iii) imbalanced allelic expression (RT-PCR in combination with other techniques such as pyrosequencing, SNuPE or SNaPshot) [18, 56, 71–75] and (iv) and to discriminate *PMS2* variants from those mapping to *PMS2* pseudogenes [76, 77]. RNA splicing analysis may also help illuminating genotype-phenotype correlations as reported by Sjursen and colleagues who described the identification of a Turcot syndrome patient homozygous for a *PMS2* splicing mutation (*PMS2* c.989-1G>T) but having a phenotype milder than expected [58]. RT-PCR analysis revealed that *PMS2* c.989-1G>T caused the production of two aberrant transcripts, one lacking the 156 nucleotide-long exon 10, and the other merely lacking its first 27 nucleotides (judged as probably less detrimental, which provided a rational explanation for the atypical phenotype).

It is anticipated that in the future, whole or targeted RNA-seq, will become a reality in molecular diagnostic laboratories, especially with the implementation of new approaches allowing long sequencing reads and single-cell analysis [68, 69]. Still, important efforts are expected in the field of bioinformatics in order to improve both RNA splicing predictions and RNA-seq data processing and analysis (including qualitative and quantitative aspects of these approaches). Moreover, further studies will be needed to determine the sensitivity and specificity of the different RNA splicing-dedicated methods. Other open questions relate to the characterization of alternative splicing patterns in different tissues or in a same tissue exposed to different external stimuli, the biological role of alternative isoforms, and the choice of the most relevant tissues to be analyzed for detecting disease-causing RNA splicing defects, such as those increasing genetic predispositions to CRC. Adequate RNA can in principle be extracted directly from cell culture, blood (heparin, citrate, or ethylenediaminetetraacetic acid), or tissue samples, provided that these are not kept under nonphysiological conditions and are processed on the same day. If the laboratory setup or other circumstances prevent the long-term or short-term culture of lymphocytes, RNA stabilizing agents or commercial kits like

RNAlater (QIAGEN) or PAXgene (PreAnalytiX) are recommended. Although these approaches are not as costly or time-consuming as cell cultures, the degradation of mRNA transcripts harboring premature termination codons (PTCs) caused by the sophisticated cellular quality control mechanism called NMD is likely to obscure results. Briefly, PTC-harboring transcripts are recognized during the "pioneer round of translation" and subsequently degraded, which helps preventing dominant-negative effects such as the incorporation of a misfolded protein in a multi-protein complex or gain of function effects.

Even if this cellular surveillance mechanism is not perfect in recognizing all PTCs, the vast majority of PTC-carrying transcripts are degraded and thus not detectable in patient-derived RNA. Consequently, NMD can be a major source of error, a fact which, depending on the strategy used, must be taken into account when analyzing RNA.

The long-term or short-term cultivation of mononuclear peripheral blood cells, although comparatively time-consuming and laborious, has many technical advantages over the direct preparation of RNA from tissue samples. Short-term lymphocyte cultures and long-term cell cultures from Epstein-Barr virus (EBV)-immortalized white blood cells can be used with equal results; however, the latter is likely to be found in only a few laboratories, due to regulatory restrictions and the considerable operating expenses involved. Compared to sampling fresh blood or tissue, the quantity and quality of RNA from cell cultures is generally higher, and NMD inhibition can be performed. In principle, there are two equally efficient substances which have been demonstrated to reliably block NMD in cell cultures: cycloheximide and puromycin. Both of these antibiotics inhibit translation at the eukaryotic ribosome, including the pioneer round of translation, with an impact on NMD [78].

In analyzing RNA from fresh blood, cultivated white blood cells, or minigene constructs transiently expressed in cell lines for genes involved in CRC syndromes, one can wonder if they recapitulate the effects produced in disease-affected tissues. By virtue of their integral role in DNA repair, cell cycle control, cellular differentiation, and genome maintenance, most genes associated with CRC syndromes are expressed ubiquitously, especially in quickly dividing tissues like white blood cells. In this regard, peripheral blood mononuclear cells (PBMCs) are well suited for RNA studies of these genes. It is nevertheless crucial to bear in mind that this is valid only for splicing events at constitutive exons, where the splicing machinery is guided and regulated primarily by the consensus DNA motifs of splice sites [20]; these exons are generally expected to be equally spliced in all tissues.

By contrast, exons affected by alternative splicing—that is, cassette exons skipped in certain isoforms—are critically regulated by a finely tuned system of tissue-specific splicing factors and splicing regulatory proteins such as the aforementioned exonic or intronic splicing enhancers and silencers. Tissue-specific differences in splicing patterns are well documented where RNA studies have been performed in different cell lines or tissues, but these differences mainly affect alternatively spliced exons. Consequently, these studies suggest a high overall consistency of results as defined by the joint detection of the main aberrant transcript [26, 67, 79]. The differences observed between cell lines, patient-derived RNA, and minigene constructs mainly affect additional alternative/aberrant transcripts or variations of intensity between distinct alternative splicing products. The European Mismatch Repair Working Group is currently formulating consensus proposals for a standardized protocol regarding cDNA analysis and the investigation of the effect of MMR variants on RNA splicing.

Expert groups have formulated recommendations for the interpretation and classification of sequence variants for LS-associated genes (International Society for Gastrointestinal Tumors, InSiGHT) [6] and for the two breast cancer susceptibility genes *BRCA1* and *BRCA2* (Evidence-Based Network for the Interpretation of Germline Mutant Alleles (ENIGMA) Consortium) [65], which advocate standardized RNA testing of all suspected splice-altering variants in order to unequivocally assess the nature of the pathogenic effect.

Many laboratories routinely use reverse transcriptase (RT) PCR-amplified cDNA fragments from fresh blood collected into PAXgene tubes (PAXgene RNA), or lymphocyte cultures to assess mRNA expression levels and to detect splicing aberrations. RT-PCR products are visualized on agarose gels to determine splicing patterns and to estimate the level of mRNA expression. Subsequent cloning and sequencing of alternate transcripts can verify splicing aberrations. This is a convenient strategy for confirming or excluding pathogenic splice defects. If the variant allele tested is found to produce only transcripts with a PTC or an in-frame deletion that disrupts a validated physiologically important domain, the variant can be reliably classified as pathogenic [6, 7, 65].

Promoter variants which are suspected to disrupt a regulatory element, like a transcription factor binding site, can reliably be analyzed by quantitative reverse transcription PCR (RT-qPCR) or allele-specific expression (ASE; see next paragraph). RT-qPCR enables reliable detection and quantitative measurement of products generated during each cycle of PCR process and is a valuable tool to assess the expression levels of a gene.

Reporter assays measure the activity of a promoter and are commonly used to study gene expression at the transcriptional level. Typically a wild type (WT) promoter sequence and the corresponding sequence containing the variant of interest are cloned in an expression vector which is thereafter transiently expressed in cell culture. The activity of the promoter can be assessed by measurement of reporter expression (usually luciferase) [80, 81].

The determination of allele-specific expression (ASE) is a powerful tool for assessing the relevance of suspected pathogenic alleles and can be performed using RNA isolated from fresh blood, PAX RNA, or cultivated lymphocytes. This approach is useful without prior knowledge of the underlying cause of a pathogenic effect, e.g., if no causative variant was identified by DNA testing due to deep intronic localization, promotor methylation, genomic inversion, translocation, etc. In single-nucleotide extension assays such as SNuPE, SNaPshot, and pyrosequencing or in MALDI-ToF mass spectrometry, ASE analysis takes advantage of a previously detected germline exonic single-nucleotide variant (SNV) as a proxy for allelic expression. This method can determine if both alleles are expressed equally or differently compared to WT control samples.

Minigene constructs are ex vivo systems in which variants can be functionally tested in a monoallelic manner, even without patient RNA. This involves the PCR amplification of patient DNA or, alternatively, the de novo construction via site-directed mutagenesis of a genomic fragment encompassing the variant of interest (preferably the entire exon) along with flanking intronic sequences, which is then cloned into a minigene system. After transient expression of these vectors in cell culture, possible differences in splicing patterns between WT transcripts and transcripts derived from the vector carrying the variant can be assessed by RT-PCR and sequencing [30, 67, 73, 79, 82]. Although potentially prone to the influence of tissue-specific splicing factors expressed in the corresponding cell lines, minigene analysis shows excellent conformity with analysis of patient-derived RNA [45]. Minor differences are observed in alternatively spliced exons which do not affect the general interpretation.

7 In Vitro Protein Functional Assays

Ideally, demonstrating that the protein encoded by the variant allele either maintains or loses the functional properties of the WT isoform should be compelling evidence for its clinical interpretation. The reality is that there are no standardized functional assays for hereditary CRC. In addition, most of the genes involved in CRC predisposition have multiple functional domains and can be involved in different cellular pathways, some of which may not be related to tumorigenesis.

In vitro assays have been developed for DNA repair genes, namely, those involved in MMR and base excision repair (BER), originally in prokaryotes, and subsequently in different eukaryotic species.

There are a number of different MMR assays that test repair activity, protein stability, interaction with partner proteins, cellular localization, resistance to alkylating agents, as well as other functions specific to single components of the MMR machinery. Some of these these tests use different artificial substrates and recombinant MMR proteins and can be performed in different cell types, including *S. cerevisiae* and human cells, or in cell-free systems [6, 83, 84]. They are available only in highly specialized laboratories and are currently not incorporated in routine diagnostic activities. In addition, their output is on a quantitative scale (i.e., % of repair compared to wild type), and there is interlaboratory variability in the results of assays testing the same properties [6].

Even less is known about the accuracy of in vitro assays for BER and polymerase proofreading activity. Although tests have been developed for *MUTYH*, they have been applied to a limited number of variants. Like MMR genes, a number of assays are available in different laboratories, and different functional properties can be investigated (Table 18.3).

Therefore, there is currently no single assay that can be used for the purpose of clinical interpretation of genetic variations in the field of hereditary CRC predisposition. In general, tests performed on mammalian systems are preferred over those

Table 18.3 Functional assays for mismatch repair and base excision repair proteins

Assay	References
Mismatch repair (MLH1, MSH2, MSH6, PMS2)	
Complementation of repair activity on artificial substrates: *a. in yeast; b. in mammalian cells*	[85–90]
Repair activity in cell-free systems	[91]
Complementation of repair activity measuring mutation rates at endogenous loci (*HPRT*; microsatellites) in cell lines	[92]
Cellular tolerance to methylating agents	[93–95]
Protein expression and stability	[96–102]
Cellular localization	[97, 102–105]
Protein-protein interactions	[106–108]
Protein-DNA binding	[109, 110]
ATPase activity, ATP/ADP cycling, ATP-induced conformational changes	[111, 112]
Base excision repair (MUTYH)	
Complementation of repair activity: *a. in E. coli; b. in mammalian cells*	[113–115]
In vitro DNA glycosylase activity	[114–117]
Protein expression	[113, 116]
Cellular localization	[113, 116]
Sensitivity to oxidative damage	[113]

in yeast or bacteria, since the conditions are more similar to those occurring in vivo in human cells. For MMR genes, it has been recommended that an assay be considered as evidence for variant classification when concordant results are obtained from two independent laboratories assessing the same function. Furthermore, multiple properties must be examined: for instance, a protein can be unstable but able to repair mismatches in vitro when expressed at levels that are, however, presumably much higher than in vivo [6]. Hence, in order to consider a variant proficient, values corresponding to the WT range must be obtained for all its different functional properties.

8 In Silico Prediction Tools

In the last two decades, a number of tools for the prediction of functional consequences have been developed to assist in the biological and clinical interpretation of DNA variant significance [7]. In this section we refer to the programs that assess the potential effects of amino acid substitutions. Importantly, their accuracy, tested versus a set of well-defined controls (i.e., variants of established pathogenicity or neutrality), is estimated between 65 and 80% [118], and specificity is particularly low, causing an excess of false positives (i.e., neutral missense changes predicted as deleterious) [119].

Due to these caveats, they should be considered as an accessory supporting source of evidence for clinical interpretation, when classification is achieved using other data. In addition, since these tools can perform differently with the same variant, depending on the gene and the protein sequence, it is advisable to use more than one program and to consider the outputs from different programs as a single piece of evidence: concordant results for pathogenicity or neutrality across two or more softwares can be used as supporting information, while discordant results are not informative [7, 120].

As discussed below, results from in silico predictions can be incorporated in multifactorial Bayesian models.

9 Multifactorial Analysis

All of the abovementioned characteristics provide qualitative clues for variant interpretation. They can also be incorporated in multifactorial Bayesian algorithms when their specificities and sensitivities have been calibrated against a robust set of reference variants of established significance. These algorithms are based on estimates of likelihood ratios (LRs) that compare for each component the probability of the observed data assuming that the variant is pathogenic versus the hypothesis of non-pathogenicity (i.e., for the MSI-H status: % MSI-H in tumors from pathogenic variant carriers/% MSI-H in tumors from noncarriers). LRs derived for each point of evidence are then cumulated, and a posterior probability of pathogenicity is calculated.

This approach has been initially developed for the *BRCA1* and *BRCA2* genes [2] and subsequently applied, with appropriate modifications, to the MMR genes. The MMR multifactorial model uses prior probabilities derived either from in silico predictions with the programs MAPP [121] and PolyPhen-2.1 [122] for potential missense changes or from values obtained on *BRCA1/BRCA2* for intronic substitutions. LR calculations are then performed for segregation analysis, family history, and tumor molecular pathology data, specifically MSI, IHC, and *BRAF* mutation status [51].

Multifactorial analysis has the advantage of providing quantitative estimates that can be easily used for clinical decisions. Although this is very useful for clinicians, the model still needs improvements to obtain more accurate assessments for the components that are already incorporated and LRs from additional datasets currently not included, such as functional studies.

10 Systems for Variant Classification

The above qualitative and quantitative evidences are used to classify gene variants for use in the clinical setting. There are two main classification systems available today: one has been devised specifically for cancer predisposition genes by a working group of the International Agency for Cancer Research (IARC) [123]; the other one is the general system developed by a joint effort of the American College of Medical Genetics and Genomics (ACMG) and the Association for Molecular

Pathology (AMP) [7]. Both use five categories, defined by qualitative terms only for ACMG/AMP and also by numbers for IARC, ranging from pathogenic (IARC Class 5) to benign/nonpathogenic (IARC Class 1). Intermediate classes include the following categories: likely pathogenic (Class 4), variants of uncertain significance (VUSs; Class 3), and likely benign/nonpathogenic (Class 2). For Class 4 and Class 2 variants, clinical advice is the same as for Class 5 and Class 1, respectively. Class 3 includes variants for which available information has not been sufficient to establish their clinical relevance and are thus non-actionable clinically.

Classification can be achieved either by a combination of qualitative data or by multifactorial analysis. The latter is the most reliable approach, but quantitative models have been built only for a very limited number of genes so far. In the field of hereditary CRC, a Bayesian algorithm has been developed for the MMR genes only.

In the ACMG/AMP system, qualitative components are subdivided based on the strength of evidence: stand-alone, very strong, strong, moderate, or supporting (in decreasing order of strength). The only stand-alone criterion is allele population frequency > 5%, allowing classification as benign.

The IARC system does not provide qualitative criteria and refers to gene-specific recommendations, such as those devised by the InSiGHT Variant Interpretation Committee (VIC) [6]. The InSiGHT MMR rules require that concordant evidence be available pertaining to both the clinical and the functional components of classification in order to assign a variant to a clinically actionable class (5, 4, 2, or 1). Sequence-based information may be used as a stand-alone criterion for variants that have a very high prior probability of pathogenicity (i.e., nonsense substitutions, with the caveats mentioned above in “Characteristics of the DNA sequence”).

The InSiGHT criteria for MMR genes have been developed by an international multidisciplinary panel of experts and are subject to periodic revisions based on novel findings that may lead to a refinement of the interpretation rules. Their use for classification of MMR variants is therefore strongly recommended.

In the absence of specific criteria, ACMG/AMP recommendations can be used for other hereditary CRC genes, having in mind that, since these are nonspecific and less robust, the likelihood of misclassification may be higher.

From the practical standpoint, health professionals who want to have information on the clinical significance of DNA sequence variants can consult online databases. The InSiGHT website contains information on hereditary CRC genes, including the classifications of >2400 MMR gene variants and the underlying evidence for each of them (https://www.insight-group.org/variants/databases/). ClinVar, hosted by the National Center for Biotechnology Information (https://www.ncbi.nlm.nih.gov/clinvar/), is a public archive of classification reports of different complexity, ranging from the representation of an allele and its interpretation to the classifications of expert panels, including the InSiGHT MMR VIC. It archives interpretations on any gene, but it does not curate submitted information nor does it perform interpretations. Therefore, the submissions must be critically assessed, checking whether they are concordant or not when there are multiple contributions for the same variant and verifying the level of evidence (i.e., single variant with no clinical information or classification of expert panel).

References

1. Gonzaga-Juaregui C, Lupski JR, Gibbs RA. Human genome sequencing in health and disease. Annu Rev Med. 2012;63:35–61. https://doi.org/10.1146/annurev-med-051010-162644.
2. Goldgar DE, Easton DF, Deffenbaugh AM, Monteiro AN, Tavtigian SV, Couch FJ, Breast Cancer Information Core (BIC) Steering Committee. Integrated evaluation of DNA sequence variants of unknown clinical significance: application to *BRCA1* and *BRCA2*. Am J Hum Genet. 2004;75:535–44.
3. Møller P, Seppälä T, Bernstein I, Holinski-Feder E, Sala P, Evans DG, et al. Cancer incidence and survival in lynch syndrome patients receiving colonoscopic and gynaecological surveillance: first report from the prospective lynch syndrome database. Gut. 2017;66:464–72. https://doi.org/10.1136/gutjnl-2015-309675.
4. Møller P, Seppälä T, Bernstein I, Holinski-Feder E, Sala P, Evans DG, et al. Incidence of and survival after subsequent cancers in carriers of pathogenic MMR variants with previous cancer: a report from the prospective lynch syndrome database. Gut. 2017;66:1657–64. https://doi.org/10.1136/gutjnl-2016-311403.
5. Wimmer K, Kratz CP, Vasen HF, Caron O, Colas C, Entz-Werle N, et al. Diagnostic criteria for constitutional mismatch repair deficiency syndrome: suggestions of the European consortium 'care for CMMRD' (C4CMMRD). J Med Genet. 2014;51:355–65. https://doi.org/10.1136/jmedgenet-2014-102284.
6. Thompson BA, Spurdle AB, Plazzer JP, Greenblatt MS, Akagi K, Al-Mulla F, et al. Application of a five-tiered scheme for standardized classification of 2,360 unique mismatch repair gene variants lodged on the InSiGHT locus-specific database. Nat Genet. 2014;46:107–15. https://doi.org/10.1038/ng.2854.
7. Richards S, Aziz N, Bale S, Bick D, Das S, Gastier-Foster J, et al. ACMG Laboratory Quality Assurance Committee. Standards and guidelines for the interpretation of sequence variants: a joint consensus recommendation of the American College of Medical Genetics and Genomics and the Association for Molecular Pathology. Genet Med. 2015;17:405–24.
8. Genome Aggregation Database (gnomAD). 2016. http://gnomad.broadinstitute.org/. Accessed 17 Mar 2018.
9. Stevens KN, Vachon CM, Couch FJ. Genetic susceptibility to triple-negative breast cancer. Cancer Res. 2013;73:2025–30. https://doi.org/10.1158/0008-5472.
10. Zugazagoitia J, Pérez-Segura P, Manzano A, Blanco I, Vega A, Custodio A, et al. Limited family structure and triple-negative breast cancer (TNBC) subtype as predictors of BRCA mutations in a genetic counseling cohort of early-onset sporadic breast cancers. Breast Cancer Res Treat. 2014;148:415–21. https://doi.org/10.1007/s10549-014-3167-4.
11. Lucci-Cordisco E, Risio M, Venesio T, Genuardi M. The growing complexity of the intestinal polyposis syndromes. Am J Med Genet A. 2013;161A:2777–87. https://doi.org/10.1002/ajmg.a.36253.
12. Lucci-Cordisco E, Boccuto L, Neri G, Genuardi M. The use of microsatellite instability, immunohistochemistry and other variables in determining the clinical significance of MLH1 and MSH2 unclassified variants in lynch syndrome. Cancer Biomark. 2006;2:11–27.
13. Van Puijenbroek M, Nielsen M, Tops CM, Halfwerk H, Vasen HF, Weiss MM, et al. Identification of patients with (atypical) *MUTYH*-associated polyposis by KRAS2 c.34G > T prescreening followed by *MUTYH* hotspot analysis in formalin-fixed paraffin-embedded tissue. Clin Cancer Res. 2008;14:139–42. https://doi.org/10.1158/1078-0432.CCR-07-1705.
14. Weren RD, Ligtenberg MJ, Kets CM, de Voer RM, Verwiel ET, Spruijt L, et al. A germline homozygous mutation in the base-excision repair gene NTHL1 causes adenomatous polyposis and colorectal cancer. Nat Genet. 2015;47:668–71. https://doi.org/10.1038/ng.3287.
15. Briggs S, Tomlinson I. Germline and somatic polymerase ε and δ mutations define a new class of hypermutated colorectal and endometrial cancers. J Pathol. 2013;230:148–53. https://doi.org/10.1002/path.4185.
16. Jansen AM, van Wezel T, van den Akker BE, Ventayol Garcia M, Ruano D, Tops CM, et al. Combined mismatch repair and *POLE/POLD1* defects explain unresolved suspected

lynch syndrome cancers. Eur J Hum Genet. 2016;24:1089–92. https://doi.org/10.1038/ejhg.2015.252.
17. Howitt BE, Shukla SA, Sholl LM, Ritterhouse LL, Watkins JC, Rodig S, Stover E, Strickland KC, D'Andrea AD, Wu CJ, Matulonis UA, Konstantinopoulos PA. Association of olymerase e-mutated and microsatellite-instable endometrial cancers with neoantigen load, number of tumor-infiltrating lymphocytes, and expression of PD-1 and PD-L1. JAMA Oncol. 2015;1:1319–23. https://doi.org/10.1001/jamaoncol.2015.2151.
18. Tricarico R, Kasela M, Mareni C, Thompson BA, Drouet A, Staderini L, et al. Assessment of the InSiGHT interpretation criteria for the clinical classification of 24 MLH1 and MSH2 gene variants. Hum Mutat. 2017;38:64–77. https://doi.org/10.1002/humu.23117.
19. Baralle D, Lucassen A, Buratti E. Missed threads. The impact of pre-mRNA splicing defects on clinical practice. EMBO Rep. 2009;10:810–6. https://doi.org/10.1038/embor.2009.170.
20. Baralle D, Buratti E. RNA splicing in human disease and in the clinic. Clin Sci (Lond). 2017;131:355–68. https://doi.org/10.1042/CS20160211.
21. Cartegni L, Chew SL, Krainer AR. Listening to silence and understanding nonsense: exonic mutations that affect splicing. Nat Rev Genet. 2002;3:285–98.
22. Ward AJ, Cooper TA. The pathobiology of splicing. J Pathol. 2010;220:152–63. https://doi.org/10.1002/path.2649.
23. Klamt B, Koziell A, Poulat F, Wieacker P, Scambler P, Berta P, Gessler M. Frasier syndrome is caused by defective alternative splicing of WT1 leading to an altered ratio of WT1 +/-KTS splice isoforms. Hum Mol Genet. 1998;7:709–14.
24. Park SA, Ahn SI, Gallo J-M. Tau mis-splicing in the pathogenesis of neurodegenerative disorders. BMB Rep. 2016;49:405–13.
25. Spurdle AB, Couch FJ, Hogervorst FBL, Radice P, Sinilnikova OM, IARC Unclassified Genetic Variants Working Group. Prediction and assessment of splicing alterations: implications for clinical testing. Hum Mutat. 2008;29:1304–13. https://doi.org/10.1002/humu.20901.
26. Houdayer C, Caux-Moncoutier V, Krieger S, Barrois M, Bonnet F, Bourdon V, et al. Guidelines for splicing analysis in molecular diagnosis derived from a set of 327 combined in silico/in vitro studies on *BRCA1* and *BRCA2* variants. Hum Mutat. 2012;33:1228–38. https://doi.org/10.1002/humu.22101.
27. Di Giacomo D, Gaildrat P, Abuli A, Abdat J, Frébourg T, Tosi M, Martins A. Functional analysis of a large set of BRCA2 exon 7 variants highlights the predictive value of hexamer scores in detecting alterations of exonic splicing regulatory elements. Hum Mutat. 2013;34:1547–57. https://doi.org/10.1002/humu.22428.
28. Erkelenz S, Theiss S, Otte M, Widera M, Peter JO, Schaal H. Genomic HEXploring allows landscaping of novel potential splicing regulatory elements. Nucleic Acids Res. 2014;42:10681–97. https://doi.org/10.1093/nar/gku736.
29. Xiong HY, Alipanahi B, Lee LJ, Bretschneider H, Merico D, Yuen RK, et al. RNA splicing. The human splicing code reveals new insights into the genetic determinants of disease. Science. 2015;347:1254806. https://doi.org/10.1126/science.1254806.
30. Soukarieh O, Gaildrat P, Hamieh M, Drouet A, Baert-Desurmont S, Frébourg T, et al. Exonic splicing mutations are more prevalent than currently estimated and can be predicted by using in Silico tools. PLoS Genet. 2016;12:e1005756. https://doi.org/10.1371/journal.pgen.1005756.
31. Teraoka SN, Telatar M, Becker-Catania S, Liang T, Onengüt S, Tolun A, et al. Splicing defects in the ataxia-telangiectasia gene, *ATM*: underlying mutations and consequences. Am J Hum Genet. 1999;64:1617–31.
32. Ars E, Serra E, García J, Kruyer H, Gaona A, Lázaro C, Estivill X. Mutations affecting mRNA splicing are the most common molecular defects in patients with neurofibromatosis type 1. Hum Mol Genet. 2000;9:237–47.
33. Lim KH, Ferraris L, Filloux ME, Raphael BJ, Fairbrother WG. Using positional distribution to identify splicing elements and predict pre-mRNA processing defects in human genes. Proc Natl Acad Sci U S A. 2011;108:11093–8. https://doi.org/10.1073/pnas.1101135108.

34. Aretz S, Uhlhaas S, Sun Y, Pagenstecher C, Mangold E, Caspari R, et al. Familial adenomatous polyposis: aberrant splicing due to missense or silent mutations in the APC gene. Hum Mutat. 2004;24:370–80.
35. Auclair J, Busine MP, Navarro C, Ruano E, Montmaigne G, Desseigne F, et al. Systematic mRNA analysis for the effect of MLH1 and MSH2 missense and silent mutations on aberrant splicing. Hum Mutat. 2006;27:145–54.
36. Adam R, Spier I, Zhao B, Kloth M, Marquez J, Hinrichsen I, et al. Exome sequencing identifies Biallelic *MSH3* Germline mutations as a recessive subtype of colorectal adenomatous polyposis. Am J Hum Genet. 2016;99:337–51. https://doi.org/10.1016/j.ajhg.2016.06.015.
37. Plaschke J, Linnebacher M, Kloor M, Gebert J, Cremer FW, Tinschert S, et al. Compound heterozygosity for two *MSH6* mutations in a patient with early onset of HNPCC-associated cancers, but without hematological malignancy and brain tumor. Eur J Hum Genet. 2006;14:561–6.
38. Dallosso AR, Dolwani S, Jones N, Jones S, Colley J, Maynard J, et al. Inherited predisposition to colorectal adenomas caused by multiple rare alleles of MUTYH but not OGG1, NUDT1, NTH1 or NEIL 1, 2 or 3. Gut. 2008;57:1252–5. https://doi.org/10.1136/gut.2007.145748.
39. Pin E, Pastrello C, Tricarico R, Papi L, Quaia M, Fornasarig M, et al. MUTYH c.933+3A>C, associated with a severely impaired gene expression, is the first Italian founder mutation in MUTYH-associated polyposis. Int J Cancer. 2013;132:1060–9. https://doi.org/10.1002/ijc.27761.
40. Borràs E, Pineda M, Cadiñanos J, Del Valle J, Brieger A, Hinrichsen I, et al. Refining the role of *PMS2* in lynch syndrome: germline mutational analysis improved by comprehensive assessment of variants. J Med Genet. 2013;50:552–63. https://doi.org/10.1136/jmedgenet-2012-101511.
41. Pachlopnik Schmid J, Lemoine R, Nehme N, Cormier-Daire V, Revy P, Debeurme F, et al. Polymerase ε1 mutation in a human syndrome with facial dysmorphism, immunodeficiency, livedo, and short stature ("FILS syndrome"). J Exp Med. 2013;209:2323–30. https://doi.org/10.1084/jem.20121303.
42. Agrawal S, Pilarski R, Eng C. Different splicing defects lead to differential effects downstream of the lipid and protein phosphatase activities of *PTEN*. Hum Mol Genet. 2005;14:2459–68.
43. Suphapeetiporn K, Kongkam P, Tantivatana J, Sinthuwiwat T, Tongkobpetch S, Shotelersuk V. PTEN c.511C>T nonsense mutation in a BRRS family disrupts a potential exonic splicing enhancer and causes exon skipping. Jpn J Clin Oncol. 2006;36:814–21.
44. Papp J, Kovacs ME, Solyom S, Kasler M, Børresen-Dale A-L, Olah E. High prevalence of germline STK11 mutations in Hungarian Peutz-Jeghers syndrome patients. BMC Med Genet. 2010;11:169. https://doi.org/10.1186/1471-2350-11-169.
45. van der Klift HM, Jansen AML, van der Steenstraten N, Bik EC, Tops CMJ, Devilee P, Wijnen JT. Splicing analysis for exonic and intronic mismatch repair gene variants associated with lynch syndrome confirms high concordance between minigene assays and patient RNA analyses. Mol Genet Genomic Med. 2015;3:327–45. https://doi.org/10.1002/mgg3.145.
46. Trojan J, Plotz G, Brieger A, Raedle J, Meltzer SJ, Wolter M, Zeuzem S. Activation of a cryptic splice site of PTEN and loss of heterozygosity in benign skin lesions in Cowden disease. J Invest Dermatol. 2001;117:1650–3.
47. Reifenberger J, Rauch L, Beckmann MW, Megahed M, Ruzicka T, Reifenberger G. Cowden's disease: clinical and molecular genetic findings in a patient with a novel PTEN germline mutation. Br J Dermatol. 2003;148:1040–6.
48. Kaufmann A, Vogt S, Uhlhaas S, Stienen D, Kurth I, Hameister H, et al. Analysis of rare *APC* variants at the mRNA level: six pathogenic mutations and literature review. J Mol Diagn. 2009;11:131–9. https://doi.org/10.2353/jmoldx.2009.080129.
49. Sharp A, Pichert G, Lucassen A, Eccles D. RNA analysis reveals splicing mutations and loss of expression defects in MLH1 and BRCA1. Hum Mutat. 2004;24:272.
50. Yan H, Papadopoulos N, Marra G, Perrera C, Jiricny J, Boland CR, et al. Conversion of diploidy to haploidy. Nature. 2000;403:723–4.

51. Thompson BA, Goldgar DE, Paterson C, Clendenning M, Walters R, Arnold S, et al. A multifactorial likelihood model for MMR gene variant classification incorporating probabilities based on sequence bioinformatics and tumor characteristics: a report from the Colon Cancer family registry. Hum Mutat. 2013;34:200–9. https://doi.org/10.1002/humu.22213.
52. Celebi JT, Wanner M, Ping XL, Zhang H, Peacocke M. Association of splicing defects in *PTEN* leading to exon skipping or partial intron retention in Cowden syndrome. Hum Genet. 2000;107:234–8.
53. Tao H, Shinmura K, Hanaoka T, Natsukawa S, Shaura K, Koizumi Y, et al. A novel splice-site variant of the base excision repair gene MYH is associated with production of an aberrant mRNA transcript encoding a truncated MYH protein not localized in the nucleus. Carcinogenesis. 2004;25:1859–66.
54. Abed AA, Günther K, Kraus C, Hohenberger W, Ballhausen WG. Mutation screening at the RNA level of the *STK11/LKB1* gene in Peutz-Jeghers syndrome reveals complex splicing abnormalities and a novel mRNA isoform (STK11 c.597(insertion mark)598insIVS4). Hum Mutat. 2001;18:397–410.
55. Spier I, Horpaopan S, Vogt S, Ulhaas S, Morak M, Stienen D, et al. Deep intronic *APC* mutations explain a substantial proportion of patients with familial or early-onset adenomatous polyposis. Hum Mutat. 2012;33:1045–50. https://doi.org/10.1002/humu.22082.
56. Nieminen TT, Pavicic W, Porkka N, Kankainen M, Järvinen HJ, Lepistö A, Peltomäki P. Pseudoexons provide a mechanism for allele-specific expression of *APC* in familial adenomatous polyposis. Oncotarget. 2016;7:70685–98. https://doi.org/10.18632/oncotarget.12206.
57. Clendenning M, Buchanan DD, Walsh MD, Nagler B, Rosty C, Thompson B, et al. Mutation deep within an intron of *MSH2* causes lynch syndrome. Familial Cancer. 2011;10:297–301. https://doi.org/10.1007/s10689-011-9427-0.
58. Sjursen W, Bjørnevoll I, Engebretsen LF, Fjelland K, Halvorsen T, Myrvold HE. A homozygote splice site PMS2 mutation as cause of Turcot syndrome gives rise to two different abnormal transcripts. Familial Cancer. 2009;8:179–86. https://doi.org/10.1007/s10689-008-9225-5.
59. Liu Q, Thompson BA, Ward RL, Hesson LB, Sloane MA. Understanding the pathogenicity of noncoding mismatch gepair gene promoter variants in lynch syndrome. Hum Mutat. 2016;37:417–26. https://doi.org/10.1002/humu.22971.
60. Yan H, Jin H, Xue G, Mei Q, Ding F, Hao L, Sun SH. Germline hMSH2 promoter mutation in a Chinese HNPCC kindred: evidence for dual role of LOH. Clin Genet. 2007;72:556–61.
61. Kadiyska TK, Todorov TP, Bichev SN, Vazharova RV, Nossikoff AV, Savov AS, et al. *APC* promoter 1B deletion in familial polyposisDOUBLEHYPHENimplications for mutation-negative families. Clin Genet. 2014;85:452–7. https://doi.org/10.1111/cge.12210.
62. Lin Y, Lin S, Baxter MD, Lin L, Kennedy SM, Zhang Z, et al. Novel APC promoter and exon 1B deletion and allelic silencing in three mutation-negative classic familial adenomatous polyposis families. Genome Med. 2015;7:42. https://doi.org/10.1186/s13073-015-0148.
63. Tutlewska K, Lubinski J, Kurzawski G. Germline deletions in the EPCAM gene as a cause of lynch syndrome - literature review. Hered Cancer Clin Pract. 2013;11:9. https://doi.org/10.1186/1897-4287-11-9.
64. Diederichs S, Bartsch L, Berkmann JC, Fröse K, Heitmann J, Hoppe C, et al. The dark matter of the cancer genome: aberrations in regulatory elements, untranslated regions, splice sites, non-coding RNA and synonymous mutations. EMBO Mol Med. 2016;8:442–57. https://doi.org/10.15252/emmm.201506055.
65. ENIGMA Consortium. https://enigmaconsortium.org/wp-content/uploads/2017/12/ENIGMA_Rules_2017-06-29.pdf. Accessed 16 Mar 2018.
66. Thompson BA, Martins A, Spurdle AB. A review of mismatch repair gene transcripts: issues for interpretation of mRNA splicing assays. Clin Genet. 2015;87:100–8. https://doi.org/10.1111/cge.12450.
67. Tournier I, Vezain M, Martins A, Charbonnier F, Baert-Desurmont S, Olschwang S, et al. A large fraction of unclassified variants of the mismatch repair genes MLH1 and MSH2 is associated with splicing defects. Hum Mutat. 2008;29:1412–24. https://doi.org/10.1002/humu.20796.

68. Conesa A, Madrigal P, Tarazona S, Gomez-Cabrero D, Cervera A, McPherson A, et al. A survey of best practices for RNA-seq data analysis. Genome Biol. 2016;17:13. https://doi.org/10.1186/s13059-016-0881-8.
69. Saliba A-E, Westermann AJ, Gorski SA, Vogel J. Single-cell RNA-seq: advances and future challenges. Nucleic Acids Res. 2014;42:8845–60. https://doi.org/10.1093/nar/gku555.
70. Liu Q, Hesson LB, Nunez AC, Packham D, Williams R, Ward RL, Sloane MA. A cryptic paracentric inversion of MSH2 exons 2-6 causes lynch syndrome. Carcinogenesis. 2016;37:10–7. https://doi.org/10.1093/carcin/bgv154.
71. De Lellis L, Aceto GM, Curia MC, et al. Integrative analysis of hereditary nonpolyposis colorectal cancer: the contribution of allele-specific expression and other assays to diagnostic algorithms. PLoS One. 2013;8:e81194. https://doi.org/10.1371/journal.pone.0081194.
72. Hesson LB, Packham D, Kwok C-T, Nunez AC, Ng B, Schmidt C, et al. Lynch syndrome associated with two MLH1 promoter variants and allelic imbalance of MLH1 expression. Hum Mutat. 2015;36:622–30. https://doi.org/10.1002/humu.22785.
73. Lastella P, Surdo NC, Resta N, Guanti G, Stella A. In silico and in vivo splicing analysis of *MLH1* and *MSH2* missense mutations shows exon- and tissue-specific effects. BMC Genomics. 2006;7:243.
74. Kwok C-T, Ward RL, Hawkins NJ, Hitchins MP. Detection of allelic imbalance in MLH1 expression by pyrosequencing serves as a tool for the identification of germline defects in lynch syndrome. Familial Cancer. 2010;9:345–56. https://doi.org/10.1007/s10689-009-9314-0.
75. Santibanez Koref M, Wilson V, Cartwright N, Cunnington MS, Mathers JC, et al. MLH1 differential allelic expression in mutation carriers and controls. Ann Hum Genet. 2010;74:479–88. https://doi.org/10.1111/j.1469-1809.2010.00603.x.
76. Etzler J, Peyrl A, Zatkova A, Schildhaus H-U, Ficek A, Merkelbach-Bruse S, et al. RNA-based mutation analysis identifies an unusual MSH6 splicing defect and circumvents PMS2 pseudogene interference. Hum Mutat. 2008;29:299–305.
77. van der Klift HM, Mensenkamp AR, Drost M, Bik EC, Vos YJ, et al. Comprehensive mutation analysis of PMS2 in a large cohort of probands suspected of lynch syndrome or constitutional mismatch repair deficiency syndrome. Hum Mutat. 2016;37:1162–79. https://doi.org/10.1002/humu.23052.
78. Nasif S, Contu L, Mühlemann O. Beyond quality control: the role of nonsense-mediated mRNA decay (NMD) in regulating gene expression. Semin Cell Dev Biol. 2018;75:78–87. https://doi.org/10.1016/j.semcdb.2017.08.053.
79. Bonnet C, Krieger S, Vezain M, Rousselin A, Tournier I, Martins A, et al. Screening BRCA1 and BRCA2 unclassified variants for splicing mutations using reverse transcription PCR on patient RNA and an ex vivo assay based on a splicing reporter minigene. J Med Genet. 2008;45:438–46. https://doi.org/10.1136/jmg.2007.056895.
80. Ward RL, Dobbins T, Lindor NM, Rapkins RW, Hitchins MP. Identification of constitutional *MLH1* epimutations and promoter variants in colorectal cancer patients from the Colon Cancer family registry. Genet Med. 2013;15:25–35. https://doi.org/10.1038/gim.2012.91.
81. Waidmann MS, Bleichrodt FS, Laslo T, Riedel CU. Bacterial luciferase reporters: the Swiss army knife of molecular biology. Bioeng Bugs. 2011;2:8–16. https://doi.org/10.4161/bbug.2.1.13566.
82. Gaildrat P, Krieger S, Théry JC, Killian A, Rousselin A, Berthet P, et al. The BRCA1 c.5434C->G (p.Pro1812Ala) variant induces a deleterious exon 23 skipping by affecting exonic splicing regulatory elements. J Med Genet. 2010;47:398–403. https://doi.org/10.1136/jmg.2009.074047.
83. Shimodaira H, Filosi N, Shibata H, Suzuki T, Radice P, Kanamaru R, et al. Functional analysis of human MLH1 mutations in Saccharomyces cerevisiae. Nat Genet. 1998;19:384–9.
84. Nyström-Lahti M, Perrera C, Räschle M, Panyushkina-Seiler E, Marra G, Curci A, et al. Functional analysis of *MLH1* mutations linked to hereditary nonpolyposis colon cancer. Genes Chromosomes Cancer. 2002;33:160–7.
85. Trojan J, Zeuzem S, Randolph A, Hemmerle C, Brieger A, Raedle J, Plotz G, Jiricny J, Marra G. Functional analysis of hMLH1 variants and HNPCC-related mutations using a human expression system. Gastroenterology. 2002;122:211–9.

86. Kondo E, Suzuki H, Horii A, Fukushige S. A yeast two-hybrid assay provides a simple way to evaluate the vast majority of hMLH1 germ-line mutations. Cancer Res. 2003;63:3302–8.
87. Plotz G, Welsch C, Giron-Monzon L, Friedhoff P, Albrecht M, Piiper A, et al. Mutations in the MutSalpha interaction interface of MLH1 can abolish DNA mismatch repair. Nucleic Acids Res. 2006;34:6574–86.
88. Ollila S, Dermadi Bebek D, Jiricny J, Nystrom M. Mechanisms of pathogenicity in human *MSH2* missense mutants. Hum Mutat. 2008;29:1355–63. https://doi.org/10.1002/humu.20893.
89. Drost M, Zonneveld JB, van Hees S, Rasmussen LJ, Hofstra RM, de Wind N. A rapid and cell-free assay to test the activity of lynch syndrome-associated MSH2 and MSH6 missense variants. Hum Mutat. 2012;33:488–94. https://doi.org/10.1002/humu.22000.
90. Wielders EA, Dekker RJ, Holt I, Morris GE, te Riele H. Characterization of *MSH2* variants by endogenous gene modification in mouse embryonic stem cells. Hum Mutat. 2011;32:389–96. https://doi.org/10.1002/humu.21448.
91. Marra G, D'Atri S, Yan H, Perrera C, Cannavo E, Vogelstein B, Jiricny J. Phenotypic analysis of hMSH2 mutations in mouse cells carrying human chromosomes. Cancer Res. 2001;61:7719–21.
92. Blasi MF, Ventura I, Aquilina G, Degan P, Bertario L, Bassi C, et al. A human cell-based assay to evaluate the effects of alterations in the MLH1 mismatch repair gene. Cancer Res. 2006;66:9036–44.
93. Mastrocola AS, Heinen CD. Lynch syndrome-associated mutations in *MSH2* alter DNA repair and checkpoint response functions in vivo. Hum Mutat. 2010;31:E1699–708. https://doi.org/10.1002/humu.21333.
94. Takahashi M, Shimodaira H, Andreutti-Zaugg C, Iggo R, Kolodner RD, Ishioka C. Functional analysis of human MLH1 variants using yeast and in vitro mismatch repair assays. Cancer Res. 2007;67:4595–604.
95. Belvederesi L, Bianchi F, Galizia E, Loretelli C, Bracci R, Catalani R, Amati M, Cellerino R. *MSH2* missense mutations and HNPCC syndrome: pathogenicity assessment in a human expression system. Hum Mutat. 2008;29:E296–309. https://doi.org/10.1002/humu.2087.
96. Perera S, Bapat B. The MLH1 variants p.Arg265Cys and p.Lys618Ala affect protein stability while p.Leu749Gln affects heterodimer formation. Hum Mutat. 2008;29:332. https://doi.org/10.1002/humu.9523.
97. Borràs E, Pineda M, Blanco I, Jewett EM, Wang F, Teulé A, et al. *MLH1* founder mutations with moderate penetrance in Spanish lynch syndrome families. Cancer Res. 2010;70:7379–91. https://doi.org/10.1158/0008-5472.
98. Hardt K, Heick SB, Betz B, Goecke T, Yazdanparast H, Küppers R, et al. Missense variants in hMLH1 identified in patients from the German HNPCC consortium and functional studies. Familial Cancer. 2011;10:273–84. https://doi.org/10.1007/s10689-011-9431-4.
99. Hinrichsen I, Brieger A, Trojan J, Zeuzem S, Nilbert M, Plotz G. Expression defect size among unclassified MLH1 variants determines pathogenicity in lynch syndrome diagnosis. Clin Cancer Res. 2013;19:2432–41. https://doi.org/10.1158/1078-0432.CCR-12-3299.
100. Borràs E, Pineda M, Brieger A, Hinrichsen I, Gómez C, Navarro M, et al. Comprehensive functional assessment of *MLH1* variants of unknown significance. Hum Mutat. 2012;33:1576–88. https://doi.org/10.1002/humu.22142.
101. Raevaara TE, Korhonen MK, Lohi H, Hampel H, Lynch E, Lönnqvist KE, et al. Functional significance and clinical phenotype of nontruncating mismatch repair variants of *MLH1*. Gastroenterology. 2005;129:537–49.
102. Gassman NR, Clodfelter JE, McCauley AK, Bonin K, Salsbury FR Jr, Scarpinato KD. Cooperative nuclear localization sequences lend a novel role to the N-terminal region of MSH6. PLoS One. 2011;6:e17907. https://doi.org/10.1371/journal.pone.0017907.
103. Belvederesi L, Bianchi F, Loretelli C, Bracci R, Cascinu S, Cellerino R. Sub-cellular localization analysis of MSH6 missense mutations does not reveal an overt *MSH6* nuclear transport impairment. Familial Cancer. 2012;11:675–80. https://doi.org/10.1007/s10689-012-9558-y.

104. Guerrette S, Wilson T, Gradia S, Fishel R. Interactions of human hMSH2 with hMSH3 and hMSH2 with hMSH6: examination of mutations found in hereditary nonpolyposis colorectal cancer. Mol Cell Biol. 1998;18:6616–23.
105. Guerrette S, Acharya S, Fishel R. The interaction of the human MutL homologues in hereditary nonpolyposis colon cancer. J Biol Chem. 1999;274:6336–41.
106. Yuan ZQ, Gottlieb B, Beitel LK, Wong N, Gordon PH, Wang Q, et al. Polymorphisms and HNPCC: PMS2-MLH1 protein interactions diminished by single nucleotide polymorphisms. Hum Mutat. 2002;19:108–13.
107. Clark AB, Cook ME, Tran HT, Gordenin DA, Resnick MA, Kunkel TA. Functional analysis of human MutS alpha and MutS beta complexes in yeast. Nucleic Acids Res. 1999;27:736–42.
108. Drotschmann K, Clark AB, Tran HT, Resnick MA, Gordenin DA, Kunkel TA. Mutator phenotypes of yeast strains heterozygous for mutations in the MSH2 gene. Proc Natl Acad Sci U S A. 1999;96:2970–5.
109. Iaccarino I, Marra G, Dufner P, Jiricny J. Mutation in the magnesium binding site of hMSH6 disables the hMutSalpha sliding clamp from translocating along DNA. J Biol Chem. 2000;275:2080–6.
110. Heinen CD, Wilson T, Mazurek A, Berardini M, Butz C, Fishel R. HNPCC mutations in hMSH2 result in reduced hMSH2-hMSH6 molecular switch functions. Cancer Cell. 2002;1:469–78.
111. Molatore S, Russo MT, D'Agostino VG, Barone F, Matsumoto Y, Albertini AM, et al. *MUTYH* mutations associated with familial adenomatous polyposis: functional characterization by a mammalian cell-based assay. Hum Mutat. 2010;31:159–66. https://doi.org/10.1002/humu.21158.
112. Komine K, Shimodaira H, Takao M, Soeda H, Zhang X, Takahashi M, Ishioka C. Functional complementation assay for 47 MUTYH variants in a MutY-disrupted Escherichia coli strain. Hum Mutat. 2015;36:704–11. https://doi.org/10.1002/humu.22794.
113. Shinmura K, Kato H, Goto M, Yamada H, Tao H, Nakamura S, Sugimura H. Functional evaluation of nine missense-type variants of the human DNA Glycosylase enzyme MUTYH in the Japanese population. Hum Mutat. 2016;37:350–3. https://doi.org/10.1002/humu.22949104.
114. Ali M, Kim H, Cleary S, Cupples C, Gallinger S, Bristow R. Characterization of mutant MUTYH proteins associated with familial colorectal cancer. Gastroenterology. 2008;135:499–507. https://doi.org/10.1053/j.gastro.2008.04.035.
115. D'Agostino VG, Minoprio A, Torreri P, Marioni I, Bossa C, Petrucci TC, et al. Functional analysis of MUTYH mutated proteins associated with familial adenomatous polyposis. DNA Repair. 2010;9:700–7. https://doi.org/10.1016/j.dnarep.2010.03.008.
116. Ou J, Niessen RC, Lützen A, Sijmons RH, Kleibeuker JH, de Wind N, et al. Functional analysis helps to clarify the clinical importance of unclassified variants in DNA mismatch repair genes. Hum Mutat. 2007;28:1047–54.
117. Rasmussen LJ, Heinen CD, Royer-Pokora B, Drost M, Tavtigian S, Hofstra RM, de Wind N. Pathological assessment of mismatch repair gene variants in lynch syndrome: past, present, and future. Hum Mutat. 2012;33:1617–25. https://doi.org/10.1002/humu.22168.
118. Thusberg J, Olatubosun A, Vihinen M. Performance of mutation pathogenicity prediction methods on missense variants. Hum Mutat. 2011;32:358–68. https://doi.org/10.1002/humu.21445.
119. Choi Y, Sims GE, Murphy S, Miller JR, Chan AP. Predicting the functional effect of amino acid substitutions and indels. PLoS One. 2012;7:e46688. https://doi.org/10.1371/journal.pone.0046688.
120. Chan PA, Duraisamy S, Miller PJ, Newell JA, McBride C, Bond JP, et al. Interpreting missense variants: comparing computational methods in human disease genes *CDKN2A*, *MLH1*, *MSH2*, *MECP2*, and tyrosinase (*TYR*). Hum Mutat. 2007;28:683–93.
121. Stone EA, Sidow A. Physicochemical constraint violation by missense substitutions mediates impairment of protein function and disease severity. Genome Res. 2005;15:978–86.

122. Adzhubei I, Jordan DM, Sunyaev SR. Predicting functional effect of human missense mutations using PolyPhen-2. Curr Protoc Hum Genet. 2013. https://doi.org/10.1002/0471142905.hg0720s76.
123. Plon SE, Eccles DM, Easton D, Foulkes WD, Genuardi M, Greenblatt MS, et al. Sequence variant classification and reporting: recommendations for improving the interpretation of cancer susceptibility genetic test results. Hum Mutat. 2008;29:1282–91. https://doi.org/10.1002/humu.20880.

Chapter 19
Prediction Models for Lynch Syndrome

Fay Kastrinos, Gregory Idos, and Giovanni Parmigiani

Abstract Numerous strategies are currently available for the identification of individuals and families with Lynch syndrome that have evolved considerably over time. Prediction models for Lynch syndrome can quantify an individual's risk of carrying a germline mismatch repair gene mutation and help clinicians decide who should be referred for further genetic risk assessment and/or genetic testing. In this chapter, we review the main prediction models developed for the identification of individuals at risk for Lynch syndrome with a focus on their specific features, performance measures as assessed by several validation studies, comparison with other clinical and molecular strategies for the diagnosis of Lynch syndrome, and their implementation and potential uses in clinical practice. We also introduce a new prediction model that provides prospective cancer risk estimates for individuals with MMR gene mutations based on comprehensive literature reviews. Lastly, we address the future considerations related to the use of clinical prediction models, including the impact of next-generation DNA sequencing technologies and the increased uptake of simultaneous testing of multiple genes (multigene panel testing) associated with inherited cancer susceptibility.

F. Kastrinos (✉)
Herbert Irving Comprehensive Cancer Center, Columbia University Medical Center, New York, NY, USA

Division of Digestive and Liver Diseases, Columbia University Medical Center, New York, NY, USA
e-mail: fk18@columbia.edu

G. Idos
Department of Medicine, Division of Gastrointestinal and Liver Disease, University of Southern California, Los Angeles, CA, USA

Norris Comprehensive Cancer Center, University of Southern California, Los Angeles, CA, USA

G. Parmigiani
Department of Biostatistics and Computational Biology, Dana-Farber Cancer Institute, Boston, MA, USA

Department of Biostatistics, Harvard Medical School, Boston, MA, USA

L. Valle et al. (eds.), *Hereditary Colorectal Cancer*,
https://doi.org/10.1007/978-3-319-74259-5_19

Keywords Lynch syndrome prediction models · MMRPredict · MMRPro · PREMM5 · PREMM · Ask2me · Discrimination · Calibration · Decision curve analysis · Clinical usefulness · Molecular tumor testing · Implementation of prediction models

1 Introduction

Lynch syndrome is the most common inherited colorectal cancer syndrome and is associated with germline mutations in the four mismatch repair (MMR) genes—*MLH1*, *MSH2*, *MSH6*, and *PMS2*—or in *EPCAM,* a promoter that initiates reading of the *MSH2* gene. The prevalence of Lynch syndrome is estimated at nearly 1/300 in the general population [1]. Individuals with Lynch syndrome not only have a 20–80% increased risk of developing colorectal cancer but also additional cancers, including those of the uterus, ovaries, stomach, small intestines, pancreas, urinary tract, brain, and cutaneous sebaceous glands [2–8]. In turn, early identification of individuals with pathogenic MMR gene variants is important as it allows for implementation of cancer prevention strategies such as intensified screening and surveillance, risk-reducing surgeries, or chemoprevention [9–14].

Numerous approaches for the identification of individuals and families with Lynch syndrome are available and have evolved considerably over time. Original strategies to select individuals for germline MMR testing were based on fulfillment of clinical criteria related to personal and family history of young-onset colorectal cancer and/or other malignancies associated with Lynch syndrome. These criteria included the Amsterdam criteria and the Bethesda guidelines [15–17]. Subsequently, molecular testing of tumors for evidence of microsatellite instability (MSI) and/or loss of the protein expression of the MMR genes on immunohistochemical (IHC) analyses was recommended as a more effective approach to evaluate individuals with colorectal cancer for Lynch syndrome, given its improved sensitivity and specificity compared to clinical criteria [2–4]. Current guidelines include a universal approach to molecular testing, where MSI and/or IHC testing is conducted in all colorectal cancers regardless of age at diagnosis or family history criteria, followed by germline genetic testing for those with abnormal tumor testing results [2–4]. Clinical prediction models are also available to quantify the risk of detecting a mutation associated with Lynch syndrome based on personal and family history and help clinicians decide who should be referred for further genetic risk assessment and/or genetic testing [18–21].

In this chapter, we review the main prediction models developed for the identification of individuals at risk for Lynch syndrome, focusing on their specific features and performance measures as assessed in several validation studies, compare the models with other clinical and molecular strategies for the diagnosis of Lynch syndrome, and discuss their implementation and potential uses in clinical practice. We also introduce a new prediction model that provides prospective cancer risk estimates for individuals with MMR gene mutations based on comprehensive literature reviews. Lastly, we discuss the future of clinical prediction models, including the potential impact of next-generation DNA sequencing technologies and the increased availability and uptake of panel testing, which offer simultaneous testing of multiple genes associated with inherited cancer susceptibility.

2 Identification of Individuals with Lynch Syndrome and the Rationale for Prediction Models

While multiple options are available for the identification of patients and families with Lynch syndrome, the optimal strategy has been debated and referral for genetic evaluation among individuals at increased risk for Lynch syndrome remains a challenge. Even in families with a known pathogenic MMR gene mutation, the rates of cascade testing in at-risk relatives who are unaffected by cancer are low [22]. Implementation of any strategy proven to be effective is critically important to maximize the diagnosis of Lynch syndrome carriers, including those who are young and unaffected by cancer as they stand to benefit the most from an early diagnosis of Lynch syndrome.

The initial approach for the identification of individuals at high risk for an inherited susceptibility to colorectal cancer were the Amsterdam criteria. They were originally developed by a consensus of experts for research purposes to distinguish families suspected of having hereditary nonpolyposis colorectal cancer and determine the prevalence of MMR gene mutations. The Bethesda guidelines were subsequently developed as a broader risk assessment tool to identify patients whose tumors should be tested for MSI; the guidelines were also revised to include extracolonic malignancies associated with Lynch syndrome, extend the ages of cancer diagnoses, and add histopathologic characteristics of the tumor. The application of these clinical criteria is quite complex in routine clinical practice, and the presence of personal and family cancer history is weighed similarly in both the Amsterdam and Bethesda guidelines. Furthermore, these clinical criteria lack sensitivity for identification of individuals with Lynch syndrome: the Amsterdam may miss up to 50% of mutation carriers, and the Bethesda guidelines may miss up to 30% of mutation carriers [23–25]. Development of quantitative prediction models was fueled by the need for more accurate risk assessment based on personal and familial cancer history, compared to that obtained through the Amsterdam and revised Bethesda guidelines. Studies have consistently shown suboptimal assessment of family cancer history and genetics referrals among different healthcare professionals [26, 27]. An additional goal has been to provide healthcare providers with tools that could be more widely implemented in the systematic evaluation of candidates for genetic referral and testing [18–21].

Given the shortcomings of the clinical criteria and in light of the known hallmark feature of MSI in tumors associated with Lynch syndrome, there is ample evidence to support universal tumor testing of all newly diagnosed colorectal cancers for MSI and/or protein expression of the relevant MMR genes by IHC. Results from the latter can also guide gene-specific germline testing [2–4]. From a clinical perspective, recognizing the heterodimeric partners *MSH2-MSH6* and *MLH1-PMS2* helps identify the causal mutations in Lynch syndrome by IHC. However, approximately 15% of sporadic colorectal cancer cases exhibit MSI due mainly to somatic hypermethylation of the *MLH1* promoter. Additional testing for *BRAF* mutations and *MLH1* promoter analyses on tumor tissue is needed to limit unnecessary genetic evaluations for Lynch syndrome [4, 28]. Despite the recommendation for universal tumor testing in newly diagnosed colorectal cancer cases, a US survey-based study noted limited and/or variable implementation by cancer centers; [29] barriers may be related to limited availability and/or uptake of genetic counseling services and associated costs or inconsistent reimbursement for molecular tumor testing, in addition to the lack of infrastructure to handle interpretation and disclosure of results.

Due to the aforementioned limitations related to clinical and clinicopathological approaches for the systematic evaluation of individuals at risk for Lynch syndrome, quantification of risk based on prediction models offers alternative or complementary means for Lynch syndrome assessment. The numerical estimates provided by the prediction models can be helpful in communicating to patients and at-risk relatives the risk of carrying a pathogenic MMR gene mutation and its implications for cancer risks. Furthermore, use of prediction models can be more widely implemented than the existing clinical or clinicopathological approaches as the pool of individuals at risk for Lynch syndrome consists mainly of those unaffected by cancer.

3 Development of Prediction Models

3.1 *Historical Perspective: The Leiden and Amsterdam-Plus Models*

The Leiden model was developed in 1998 and was the first Lynch syndrome risk prediction tool for the identification of *MLH1* and *MSH2* gene mutation carriers [30]. This multivariable logistic regression model was developed from 184 unrelated families at high risk of familial colorectal cancer, with 47 mutation carriers (28 *MLH1*, 19 *MSH2*). Risk estimates were based on the fulfillment of the Amsterdam criteria, presence of endometrial cancer in the family, and mean age at colorectal cancer diagnosis. In 2004, the Amsterdam-plus model was introduced. It was trained on 250 kindreds from familial cancer registries, 34 (14%) of whom had mutations in *MLH1* ($n = 25$), *MSH2* ($n = 8$), or *MSH6* ($n = 1$) [31]. In addition to the Amsterdam criteria, the model included the following five variables: number of relatives with colorectal and endometrial cancers, number of relatives with more than one colorectal cancer, mean ages at colorectal and endometrial cancer diagnosis in affected relatives, and number of relatives with five or more adenomas. Both models were developed using relatively small, selected populations derived from high-risk familial cancer registries and were not externally validated, which limited their generalizability to other settings and their wide adoption in clinical practice.

4 Currently Recommended Lynch Syndrome Prediction Models

In 2006, three prediction models were introduced to quantify an individual's probability of carrying a MMR gene mutation most commonly associated with Lynch syndrome. These models are MMRPredict, MMRPro, and PREMM$_{1,2}$ (Prediction of Mismatch Repair Gene Mutations in *MLH1* and *MLH2*) [20, 21, 32]. The latter model has undergone two subsequent expansions to include prediction of *MSH6* gene mutations (PREMM$_{1,2,6}$) [19], and most recently *PMS2* and *EPCAM* (updated to PREMM$_5$), thereby accounting for all five germline mutations associated with Lynch syndrome [18]. PREMM$_5$ will replace all preceding iterations of the PREMM model. While the overall purpose of developing these models were the same, there are important differences, including the genes considered, the populations where they were trained (particularly with regard to the total number of mutation carriers), and the statistical methodology used. Table 19.1 provides a comparison of the recent Lynch syndrome prediction models.

4.1 MMRPro

The MMRPro model was developed to evaluate an individual's probability of carrying an *MLH1*, *MSH2*, and/or *MSH6* gene mutation and used published values for MMR mutation prevalence and penetrance to calculate the predicted risk [21]. Unlike MMRPredict and PREMM, risk prediction estimates are based on a Bayesian approach and Mendelian inheritance laws. External validation was performed by the investigators involved in its development, in 279 patients recruited through familial colorectal cancer registries enriched with Lynch syndrome families where the mutation prevalence of any MMR gene was 43% (121/279) and included 51 *MLH1*, 63 *MSH2*, and 7 *MSH6* gene mutation carriers. The model includes data for the individual being evaluated and for each first-degree relative (FDR) and second-degree relative (SDR) as related to the presence of colorectal and/or endometrial cancer, age at diagnosis, and current age or age at last follow-up for those unaffected by these cancers. It was subsequently extended to handle pedigrees of arbitrary size. Data on relatives who are unaffected by cancer is also utilized to improve accuracy of risk prediction. The MMRPro model does not take into account the presence of multiple colorectal cancers in the proband. Among extracolonic cancers associated with Lynch syndrome, it only considers endometrial cancer. There are a number of unique features of the MMRPro model including its ability to (1) incorporate molecular tumor testing results including MSI and IHC testing, (2) calculate the residual probability of finding a mutation if molecular tumor testing is negative, and (3) provide estimates of future colorectal and endometrial cancer risks for unaffected individuals (including known mutation carriers), untested individuals, and individuals in whom no mutation is found. With emerging data on the prevalence and penetrance of MMR genes since the model's introduction, the investigators are currently updating the model to continue improving risk prediction. The MMRPro model is accessible at http://bayesmendel.dfci.harvard.edu.

Table 19.1 Prediction models for the identification of mismatch repair gene mutation carriers

Prediction model	Ascertainment	# Individuals tested	Outcome	Method	Molecular testing included	Predictors	Strengths	Limitations/special considerations
MMRPredict [20]	Derivation: population-based (limited to CRC patients <55y)	870	Overall estimate *MLH1*, *MSH2*, *MSH6*	Two-stage evaluation: Multivariate logistic regression analysis and MSI/IHC data to refine carrier's prediction	YES	Proband: age, gender, CRC tumor location, multiple CRC s Family: CRC age (dichotomized at 50 years), endometrial cancer in first-degree relative)	Population-based cohort; overall estimate for the MMR genes refinement of prediction with molecular tumor data; genetic evaluation/testing when predicted risk ≥5%	Developed and validated in a young-onset CRC population; extracolonic Lynch-associated tumors other than endometrial not included; poor discrimination and calibration in large-scale validation studies [33]
	Validation: population-based (limited to CRC patients <45 years)	155						
MMRPro [21]	Derivation: Population and clinic-based	N/A	Gene-specific estimate *MLH1*, *MSH2*, *MSH6*	Mendelian and Bayesian analysis. Accounts for family size and unaffected individuals	YES	Proband and family: CRC and endometrial cancer status, age at dx, relation to the proband, current age or at last follow-up, includes MSI/IHC data, post-hoc risk estimate based on germline testing result	Offers pre- and post-sequencing gene-specific estimates; accounts for unaffected relatives and family size; considers molecular tumor data; genetic evaluation/testing when predicted risk ≥5%; offers risk prediction of developing cancer in unaffected members; http://bayesmendel.dfci.harvard.edu	Time-consuming process with pedigree drawing; extracolonic Lynch-associated neoplasms other than endometrial cancer not included; good discrimination and fair calibration in large-scale validation studies [33]
	Validation: clinic-based	279						
PREMM$_{1,2,6}$ [19]	Derivation: clinic-based	4538	Gene-specific estimate *MLH1*, *MSH2*, *MSH6*	Logistic regression analysis	NO	Proband: gender, number of CRC, other Lynch-associated tumors, youngest ages at cancer diagnoses Family: age and number of first- and second-degree relatives with CRC and other Lynch-associated tumors	Provides gene-specific estimates and individualized risk prediction; genetic evaluation/testing when predicted risk ≥5%; provides clinical applicability at different cut offs; easy to use	Molecular tumor data not incorporated; developed in a cohort with heightened risk; family size and unaffected individuals are not considered; good discrimination and good calibration in large-scale validation studies [33]
	Validation: population and clinic-based	1827						
PREMM$_5$ [18]	Derivation: clinic-based	18,734	Overall estimate *MLH1*, *MSH2/EPCAM*, *MSH6*, *PMS2*	Logistic regression analysis	NO	Proband: age at time of genetic testing, gender, number of CRC, other Lynch-associated tumors, youngest ages at cancer diagnoses Family: age and number of first- and second-degree relatives with CRC and other Lynch-associated tumors	Provides *PMS2* and *EPCAM* prediction; genetic evaluation/testing when predicted risk ≥2.5%; largest development cohort; easy to use; http://premm.dfci.harvard.edu/	Developed in a cohort with 40% individuals unaffected by cancer; molecular tumor data not incorporated; family size not considered
	Validation: unselected CRC cases	1058						

CRC colorectal cancer, *IHC* immunohistochemistry, *MSI* microsatellite instability, *N/A*not available

4.2 *MMRPredict*

The MMRPredict model was developed from data on 870 unselected, population-based cases of colorectal cancer diagnosed under the age of 55 years and uses logistic regression methodology, similar to the PREMM models [20]. The mutation prevalence was 4% and included mutations in *MLH1* ($n = 15$), *MSH2* ($n = 16$), and *MSH6* ($n = 7$). The model provides an overall likelihood of carrying a mutation in *MLH1*, *MSH2,* or *MSH6*, but does not provide risk estimates for each gene. MMRPredict's estimates are derived from information obtained in two stages. The first stage involves clinical data for the proband such as gender, age at colorectal cancer diagnosis, location of colorectal cancer (proximal versus distal), multiple colorectal cancers (synchronous or metachronous), and family history limited to FDRs and the presence and age(s) of colorectal and/or endometrial cancer diagnoses. To refine the risk estimates based on personal and family cancer history, the second stage incorporates tumor molecular diagnostic information including MSI and IHC testing results. MMRPredict does not include extracolonic cancer history, does not take into account the number of relatives affected with colorectal or endometrial cancer, and limits family history to FDRs. The model was validated in an independent, retrospective series of patients with colorectal cancer prior to 45 years. Since MMRPredict was developed and validated in patients diagnosed before age 55 and 45 years, respectively, its generalizability to older individuals with colorectal cancer is less well characterized. Lastly, it does not generate risk estimates for probands without colorectal cancer and does not account for personal history of extracolonic Lynch syndrome-associated cancers (including endometrial cancer) in the proband.

4.3 *PREMM$_5$*

The PREMM$_5$ model was introduced in 2017 and is the only prediction model to provide risk estimation for all five Lynch syndrome-associated genes, including *PMS2* and *EPCAM* [18]. The original model was PREMM$_{1,2}$ which estimated *MLH1* and *MSH2* carrier probabilities [32]. This model was later expanded to PREMM$_{1,2,6}$ to include *MSH6* carrier probabilities [19]. PREMM$_5$ was developed using multivariable polytomous logistic regression. The training cohort includes genotype and phenotypic data from 18,734 individuals who underwent genetic testing through a commercial laboratory, based on either personal or family history of cancer. To date, this cohort includes the largest number of unrelated gene mutation carriers used for model development. Mutation prevalence was 5% (1000/18,734) with 306 *MLH1*, 354 *MSH2*, 177 *MSH6*, 141 *PMS2*, and 22 *EPCAM* carriers. Proband specific variables include gender, age at genetic testing, the occurrence and age at colorectal cancer diagnosis (including multiple colorectal cancer diagnoses), endometrial cancer, and other Lynch syndrome-associated cancers (specifically cancers of the ovary, stomach, kidney, ureter, bile duct, small bowel, brain (glioblastoma multiforme), pancreas, or sebaceous gland). Variables related to family members are limited to FDR and SDR cancer histories and include the number of relatives with colorectal cancer, endometrial cancer, or other Lynch syndrome-associated cancers as well as the minimum age at diagnosis of each cancer among relatives. The model does not include molecular tumor data in risk prediction or data on unaffected family members and family size. The $PREMM_5$ model was externally validated in an independent cohort of 1058 subjects with colorectal cancer from a single institution registry, who were recruited without preselection for high-risk features of Lynch syndrome (e.g., age at diagnosis, personal/family history of cancer, or tumor MSI/MMR deficiency) and performance metrics were similar between the development and validation cohorts. The investigators also compared performance of $PREMM_5$ to

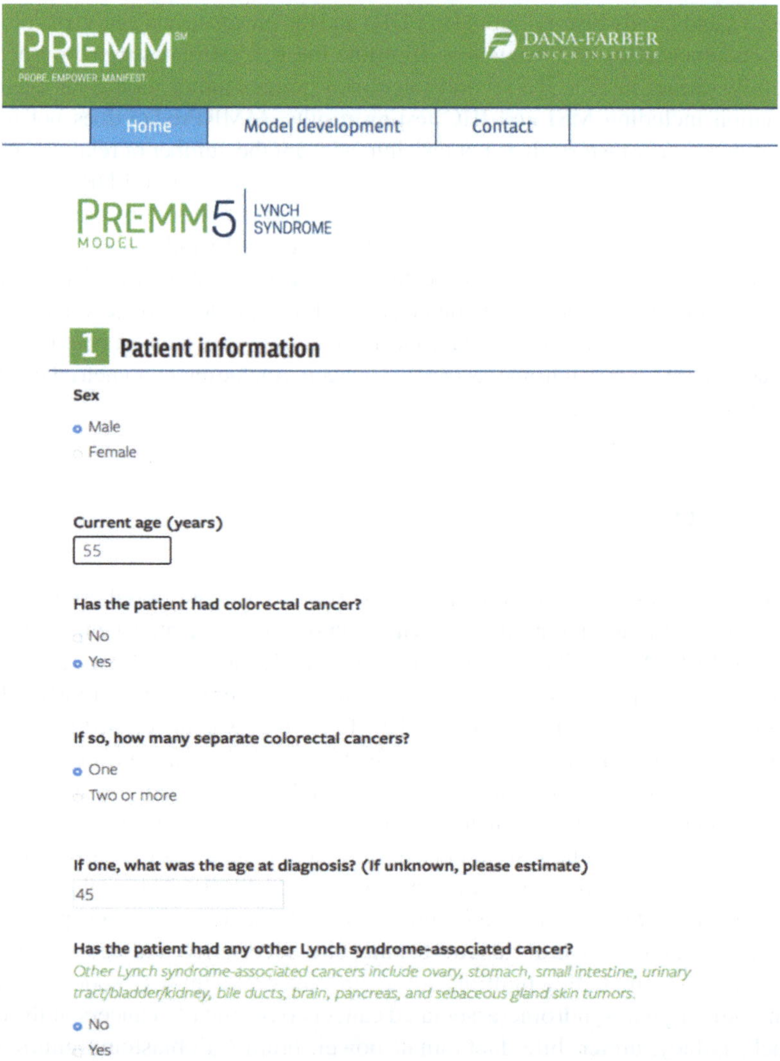

Fig. 19.1 (**a**) Risk assessment using PREMM5: http://premm.dfci.harvard.edu. (**b**) Calculation of overall mutation probability through PREMM5: http://premm.dfci.harvard.edu

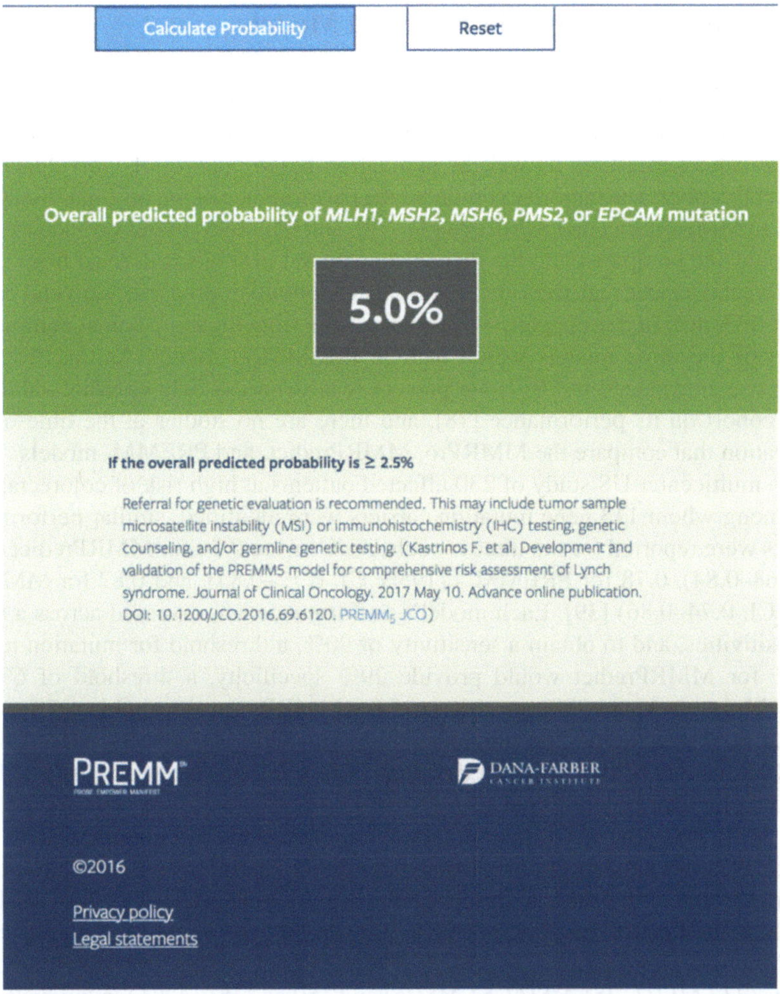

Fig. 19.1 (continued)

$PREMM_{1,2,6}$ using receiver operating characteristic curves, calibration, and reclassification analysis and reported over-prediction with $PREMM_{1,2,6}$. As a result they propose that $PREMM_5$ replace $PREMM_{1,2,6}$ in clinical practice [18]. In addition, analyses also support genetic evaluation and/or testing for individuals with a predicted risk score of 2.5% or greater.The $PREMM_5$ model is accessible via an easy to use web-based tool for healthcare providers (http://premm.dfci.harvard.edu/). Figure 19.1 provides a screenshot view of the online $PREMM_5$ risk calculator with a sample risk estimate and recommendation.

5 Validation of Clinical Prediction Models

A number of studies have compared the performance and accuracy of the Lynch syndrome models in diverse populations, including those derived from high-risk familial cancer registries as well as population-based cohorts of individuals with colorectal cancer. The majority compared the performance of the original $PREMM_{1,2}$ model to MMRPredict and MMRPro [34–39], and only two studies provide external validation and comparison to the $PREMM_{1,2,6}$ model in subjects derived from familial colorectal cancer registries and in unselected, population-based colorectal cancer cohorts [33, 40]. In this chapter, we present results from the more recent comparison studies of the three models which include $PREMM_{1,2,6}$ model. As the $PREMM_5$ model was introduced in 2017, we present results on the only external validation study cohort on its performance [18], and there are no studies at the time of this publication that compare the MMRPro, MMRPredict, and $PREMM_5$ models.

In a multicenter US study of 230 affected patients at high risk of colorectal cancer, among whom 113 gene mutation carriers were identified, similar performance metrics were reported for the three models; AUCs were 0.76 for MMRPredict (95% CI, 0.68–0.84), 0.78 for $PREMM_{1,2,6}$ (95% CI, 0.72–0.84), and 0.82 for MMRPro (95% CI, 0.74–0.86) [39]. Each model's performance was assessed across a range of sensitivities, and to obtain a sensitivity of 90%, a threshold for mutation testing of 4% for MMRPredict would provide 29% specificity, a threshold of 6% for $PREMM_{1,2,6}$ would be 38% specific, and for MMRPro, a threshold of 7% would provide 36% specificity. The previous validation studies comparing $PREMM_{1,2}$ to MMRPredict and MMRPro yielded similar results among selected patients at high-risk for colorectal cancer [35–37].

In the largest reported validation study comparing the three models, data from colorectal cancer patients enrolled through six clinic-based and five population-based registries from North America, Europe, and Australia were used to calculate predicted probabilities of pathogenic *MLH1*, *MSH2*, or *MSH6* gene mutations by each model [33]. Mutations were detected in 539 of 2304 (23%) individuals from the clinic-based cohorts (237 *MLH1*, 251 *MSH2*, 51 *MSH6*) and 150 of 3451 (4.4%) individuals from the population-based cohorts (47 *MLH1*, 71 *MSH2*, 32 *MSH6*). Discrimination was similar for both the clinic and population-based data with AUCs of 0.76 vs 0.77 for MMRPredict, 0.82 vs 0.85 for MMRPro, and 0.85 vs 0.88 for $PREMM_{1,2,6}$. Calibration, as measured by the observed versus expected ratio, followed a similar pattern as discrimination for the three models. Calibration for MMRPredict was 0.38 for clinic and 0.31 for population-based data, whereas MMRPro performed better (0.62 and 0.36, respectively) and more satisfactory results were observed for $PREMM_{1,2,6}$ (1.0 and 0.70 for clinic and population-based data, respectively). The investigators also report on a novel approach to assess performance of prediction models called clinical usefulness which is based on decision curve analyses. This approach offers important information beyond the standard performance metrics of discrimination and calibration and allows for the estimation of the net number of carriers identified by each model over different risk thresholds to select cases for further testing while penalizing for the number of patients receiving unnecessary testing. The numbers of identified carriers and those having unnecessary testing are also used in sensitivity and specificity calculations and are incorporated in the calculation of the net benefit. With thresholds of 5% or greater, MMRPro and $PREMM_{1,2,6}$ are clinically useful in clinic-based cohorts; $PREMM_{1,2,6}$ had an appreciable net benefit in the population-based cohorts as captured by its better calibration than MMRPro or MMRPredict. While all models overestimated the probability of being a carrier among population-based cases, they most often deviated in predictions under 5%, which has had limited clinical significance so far, because germline testing has not been recommended in patients with predicted probabilities under 5%. However, the authors concluded that consideration can be given to a lower threshold in the future, if costs of mutation analysis decrease further or if multigene panel testing based on next-generation DNA sequencing becomes incorporated into clinical practice as the standard of care.

Similar results were observed in an earlier study of an unselected, population-based colorectal cancer cohort [37] of 725 subjects diagnosed before age 75 years (18 MMR gene mutation carriers), where all the models overestimated MMR gene mutation carrier status by 2.1–4.3-fold. The investigators corrected the prediction estimates for bias introduced by family size and age structure on MMRPredict and $PREMM_{1,2}$ (MMRPro internally accounts for this already), and improvement in discriminating carriers from noncarriers was noted for both models.

In the only validation study to involve the $PREMM_5$ model, the discriminative ability in discerning mutation carriers from noncarriers in both the development (n = 18,734) and external validation (n = 1058) cohorts was similar with AUCs of 0.81 (95% CI:0.79–0.82) and 0.83 (95% CI:0.75–0.92), respectively [18]. The polytomous multivariable model showed good discrimination for *MLH1* (AUC 0.89, 95% CI:0.87–0.91), *MSH2/EPCAM* (AUC 0.84, 95% CI:0.82–0.86), and *MSH6* (AUC 0.76, 95% CI:0.73–0.79) but less for *PMS2* (AUC 0.64, 95% CI:0.60–0.68). As a result, the $PREMM_5$ model provides overall prediction of any germline mutation based on multivariable logistic regression analyses and does not provide gene-specific risk estimates. At the currently recommended 5% threshold to pursue genetic testing, 721/1000 carriers would be identified using $PREMM_5$. At a 2.5% threshold, 894/1000 carriers would be identified, but with lower specificity. The number needed to test to identify one carrier at 5% and 2.5% were 7 and 11 individuals, respectively, which represent a substantial decrease from the 19 needed to test if $PREMM_5$ was not used. Between 2.5% and 10%, the NPV was 97% to 99% of individuals correctly identified as mutation negative. By decision curve analysis, the clinical impact of $PREMM_5$ in identifying individuals who should undergo germline testing was observed at thresholds ≥2.5% and was superior to testing all subjects. $PREMM_5$ had minimal clinical impact at thresholds below 2.5%, since few individuals would be excluded from genetic testing, close to a test-all approach.

6 Performance of Prediction Models Compared to Clinical Criteria and Molecular Tumor Testing

The ability of the Lynch syndrome prediction models to identify gene mutation carriers has been compared to existing clinical criteria. There is ample evidence that each of the models has superior performance characteristics in terms of sensitivity, specificity, and positive and negative predictive values. This supports using the models rather than the existing clinical guidelines for the diagnosis and evaluation for Lynch syndrome [20, 21, 32, 34–37].

One study compared the performance of the $PREMM_{1,2,6}$ model to molecular tumor testing [41] in 1651 patients with colorectal cancer recruited through an international consortium of population and clinic-based family registries. The prevalence of mutation carriers was 14% (239/2651), and the AUCs for $PREMM_{1,2,6}$, IHC, and MSI were 0.90, 0.82, and 0.78, respectively. The strategy which most improved the $PREMM_{1,2,6}$ model's discriminative ability among both population and clinic-based cases was adding IHC tumor testing; the AUC improved to 0.94 in the overall and population-based cohorts and 0.92 in the clinic-based cohort. MSI testing added to the combination of $PREMM_{1,2,6}$ + IHC provided no additional discrimination. The proband's age at colorectal cancer diagnosis impacted the discriminative ability of each strategy with every 10-year increase in the initial age of colorectal cancer diagnosis. IHC's performance decreased to AUC of 0.85 for colorectal cancer diagnosed by 50 years, 0.84 for diagnosis by 60 years, and 0.82 for diagnosis by 70 years. In contrast, $PREMM_{1,2,6}$'s performance increased slightly with every 10-year increase in age of colorectal cancer diagnosis: AUC of 0.87 to 0.88 to 0.90 for diagnoses by 50, 60, and 70 years, respectively. Similar to IHC, MSI testing had AUC of 0.83 for colorectal cancer diagnosed by ages 50 and 60 years, which decreased to 0.81 for diagnosis by 70 years.

7 Prediction Models as a First-Line Option in the Identification of Lynch Syndrome

Based on the aforementioned evidence in support of the prediction models for the identification of individuals at risk for Lynch syndrome, the National Comprehensive Cancer Network and a number of professional societies, including the Multi-Society Task Force on Colorectal Cancer, include the three Lynch syndrome models as a first-line option in screening for Lynch syndrome [2, 3, 42]. The recommendation is that germline testing be considered when prediction scores using MMRPro, MMRPredict, and $PREMM_{1,2,6}$ are ≥5%. Risk assessment using the prediction models should also be the strategy of choice when tumor testing is not available or feasible.

8 Prediction Models and Cost-Effective Strategies for the Identification of Lynch Syndrome

A number of cost-effectiveness analyses compare different strategies for identifying MMR gene mutation carriers among patients with colorectal cancer. These comparisons include prediction model estimates [43–45]. A Markov modeling analysis examined clinical criteria (Amsterdam and Bethesda guidelines), the three prediction models (MMRPro, MMRPredict, and $PREMM_{1,2,6}$), tumor testing or up-front germline mutation testing followed by directed screening and risk-reducing surgery [43]. When clinical criteria were met or prediction models generated a 5% or greater likelihood of carrying a MMR gene mutation, IHC testing followed by germline testing was offered or germline testing was directly pursued. Tumor testing strategies were more costly than clinical criteria and prediction model strategies, assuming perfect implementation of all strategies. However, with decreased implementation rates of clinical criteria compared with tumor testing, the latter became more cost-effective. The most cost-effective strategy to evaluate for Lynch syndrome among newly diagnosed patients with colorectal cancer diagnosed before age 70 years was IHC testing (plus *BRAF* mutation testing for *MLH1* protein loss), followed by targeted MMR gene sequencing; an incremental cost-effectiveness ratio (ICER) of $36,200 per life year gained (LYG) resulted from this strategy. However, the critical determinant of cost-effectiveness of any strategy was highly dependent on the number of relatives per proband who underwent germline testing given the opportunities for cancer risk reduction in these individuals.

Another study compared the effectiveness and cost-effectiveness of 21 screening strategies for the identification of individuals with Lynch syndrome and supported the use of prediction models as a first-line strategy [44]. The most cost-effective approach in a three-step sequential strategy was one that began with use of the $PREMM_{1,2,6}$ model, followed by IHC testing and germline analysis, yielding an ICER of $35,000 per LYG as compared to another favorable, albeit higher ICER of $47,000 per LYG for IHC testing up-front when use of prediction models was excluded. The study assumed perfect implementation of the proposed strategies, including the universal application of prediction models. The investigators concluded that more widespread implementation of prediction models to systematically assess family cancer history in screening for Lynch syndrome could spare considerable societal resources that would be incurred with molecular tumor testing. The exception for when IHC tumor testing should be used as first-line approach was when the assumptions made in the analysis were not upheld in clinical situations, including when family history was unattainable, incomplete, or family size was small [44].

A cost-effective analysis examined screening approaches for Lynch syndrome among individuals *without* cancer in the general population [45]. In a simulation-based analysis using the $PREMM_{1,2,6}$ model to detect Lynch syndrome carriers and their at-risk relatives, integrated models of colorectal and endometrial cancers with a multi -generation family history were developed to predict health and economic outcomes of 20 primary screening strategies (with a wide range of compliance levels). These strategies included different screening ages for starting risk assessment and different risk thresholds above which to recommend genetic testing. For each strategy, 100,000 simulated individuals representative of the US population were followed from age 20 years, and the outcomes were compared with current practice. Risk assessment starting at ages 25, 30, or 35 years, followed by genetic testing of those with $PREMM_{1,2,6}$ risks estimates exceeding 5%, reduced colorectal and endometrial cancer incidence in Lynch syndrome carriers by approximately 12.4% and 8.8%, respectively. Of note, genetic testing was equally cost-effective at a threshold of 2.5% with slightly higher costs but with more lives saved. For a population of 100,000 individuals with 392 mutation carriers, this strategy increased quality-adjusted life years (QALY) by approximately 135 with an average cost-effectiveness ratio of $26,000 per QALY. The cost-effectiveness of screening for MMR gene mutations starting at 25, 30, or 35 years was comparable to currently well-accepted cancer screening activities for colorectal, cervical, and breast cancer and these results support risk assessment of unaffected individuals for Lynch syndrome based on their family cancer history using $\mathrm{PREMM}_{1,2,6}$.

9 Summary of Comparison of Models

The MMRPro, MMRPredict, and PREMM_5 models all provide a quantitative assessment of the risk of being a MMR gene mutation carrier. The decision to pursue use of one model over another may be related to the patient population that is being evaluated (such as whether the individual is affected by cancer or not), and the resources available to healthcare providers to perform systematic genetic risk assessment effectively and efficiently in relation to their particular clinical setting. Preference for one prediction model over another should also consider implementation and cost, in addition to predictive performance. Validation studies show that the PREMM and MMRPro models have similar ability to discriminate gene mutation carriers from noncarriers, while MMRPredict has suboptimal performance. The populations in which the models were validated brings to light that their specific characteristics may impact the accuracy of their risk estimates and help healthcare providers select which may be more appropriate to use in their respective clinical settings.

MMRPro's predictions account for family size and unaffected relatives, the possibility of including molecular tumor data in the risk analysis, and the option of predicting gene mutation carrier status following germline testing. The major limitation in the widespread use of MMRPro in routine practice is the need to input the entire pedigree which is time consuming. Its best use at the current time is likely to be as a genetic counseling tool in a specialized high-risk clinic or research setting. PREMM_5's major advantage is that it is easy to use, is the only model to include prediction for the *PMS2* and *EPCAM* genes, and includes risk prediction based on personal and family cancer history up to second-degree relatives for a broad spectrum of Lynch syndrome related extracolonic cancers. However, the model does not take into account family size, does not incorporate tumor testing results, or provide post hoc risk estimates based on gene sequencing results. Given the ease with which one can use the PREMM_5 model, it may be best utilized by healthcare providers whose aim is primarily to identify patients who should be referred for genetic evaluation and is likely to be most useful in the pretesting decision-making process. MMRPredict was developed in a patient population with young-onset colorectal cancer with diagnoses at 55 years and younger and can only be applied to individuals with colorectal cancer. Its generalizability is limited because of this, and with the increased prevalence of mutation carriers diagnosed over age 55 years, MMRPredict could provide less accurate results when used to evaluate older individuals affected by colorectal cancer and families with Lynch syndrome-associated cancers.

10 The Ask2me Knowledge Management and Decision Support Tool: Gene-Specific Prediction of Associated Cancer Risks in Identified Carriers

Advances in genetic sequencing technologies have led to the discovery of numerous new genes implicated in hereditary cancers beyond the limited few that are related to well-defined clinical syndromes such as Lynch syndrome. As a result, multigene panel testing has emerged and is increasingly being used by providers. Multigene panel testing can identify germline mutation carriers by simultaneously testing for multiple genes of moderate and high penetrance, with the ability to test from 25 to 300 cancer susceptibility genes at a time [46]. As a result, consideration for genetic testing in individuals with hereditary susceptibility to colorectal cancer can extend beyond Lynch syndrome and at a much lower cost than was required to test for the MMR genes just a few years ago.

As the evidence for additional genes associated with colorectal and other gastrointestinal cancers continues to rapidly emerge, so does the number of potentially relevant gene-cancer associations. Thus quantifiable estimates related to lifetime cancer risks associated with specific, pathogenic gene mutations are critical to personalize cancer prevention strategies for individuals who are found to carry deleterious mutations. Currently, genetic testing reports from commercial laboratories include general information about the associated cancer risks, such as a lifetime risk or a relative risk compared to the general population and recommendations and/or considerations for clinical management. However, it is often more helpful to personalize and refine cancer risk prediction further to better guide screening and other cancer prevention strategies. As an example in the case of Lynch syndrome, the individual identified with a pathogenic *PMS2* gene mutation at young age has about a 22% lifetime risk of developing colorectal cancer [47]. However, when evaluated at the age of 70 years old, this individual's chance for developing colorectal cancer is far smaller, close to 5%, as the majority of diagnoses in this mutation group have been observed to occur earlier than 70 years of age.

The All Syndromes Known to Man Evaluator, or Ask2me, is a knowledge management and decision support tool that provides personalized absolute risk for carriers of germline mutations in genes commonly tested in commercial panels [48]. It is currently web-based and available free at https:// ask2me.org. Ask2me attempts to address the multiple challenges related to cancer risk estimation and interpretation in inherited conditions with an increased susceptibility to the development of malignancy. One of the challenges in this field is that information on risk is dispersed over a number of studies, the quality of the studies is uneven, and published results seldomly include absolute risk estimates directly applicable to patient care [49].

Ask2me provides a single tool for healthcare providers and researchers to access data from high-quality studies, in a format directly usable for clinical decisions. As most studies do not report the penetrance risk estimates directly, (but rather odd ratios (OR), hazard ratios (HR), relative risks (RR), standardized incidence ratios (SIR), and cumulative risk (CR) estimates) Ask2me estimates the penetrance from these measures and other population sources such as the SEER (Surveillance, Epidemiology, and End Results) program [50], using statistical approaches developed specifically for this purpose. Ask2me presents results through a web-based interface for healthcare providers, which allows users to select gene, gender, age, prior surgery, and prior cancer. After entering this information, the provider is provided with patient-specific risk in figures and tables and a direct link to the study from which the risk estimates were obtained (Fig. 19.2). For each of 65 gene-cancer

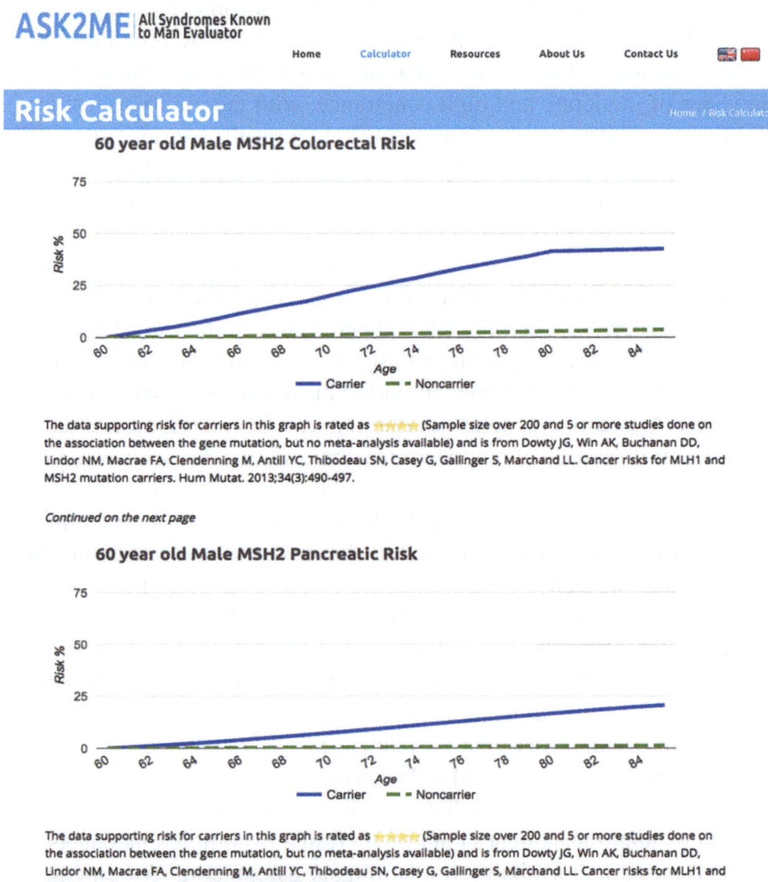

Fig. 19.2 (**a**) Illustration of Ask2me lifetime cancer risk calculation for a 60-year-old carrier of an *MSH2* pathogenic mutation. (**b**) Illustration of Ask2me summary of management recommendations for 60-year-old carrier of *MSH2* pathogenic mutation

Management

Management options and guidelines have been published by 4 groups. This table shows the management suggestions from these groups. We only reproduce here the guidelines as published. We are not making management recommendations. We suggest you use your clinical judgment and your knowledge of the patient in determining the best management strategy.

Intervention	NCCN	Esmo	Tung	Graffeo
Central Nervous System				
Physical/ Neurological Exam	Start at 25- 30, annually	Annually	NA	Start at 25- 30, annually
Colon and Rectum				
Colonoscopy	Start at 20- 25, repeat q 1- 2y (Or 2- 5y prior to earliest colorectal cancer)	Start at 20- 25, annually	NA	Start at 20- 25, annually (Or 2- 5y prior to earliest colorectal cancer)
Reproductive System				
Genetic Testing	At reproductive age. Consider genetic testing of a partner of a mutation carrier to inform reproductive decision making*	NA	NA	NA
Pre-implantation Genetic Diagnosis	At reproductive age. Advise about options, discuss the known risks, limitations and benefits.	NA	NA	NA
Skin				
Dermatological Exam	NA	NA	NA	Annually
Stomach				
EGD with extended duodenoscopy	Start at 30- 35, repeat q 3-5y. Treat H. pylori	NA	NA	Start at 30- 35, repeat q 2- 3y. Treat H. pylori
Urothelium				
Urinalysis	Start at 30- 35, annually	NA	NA	Start at 30- 35, annually

*Biallelic mutations may be associated with rare autosomal recessive conditions. Thus, consideration would be given to carrier testing the partner for mutations in the same gene if it would inform reproductive assessment and management.

Fig. 19.2 (continued)

associations currently assessed, risk estimates are presented by gene, cancer, and gender and age of the person being counseled. In clinical terms, these curves provide absolute risk estimates that are the foundation of decision support. It is anticipated that future cancer screening and surveillance recommendations will be tailored to account for gene-specific variability in penetrance, in addition to the individual's age. At present, the implementation of gene-specific guidelines for the initiation and surveillance of colorectal cancer and other extracolonic cancers by specific MMR gene alteration is not currently supported until additional data is available.

The architecture of Ask2me involves four aspects: (1) a structured database and data curation methodology, (2) quality assessment of individual studies, (3) risk estimation, and (4) presentation of risk in an intuitive visualization specific to the patient. The database is assembled using comprehensive review approaches and stores published results in a computable form. Each entry undergoes quality assessment to (1) select a single, sufficiently reliable, study to be used for the risk estimation for a specific gene-cancer association or (2) conclude that no study is of sufficient quality and detail to provide risk estimates. Ask2me uses a ranking system to assess the quality of published studies for specific gene-cancer associations. Unless the selected study is itself a meta-analysis, a major limitation of this approach is that it does not currently integrate information across relevant publications; if more than one study has a similar ranking, Ask2me currently reports the study with the larger sampler size.

Ask2me is in its early stages and continues to be expanded upon and refined. Current limitations of its implementation include that only a fraction of the relevant cancer-gene combinations is covered; a single source is used for each cancer-gene combination; a specific gene mutation may have different implications on risk, which have yet to be addressed.

11 Implementation of Clinical Risk Assessment Strategies and Prediction Models for the Identification of Lynch Syndrome

Given the diverse clinical settings in which an individual can be evaluated for Lynch syndrome, prediction models are a feasible and useful screening strategy that can ultimately impact the clinical management and cancer prevention recommendations for those identified as gene mutation carriers, regardless of whether they are affected with colorectal cancer or not. The National Comprehensive Cancer Network and the US Multi-Society Task Force on Colorectal Cancer support the widespread implementation of risk prediction models for the identification of individuals at high-risk for Lynch syndrome who would benefit from referral for genetic counseling and testing [2, 42]. Such an approach could address the difficulties that healthcare providers have in obtaining an accurate family cancer history due to time and resource constraints [26, 51, 52]. Studies have consistently shown that the frequency of systematic genetic risk assessment based on personal and family history of cancer and referral for the genetic evaluation of hereditary colorectal cancer syndromes in routine clinical practice is underutilized.

In addition to the aforementioned Lynch syndrome prediction models, another strategy recommended by the US National Colorectal Cancer Roundtable and the Multi-Society Task Force on Colorectal Cancer is the implementation of a simple three-question Colorectal Cancer Risk Assessment Tool for the identification of individuals at a potentially increased risk of an inherited predisposition who merit more detailed assessment of personal and family cancer history [53]. The risk assessment tool was validated in a prospective cohort of 5335 patients referred for outpatient colonoscopy at a large community gastroenterology private practice where 20% (n = 1069) were categorized as high risk for an inherited colorectal cancer syndrome, and the tool achieved an overall cumulative sensitivity of 77%.

Furthermore, the risk assessment tool accurately identified 95% of the individuals with germline MMR gene mutations associated with Lynch syndrome. A subsequent feasibility study integrated the three-question Colorectal Cancer Risk Assessment Tool into the electronic health records system of a private community-based gastroenterology practice to screen all patients referred for colonoscopy for an inherited predisposition to the development of colorectal cancer. Among 6031 patients who underwent colonoscopy, 14% (n = 848) were identified as high-risk based on the Colorectal Cancer Risk Assessment Tool, of which 9% (n = 77) were referred for genetics evaluation [54].

A recent study implemented the $PREMM_{1,2,6}$ model and the aforementioned Colorectal Cancer Risk Assessment Tool into the routine evaluation of individuals presenting for outpatient colonoscopy at an academic tertiary care center [55]. Subjects were screening for inherited colorectal cancer risk and Lynch syndrome in two stages: (1) use of the Colorectal Cancer Risk Assessment Tool (expanded to five question to improve specificity) and (2) those identified in stage 1 were evaluated with the $PREMM_{1,2,6}$ prediction model. Among 700 individuals evaluated with the expanded Colorectal Cancer Risk Assessment Tool and $PREMM_{1,2,6}$, 10% (n = 69) were identified as high-risk and eligible for genetic evaluation. Among these high-risk individuals, 33% (n = 23) pursued genetic evaluation and 10% (n = 7/69) were identified as carriers of a germline mutation associated with colorectal cancer.

Additional studies demonstrate the feasibility of integrating Lynch syndrome risk prediction models into community-based ambulatory care settings. In a study from a large gastroenterology practice and endoscopy facility, 3134 individuals completed a self-administered version of the $PREMM_{1,2,6}$ model prior to their office visit or colonoscopy procedure [56]. Individuals with a $PREMM_{1,2,6}$ score of 5% or greater, (n = 177, 5.6%) underwent genetic counseling, and of those who pursued genetic testing, 2.1% (n = 3/146) were found to carry a germline MMR gene conferring Lynch syndrome. Surveys of patient perspectives reported that 98% of those who underwent testing understood the information provided to them for hereditary cancer, and 85% felt that the assessment had an impact on their clinical care. From a provider perspective, 82% of the healthcare providers (ten gastroenterologists and one nurse practitioner) reported that use of the $PREMM_{1,2,6}$ model for hereditary cancer risk assessment improved the care of patients and clinically impacted their treatment and management decisions, and 100% felt satisfied with the integration of hereditary risk assessment and genetic testing into their practice.

Overall, these feasibility studies support the implementation of routine risk assessment for Lynch syndrome in diverse clinical settings, including both academic tertiary care and large community-based ambulatory care centers. These results suggest that implementation of evidence-based Lynch syndrome risk prediction models and assessment tools can achieve a balance between reliability and ease of use and integration, an important consideration in primary care settings. Additional studies are needed to evaluate the outcomes related to the performance of Lynch syndrome prediction models and their impact in the identification and clinical management of gene mutation carriers.

12 Future Considerations for the Identification and Personalized Clinical Management of Lynch Syndrome and the Role of Prediction Models

With decreasing costs related to germline genetic testing and the increased uptake of multigene panel testing, additional studies to optimize and integrate inherited cancer risk assessment tools and prediction models into routine clinical care are essential to enhance the identification of individuals with Lynch syndrome. Furthermore, information from multigene panel testing will allow for an improved understanding of the spectrum of Lynch syndrome-associated cancers and their respective lifetime risk, which ultimately influence recommendations for cancer screening and surveillance. Based on available evidence, the $PREMM_5$ and MMRPro models are effective strategies to identify individuals at high risk for Lynch syndrome, and their systematic implementation can be considered in routine clinical care and at various stages of cancer risk assessment and prevention.

The individuals that benefit the most from the early identification of Lynch syndrome are those who are unaffected by cancer as they can participate in screening and other prevention strategies to remain cancer-free. Currently, cascade testing is low among healthy, at-risk relatives in families with known MMR genes; the diagnosis of Lynch syndrome is often made in an individual with colorectal or endometrial cancer who had abnormal molecular tumor testing results that prompted germline testing, but relatives do not partake in genetic testing and Lynch syndrome remains undiagnosed. When a family history of cancer is present, the quantifiable estimates provided by prediction models simplify the risk assessment process, making it easier for patients to understand risk and can aide them in the decision-making process regarding genetic evaluation and/or surveillance strategies for colorectal and other Lynch syndrome-associated cancers. Additional studies to better elucidate the performance of the prediction models among persons without cancer are underway, and implementation of these models in preventive care settings is crucial. There is an ongoing need to expand genetic risk assessment and refine management decision tools through the use of prediction models given the rapid advances made in DNA sequencing technologies and the need to personalize cancer care among individuals with an inherited predisposition to the development of malignancy.

References

1. Win AK, Jenkins MA, Dowty JG, et al. Prevalence and penetrance of major genes and polygenes for colorectal cancer. Cancer Epidemiol Biomarkers Prev. 2017;26:404–412
2. Giardiello FM, Allen JI, Axilbund JE, et al. US Multi-Society Task Force on Colorectal Cancer. Guidelines on genetic evaluation and management of Lynch syndrome: a consensus statement by the US Multi-Society Task Force on colorectal cancer. Gastroenterology. 2014;147:502–26.
3. Syngal S, Brand RE, Church JM, et al. ACG clinical guideline: genetic testing and management of hereditary gastrointestinal cancer syndromes. Am J Gastroenterol. 2015;110:223–62.

4. Jasperson KW, Tuohy TT, Neklason DW, et al. Hereditary and familial colon cancer. Gastroenterology. 2010;138:2044–58.
5. Jenkins MA, Baglietto L, Dowty JG, et al. Cancer risks for mismatch repair gene mutation carriers: a population-based early onset case-family study. Clin Gastroenterol Hepatol. 2006;4:489–98.
6. Stoffel E, Mukherjee B, Raymond VM, et al. Calculation of risk of colorectal and endometrial cancer among patients with Lynch syndrome. Gastroenterology. 2009;137:1621–7.
7. Engel C, Loeffler M, Steinke V, et al. Risks of less common cancers in proven mutation carriers with Lynch syndrome. J Clin Oncol. 2012;30:4409–15.
8. Win AK, Young JP, Lindor NM, et al. Colorectal and other cancer risks for carriers and noncarriers from families with a DNA mismatch repair gene mutation: a prospective cohort study. J Clin Oncol. 2012;30:958–64.
9. Jarvinen HJ, Aarnio M, Mustonen H, et al. Controlled 15-year trial on screening for colorectal cancer in families with hereditary nonpolyposis colorectal cancer. Gastroenterology. 2000;118:829–34.
10. de Jong AE, Hendiks YM, Kleibeuker JH, et al. Decrease in mortality in Lynch syndrome families because of surveillance. Gastroenterology. 2006;130:665–71.
11. Vasen HF, Abdirahman M, Brohet R, et al. One to 2- year surveillance intervals reduce risk of colorectal cancer in families with Lynch syndrome. Gastroenterology. 2010;138:2300–6.
12. Lindor NM, Petersen GM, Hadley DW, et al. Recommendations for the care of individuals with an inherited predisposition to Lynch syndrome: a systematic review. JAMA. 2006;296:1507–17.
13. Vasen HF, Blanco I, Aktan-Collan K, et al. Revised guidelines for the clinical management of Lynch syndrome (HNPCC): recommendations by a group of European experts. Gut. 2013;62:812–23.
14. Ouakrim AD, Dashti SG, Buchanan DD, et al. Aspirin, ibuprofen, and the risk of colorectal cancer in Lynch syndrome. J Natl Cancer Inst. 2015;107. https://doi.org/10.1093/jnci/djv170.
15. Park JG, Vasen HF, Park KJ, et al. Suspected hereditary non-polyposis colorectal cancer: International Collaborative Group on Hereditary Non-Polyposis Colorectal Cancer (ICG-HNPCC) criteria and results of genetic diagnosis. Dis Colon Rectum. 1999;42:710–5.
16. Umar A, Boland CR, Terdiman JP, et al. Revised Bethesda guidelines for hereditary nonpolyposis colorectal cancer (Lynch syndrome) and microsatellite instability. J Natl Cancer Inst. 2004;96:261–8.
17. Rodriguez-Bigas MA, Boland CR, Hamilton SR, et al. A National Cancer Institute workshop on hereditary nonpolyposis colorectal cancer syndrome: meeting highlights and Bethesda guidelines. J Natl Cancer Inst. 1997;89:1758–62.
18. Kastrinos F, Uno H, Ukaegbu C, et al. Development and validation of the $PREMM_5$ model for comprehensive risk assessment of Lynch syndrome. J Clin Oncol. 2017;35:2165–72.
19. Kastrinos F, Steyerberg E, Mercado R, et al. The $PREMM_{1,2,6}$ model predicts risk of germline *MLH1* , *MSH2* , and *MSH6* germline mutations based on cancer history. Gastroenterology. 2011;140:73–81.
20. Barnetson RA, Tenesa A, Farrington SM, et al. Identification and survival of carriers of mutations in DNA mismatch repair genes in colon cancers. N Engl J Med. 2006;354:2751–63.
21. Chen S, Wang W, Lee S, et al. Prediction of germline mutations and cancer risk in the Lynch syndrome. JAMA. 2006;296:1479–87.
22. Hampel H. Genetic counseling and cascade genetic testing in Lynch syndrome. Familial Cancer. 2016;15:423–7.
23. Hampel H, Frankel WL, Martin E, et al. Screening for the Lynch syndrome (hereditary nonpolyposis colorectal cancer). N Engl J Med. 2005;352:1851–60.
24. Julié C, Trésallet C, Brouquet A, et al. Identification in daily practice of patients with Lynch syndrome (hereditary nonpolyposis colorectal cancer): revised Bethesda guidelines-based approach versus molecular screening. Am J Gastroenterol. 2008;103:2825–35.
25. Pérez-Carbonell L, Ruiz-Ponte C, Guarinos C, et al. Comparison between universal molecular screening for Lynch syndrome and revised Bethesda guidelines in a large population-based cohort of patients with colorectal cancer. Gut. 2012;61:865–72.

26. Grover S, Stoffel EM, Bussone L, et al. Physician assessment of family cancer history and referral for genetic evaluation in colorectal cancer patients. Clin Gastroenterol Hepatol. 2004;2:813–9.
27. Flynn BS, Wood ME, Ashikaga T, et al. Primary care physicians' use of family history for cancer risk assessment. BMC Fam Pract. 2010;11:45.
28. Parsons MT, Buchanan DD, Thompson B, et al. Correlation of tumour BRAF mutations and MLH1 methylation with germline mismatch repair (MMR) gene mutation status: a literature review assessing utility of tumour features for MMR variant classification. J Med Genet. 2012;49:151–7.
29. Beamer LC, Grant ML, Espenschied CR, et al. Reflex immunohistochemistry and microsatellite instability testing of colorectal tumors for Lynch syndrome among US cancer programs and follow-up of abnormal results. J Clin Oncol. 2012;30:1058–63.
30. Wijnen JT, Vasen HF, Khan PM, et al. Clinical findings with implications for genetic testing in families with clustering of colorectal cancer. N Engl J Med. 1998;339:511–8.
31. Lipton LR, Johnson V, Cummings C, et al. Refining the Amsterdam Criteria and Bethesda Guidelines: testing algorithms for the prediction of mismatch repair mutation status in the familial cancer clinic. J Clin Oncol. 2004;22:4934–43.
32. Balmaña J, Stockwell DH, Steyerberg EW, et al. Prediction of *MLH1* and *MSH2* mutations in Lynch syndrome. JAMA. 2006;296:1469–78.
33. Kastrinos F, Ojha RP, Leenen C, et al. Comparison of prediction models for Lynch syndrome among individuals with colorectal cancer. J Natl Cancer Inst. 2015;108(2). pii: djv308.
34. Balaguer F, Balmaña J, Castellví-Bel S, et al. Validation and extension of the PREMM1,2 model in a population-based cohort of colorectal cancer patients. Gastroenterology. 2008;134:39–46.
35. Balmaña J, Balaguer F, Castellví-Bel S, et al. Comparison of predictive models, clinical criteria and molecular tumor screening for the identification of patients with Lynch syndrome in a population-based cohort of colorectal cancer patients. J Med Genet. 2008;45:557–63.
36. Monzon JG, Cremin C, Armstrong L, et al. Validation of predictive models for germline mutations in DNA mismatch repair genes in colorectal cancer. Int J Cancer. 2010;126:930–9.
37. Green RC, Parfrey PS, Woods MO, et al. Prediction of Lynch syndrome in consecutive patients with colorectal cancer. J Natl Cancer Inst. 2009;101:331–40.
38. Tresallet C, Brouquet A, Julié C, et al. Evaluation of predictive models in daily practice for the identification of patients with Lynch syndrome. Int J Cancer. 2012;130:1367–77.
39. Pouchet CJ, Wong N, Chong G, et al. A comparison of models used to predict MLH1, MSH2 and MSH6 mutation carriers. Ann Oncol. 2009;20:681–8.
40. Khan O, Blanco A, Conrad P, et al. Performance of Lynch syndrome predictive models in a multi-center US referral population. Am J Gastroenterol. 2011;106:1822–7.
41. Kastrinos F, Steyerberg EW, Balmaña J, et al. Comparison of the clinical prediction model PREMM1,2,6 and molecular testing for the systematic identification of Lynch syndrome in colorectal cancer. Gut. 2013;62:272–9.
42. National Comprehensive Cancer Network Guidelines Version 1.2017 Genetic/Familial High Risk Assessment: Colorectal. MS-15; Retrieved from https://www.nccn.org/professionals/physician_gls/pdf/genetics_colon.pdf. Accessed 3 Aug 2017.
43. Ladabaum U, Wang G, Terdiman J, et al. Strategies to identify the Lynch syndrome among patients with colorectal cancer: a cost-effectiveness analysis. Ann Intern Med. 2011;155:69–79.
44. Barzi A, Sadeghi S, Kattan MW, et al. Comparative effectiveness of screening strategies for Lynch syndrome. J Natl Cancer Inst. 2015;107(4):dvj005.
45. Dinh TA, Rosner BI, Atwood JC, et al. Health benefits and cost-effectiveness of primary genetic screening for Lynch syndrome in the general population. Cancer Prev Res. 2011;4:9–22.
46. Plichta JK, Griffin M, Thakuria J, et al. What's new in genetic testing for cancer susceptibility? Oncology (Williston Park). 2016;30:787–99.
47. ten Broeke SW, Nielsen M. A *PMS2*-specific colorectal surveillance guide. Genet Med. 2015;17:684.
48. Braun D, Yang J, Griffin M, et al. A clinical decision support tool to predict cancer risk for commonly tested cancer-related germline mutations. Manuscript under review.

49. Strande NT, Riggs ER, Buchanan AH, et al. Evaluating the clinical validity of gene-disease associations: an evidence-based framework developed by the clinical genome resource. Am J Hum Genet. 2017;100:895–906.
50. Cronin KA, Ries LA, Edwards BK. The Surveillance, Epidemiology, and End Results (SEER) Program of the National Cancer Institute. Cancer. 2014;120(Suppl 23):3755–7.
51. Drohan B, Ozanne EM, Hughes KS. Electronic health records and the management of women at high risk of hereditary breast and ovarian cancer. Breast J. 2009;15(Suppl 1):S46–55.
52. Doerr M, Teng K. Family history: still relevant in the genomics era. Cleve Clin J Med. 2012;79:331–6.
53. Kastrinos F, Allen JI, Stockwell DH, et al. Development and validation of a colon cancer risk assessment tool for patients undergoing colonoscopy. Am J Gastroenterol. 2009;104:1508–18.
54. Gunaratnam NT, Akce M, Al Natour R, et al. Screening for cancer genetic syndromes with a simple risk-assessment tool in a community-based open-access colonoscopy practice. Am J Gastroenterol. 2016;111:589.
55. Guivatchian T, Koeppe ES, Baker JR, et al. Family history in colonoscopy patients: feasibility and performance of electronic and paper-based surveys for colorectal cancer risk assessment in the outpatient setting. Gastrointest Endosc. 2017;86:684-691.
56. Luba DG, DiSario JA, Rock C, et al. Community practice implementation of a self-administered version of $PREMM_{1,2,6}$ to assess risk for Lynch syndrome. Clin Gastroenterol Hepatol. 2018;16:49–58.

Chapter 20
Surveillance Guidelines for Hereditary Colorectal Cancer Syndromes

Neda Stjepanovic, Leticia Moreira, Judith Balmaña, and Joan Brunet

Abstract The identification of hereditary colorectal cancer syndromes allows the prevention of colorectal and related extracolonic cancers and the possibility of genetic counseling to family members. The management of these syndromes requires a multidisciplinary approach, including counseling and genetic testing, screening recommendations, prevention options, and treatment strategies. Gene-specific risk estimations are leading to adapt surveillance recommendations for some Lynch and polyposis patients. New techniques such as chromoendoscopy are being incorporated to screening procedures in order to increase adenoma detection. This chapter reviews the surveillance guidelines of the most common hereditary colorectal syndromes, the types of recommendation, and the quality of evidence for each one.

Keywords Surveillance · Prevention · Screening · Guidelines

1 Introduction

Colorectal cancer (CRC) is the most common gastrointestinal neoplasia. Inherited factors account for approximately 5% of all CRC cases. The identification of hereditary syndromes allows the prevention of colorectal and related extracolonic cancers and the

N. Stjepanovic · J. Balmaña (✉)
Department of Medical Oncology, Hospital Universitari Vall d'Hebron, VHIO, Barcelona, Spain
e-mail: jbalmana@vhio.net

L. Moreira
Department of Gastroenterology, Hospital Clínic, Centro de Investigación Biomédica en Red en Enfermedades Hepáticas y Digestivas (CIBERehd), Institut de Investigació August Pi i Sunyer (IDIBAPS), Barcelona, Spain

J. Brunet (✉)
Hereditary Cancer Program, Catalan Institute of Oncology, Centro de Investigación Biomédica en Red de Cáncer (CIBEROnc), Institut d'Investigació Biomèdica de Girona (IdIBGi), Girona, Spain
e-mail: jbrunet@iconcologia.net

L. Valle et al. (eds.), *Hereditary Colorectal Cancer*,
https://doi.org/10.1007/978-3-319-74259-5_20

possibility of genetic counseling to family members. The management of these syndromes requires a multidisciplinary approach, including counseling and genetic testing, screening recommendations, prevention options, and treatment strategies.

The aim of this chapter is to review the surveillance guidelines of the most common CRC hereditary syndromes. The types of recommendation and quality of evidence in each syndrome are summarized in Table 20.1.

1.1 Lynch Syndrome

Lynch syndrome (LS) is caused by a mutation in one of the mismatch repair genes: *MLH1*, *MSH2*, *MSH6*, or *PMS2* and is characterized by an increased risk of CRC, endometrial, ovarian, stomach, small bowel, pancreatic, urinary tract, biliary tract, and central nervous system (usually glioblastoma) cancer.

For individuals with LS, prevention and early detection of associated cancers by active surveillance can improve quality of life and increased survival [1]. Historically, surveillance recommendations have been universal for all individuals with LS, regardless of the mutated gene. In light of recently available information regarding genotype-phenotype correlation for LS patients, surveillance could be adapted according to the gene mutated, mutation origin, and family history of cancer.

1.1.1 Colorectal Surveillance

Periodic surveillance with colonoscopy in individuals with LS has proven to be effective, allowing identification and resection of polyps and early stage CRC [2].

Surveillance with colonoscopies performed every 3 years has shown a reduction of CRC incidence by 62% and a reduction of CRC mortality by 66% [2–4]. More frequent screening has been associated with earlier stage of CRC at diagnosis [5–8] and up to 72% decrease in CRC mortality [9].

Due to an accelerated adenoma-carcinoma sequence in LS [10], CRC in this group of patients has been observed within a 3-year interval after the last normal colonoscopy and with a less favorable stage if the time from last surveillance was superior to 2 years [11–13]. With systematic colonoscopies performed every 2 years, the incidence of CRC was only 2%, as reported in a recent prospective observational study [14]. Therefore, colonoscopies every 1–2 years have become a widely accepted prevention strategy for individuals with LS (Table 20.2).

An increased risk of CRC in individuals with LS is observed from age 30, irrespective of the gene mutated [15]. Therefore, the onset of colorectal surveillance is generally accepted at the age of 20–25 years or 10 years prior to the youngest CRC diagnosis in the family (Table 20.2). For *MLH1* and *MSH2* carriers, an estimated cumulative risk of CRC is 40% and 48% by age 70 years, respectively, with approximately 1% of carriers being diagnosed with CRC in their 20s [16]. In contrast, in carriers of deleterious mutations in *MSH6* and *PMS2* genes, the cumulative risk of

Table 20.1 Colorectal cancer hereditary syndrome surveillance: strength of recommendation and quality of supporting evidence

Syndrome	Cancer risk	Surveillance indication	Strength of recommendation/quality of supporting evidence
Lynch syndrome [25, 26, 35, 42, 52, 86, 87]	Colorectum	Absolute	Strong recommendation/ moderate quality of evidence
	Endometrium/ovary	Consider	Conditional recommendation/low quality of evidence
	Stomach	Conditional (family history, high-incidence countries)	Weak and conditional recommendation/very low quality of evidence
	Other associated neoplasia (small bowel, pancreas, urinary and biliary tract, skin, brain)	Not recommended (consider if family history)	Conditional recommendation/low quality of evidence
Familial adenomatous polyposis [26, 50, 52]	Colorectum	Absolute	Strong recommendation/ moderate quality of evidence
	Stomach/duodenum	Absolute	Strong recommendation/ low quality of evidence
	Thyroid	Consider	Moderate recommendation/low quality of evidence
	Liver (hepatoblastoma)	Conditional (family history)	Conditional recommendation/ very low quality of evidence
	Desmoid tumors	Conditional (family history, site of *APC* mutation)	Conditional recommendation/ low quality of evidence
MUTYH-associated polyposis [26, 50, 52]	Colorectum	Absolute	Strong recommendation/ low quality of evidence
	Stomach/Duodenum	Consider	Moderate recommendation/low quality of evidence
Juvenile polyposis [26, 73, 75]	Colorectum	Consider	Strong recommendation/ very low quality of evidence
	Stomach	Consider	Strong recommendation/ very low quality of evidence
	Small bowel	Consider	Weak recommendation/ very low quality of evidence

(continued)

Table 20.1 (continued)

Syndrome	Cancer risk	Surveillance indication	Strength of recommendation/quality of supporting evidence
Peutz-Jeghers syndrome [26, 35, 76, 78]	Colorectum	Absolute	Strong recommendation/ low quality of evidence
	Stomach	Absolute	Strong recommendation/ low quality of evidence
	Small bowel	Consider	Moderate recommendation/low quality of evidence
	Pancreas	Consider	Moderate recommendation/very low quality of evidence
	Breast	Absolute	Strong recommendation/ low quality of evidence
	Endometrium/cervix/ ovarium	Consider	Weak recommendation/ very low quality of evidence
	Testes	Consider	Weak recommendation/ very low quality of evidence
Serrated polyposis syndrome [26, 89]	Colorectum	Consider	Conditional recommendation/ low quality of evidence
Biallelic mismatch repair deficiency syndrome [85, 86]	Brain	Consider	Weak recommendation/ low quality of evidence
	Upper gastrointestinal tract	Consider	Weak recommendation/ very low quality of evidence
	Lower gastrointestinal tract	Consider	Weak recommendation/ low quality of evidence
	Non-Hodgkin lymphoma/ other lymphoma	Consider	Weak recommendation/ very low quality of evidence
	Leukemia	Consider	Weak recommendation/ very low quality of evidence
	Endometrium	Consider	Weak recommendation/ very low quality of evidence
	Urinary tract	Consider	Weak recommendation/ very low quality of evidence

Table 20.2 Surveillance guidelines in Lynch syndrome

Tumor site	Examination	*MALLORCA* group 2013 [25]		*ESMO* 2013 [52]		*SEOM* 2015 [88]		*ACG* 2015 [26]		*NCCN* 2016 [90]	
		Age (y)	Interval (y)	Age (y)	Interval (y)	Age (y)	Interval (y)	Age (y)	Interval (y)	Age (y)	Interval (y)
Colorectum	**Colonoscopy**	20–25	1–2	20–25	1–2	25[a]	1–2	20–25	1–2	20–25[b]	1–2
						40	1				
						30–35[c]	2–3				
						35–40[d]	2–3				
Uterus	**TV-ultrasound**	35–40	1–2	30–35	1	30–35	1	30–35	1	Physician discretion	
	Aspiration biopsy									Optional	1
Ovaries	**CA125**			30–35	1	30–35	1				
Stomach	**UGI endoscopy**	30–35[e]	1–2	N/A[e]	1–3	30–35[f]	3–5	30–35[g]	3–5[g]	30–35[h]	3–5
	HP eradication	>25		N/A				N/A		N/A	
Urinary tract	**Urine cytology**	30–35[i]	N/A			25–30[j]	1–2			30–35	1
	Urine ultrasound					25–30[j]	1–2				
CNS	**Neurological examination**									25–30	1

ACG American College of Gastroenterology, *CNS* central nervous system, *ESMO* European Society for Medical Oncology, *HP Helicobacter pylori*, *NCCN* National Comprehensive Cancer Network, *SEOM* Spanish Society of Medical Oncology, *TV-ultrasound* transvaginal ultrasound, *UGI* upper gastrointestinal, *y* years

[a]Or 5 years prior to the earliest CRC, if diagnosis <25 years

[b]Or 2–5 years prior to the earliest CRC, if diagnosis <25 years

[c]For *MSH6* carriers, start surveillance at age 30–35 years or 10 years prior to the earliest CRC diagnosis

[d]For *PMS2* carriers, start surveillance at age 35–40 years in the absence of early-onset CRC

[e]In high-incidence countries

[f]If family history of gastric cancer

[g]Baseline endoscopy with biopsies at 30–35 years and if family history repeat every 3–5 years

[h]In Asian population

[i]For *MSH2* carriers (research)

[j]If family history of urinary tract cancer

CRC has been estimated at 10–22%, and CRC is very rarely diagnosed before age 40 [1, 15, 17, 18]. Therefore gene-specific surveillance may be considered for *MSH6* and *PMS2* carriers and endoscopic surveillance postponed until age 30 years (Table 20.2), unless there is family history of early-onset cancer. This gene-specific surveillance approach is controversial and has not been evaluated in clinical studies.

Standard colonoscopy has limitations for detection of flat adenomas, which are usually located in the proximal colon and have a high risk of malignant transformation [19]. Various endoscopic techniques that enhance the visualization of small and flat adenomas by using a dye spray are being developed in order to improve the yield of CRC surveillance. Chromoendoscopy with indigo carmine or methylene blue added to the standard colonoscopy has shown to be significantly more effective than colonoscopy alone in LS individuals with adenoma detection rate of 41% vs. 23% [20]. Nevertheless, there are no randomized controlled trials comparing standard colonoscopy with chromoendoscopy.

1.1.2 Gastric Surveillance

The estimated risk of gastric cancer in individuals with LS is as high as 13% [21], with significant variability depending on mutation type, ethnicity, and place of residence. Particularly high risk of gastric cancer has been reported in individuals with mutations in *MLH1 (5–18%)* or *MSH2 (2–9%)* genes [1, 21, 22]. Korea and Japan are considered high-risk population with up to 30% of lifetime risk of gastric cancer in LS patients [23]. There is no clear evidence to support endoscopic surveillance in all LS patients [24], while identification and eradication of *Helicobacter pylori* are widely considered. Some groups recommend gastroscopies every 1–3 years in regions with an increased prevalence of gastric cancer or in those families with history of gastric neoplasms, starting at the age of 30–35 [25]. Recent ACG guidelines even consider a baseline endoscopy with biopsy at age 30–35 [26], as described in Table 20.2.

1.1.3 Small Bowel Surveillance

The risk of small bowel cancer ranges from 3% to 5%, being more frequent in the duodenum (43%) and jejunum (33%) than in the ileum (7%) [27–29]. In one observational study of 35 LS patients, findings in the small bowel were present in 9% of cases, including only one jejunal carcinoma and two jejunal adenomas, while additional 14% of patients had images of uncertain clinical relevance, which prompted further invasive investigations [30]. Therefore, routine surveillance of the small bowel in LS is not considered to be cost-efficient [31].

1.1.4 Pancreatic Surveillance

Cumulative risk of pancreatic cancer in individuals with LS is up to 4% by age 70 years [32–34]. An international pancreas consensus panel based on expert opinion recommended considering annual magnetic resonance and/or endoscopic ultrasound surveillance in individuals with LS and one first-degree relative affected with pancreatic cancer [35]. These recommendations have not been included in the LS guidelines and more supporting evidence is needed before introducing routine pancreatic cancer surveillance (Table 20.2).

1.1.5 Gynecological Surveillance

The cumulative risk of endometrial cancer in women with Lynch syndrome is 39–50% [36]. As with CRC, the risk varies depending on the gene mutated with up to 54% in *MLH1/MSH2* carriers, 71% in *MSH6* carriers, and 15% in *PMS2* carriers [26].

Surveillance with transvaginal ultrasound and endometrial sampling has been evaluated in observational studies [37–43]. Transvaginal ultrasound has shown poor sensitivity and specificity for the diagnosis of endometrial cancer in this population [37, 40], while endometrial sampling could identify patients with premalignant endometrial lesions or asymptomatic endometrial carcinomas [38–40]. Still, survival benefit from endometrial cancer surveillance has not been observed.

Several guidelines contemplate annual gynecological examination with transvaginal ultrasound and aspiration biopsy, starting at 30–35 years (Table 20.2). The most recent update of the NCCN guideline leaves the indication of screening to physician's discretion, although no specific recommendations are made based on the genetic condition.

Estimates of the cumulative lifetime risk of ovarian cancer in LS patients ranges from 3% to 22% [26]. Transvaginal ultrasound and serum CA125 testing have not shown to be sensitive or specific for detection of ovarian cancer in LS patients [41, 44, 45]. Currently, no studies on the effectiveness of ovarian screening are available for women with LS.

Given the high incidence of endometrial cancer, the moderate incidence of ovarian cancer and the low specificity of surveillance methods, prophylactic surgery (i.e., hysterectomy and bilateral oophorectomy) is accepted in postmenopausal LS patients and premenopausal women who have completed their reproductive desire (Table 20.2).

1.1.6 Urinary Tract Surveillance

Estimates of the lifetime risk of urinary tract cancer in LS range from 1% to 7%, with greater risk among MSH2 carriers (7%), compared to MLH1 (3%) and MSH6 (2%) [46]. Urinary surveillance with cytology in LS families found a poor sensitivity (29%) in diagnosing cancer in asymptomatic individuals, while numerous false positive results required further invasive diagnostic techniques [47]. Despite this, the 2017 edition of the NCCN guidelines includes consideration of cytology beginning at 30–35 years, taking into account the simplicity and the low cost of the test [48]. The benefit of the ultrasound screening is unknown and has only been endorsed by the SEOM guidelines starting at age 25–30 in the presence of a family history of urinary tract cancers (Table 20.2).

2 Adenomatous Polyposis Syndromes

The presence of numerous colorectal adenomas can be associated with different gastrointestinal polyposis syndromes, among which familial adenomatous polyposis (FAP) and *MUTYH*-associated polyposis (MAP) are the most common ones. In patients with adenomatous polyposis syndromes, colorectal surveillance allows for prevention of CRC and improves their prognosis [49] (Table 20.1).

2.1 Familial Adenomatous Polyposis

Germline mutations in the *APC* gene are inherited in an autosomal dominant fashion and are associated with FAP. This disorder is characterized by the presence of numerous colorectal adenomas, the classical form characterized by more than 100 adenomas along the entire colon, with a nearly 100% risk of CRC before age 40 years, and the attenuated form having between 10 and 100 adenomas, preferentially localized in the right colon and with a later onset.

It is associated with a broad spectrum of extracolonic tumors, including hepatoblastoma, duodenal, pancreatic, thyroid, and brain cancer. The most common extracolonic manifestations in FAP patients are upper gastrointestinal polyps (stomach, duodenum, and periampullary region). There are also benign extracolonic manifestations, including the congenital hypertrophy of the retinal pigment epithelium (CHRPE) (70–80%), epidermoid cysts (50%), fibromas (25–50%), dental abnormalities (79–90%), osteomas (50–90%), and desmoid tumors (10–15%) [50, 51].

Surveillance should be recommended to all mutation carriers as well as members of any given family in which the causative germline mutation could not be identified.

2.1.1 Colorectal Surveillance

The goal of colorectal surveillance is to prevent CRC [52]. There are several studies demonstrating that surveillance reduces significantly CRC development and mortality [49, 53, 54]. This management includes both endoscopic polypectomy and

Table 20.3a Surveillance guidelines for classical familial adenomatous polyposis syndrome

Tumor site	Examination	*ESMO* 2013 [52]		*ACG* 2015 [26]		*NCCN* 2016 [90]	
		Age (y)	Interval (y)	Age (y)	Interval (y)	Age (y)	Interval (y)
Colorectum	**Sigmoidoscopy**	12–14	2[a]	10–15	1–2		
	Colonoscopy	Once polyps are detected	1	10–15	1–2	10–15	1
Duodenum	**UGI endoscopy**[b]	25–30[c]	1–5[d]	25–30	1–5[d]	20–25	1–5[d]
Thyroid	**Cervical palpation**	25–30	1	Late teens	1	Late teens	1
	Cervical US						
Hepatoblastoma	**Abdominal US**			Infancy[e]	6 m	Infancy[f]	3–6 m
	Serum alpha-fetoprotein						
Desmoid	**CT/MRI**	If family history and site of *APC* mutation				After colectomy	1–3[g]
	Abdominal palpation			N/A	1	N/A	1

ACG American College of Gastroenterology, *ESMO* European Society for Medical Oncology, *NCCN* National Comprehensive Cancer Network, *UGI* upper gastrointestinal, *US* ultrasound, *y* years
[a]Every 2 years until adenomas are detected, then annually
[b]Front view and side view
[c]Or when colorectal polyps are diagnosed
[d]Based on Spigelman stage
[e]Until 7 years old. Consider family history
[f]Until 5 years old. Consider family history
[g]Every 1–3 years after colectomy; every 5–10 years if family history

surgery. Based on the risk of CRC before 20 years old is up to 1.5% [50], flexible sigmoidoscopy or colonoscopy should be carried out every 2 years, starting at age 10–14 years [50]. Once adenomas are detected, total colonoscopy should be performed annually until colectomy is planned (usually before 25 years old, depending on the size, dysplasia, and number of polyps) [50] (Tables 20.3a, 20.3b, and 20.3c). After surgery, annual endoscopic follow-up is recommended for the rectal remnant due to the risk of developing rectal cancer (up to 30% of the cases), as well as reservoir endoscopic surveillance given the high risk of developing adenomas and advanced neoplasia (up to 60% of the cases) [55–57].

Management of attenuated FAP is commonly endoscopic, reserving surgery to those cases not suitable to endoscopic control. In attenuated FAP (AFAP) cases,

Table 20.3b Surveillance guidelines for attenuated familial adenomatous polyposis syndrome

Tumor site	Examination	*ESMO* 2013 [52] Age (y)	Interval (y)	*ACG* 2015 [26] Age (y)	Interval (y)	*NCCN* 2016 [90] Age (y)	Interval (y)
Colorectum	**Colonoscopy**	18–20	1–2[a]	18–20	1–2 [a]	Late teens	2–3
Duodenum	**UGI endoscopy**[b]	25–30[c]	1–5[d]	25–30	1–5[d]	20–25	1–5[d]
Thyroid	**Cervical palpation**	25–30	1	25–30	1	Late teens	1
	Cervical US						
Hepatoblastoma	**Abdominal US**			Infancy[e]	6 m		
	Serum alpha-fetoprotein						
Desmoid	**CT/MRI**	If family history and site of *APC* mutation				After colectomy	1–3[g]
	Abdominal palpation			N/A	1[f]	N/A	1

ACG, American College of Gastroenterology, *ESMO* European Society for Medical Oncology, *m* months, *NCCN* National Comprehensive Cancer Network, *UGI* upper gastrointestinal, *US* ultrasound, *y* years
[a]Every 2 years until adenomas are detected, then annually
[b]Front view and side view
[c]Or when colorectal polyps are diagnosed
[d]Based on Spigelman stage
[e]Until 7 years old
[f]If family history of desmoid tumors
[g]Every 1–3 years after colectomy; every 5–10 years if family history

Table 20.3c Surveillance guidelines for *MUTYH*-associated polyposis syndrome

Tumor site	Examination	*ESMO* 2013 [52] Age (y)	Interval (y)	*ACG* 2015 [26] Age (y)	Interval (y)	*NCCN* 2016 [90] Age (y)	Interval (y)
Colorectum	**Colonoscopy**	18–20	1–2[a]	25–30	1–2 [a]	Late teens	2–3
Duodenum	**UGI endoscopy**[b]	25–30[c]	1–5[d]	30–35	1–5[d]	30–35	1–5[d]
Thyroid	**Cervical palpation**			25–30	1		
	Cervical US						

ACG American College of Gastroenterology, *ESMO* European Society for Medical Oncology, *NCCN* National Comprehensive Cancer Network, *UGI* upper gastrointestinal, US ultrasound, *y* years
[a]Every 2 years until adenomas are detected, then annually
[b]Front view and side view
[c]Or when colorectal polyps are diagnosed
[d]Based on Spigelman stage

colonoscopy is recommended instead of sigmoidoscopy every 1–2 years, starting at the age of 18–20 years. Once adenomas are detected, colonoscopy should be carried out annually [50] (Tables 20.3a, 20.3b and 20.3c).

The use of additional endoscopic techniques, such as chromoendoscopy, is limited due to the high number of detected polyps with conventional colonoscopy, although it could be useful to identify additional lesions in AFAP patients, especially for planning the best management and the type of surgery [58].

2.1.2 Small Bowel Surveillance

Up to 90% of FAP patients develop duodenal adenomas. Duodenal cancer is the second cause of cancer death in this disease, with a cumulative lifetime risk of 5% [59].

The treatment and surveillance approach of duodenal polyps is based on the Spigelman's classification, considering the number of polyps, size, histology, and dysplasia (Table 20.4) [60, 61]. Stage I indicates mild duodenal polyposis, whereas stages III–IV indicate severe duodenal disease, with an associated duodenal cancer risk up to 36%. Approximately 10–20% of the cases are classified as stage IV.

Management of severe duodenal disease is challenging, with a high rate of adenoma recurrence (>50%) and complications (such as hemorrhage, intestinal perforation, or acute pancreatitis) [62]. Therefore, a common consensus is to remove adenomas with high-grade dysplasia or larger than 10 mm. In most of the cases, duodenal adenomas are controlled by endoscopy, reserving surgery (including duodenotomy with polypectomy, pancreas-sparing duodenectomy, and duodenal-pancreatectomy) to some advanced cases [59, 62].

It is recommended an additional endoscopic assessment with a side-viewing endoscope for correct visualization of the papilla, especially in patients with Spigelman's stages III and IV, and, if the papilla is involved, perform an endoscopic

Table 20.4 Spigelman's classification [60, 61]

Findings by duodenoscopy	**1 point**	**2 points**	**3 points**
N° of polyps	<4	5–20	>20
Size (mm)	<4	5–10	>10
Histology	Tubular	Tubulovillous	Villous
Dysplasia	Mild	Moderate	Severe
Spigelman stage	**Total points**	**Surveillance**	
0	0	Every 4–5 years	
I	1–4	Every 2–3 years	
II	5–6	Every 1–3 years	
III	7–8	Every 6–12 months	
IV	9–12	Every 3–6 months. Surgical evaluation	

ultrasonography to complete locoregional evaluation. Recently it has been considered that the endoscopic capsule may play a role in the diagnosis of small bowel polyps [63].

Regarding chromoendoscopy, although it detects more duodenal lesions, it does not modify the definitive Spigelman stage and therefore the final management.

2.1.3 Stomach Surveillance

Gastric polyps are usually benign fundic gland polyps (FGP) and occur in 20% to 84% of FAP patients [64], while gastric carcinomas are rare (<1%) [65]. Gastric surveillance is performed as part of the surveillance of duodenal polyps, but biopsy or polypectomy is undertaken only for large or suspicious lesions, especially in the antrum [64, 65].

2.1.4 Thyroid Surveillance

Some FAP patients present an increased risk for papillary thyroid carcinoma (2–6% lifetime risk), with a female predominance and a pike of incidence in the third decade of life. Therefore there is expert consensus recommending thyroid palpation and annual cervical ultrasonography starting at late teenage [50] (Tables 20.3a, 20.3b, and 20.3c).

2.1.5 Hepatoblastoma Surveillance

Hepatoblastoma is a rare tumor that occurs in children with FAP usually between 6 months to 3 years of age, with an absolute risk less than 2% [66]. There is no strong evidence supporting surveillance in FAP patients, but due to the aggressiveness of this tumor, some experts recommend abdominal ultrasonography and serum alpha-fetoprotein every 3–6 months up to 5–7 years of age (Tables 20.3a, 20.3b, and 20.3c).

2.1.6 Desmoid Tumor Surveillance

Up to 15% of FAP patients develop desmoids. These lesions are related to a positive family history, abdominal surgery, and site of the mutation (codon 1444) and can occur inside the abdomen or in the abdominal wall. Based on the lack of malignant potential and high recurrence rate, surgery is reserved to cases with severe complications. Experts' consensus recommends surveillance in cases with associated risk factors, consisting in annual abdominal palpation and abdominal CT or MRI, especially after abdominal surgery (Tables 20.3a, 20.3b, and 20.3c).

2.1.7 Other Tumors

The incidence of other less common extraintestinal malignancies (pancreatic, brain, adrenal, among others) is very low, and surveillance is not currently recommended, except if there is a strong family history of any of these specific extraintestinal manifestations.

2.2 *MUTYH-Associated Polyposis*

The characteristic phenotype of MAP is of attenuated adenomatous polyposis, showing fewer than 100 adenomas and a lower risk of extracolonic manifestations in comparison to FAP. It is an autosomal recessive syndrome caused by biallelic germline mutations in the *MUTYH* gene. There are several studies supporting the variability of mutations in *MUTYH* based on geographical and ethnic differences. The most prevalent mutations in the Caucasian population are Y179C and G396D [67, 68]. Up to 30% of biallelic mutation carriers display CRC without a clear polyposis phenotype, commonly associated with early-onset CRC without mismatch repair (MMR) deficiency [67].

2.2.1 Colorectal Surveillance

Management of colorectal polyps is similar to that proposed for patients with AFAP, focused on controlling the polyps endoscopically (Tables 20.3a, 20.3b, and 20.3c). If surgery is required (total colectomy with ileorectal anastomosis, or proctocolectomy with ileal pouch and ileoanal anastomosis, if the rectum is affected), subsequent annual endoscopic surveillance is recommended [50, 52].

2.2.2 Stomach and Duodenum Surveillance

The risk of gastric cancer is 1%, and, as in FAP patients, surveillance is usually based on duodenal findings or in the family history of gastric malignancies. A recent study reported an incidence of duodenal polyposis of 17% with a lifetime risk of duodenal cancer of 4% [69].

2.2.3 Other Tumors

The incidence of other FAP-related manifestations is very low (gastric fundic gland polyp, lipomas, CHRPE, epidermoid cyst, desmoid tumor, and thyroid carcinoma) [70]; hence no extra-gastrointestinal cancer surveillance is recommended.

2.3 Polymerase Proofreading-Associated Polyposis

Recent studies have identified two different genes associated with multiple adenomas and early-onset CRC (*POLE* and *POLD1*) [71]. Nowadays, there are no specific recommendations for the management of these patients, and an intermediate approach between LS and MAP is recommended with regular colonoscopy surveillance.

3 Hamartomatous Polyposis Syndromes

These syndromes are infrequent; therefore most diagnostic criteria and surveillance recommendations are based on expert consensus (Table 20.1).

3.1 Juvenile Polyposis

It is the most common hamartomatous syndrome, with an incidence of 1 in 100,000 births [72], characterized by multiple gastrointestinal hamartomatous polyps, primarily in the colon and stomach, and an increased risk of gastrointestinal cancers. It is an autosomal dominant syndrome, 50% of cases associated with germline mutations in *SMAD4*, *BMPR1A*, or *ENG* gene [73, 74].

3.1.1 Colorectal Surveillance

Treatment consists of endoscopic polypectomy of large polyps. Surgical resection is reserved for symptomatic or complicated polyps (due to severe bleeding, bowel obstruction, or invagination). Lifetime risk for CRC is 40–50%. Colonoscopy surveillance is recommended every 1–2 years, starting at the age of 15–18 years [75] (Table 20.5).

3.1.2 Stomach Surveillance

The cumulative risk of gastric cancer is 21%. Gastroscopy is recommended every 1–3 years, starting at the age of 12–15 years [26] (Table 20.5).

3.1.3 Small Bowel Surveillance

Besides upper endoscopy, some consensus recommended surveillance with capsule endoscopy or CT/MRI enteroscopy every 1–2 years, after the age of 25 years [75].

No extra-gastrointestinal cancer surveillance is recommended.

Table 20.5 Surveillance guidelines in hamartomatous syndromes

Tumor site	Examination	*ACG* 2015 [26] Age (y)	*ACG* 2015 [26] Interval (y)	*NCCN* 2016 [90] Age (y)	*NCCN* 2016 [90] Interval (y)
Juvenile polyposis					
Colorectum	**Colonoscopy**	12–15	1–3	15	1–3[c]
Stomach	**UGI endoscopy**[a]	12–15	1–3	15	1–3[c]
Peutz-Jeghers syndrome					
Colorectum	**Colonoscopy**	8,18[b]	3	Late teens	2–3
Stomach	**UGI endoscopy**	8,18[b]	3	Late teens	2–3
Small bowel	**Video capsule endoscopy**	8,18[b]	3		
	CT or MRI			8,18*	2–3
Pancreas	**MRI or USE**	30	1–2	30–35	1–2
Breast	**MRI and/or mammogram**	25	1	25	1
Endometrium/ Ovarium/ cervix	**Pelvic exam and US**	25	1	18–20	1
Testes	**Physical exam**	Birth to teenage		Birth	1

ACG, American College of Gastroenterology, *NCCN* National Comprehensive Cancer Network, *UGI* upper gastrointestinal, *US* ultrasound, *y* years
[a]Front view and side view
[b]First procedure at 8 years old; if polyps, repeat every 3 years; if no polyps, restart at 18 years old and every 3 years
[c]Annually if polyps; if no polyps, every 2–3 years

3.2 *Peutz-Jeghers Syndrome*

It is an inherited disorder characterized by the presence of hamartoma polyps throughout the digestive tract and mucocutaneous hyperpigmentation. Polypoid lesions are of different sizes and diffusely distributed throughout the digestive tract, predominantly in the small intestine (60–90%) and colon (50–64%). The cumulative risk of developing cancer at the age of 70 is 85–90%. The most common malignancies are breast and CRC, followed by pancreas, stomach, ovaries, and sex cords [76]. It is an autosomal dominant syndrome due to germline mutations in the *STK11* gene (also known as *LKB1*) [77].

3.2.1 Colorectal Surveillance

Lifetime risk for CRC is 39%. Colonoscopy should be performed every 2–3 years, starting at the age of 18 years [76] (Table 20.5).

Treatment is endoscopic polypectomy of all polyps greater than 1.5 cm or those causing symptoms. However, it is sometimes necessary to perform a segmental bowel resection due to complications associated with chronic bleeding, intussusception, or intestinal obstruction.

3.2.2 Stomach and Small Bowel Surveillance

The estimated risk of gastric cancer is 30%, with a mean age at diagnosis of 30–40 years [78]. Lifetime risk for small bowel cancer is 13%. First gastrointestinal examination is recommended at the age of 8 years, by gastroduodenal endoscopy associated with capsule endoscopy or CT/MRI enteroscopy, every 2–3 years (Table 20.5).

3.2.3 Pancreas Surveillance

The cumulative risk of pancreatic adenocarcinomas is 36%. Although there is no evidence to support surveillance measures, some guidelines recommend endoscopic ultrasonography or MRI every 1–2 years, starting at the age of 30 years (Table 20.5) [35].

3.2.4 Breast Surveillance

The cumulative risk is 54%. Annual mammography or breast MRI is recommended, starting at the age of 25 years [79] (Table 20.5).

4 Serrated Polyposis Syndrome

Serrated polyposis syndrome (SPS) is an entity characterized by the presence of serrated polyps, mainly in the proximal colon, and an increased risk of CRC. Although suspected, it has not been possible to identify a causative germline defect. In a small proportion of patients, a biallelic *MUTYH* germline mutation has been identified, in the context of concomitant adenomatous polyposis.

Recently, a study described a CRC risk of 15% and the association of a higher risk to specific polyp characteristics, such as sessile serrated adenomas, proximal location, and presence of high-grade dysplasia [80]. Colonoscopy is recommended every 1–2 years, removing all polyps larger than 5 mm. Recent studies suggest that chromoendoscopy and narrowband imaging improve the detection rate of these polyps compared with conventional white-light endoscope [81, 82] (Table 20.6).

The recommended clinical management is with endoscopic polypectomy, reserving surgery for patients with CRC or when endoscopic polypectomy is not feasible. Subsequent proctoscopies every 6–12 months are needed for the surveillance of the remnant rectal. Extracolonic surveillance is not recommended [26].

Based on the increased relative risk of CRC in first-degree relatives compared with the general population, surveillance colonoscopy is recommended with an individualized approach taking into consideration family history and endoscopic findings (Table 20.6).

5 Biallelic Mismatch Repair Deficiency Syndrome

Patients with biallelic mutations in one of the MMR genes are usually affected with cancer during childhood, and the spectrum of cancers differs from the LS spectrum. There is a high incidence of CRC, adenomatous polyposis and small bowel tumors, hematological tumors (leukemia/ lymphoma), and brain, endometrium, and urinary tract tumors. Recently, two different expert consensus have proposed a surveillance approach acknowledging the lack of robust evidence and the need of more research [83, 84]. Recommendations are summarized in Table 20.7.

Table 20.6 Surveillance in serrated polyposis syndrome

		ACG 2015 [26]		*NCCN* 2016	
Tumor site	Examination	Age (y)	Interval (y)	Age (y)	Interval (y)
Colorectum	Colonoscopy Removing polyps >5 mm	Diagnosis	1–3	Diagnosis	1–3
		FDR: Individualize based on family history and endoscopic findings		FDR: (a) age of SPS diagnosis (b) 10 years earlier that CRC (c) 40 years old Stablish subsequent colonoscopies based on previous findings. If no polyps: Every 5y	

ACG American College of Gastroenterology, *FDR* first-degree relatives, *NCCN* National Comprehensive Cancer Network, *y* years

Table 20.7 Surveillance recommendations in biallelic mismatch repair deficiency syndrome

		European consortium 2014 [83]		US multi-society task force on colorectal cancer 2017 [84]	
Tumor site	Examination	Age (y)	Interval (y)	Age (y)	Interval (y)
Brain	**MRI**	2	0.5–1	2	0.5
UGI tract	**UGI endoscopy; capsule endoscopy**	10	1	8	1
Lower GI tract	**Ileocolonoscopy**	8	1	6	1
Non-Hodgkin lymphoma/other lymphoma	**Clinical exam; optional: abdominal ultrasound**	1	0.5	1	0.5
Leukemia	**Blood analysis**	1	0.5	1	0.5
Endometrium	**Gynecological exam, vaginal ultrasound, endometrial sampling**	20	1	20	1
Urinary tract	**Urine cytology**	20	1	10	1

GI gastrointestinal, *UGI* upper gastrointestinal, *y* years

R eferences

1. Moller P, Seppala T, Bernstein I, et al. Cancer incidence and survival in Lynch syndrome patients receiving colonoscopic and gynaecological surveillance: first report from the prospective Lynch syndrome database. Gut. 2017;66:464–72.
2. Jarvinen HJ, Aarnio M, Mustonen H, et al. Controlled 15-year trial on screening for colorectal cancer in families with hereditary nonpolyposis colorectal cancer. Gastroenterology. 2000;118:829–34.
3. Jarvinen HJ, Mecklin JP, Sistonen P. Screening reduces colorectal cancer rate in families with hereditary nonpolyposis colorectal cancer. Gastroenterology. 1995;108:1405–11.
4. Jarvinen HJ, Renkonen-Sinisalo L, Aktan-Collan K, et al. Ten years after mutation testing for Lynch syndrome: cancer incidence and outcome in mutation-positive and mutation-negative family members. J Clin Oncol. 2009;27:4793–7.
5. de Vos tot Nederveen Cappel WH, Nagengast FM, Griffioen G, et al. Surveillance for hereditary nonpolyposis colorectal cancer: a long-term study on 114 families. Dis Colon Rectum. 2002;45:1588–94.
6. Engel C, Rahner N, Schulmann K, et al. Efficacy of annual colonoscopic surveillance in individuals with hereditary nonpolyposis colorectal cancer. Clin Gastroenterol Hepatol. 2010;8:174–82.
7. Stuckless S, Green JS, Morgenstern M, et al. Impact of colonoscopic screening in male and female Lynch syndrome carriers with an MSH2 mutation. Clin Genet. 2012;82:439–45.
8. Vasen HF, Abdirahman M, Brohet R, et al. One to 2-year surveillance intervals reduce risk of colorectal cancer in families with Lynch syndrome. Gastroenterology. 2010;138:2300–6.
9. Dove-Edwin I, Sasieni P, Adams J, et al. Prevention of colorectal cancer by colonoscopic surveillance in individuals with a family history of colorectal cancer: 16 year, prospective, follow-up study. BMJ. 2005;331:1047.
10. Edelstein DL, Axilbund J, Baxter M, et al. Rapid development of colorectal neoplasia in patients with Lynch syndrome. Clin Gastroenterol Hepatol. 2011;9:340–3.
11. De Jong AE, Morreau H, Van Puijenbroek M, et al. The role of mismatch repair gene defects in the development of adenomas in patients with HNPCC. Gastroenterology. 2004;126:42–8.
12. Vasen HF, Taal BG, Nagengast FM, et al. Hereditary nonpolyposis colorectal cancer: results of long-term surveillance in 50 families. Eur J Cancer. 1995;31A:1145–8.
13. Renkonen-Sinisalo L, Aarnio M, Mecklin JP, et al. Surveillance improves survival of colorectal cancer in patients with hereditary nonpolyposis colorectal cancer. Cancer Detect Prev. 2000;24:137–42.
14. Lindberg LJ, Ladelund S, Frederiksen BL, et al. Outcome of 24 years national surveillance in different hereditary colorectal cancer subgroups leading to more individualised surveillance. J Med Genet. 2016.
15. Bonadona V, Bonaiti B, Olschwang S, et al. Cancer risks associated with germline mutations in MLH1, MSH2, and MSH6 genes in Lynch syndrome. JAMA. 2011;305:2304–10.
16. Jenkins MA, Dowty JG, Ait Ouakrim D, et al. Short-term risk of colorectal cancer in individuals with lynch syndrome: a meta-analysis. J Clin Oncol. 2015;33:326–31.
17. Senter L, Clendenning M, Sotamaa K, et al. The clinical phenotype of Lynch syndrome due to germ-line PMS2 mutations. Gastroenterology. 2008;135:419–28.
18. Baglietto L, Lindor NM, Dowty JG, et al. Risks of Lynch syndrome cancers for MSH6 mutation carriers. J Natl Cancer Inst. 2010;102:193–201.
19. Hurlstone DP, Karajeh M, Cross SS, et al. The role of high-magnification-chromoscopic colonoscopy in hereditary nonpolyposis colorectal cancer screening: a prospective "back-to-back" endoscopic study. Am J Gastroenterol. 2005;100:2167–73.
20. Rahmi G, Lecomte T, Malka D, et al. Impact of chromoscopy on adenoma detection in patients with Lynch syndrome: a prospective, multicenter, blinded, tandem colonoscopy study. Am J Gastroenterol. 2015;110:288–98.

21. Capelle LG, Van Grieken NC, Lingsma HF, et al. Risk and epidemiological time trends of gastric cancer in Lynch syndrome carriers in the Netherlands. Gastroenterology. 2010;138:487–92.
22. Win AK, Lindor NM, Young JP, et al. Risks of primary extracolonic cancers following colorectal cancer in Lynch syndrome. J Natl Cancer Inst. 2012;104:1363–72.
23. Park YJ, Shin KH, Park JG. Risk of gastric cancer in hereditary nonpolyposis colorectal cancer in Korea. Clin Cancer Res. 2000;6:2994–8.
24. Renkonen-Sinisalo L, Sipponen P, Aarnio M, et al. No support for endoscopic surveillance for gastric cancer in hereditary non-polyposis colorectal cancer. Scand J Gastroenterol. 2002;37:574–7.
25. Vasen HF, Blanco I, Aktan-Collan K, et al. Revised guidelines for the clinical management of Lynch syndrome (HNPCC): recommendations by a group of European experts. Gut. 2013;62:812–23.
26. Syngal S, Brand RE, Church JM, et al. ACG clinical guideline: genetic testing and management of hereditary gastrointestinal cancer syndromes. Am J Gastroenterol. 2015;110:223–62; quiz 263
27. Koornstra JJ. Small bowel endoscopy in familial adenomatous polyposis and Lynch syndrome. Best Pract Res Clin Gastroenterol. 2012;26:359–68.
28. Schulmann K, Brasch FE, Kunstmann E, et al. HNPCC-associated small bowel cancer: clinical and molecular characteristics. Gastroenterology. 2005;128:590–9.
29. ten Kate GL, Kleibeuker JH, Nagengast FM, et al. Is surveillance of the small bowel indicated for Lynch syndrome families? Gut. 2007;56:1198–201.
30. Saurin JC, Pilleul F, Soussan EB, et al. Small-bowel capsule endoscopy diagnoses early and advanced neoplasms in asymptomatic patients with Lynch syndrome. Endoscopy. 2010;42:1057–62.
31. Watson P, Vasen HF, Mecklin JP, et al. The risk of extra-colonic, extra-endometrial cancer in the Lynch syndrome. Int J Cancer. 2008;123:444–9.
32. Barrow E, Robinson L, Alduaij W, et al. Cumulative lifetime incidence of extracolonic cancers in Lynch syndrome: a report of 121 families with proven mutations. Clin Genet. 2009;75:141–9.
33. Kastrinos F, Stoffel EM, Balmana J, et al. Phenotype comparison of MLH1 and MSH2 mutation carriers in a cohort of 1,914 individuals undergoing clinical genetic testing in the United States. Cancer Epidemiol Biomark Prev. 2008;17:2044–51.
34. Win AK, Young JP, Lindor NM, et al. Colorectal and other cancer risks for carriers and noncarriers from families with a DNA mismatch repair gene mutation: a prospective cohort study. J Clin Oncol. 2012;30:958–64.
35. Canto MI, Harinck F, Hruban RH, et al. International Cancer of the Pancreas Screening (CAPS) Consortium summit on the management of patients with increased risk for familial pancreatic cancer. Gut. 2013;62:339–47.
36. Stoffel E, Mukherjee B, Raymond VM, et al. Calculation of risk of colorectal and endometrial cancer among patients with Lynch syndrome. Gastroenterology. 2009;137:1621–7.
37. Dove-Edwin I, Boks D, Goff S, et al. The outcome of endometrial carcinoma surveillance by ultrasound scan in women at risk of hereditary nonpolyposis colorectal carcinoma and familial colorectal carcinoma. Cancer. 2002;94:1708–12.
38. Gerritzen LH, Hoogerbrugge N, Oei AL, et al. Improvement of endometrial biopsy over transvaginal ultrasound alone for endometrial surveillance in women with Lynch syndrome. Familial Cancer. 2009;8:391–7.
39. Lecuru F, Le Frere Belda MA, Bats AS, et al. Performance of office hysteroscopy and endometrial biopsy for detecting endometrial disease in women at risk of human non-polyposis colon cancer: a prospective study. Int J Gynecol Cancer. 2008;18:1326–31.
40. Renkonen-Sinisalo L, Butzow R, Leminen A, et al. Surveillance for endometrial cancer in hereditary nonpolyposis colorectal cancer syndrome. Int J Cancer. 2007;120:821–4.
41. Rijcken FE, Mourits MJ, Kleibeuker JH, et al. Gynecologic screening in hereditary nonpolyposis colorectal cancer. Gynecol Oncol. 2003;91:74–80.
42. Schmeler KM, Lynch HT, Chen LM, et al. Prophylactic surgery to reduce the risk of gynecologic cancers in the Lynch syndrome. N Engl J Med. 2006;354:261–9.

43. Stuckless S, Green J, Dawson L, et al. Impact of gynecological screening in Lynch syndrome carriers with an MSH2 mutation. Clin Genet. 2013;83:359–64.
44. Auranen A, Joutsiniemi T. A systematic review of gynecological cancer surveillance in women belonging to hereditary nonpolyposis colorectal cancer (Lynch syndrome) families. Acta Obstet Gynecol Scand. 2011;90:437–44.
45. Chen LM, Yang KY, Little SE, et al. Gynecologic cancer prevention in Lynch syndrome/hereditary nonpolyposis colorectal cancer families. Obstet Gynecol. 2007;110:18–25.
46. Joost P, Therkildsen C, Dominguez-Valentin M, et al. Urinary tract cancer in Lynch syndrome; increased risk in carriers of MSH2 mutations. Urology. 2015;86:1212–7.
47. Myrhoj T, Andersen MB, Bernstein I. Screening for urinary tract cancer with urine cytology in Lynch syndrome and familial colorectal cancer. Familial Cancer. 2008;7:303–7.
48. Mork M, Hubosky SG, Roupret M, et al. Lynch syndrome: a primer for urologists and panel recommendations. J Urol. 2015;194:21–9.
49. Mallinson EK, Newton KF, Bowen J, et al. The impact of screening and genetic registration on mortality and colorectal cancer incidence in familial adenomatous polyposis. Gut. 2010;59:1378–82.
50. Vasen HF, Moslein G, Alonso A, et al. Guidelines for the clinical management of familial adenomatous polyposis (FAP). Gut. 2008;57:704–13.
51. Groen EJ, Roos A, Muntinghe FL, et al. Extra-intestinal manifestations of familial adenomatous polyposis. Ann Surg Oncol. 2008;15:2439–50.
52. Balmana J, Balaguer F, Cervantes A, et al. Familial risk-colorectal cancer: ESMO Clinical Practice Guidelines. Ann Oncol. 2013;24(Suppl 6 vi):73–80.
53. Gibbons DC, Sinha A, Phillips RK, et al. Colorectal cancer: no longer the issue in familial adenomatous polyposis? Familial Cancer. 2011;10:11–20.
54. Jarvinen HJ. Epidemiology of familial adenomatous polyposis in Finland: impact of family screening on the colorectal cancer rate and survival. Gut. 1992;33:357–60.
55. Friederich P, de Jong AE, Mathus-Vliegen LM, et al. Risk of developing adenomas and carcinomas in the ileal pouch in patients with familial adenomatous polyposis. Clin Gastroenterol Hepatol. 2008;6:1237–42.
56. Tajika M, Nakamura T, Nakahara O, et al. Prevalence of adenomas and carcinomas in the ileal pouch after proctocolectomy in patients with familial adenomatous polyposis. J Gastrointest Surg. 2009;13:1266–73.
57. Smith JC, Schaffer MW, Ballard BR, et al. Adenocarcinomas after prophylactic surgery for familial adenomatous polyposis. J Cancer Ther. 2013;4:260–70.
58. Matsumoto T, Esaki M, Fujisawa R, et al. Chromoendoscopy, narrow-band imaging colonoscopy, and autofluorescence colonoscopy for detection of diminutive colorectal neoplasia in familial adenomatous polyposis. Dis Colon Rectum. 2009;52:1160–5.
59. Biasco G, Pantaleo MA, Di Febo G, et al. Risk of duodenal cancer in patients with familial adenomatous polyposis. Gut. 2004;53:1547; author reply 1547
60. Spigelman AD, Williams CB, Talbot IC, et al. Upper gastrointestinal cancer in patients with familial adenomatous polyposis. Lancet. 1989;2:783–5.
61. Bulow S, Bjork J, Christensen IJ, et al. Duodenal adenomatosis in familial adenomatous polyposis. Gut. 2004;53:381–6.
62. Brosens LA, Keller JJ, Offerhaus GJ, et al. Prevention and management of duodenal polyps in familial adenomatous polyposis. Gut. 2005;54:1034–43.
63. Yamada A, Watabe H, Iwama T, et al. The prevalence of small intestinal polyps in patients with familial adenomatous polyposis: a prospective capsule endoscopy study. Familial Cancer. 2014;13:23–8.
64. Sarre RG, Frost AG, Jagelman DG, et al. Gastric and duodenal polyps in familial adenomatous polyposis: a prospective study of the nature and prevalence of upper gastrointestinal polyps. Gut. 1987;28:306–14.
65. Bianchi LK, Burke CA, Bennett AE, et al. Fundic gland polyp dysplasia is common in familial adenomatous polyposis. Clin Gastroenterol Hepatol. 2008;6:180–5.

66. Aretz S, Stienen D, Friedrichs N, et al. Somatic APC mosaicism: a frequent cause of familial adenomatous polyposis (FAP). Hum Mutat. 2007;28:985–92.
67. Balaguer F, Castellvi-Bel S, Castells A, et al. Identification of MYH mutation carriers in colorectal cancer: a multicenter, case-control, population-based study. Clin Gastroenterol Hepatol. 2007;5:379–87.
68. Grover S, Kastrinos F, Steyerberg EW, et al. Prevalence and phenotypes of APC and MUTYH mutations in patients with multiple colorectal adenomas. JAMA. 2012;308:485–92.
69. Vogt S, Jones N, Christian D, et al. Expanded extracolonic tumor spectrum in MUTYH-associated polyposis. Gastroenterology. 2009;137:1976–85 e1–10.
70. Nielsen M, Morreau H, Vasen HF, et al. MUTYH-associated polyposis (MAP). Crit Rev Oncol Hematol. 2011;79:1–16.
71. Bellido F, Pineda M, Aiza G, et al. POLE and POLD1 mutations in 529 kindred with familial colorectal cancer and/or polyposis: review of reported cases and recommendations for genetic testing and surveillance. Genet Med. 2016;18:325–32.
72. Howe JR, Sayed MG, Ahmed AF, et al. The prevalence of MADH4 and BMPR1A mutations in juvenile polyposis and absence of BMPR2, BMPR1B, and ACVR1 mutations. J Med Genet. 2004;41:484–91.
73. Latchford AR, Neale K, Phillips RK, et al. Juvenile polyposis syndrome: a study of genotype, phenotype, and long-term outcome. Dis Colon Rectum. 2012;55:1038–43.
74. Schreibman IR, Baker M, Amos C, et al. The hamartomatous polyposis syndromes: a clinical and molecular review. Am J Gastroenterol. 2005;100:476–90.
75. Dunlop MG, British Society for G, Association of Coloproctology for Great B, et al. Guidance on gastrointestinal surveillance for hereditary non-polyposis colorectal cancer, familial adenomatous polypolis, juvenile polyposis, and Peutz-Jeghers syndrome. Gut. 2002;51(Suppl 5):V21–7.
76. Beggs AD, Latchford AR, Vasen HF, et al. Peutz-Jeghers syndrome: a systematic review and recommendations for management. Gut. 2010;59:975–86.
77. Tomlinson IP, Houlston RS. Peutz-Jeghers syndrome. J Med Genet. 1997;34:1007–11.
78. van Lier MG, Westerman AM, Wagner A, et al. High cancer risk and increased mortality in patients with Peutz-Jeghers syndrome. Gut. 2011;60:141–7.
79. Kastrinos F, Syngal S. Screening patients with colorectal cancer for Lynch syndrome: what are we waiting for? J Clin Oncol. 2012;30:1024–7.
80. Carballal S, Rodriguez-Alcalde D, Moreira L, et al. Colorectal cancer risk factors in patients with serrated polyposis syndrome: a large multicentre study. Gut. 2015;65(11):1829–37.
81. Boparai KS, van den Broek FJ, van Eeden S, et al. Increased polyp detection using narrow band imaging compared with high resolution endoscopy in patients with hyperplastic polyposis syndrome. Endoscopy. 2011;43:676–82.
82. Pellise M, Diaz Tasende J, Balaguer F, et al. Technical review of advanced diagnostic endoscopy in patients at high risk of colorectal cancer. Gastroenterol Hepatol. 2012;35:278–92.
83. Vasen HF, Ghorbanoghli Z, Bourdeaut F, et al. Guidelines for surveillance of individuals with constitutional mismatch repair-deficiency proposed by the European Consortium "Care for CMMR-D" (C4CMMR-D). J Med Genet. 2014;51:283–93.
84. Durno C, Boland CR, Cohen S, et al. Recommendations on surveillance and management of Biallelic Mismatch Repair Deficiency (BMMRD) syndrome: a consensus statement by the US Multi-Society Task Force on Colorectal Cancer. Gastroenterology. 2017;30175-0(17):S0016–5085.
85. Engel C, Loeffler M, Steinke V, et al. Risks of less common cancers in proven mutation carriers with Lynch syndrome. J Clin Oncol. 2012;30:4409–15.
86. Kastrinos F, Stoffel EM. History, genetics, and strategies for cancer prevention in Lynch syndrome. Clin Gastroenterol Hepatol. 2014;12:715–27.
87. Stoffel EM, Mangu PB, Gruber SB, et al. Hereditary colorectal cancer syndromes: American Society of Clinical Oncology clinical practice guideline endorsement of the familial risk-colorectal cancer: European Society for Medical Oncology clinical practice guidelines. J Clin Oncol. 2015;33:209–17.

88. Guillen-Ponce C, Serrano R, Sanchez-Heras AB, et al. Clinical guideline seom: hereditary colorectal cancer. Clin Transl Oncol. 2015;17:962–71.
89. Boparai KS, Reitsma JB, Lemmens V, et al. Increased colorectal cancer risk in first-degree relatives of patients with hyperplastic polyposis syndrome. Gut. 2010;59:1222–5.
90. National Comprehensive Cancer Network. Genetic/Familial High-Risk Assessment: Colorectal (Version 2.2016). http://www.nccn.org/professionals/physician_gls/pdf/genetics_colon.pdf. Accessed April 6, 2017.

Chapter 21
Surgical Management of Hereditary Colorectal Cancer Syndromes

Johannes Dörner, Mahmoud Taghavi Fallahpour, and Gabriela Möslein

Abstract Due to the advances in molecular genetic diagnostics of adenomatous polyposis variants as well as nonpolyposis syndromes, identification of patients with a genetic predisposition and their at-risk relatives is becoming increasingly important in clinical practice. Knowledge of the specific risk profile is gaining significance and requires a clinically differentiated approach to correctly identify the indications for prophylactic and extended therapeutic surgery. In this chapter, decision-making and the technical details of the operation for different colorectal cancer (CRC) syndromes are outlined. Besides the more commonly known polyposis syndromes, such as familial adenomatous polyposis (FAP), surgeons should be able to clinically distinguish between attenuated and classical variants of FAP and be aware of MUTYH-associated polyposis (MAP) and the newly described polyposis polymerase proofreading-associated polyposis (PPAP), among others. Surgeons should be familiar with the specific indications and extent of surgery for prophylactic organ removal in the lower gastrointestinal tract to knowledgeably advise patients and enable them to make informed decisions. Moreover, reconstructive options after proctocolectomy and novel innovative techniques in proctectomy, such as the transanal total mesorectal excision (TaTME), are discussed.

Keywords Timing of surgery · Ileal pouch-anal anastomosis · Ileorectal anastomosis · Quality of life · Desmoid disease · Prophylactic surgery

J. Dörner
Klinik für Allgemein- und Viszeralchirurgie, HELIOS University Hospital Witten/Herdecke, Wuppertal, Germany

M. T. Fallahpour
Private University Witten/Herdecke, Witten, Germany

G. Möslein (✉)
Center for Hereditary Tumours, HELIOS University Hospital Witten/Herdecke, Wuppertal, Germany
e-mail: Gabriela.Moeslein@helios-gesundheit.de

L. Valle et al. (eds.), *Hereditary Colorectal Cancer*,
https://doi.org/10.1007/978-3-319-74259-5_21

1 Surgical Management in Polyposis Syndromes

1.1 Introduction

Since most – if not all – patients with familial adenomatous polyposis (FAP) will develop colon or rectal cancer at some point in their life, surgery remains the only definitive prophylactic option. At an early stage of polyp development, participation in chemopreventive studies should be encouraged. However, to date there is no evidence for efficient long-term polyp (cancer) management with the agents studied so far. Therefore, the question is not if but rather when and how extensive the surgery should be. As most patients are young, socially and professionally active at the time of surgery, low morbidity, good social functioning, and excellent quality of life are important goals. In the following section, we will discuss clinical and personal factors that need to be considered for optimal patient counseling as well as technical details of the procedure.

1.2 Timing of Prophylactic Surgery for Familial Adenomatous Polyposis

The optimal timing for prophylactic surgery for familial adenomatous polyposis is not well established. Most surgeons will agree that prophylactic proctocolectomy is not indicated at the time of presentation of first polyps but should be performed before cancer develops. Between both extremes, decisions are usually made based on personal or institutional practice and are based on limited scientific evidence. A recent retrospective study of 303 patients who underwent colorectal surgery for FAP determined 46, 31, and 27 years as the optimal cutoff age for predicting the development of CRC in the attenuated, sparse, and profuse phenotype, respectively [1]. However, even though genotype and family information contribute to decision-making, the individual clinical findings as well as personal patient preference should be taken into consideration. Symptoms such as bleeding, diarrhea, or obstruction may warrant timely intervention independently of polyp burden. On the other hand, surgery may be delayed in women of childbearing age since some controversial data suggests reduced fertility in female patients after ileal pouch-anal anastomosis (IPAA) [2]. Other reasons for postponing elective surgery may be in obese patients with planned weight loss or patients carrying a high risk for desmoid disease [3]. In the absence of tumor-specific symptoms, authors have based recommendation toward surgery on polyp overall burden and progression that can be monitored by repeated colonoscopy [4]. In a retrospective study, the Saint Marks group found a two to three times greater risk of cancer in patients with >1000 colorectal polyps [5]. Until recently, a staging system similar to the Spigelman score that classifies duodenal polyps in FAP patients and is used to guide decision-making [6] has been lacking. Recently, a staging system taking into account polyp burden and size has

Table 21.1 Proposed InSiGHT staging system classification and clinical interventions for colonic polyposis [7]

Stage[a]	Polyp description	Clinical intervention		Comments
0	<20 polyps, all <5 mm	A	Repeat colonoscopy in 2 years	Biopsy at baseline to confirm histology; polyp removal discretionary (not clearly indicated)
1[b]	20–200 polyps most <5 mm, none, >1 cm	B	Repeat colonoscopy in 1 year	Some would consider colectomy, especially when polyp count is high
2[b]	200–500 polyps, <10 that are >1 cm	C	Repeat colonoscopy in 1 year polypectomy preferred	Removal of large polyps clearly necessary when performed to postpone surgery. The alternative would be to consider surgery
3[b]	500–1000 polyps or any number if there are 10–50 that are >1 cm and amenable to complete polypectomy	D	Repeat colonoscopy in 6–12 months or consider colectomy	Removal of large number of larger polyps defensible, but only when there are clear reasons to delay surgery
4	>1000 polyps and/or any polyps grown to confluence and not amenable to simple polypectomy; any invasive cancer	E	Colectomy proctocolectomy clearly indicated within 3 months to a year	Any decision to delay surgery must be highly individualized and based on compelling circumstances

[a]Patients who cannot be allotted a particular stage (e.g., patients with mixed polyposis) call for an external discussion by a multidisciplinary specialty team
[b]Presence of high-grade dysplasia warrants upstaging of patient to stage 4

been proposed to provide guidance for stage-specific interventions including surgery for colorectal polyps in FAP (Table 21.1) [7]. Once validated in prospective studies, it may help guide decision-making for this patient population.

Finally, recent evidence suggests that endoscopic polyp management may be feasible and safe in patients refusing colectomy during a median follow-up of almost 4–5 years [8]; however, it may only be used to delay surgery and not as a substitute.

1.3 Indications and Surgical Technique

1.3.1 Ileorectal Anastomosis Versus Ileoanal Pouch

The extent of removal of the target organ depends mainly on the different phenotypes in FAP. Although a genotype-phenotype correlation has been described [9], the individual clinical phenotype is currently considered pivotal for surgical decision-making. In attenuated FAP (aFAP), distribution of the polyps is usually indicative, since a right-sided phenotype is common and the rectum is usually spared entirely. Therefore, an ileorectal anastomosis (IRA) with superior functional outcome [10] and similar quality of life [11] is considered appropriate for the subset of patients with aFAP (mutation in codon 0–200 or >1500) [12]. In classical FAP, due to left-sided predominance with initial polyp formation in the rectosigmoid and progression toward proximal segments of the colon, a restorative proctocolectomy with an IPAA is the treatment of choice. Not surprisingly, most cancers in patients with classical FAP occur in the rectum [13]. Some patients with classical FAP however may present without rectal polyps at a young age but usually will develop them later in life with a serious risk of rectal cancer and higher morbidity due to a second operation if primary proctocolectomy had not been performed in the first place. Also, the increased risk of desmoid development after further surgeries must be taken into account. A recent study from Finland demonstrated a 53% cumulative risk of secondary proctectomy at 30 years after colectomy with IRA, mostly due to cancer (including suspicion of cancer) or uncontrollable rectal polyposis (44% each) [14]. Therefore, in patients with a classical FAP, total proctocolectomy usually is the preferred option. The accepted standard for recommending an IPAA in FAP patients is the presence of 20 rectal polyps at the time of colectomy. However, as noted previously, the timing of prophylactic surgery is not well defined and varies widely. Predictors for the development of cancer of the rectum are the presence of more than 1000 polyps or cancer at colectomy with IRA and a mutation occurring between codons 1250 and 1500 [15–17]. In patients with a known or family history for desmoid disease, it seems advisable to postpone the operation as late as safely possible due to the established triggering effect of surgical trauma on desmoid formation [18, 19]. This recommendation however does not consider the beneficial effect of preventive medication as it predates the times when they were available. Patients with desmoids carry a high risk of failure of pouch formation if a secondary proctectomy must be performed after IRA [20] as desmoids in the mesentery may render mobilization and lengthening of the mesentery impossible. Therefore, in these patients it seems advisable to reduce the risk of secondary surgery by performing a restorative proctocolectomy with an ileoanal pouch as the definitive primary option. For classical FAP, laparoscopic restorative proctocolectomy without diverting ileostomy and a hand-sewn anastomosis or possible TaTME will probably be the best choice, leading to a comparable quality of life to the normative population [21] and eliminated cancer risk of the rectum. The factors that influence surgical decision-making are summarized in Table 21.2.

1.3.2 Alternative Restorative Options: Permanent Ileostomy or the Continent Intra-Abdominal Pouch

Besides IRA and IPAA, other restorative options exist. Total proctocolectomy (TPC) with permanent ileostomy and total proctectomy with the formation of a primary continent ileostomy (the so-called Kock pouch after its describer Nils G. Kock) [22] are alternative options that are occasionally performed in FAP patients. TPC with permanent ileostomy is performed infrequently in patients with an unacceptably low anal sphincter function, when cancer involving the sphincter is

Table 21.2 Factors influencing choice of surgery for familial adenomatous polyposis (FAP)

Disease factors	Type of mutation of the *APC* gene (classical FAP vs. aFAP/MAP) Disease phenotype (number and location of polyps, presence of rectal polyps) Presence or risk of desmoid disease Presence of cancer
Patient factors	Age Sex Family history Prior surgery Reproductive life planning Sexual function Compliance with follow-up surveillance Body image, cosmesis, acceptance of (temporary) stoma

Abbreviations: *MAP* MUTYH-associated polyposis

present or when IPAA construction is technically infeasible, for instance, due to desmoid disease with shortening of the mesentery leading to inability to advance the ileal pouch to the anus. TPC with permanent ileostomy is also occasionally chosen as a primary procedure in patients that perceive the frequent bowel movements associated with IPAA as too compromising to their lifestyle and prefer permanent ileostomy. In most of the mentioned scenarios, the continent ileostomy is a viable alternative to permanent ileostomy. It involves the construction of an intra-abdominal reservoir from the terminal ileum, which is intussuscepted to form a valve that prevents stool and gas from escaping in an uncontrolled manner. A short portion of the ileum issues from the pouch to the abdominal skin, usually on the right lower abdominal quadrant. The patient can control defecation by intubating the pouch three to five times a day, allowing the stool to escape into a toilet and eliminating the necessity for wearing an ostomy bag. Overall, quality of life (QOL) in patients with a continent ileostomy equals or surpasses patients with conventional Brooke ileostomy and the primary diagnosis of ulcerative colitis (UC) [23]. FAP patients have an overall superior outcome with ileoanal pouches. Nevertheless, in poorly functioning pouches after septic complications or fistulae, the continent ileostomy seems to be a recommendable important alternative to a terminal ileostomy, especially taking secondary complications such as acute and chronic renal failure into account.

1.3.3 Laparoscopic Versus Open Technique

The benefits of a laparoscopic approach for major colorectal surgery for benign disease are well documented, but growing evidence suggests that it may also be performed safely in rectal cancer patients with benefits in return of normal bowel function and length of hospital stay [24]. Well-documented advantages of laparoscopy in FAP include better cosmesis, faster recovery, reduction of adhesions [25], increased pregnancy rate [26], as well as faster restoration of intestinal continuity [27]. To date, the only randomized, controlled study that compares open to laparoscopic proctocolectomy with IPAA was terminated prematurely due to poor recruitment [28]. Until termination, 42 patients were randomized; there was no significant difference in the primary endpoint blood loss (laparoscopic, 261.5 ± 195.4 ml; open, 228.1 ± 119.5 ml); the secondary endpoint duration of surgery was significantly longer for the laparoscopic procedure (laparoscopic group (313.9 ± 52 min), open group (200.2 ± 53.8 min)). A randomized trial that compared open vs. laparoscopic restorative proctocolectomy with IPAA found no difference in the primary endpoint postoperative recovery in the 3 months after surgery as measured by quality of life questionnaires and in the secondary outcomes postoperative morphine requirement, morbidity, and hospital stay [29]. Operating times were significantly higher in the laparoscopic procedures (210 vs. 133 min, $p < 0.001$). Generally, laparoscopically performed proctocolectomy for FAP is safe and its percentage increasing: three in four proctocolectomies were performed laparoscopically in a recent series from Japan [30]. In our view, laparoscopic proctocolectomy should be the standard of care if no contraindications to laparoscopy are present.

1.3.4 Mesocolic Dissection Versus Total Mesorectal Excision

Avoiding pelvic autonomic nerve damage during proctectomy is of paramount importance when performing restorative proctocolectomy, specifically in young patients in a prophylactic setting [31]. When no rectal cancer is present at the time of proctectomy, not only total mesorectal excision (TME) as is the standard in rectal cancer but also close rectal dissection (CRD) is acceptable from an oncological standpoint. CRD, immediately on the rectal musculature within the mesorectal fat, may potentially lead to a reduction in injury to the autonomic nerves that lie anterolateral from the mesorectal fascia. This dissection however is technically tedious as it is not an anatomical plane and prone to bleeding that may misguide further tissue preparation, which can somewhat be mitigated by the use of a vessel sealing device [32]. Moreover, TME with the preservation of anterolateral mesorectum seems to lead to similar outcomes in terms of sexual function [33]. In a randomized clinical trial that directly compared CRD to TME, preliminary data showed a somewhat lower rate of high-grade (Clavien-Dindo Grade 3) surgical complications in the CRD group (2 of 28 vs. 10 of 31, $p = 0.027$) and more favorable outcomes on some quality of life subscales for CRD [34]. The primary outcome (pouch compliance) of the trial is yet to be reported. In that trial, the indication for proctectomy was ulcerative colitis in 50 patients and FAP in only 6 patients. For FAP patients, there may be another aspect to consider: We have identified several patients that have developed desmoids in the mesorectum that led to pouch inlet problems. Since desmoid disease generally originates from the mesentery, a CRD may reduce the risk of this complication in desmoid-prone patients. Systematic studies that have studied this effect are lacking. Another innovative technique, transanal total mesorectal excision (TaTME) [35], may provide technical advantages due to avoidance of using several stapler lines and a precise determination of the level of the anastomosis and by utilizing a circular instead of a double-stapled anastomosis. In this technique, the low pelvic mesorectum is approached via the anus using a single laparoscopic port, leading to improved preparation of the low rectum compared to the transabdominal approach. It was initially developed to improve quality of TME in mid and low rectal cancer but is increasingly used for proctectomy in benign disease, including FAP [36]. While small studies have shown TaTME to be safe and associated with a functional outcome comparable to published results after conventional laparoscopic low anterior resection for rectal cancer [37], prospective randomized studies are needed to determine long-term functional results. The advantage, clearly, is a circular anastomosis in the height of the dentate line avoiding the (even) small rectal remnant that increasingly has been identified as sequelae for future neoplastic problems leading to secondary interventions or even rectal cancer with the secondary need of proctectomy and ileostomy.

1.3.5 Maintaining the Ileocolic Blood Supply

Adequate, tension-free reach of the pouch into the pelvis is often challenging. Numerous strategies, including ileocolic vessel ligation at the origin of the superior mesenteric artery [38], have been described to increase mobility of the small bowel mesentery. At least in theory, preservation of both the circulation of the ileocolic and mesenteric vessels may improve healing of the anastomosis and even have long-term benefits of avoiding or improving inflammation in the form of pouchitis. In the event of requiring mesenteric lengthening, ligation of the ileocolic artery is safe. Alternatively, if the ileal branch of the superior mesenteric artery (SMA) is divided, preservation of the ileocolic vessels results in maintained perfusion via the SMA. We therefore recommend initial preservation of the ileocolic as well as mesenteric vessels and intraoperative determination of the main length-restricting vessel that may subsequently be divided. Prospective studies are needed to determine whether this fairly simple strategy results in improved outcomes of function, pouchitis, and early or late surgical complications [39].

1.3.6 Hand Suture Versus Double-Stapled Anastomosis

For a long time, the pouch-anal anastomosis was performed after mucosectomy and hand-sewn at the level of the dentate line, as first described by Parks and Nicholls in 1978 [40]. Conceptually, this approach removes all mucosa of the rectum and should eliminate risk of rectal neoplasia. The double-stapled anastomosis as described by Heald [41] in 1986 is easier to perform, and leads to better functional results, but is also associated with a higher risk of remaining rectal mucosa [42] with the potential of adenoma and cancer formation [43]. The short- and long-term consequences of either approach have been studied extensively, albeit mostly in patients with ulcerative colitis (UC) where inflammation of the remaining mucosa, so-called cuffitis, is an important issue. Hence, as prospective studies with sufficient follow-up are lacking, the true long-term risk of relevant neoplasia in the rectal remnant for both techniques is unknown. Taking recent publications describing a high rate of adenomas [44] into account, some skepticism concerning the general preference of double-stapled anastomosis remains. A retrospective study by the Cleveland Clinic [45] suggests that transition zone adenomas may safely be managed expectantly or with mucosectomy. Most experts probably agree that close follow-up with annual pouchoscopy is recommended to detect neoplasia in early treatable stages for all patients after IPAA, regardless of anastomosis technique. Again, the use of TaTME with a hand-sewn circular end-to-end anastomosis or stapled anastomosis may provide benefit regarding extent of proctectomy.

1.3.7 Shape and Size of Pouch

While the initial report of IPAA described a hand-sewn pouch with an s-configuration [40], the J pouch, as described by Utsunomiya in 1980 [46], is today considered the ileoanal pouch shape of choice. The J pouch is easy to construct with the use of a GIA stapler [47] and results in good functional outcomes without the need for intubation. Other pouch designs may be indicated in subgroups of patients; an S or K pouch may, for instance, be beneficial in patients that have a shortened mesenterium due to desmoid disease. Kalady reported that his standard procedure of choice at the Cleveland Clinic is the construction of an S pouch with a 2 cm outlet [3]. He claims that this configuration facilitates emptying of the pouch; however this is not supported with data. The total size of the pouch does not necessarily need to be correlated with good functioning, since smaller pouches perform as well as larger pouches and may even lead to fewer inlet problems [48]. A Swedish group reported better results for the K than for the J pouch in a large group of patients [49]. However, as in many studies comparing other pouch designs, only a small percentage of patients had FAP as diagnosis. The optimal pouch design for patients receiving IPAA for FAP remains a matter of debate with the J pouch being considered the standard choice being challenged by proponents of other designs that may be preferred in special settings. Despite equal length of pouch limbs at the time of surgery – regardless of the pouch design – later volume appears to depend on a variety of not understood influencing factors. Some of these may correlate to postoperative complications such as pelvic sepsis or fistulae. Clearly prospective studies in polyposis patients are warranted to address these important issues that are essential for QOL in patients with a prophylactic versus an oncological setting.

1.3.8 Protective Ileostomy (One-Stage Versus Two-Stage IPAA)

Many institutions perform a protective diverting loop ileostomy at the time of IPAA to minimize the substantial risk of pelvic sepsis and functional impairment due to anastomotic leakage [3, 50, 51]. However, many studies have shown the feasibility of a one-stage approach with similar rates of postoperative complications such as pelvic sepsis, anastomotic stricture, and a shorter duration of hospital stay [52]. The observation that ulcerative colitis was associated with significantly higher rates of pouch-related septic complications (PRSC) compared to FAP gives further support to the omission of a diverting ileostomy in IPAA for FAP [53]. Not surprisingly, the same study found a higher risk for PRSC in patients where anastomotic tension had occurred, supporting the use of diverting ileostomy in selected cases with patient- or procedure-related risk factors for anastomotic failure, such as steroid intake, malnutrition, and anemia or intraoperative complications. If a desmoid-prone patient requires IPAA, a one-stage procedure is advised since it is well-known that surgical trauma triggers the formation of desmoids. We performed a retrospective analysis of our own patients with IPAA for FAP (10/2005–10/2011) with a minimal follow-up of 12 months after proctocolectomy or ileostomy closure. The decision to perform an ileostomy was taken intraoperatively by the surgeon based on intraoperative factors such as tension on the anastomosis. A total of 115 patients (52 male, 63 female) were included, and 97 received and 18 did not receive an ileostomy. Follow-up was performed at our institution. There was a trend toward fewer ileostomies at the end of the treatment period. Twenty-one out of 97 patients that had ileostomy developed an abdominal wall desmoid at or close to the ileostomy site; 11 of these additionally developed mesenteric desmoids. None of the 18 patients without ileostomy developed abdominal desmoids in the observation period. Furthermore, depending on individual anatomy, building an ileostomy may lead to increased tension on the pouch and the pouch-anal anastomosis. A so-called ghost or virtual ileostomy (VI) may be a good compromise between unnecessary ileostomy formation and surgeons' peace of mind. In this recently described technique [54], a vascular loop is passed around the terminal ileum, exteriorized through the abdominal wall, and securely fixed to the skin to allow easy secondary ileostomy construction under local anesthesia and without relaparotomy in the event of an anastomotic complication. In most patients where diverting ileostomy is not needed, the vessel may be removed easily at the bedside. A randomized controlled trial compared laparoscopic anterior rectal resection with GI and without ileostomy [55]. Patients with VI had lower severity of anastomotic leakage and a shorter hospital stay. More studies are needed to prospectively compare virtual ileostomy to conventional ileostomy.

1.3.9 Surgical Management of Desmoid Disease

In patients with a known or family history of desmoid disease, it is advisable to delay prophylactic surgery as late as safely possible. This recommendation is due to the known triggering effect of surgical trauma on desmoid growth, and all FAP patients are potentially at risk of desmoid formation. However, novel chemopreventive options may modify this recommendation in the future. As we have outlined, many patients that receive ileorectal anastomosis as a first procedure require secondary proctectomy due to rectal neoplasia. In desmoid-prone patients, a secondary operation not only increases the risk of desmoid growth, but there is also a substantial risk of failure to construct a pelvic pouch if desmoids are already present. Therefore, we recommend definitive proctocolectomy and pouch surgery as the initial procedure [18]. Asymptomatic mesenteric desmoids are present prior to surgery in about 3% of patients with FAP [56]. They will only in some cases progress, and chemopreventive options exist. Resection will almost invariably result in promotion or triggering of new desmoid growth that impacts the vascularization of a small bowel segment. Thus, we recommend to surgically ignore asymptomatic desmoids, even if of larger size and proceed with a planned pouch formation. We advocate to discuss with patients the option of a low-dose antiestrogen therapy in combination with sulindac as an effective off-label chemopreventive option in these cases postsurgery, as for patients with a known family history of desmoid tumors. We have prospectively evaluated 21 patients at our institution with this strategy and discontinued medication if an MRI at 1 year after surgery showed absence of visible desmoid. Only one patient from a high-risk family developed desmoid disease with this strategy and was subsequently treated successfully with high-dose treatment [57].

1.3.10 Surgery for Duodenal Disease in FAP

In the presence of Spigelman stage 4 duodenal polyps, a prophylactic, pancreas-sparing duodenectomy is recommended [58], since duodenal carcinoma is the second leading cause of death in FAP after CRC [59] and stage 4 duodenal disease is associated with a 36% risk of duodenal cancer [60]. Preserving the head of the pancreas has advantages compared to more radical procedures such as the Whipple procedure in terms of morbidity and long-term function [61, 62]. In a recent randomized double-blind study in patients with FAP, the use of sulindac (150 mg, twice daily) and erlotinib (75 mg) daily compared with placebo resulted in a significantly lower duodenal polyp burden after 6 months [63]. The use of sulindac and erlotinib was associated with an acne-like rash in 87% of patients compared to only 20% of patients treated with placebo. Grade 3 adverse events were uncommon (2 in 92 patients). Further studies with longer follow-up are needed to determine whether the observed effects will lead to improved clinical outcomes.

2 Surgical Management for Nonpolyposis Syndromes

2.1 Introduction

The surgical management of CRC in patients with a clinical diagnosis of hereditary nonpolyposis colorectal cancer (HNPCC) or confirmed Lynch syndrome needs to be highly individualized. Due to the known risk of synchronous and metachronous cancer, most surgeons familiar with the treatment of HNPCC favor an extended resection at the time of diagnosis of CRC. Age at diagnosis, tumor stage and location, comorbidities, but also gene and gender as well as patient preference must be considered in order to determine the optimal surgical strategy for every patient. A recent study suggests that the mutated gene has a major role in risk determination for subsequent cancers in Lynch-associated CRC patients [64]. Pathogenic *MSH6* carriers have a lower risk of developing secondary cancers compared to mutation carriers in *MLH1* and *MSH2*. If the exact mutation is known, treating surgeons can estimate the individual risk of a patient to develop secondary cancer in Lynch-associated CRC patients using a risk calculator that is available at http://lscarisk.org (see pictures 1–4 for examples). To fully understand the impact of the underlying condition and make an informed decision, Lynch-associated cancer should optimally be diagnosed prior

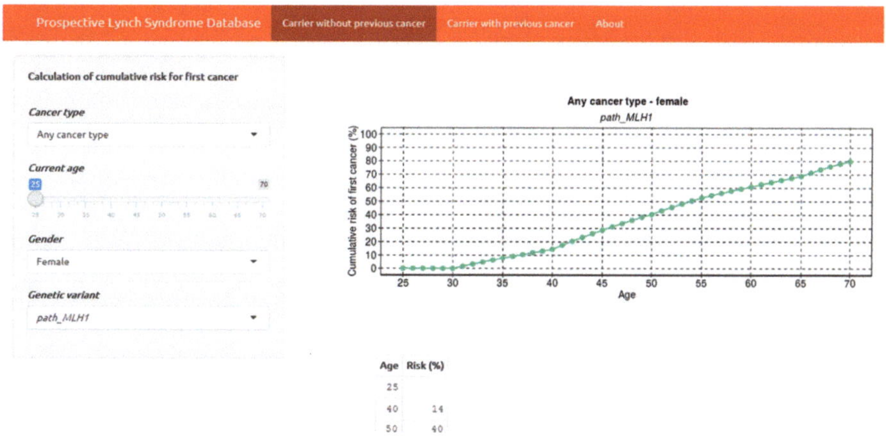

Fig. 21.1 Calculation of the risk for any cancer for a 25-year-old female without previous cancer with a pathogenic *MLH1* mutation

to cancer surgery in the first place. Unfortunately, Lynch syndrome caused by a germline mutation in one of the known mismatch repair (MMR) genes is underdiagnosed if clinical criteria (Amsterdam and Bethesda criteria) are used to select for patients. In other countries, such as the UK, guidelines were recently (February 2017) released for reflex (systematic) testing of all CRC regardless even of age. Screening for the condition with immunohistochemical (IHC) staining of the MMR proteins or microsatellite instability (MSI) testing is now required [65–67]. There is growing evidence and expert consensus that IHC staining or MSI testing for screening in all CRC and endometrial cancer patients, irrespective of age and family history, should be performed. Many experts even argue to perform extended gene panel testing in all or at least in all younger patients with CRC [68, 69]. In some countries including the UK, national guidelines now recommend MSI screening in all CRC patients, and others are likely to follow. Importantly, from the surgical point of view, this screening should be performed prior to surgery using tumor biopsy material to allow for informed decision-making regarding individualized surgery. This strategy has been shown to be feasible and even superior to analysis of the surgical resection specimen, especially in patients where the tumor had been subjected to neoadjuvant chemo- and/or radiotherapy [70, 71]. As outlined, the diagnosis of Lynch-associated CRC prior to surgery optimally would allow determining extent of surgery according to disease and patient factors. There are no randomized studies suggesting that Lynch patients that undergo extended surgery have a survival advantage compared to patients undergoing segmental oncologic resection. Retrospective studies have demonstrated that patients undergoing extended procedures will develop less metachronic cancers and will undergo less subsequent procedures for CRC [72]. In females, abdominal hysterectomy and bilateral salpingo-oophorectomy should be considered, either at the time of surgery for CRC or as a risk-reducing procedure after the completion of childbearing.

Figures 21.1 and 21.2, show examples of risk calculation based on gene and gender (www.lscarisk.org).

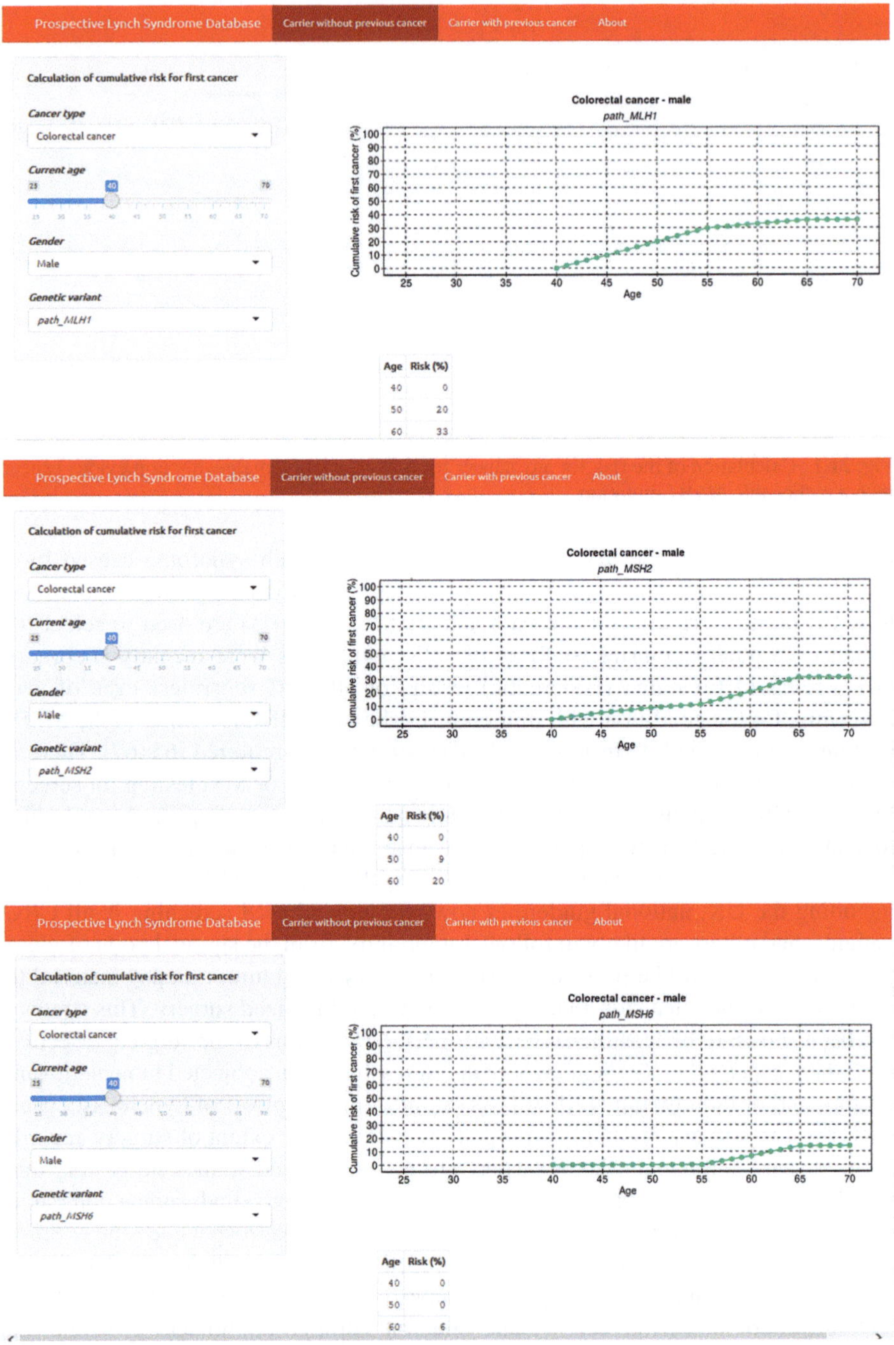

Fig. 21.2 Calculation of the risk for colorectal cancer for a 40-year-old male without previous cancer with a pathogenic mutation in *MLH1*, *MSH2*, and *MSH6*, respectively

2.2 *Management of the Newly Diagnosed Patient with Colorectal Cancer*

Most newly diagnosed CRCs in patients with Lynch syndrome present with a cancer proximal to the splenic flexure. But rectal as well as left colon cancers are frequently the sentinel cancer. Synchronous CRCs in HNPCC (clinical criteria) and Lynch syndrome (identified MMR mutation) have been reported to be present in 6–18% [73]. The cumulative incidences for any subsequent cancer from ages 40 to 70 have been reported to be 73% for pathogenic *MLH1* carriers, 76% for pathogenic *MSH2* carriers, and 52% for pathogenic *MSH6* carriers, and the cumulative incidences for CRC were 46%, 48%, and 23%, respectively [64]. The diagnostic workup for patients with colorectal cancer should include a complete pretreatment evaluation to clinically stage the tumor. If a familial colorectal cancer is suspected, screening for Lynch syndrome using IHC or MSI testing of the tumor biopsy material should be promptly initiated. If the screening turns out positive, germline mutation testing in the MMR genes should be performed to guide further management. In the future, tumor panel testing using a gene panel for cancer predisposition genes in all CRC patients may help identify any relevant gene mutations that have been shown to be present in about 10% of unselected CRC patients [69]. Pretreatment workup for any CRC must include all recommended parameters for sporadic cancer.

2.3 *Colon*

Because of the increased incidence of metachronous CRC in Lynch syndrome patients, a total abdominal colectomy with an ileorectal anastomosis (IRA) has been recommended as the procedure of choice at presentation of a primary colon cancer. Until now, studies showing a survival benefit of total vs. extended colectomy are lacking [74]. However, several retrospective studies have shown that extended resection significantly reduces the risk of metachronous colon cancer [72, 75]. Several mathematical models predict benefits of extended surgery including higher life expectancy especially in younger patients [76, 77]. However, the predicted benefit is only small or inexistent in older patients [78]. Therefore, the benefit of total colectomy must be weighed against the disadvantages of extended surgery. These include mainly defecation-related issues such as increased stool frequency of three to five bowel movements per 24 h [79] and social impact, while quality of life was similar in patients that received segmental vs. total colectomy [80]. Most patients eventually adapt to the change in bowel habits. Although IRA is a more extensive procedure compared to segmental colectomy, morbidity and mortality are low [79]. Importantly, IRA does not prevent rectal cancer that occurs in approximately 8–18% of patients during a median follow-up of 8–13 years after surgery for colon cancer [81–83]. Based on these observations, Cirillo et al. propose to perform total proctocolectomy with IPAA in Amsterdam-positive patients with a first-degree family history of rectal cancer [81]. Another option that may be discussed with patients concerned about functional outcomes after total colectomy is subtotal colectomy with ileosigmoid anastomosis (ISA). This procedure combines the advantages of extended colon surgery with a better functional outcome. Studies comparing IRA with IRA or segmental colectomy are lacking. We recently asked a group of experts (n = 73) for which type of surgery they would opt in the hypothetical event of receiving a diagnosis of a stage 1 or 2 right colon cancer with a Lynch-associated mutation at the age of 35 years. 32.9% would prefer subtotal colectomy with ISA, and 26% would elect for a segmental resection, 24.7% for total colectomy with IRA, and 13,7 for a total proctocolectomy with IPAA. Irrespective of performed surgery, patients will continue to need endoscopic surveillance of the remainder rectum and colon at risk.

2.4 Rectum

Like sporadic rectal cancer, treatment options in hereditary rectal cancer depend largely on the location of the tumor and its clinical stage. These options include local excision (rarely, and only in carefully selected patients), low anterior resection, abdominoperineal resection (APR) in case of sphincter involvement anorectal extirpation and end colostomy. In the setting of a hereditary disposition and in analogy to FAP, a restorative proctocolectomy with IPAA may be discussed. Results of a watch-and-wait strategy following complete pathologic remission with radiochemotherapy as reported by Habr-Gama [84] for sporadic rectal cancer have not been published for familial rectal cancer. In the absence of data, this interesting strategy for well-selected patients cannot be recommended in Lynch-associated rectal cancer. Restorative proctocolectomy theoretically eliminates the colonic and rectal cancer risk. The experience with this procedure in rectal cancer is scarce. However, comparable to patients with FAP, patients with Lynch-associated rectal cancer would need to undergo surveillance for the pouch, as neoplasia may, albeit rarely, form in the anal canal, the pouch-anal anastomosis, and even the ileal pouch. The risk of metachronous colon cancer after proctectomy for HNPCC was reported to be 17% (median duration after index colorectal cancer diagnosis, 203 months; range, 27–373 months) [85] and 15.2% (mean duration after proctectomy, 6 years; range, 3.5–16 years) [86], respectively. In total, 51.5% of the patients of the series from the Cleveland Clinic developed high-risk colonic adenoma or cancer after a median follow-up of 101.7 months after rectal resection with or without proctectomy. So, given this considerable risk of metachronous colonic neoplasia in LS patients, the option of proctocolectomy with IPAA should be discussed at the time of rectal cancer. However, as in determining the optimal extent of resection in hereditary colon cancer, other patient and disease factors need to be considered. The functional results of IPAA in LS should be compared to the very good functional outcomes in FAP versus ulcerative colitis with less pouchitis and fistula formation among others. The increased frequency of bowel movements and the other well-known functional constraints must be individually weighed by an informed patient versus the benefit in oncological outcome [10, 87].

Finally, all patients undergoing segmental or extended procedures for rectal cancer will be recommended to further pursue close endoscopic surveillance for early detection of further neoplasia.

2.5 The Asymptomatic Gene Mutation Carrier

2.5.1 Patients Managed with Segmental Resection

There is no evidence supporting completion colectomy in an asymptomatic patient that had previously been treated by segmental colectomy. These patients usually have received limited surgery either because the diagnosis of Lynch syndrome was unknown at the time of surgery or due to patient or physician preference. Treatment options include completion colectomy with ileorectal or ileosigmoid anastomosis in selected cases, surveillance, and chemoprevention. The recommended interval for colonoscopic surveillance is every 1–2 years [88]. In the CAPP2 trial, 600 mg aspirin per day for a mean duration of 25 months reduced cancer incidence after 55,7 months in carriers of hereditary colorectal cancer [89]. A follow-up study, the CAPP3 trial, is underway to determine the optimal dose and duration of aspirin treatment in mutation carriers [90].

2.5.2 Asymptomatic Mutation Carriers Without Previous CRC

Prophylactic colectomy should not be performed generally but may be offered to mutation carriers in whom colonoscopic surveillance is not technically feasible, who refuse to undergo regular colonoscopy, or who develop numerous polyps (see below). It may also be considered in patients with a disabling psychological impact due to anxiety of developing colorectal cancer. However, as mentioned earlier, patients will need to continue regular endoscopic surveillance, albeit with a lesser impact both regarding bowel preparations as well as the endoscopic procedure itself, since flexible sigmoidoscopy is much easier to perform with less associated risk than a complete colonoscopy.

2.5.3 Presence of Adenomas in the Gene Mutation Carrier

In Lynch syndrome, the adenoma to carcinoma sequence is thought to be accelerated compared to sporadic adenomas [91, 92], leading to carcinoma formation even if regular colonoscopy is performed [93]. Therefore, a more aggressive management compared to sporadic adenomas may be justified. The available treatment options for these patients include endoscopic polypectomy and close surveillance or surgical resection as for CRC in HNPCC. Factors to consider and to discuss with patients to inform decision for surveillance vs. surgery include size and number as well as histology of adenomas, the frequency of recurrence, the risk of interval cancer despite surveillance, and the morbidity of endoscopic and prophylactic surgical treatment.

2.6 Endometrial and Ovarian Cancer

Women diagnosed with Lynch syndrome carry an increased risk of endometrial and, to a lesser degree, ovarian cancer. The risk for women with HNPCC or Lynch syndrome to develop endometrial cancer ranges from 20% to 60% in various reports [94–96], and in some studies the risk exceeds the risk of CRC. The risk of ovarian cancer is increased to 5–12%. Obermair et al. reported that approximately 25% of women with HNPCC will develop endometrial cancer within 10 years after CRC diagnosis [97]. Equal to CRC, the risk for gynecologic cancers depends largely on the affected gene. In a recent prospective analysis of 1942 mutation carriers without previous cancer, the cumulative incidences for endometrial cancer for *MLH1*, *MSH2*, *MSH6*, and *PMS2* mutation carriers were 34%, 51%, 49%, and 24% and for ovarian cancer 11%, 15%, 0%, and 0%, respectively [93]. In patients undergoing colectomy for CRC, the opportunity to perform abdominal hysterectomy and bilateral salpingo-oophorectomy simultaneously should be discussed. In a prophylactic setting without neoplasia, abdominal hysterectomy and bilateral salpingo-oophorectomy should if possible be delayed until the completion of menopause or in premenopausal women after the completion of family planning. Patients need to be counseled about the long-term effects of early menopause including cardiovascular and skeletal effects as well as consequences for mood and sexual function [98]. Women undergoing prophylactic surgery did not develop cancer in a study including 300 women with Lynch-associated germline mutations, whereas 33% of the women that did not undergo prophylactic surgery developed endometrial and 5.5% ovarian cancer [99]. However, since HNPCC endometrial cancer has a good prognosis with a 5-year survival rate of 88% [100], prophylactic surgery might not decrease mortality. There are no prospective studies comparing prophylactic surgery for gynecologic cancers with surveillance in HNPCC patients.

2.7 Conclusions

The surgical care of patients with HNPCC and Lynch syndrome needs to be highly individualized. Disease and patient factors including pathogenic mutation and age at diagnosis need to be considered and discussed with the patient, ideally by a team specialized in the treatment of hereditary CRC. Segmental and extended (procto) colectomies are options if CRC is present but may in highly selected cases be offered to asymptomatic patients. Abdominal hysterectomy and bilateral salpingo-oophorectomy should be offered to women undergoing surgery for CRC and after family completion as a purely prophylactic measure, depending on the underlying gene affected.

References

1. Kobayashi H, Ishida H, Ueno H, et al. Association between the age and the development of colorectal cancer in patients with familial adenomatous polyposis: a multi-institutional study. Surg Today. 2017;47:690–6.
2. Rajaratnam SG, Eglinton TW, Hider P, et al. Impact of ileal pouch-anal anastomosis on female fertility: meta-analysis and systematic review. Int J Color Dis. 2011;26:1365.
3. Warrier SK, Kalady MF. Familial adenomatous polyposis: challenges and pitfalls of surgical treatment. Clin Colon Rectal Surg. 2012;25:083–9.
4. Gordon PH, Nivatvongs S. Principles and practice of surgery for the colon, rectum, and anus: CRC Press, Boca Raton, FL; 2007.
5. Debinski HS, Love S, Spigelman AD, et al. Colorectal polyp counts and cancer risk in familial adenomatous polyposis. Gastroenterology. 1996;110:1028–30.
6. Spigelman AD, Williams CB, Talbot IC, et al. Upper gastrointestinal cancer in patients with familial adenomatous polyposis. Lancet. 1989;2:783–5.
7. Lynch PM, Morris JS, Wen S, et al. A proposed staging system and stage-specific interventions for familial adenomatous polyposis. Gastrointest Endosc. 2016;84:115–125.e114.
8. Ishikawa H, Mutoh M, Iwama T, et al. Endoscopic management of familial adenomatous polyposis in patients refusing colectomy. Endoscopy. 2016;48:51–5.
9. Nieuwenhuis MH, LM M–V, Slors FJ, et al. Genotype-phenotype correlations as a guide in the management of familial adenomatous polyposis. Clin Gastroenterol Hepatol. 2007;5:374–8.
10. Soravia C, Klein L, Berk T, et al. Comparison of ileal pouch-anal anastomosis and ileorectal anastomosis in patients with familial adenomatous polyposis. Dis Colon Rectum. 1999;42:1028–33.
11. Van Duijvendijk P, Slors J, Taat C, et al. Quality of life after total colectomy with ileorectal anastomosis or proctocolectomy and ileal pouch—anal anastomosis for familial adenomatous polyposis. Br J Surg. 2000;87:590–6.
12. Bülow C, Vasen H, Järvinen H, et al. Ileorectal anastomosis is appropriate for a subset of patients with familial adenomatous polyposis. Gastroenterology. 2000;119:1454–60.
13. Stelzner F. Homingareale bei erblichen, synchronen und metachronen Rektokolonkrebsen. Chirurg. 2006;77:1056–60.
14. Koskenvuo L, Renkonen-Sinisalo L, Järvinen H, et al. Risk of cancer and secondary proctectomy after colectomy and ileorectal anastomosis in familial adenomatous polyposis. Int J Color Dis. 2014;29:225–30.
15. Bertario L, Russo A, Radice P, et al. Genotype and phenotype factors as determinants for rectal stump cancer in patients with familial adenomatous polyposis. Ann Surg. 2000;231:538–43.
16. Björk JA, Åkerbrant HI, Iselius LE, et al. Risk factors for rectal cancer morbidity and mortality in patients with familial adenomatous polyposis after colectomy and ileorectal anastomosis. Dis Colon Rectum. 2000;43:1719–25.
17. Bülow S, Bülow C, Vasen H, et al. Colectomy and ileorectal anastomosis is still an option for selected patients with familial adenomatous polyposis. Dis Colon Rectum. 2008;51:1318.
18. Durno C, Monga N, Bapat B, et al. Does early colectomy increase Desmoid risk in familial adenomatous polyposis? Clin Gastroenterol Hepatol. 2007;5:1190–4.
19. Sturt NJH, Clark SK. Current ideas in desmoid tumours. Familial Cancer. 2006;5:275–85.
20. Church JM, Xhaja X, Warrier SK, et al. Desmoid tumors do not prevent proctectomy following abdominal colectomy and ileorectal anastomosis in patients with familial adenomatous polyposis. Dis Colon Rectum. 2014;57:343–7.
21. Larson DW, Davies MM, Dozois EJ, et al. Sexual function, body image, and quality of life after laparoscopic and open ileal pouch-anal anastomosis. Dis Colon Rectum. 2008;51:392–6.
22. Kock NG. Intra-abdominal "reservoir" in patients with permanent ileostomy. Preliminary observations on a procedure resulting in fecal "continence" in five ileostomy patients. Arch Surg (Chicago, Ill 1960). 1969;99:223–31.

23. Gerber A, Apt MK, Craig PH. The improved quality of life with the Kock continent ileostomy. J Clin Gastroenterol. 1984;6:513–7.
24. Bonjer HJ, Deijen CL, Abis GA, et al. A randomized trial of laparoscopic versus open surgery for rectal cancer. N Engl J Med. 2015;372:1324–32.
25. Indar AA, Efron JE, Young-Fadok TM. Laparoscopic ileal pouch–anal anastomosis reduces abdominal and pelvic adhesions. Surg Endosc. 2009;23:174.
26. Bartels SA, D'hoore A, Cuesta MA, et al. Significantly increased pregnancy rates after laparoscopic restorative proctocolectomy: a cross-sectional study. Ann Surg. 2012;256:1045–8.
27. Fajardo AD, Dharmarajan S, George V, et al. Laparoscopic versus open 2-stage ileal pouch: laparoscopic approach allows for faster restoration of intestinal continuity. J Am Coll Surg. 2010;211:377–83.
28. Schiessling S, Leowardi C, Kienle P, et al. Laparoscopic versus conventional ileoanal pouch procedure in patients undergoing elective restorative proctocolectomy (LapConPouch Trial)—a randomized controlled trial. Langenbeck's Arch Surg. 2013;398:807–16.
29. Maartense S, Dunker MS, Slors JF, et al. Hand-assisted laparoscopic versus open restorative proctocolectomy with ileal pouch anal anastomosis: a randomized trial. Ann Surg. 2004;240:984–92.
30. Ueno H, Kobayashi H, Konishi T, et al. Prevalence of laparoscopic surgical treatment and its clinical outcomes in patients with familial adenomatous polyposis in Japan. Int J Clin Oncol. 2016;21:713–22.
31. Lindsey I, Guy R, Warren B, et al. Anatomy of Denonvilliers' fascia and pelvic nerves, impotence, and implications for the colorectal surgeon. Br J Surg. 2000;87:1288–99.
32. De Zeeuw S, Ahmed Ali U, Van Der Kolk MB, et al. Ileal pouch anal anastomosis with close rectal dissection using automated vessel sealers for ulcerative colitis: a promising alternative. Dig Surg. 2011;28:345–51.
33. Lindsey I, George BD, Kettlewell MGW, et al. Impotence after mesorectal and close rectal dissection for inflammatory bowel disease. Dis Colon Rectum. 2001;44:831–5.
34. Bartels S, Gardenbroek T, Aarts M, et al. Short-term morbidity and quality of life from a randomized clinical trial of close rectal dissection and total mesorectal excision in ileal pouch–anal anastomosis. Br J Surg. 2015;102:281–7.
35. Sylla P, Rattner DW, Delgado S, et al. NOTES transanal rectal cancer resection using transanal endoscopic microsurgery and laparoscopic assistance. Surg Endosc. 2010;24:1205–10.
36. Leo CA, Samaranayake S, Perry-Woodford ZL, et al. Initial experience of restorative proctocolectomy for ulcerative colitis by transanal total mesorectal rectal excision and single-incision abdominal laparoscopic surgery. Color Dis. 2016;18:1162–6.
37. Koedam T, Van Ramshorst G, Deijen C, et al. Transanal total mesorectal excision (TaTME) for rectal cancer: effects on patient-reported quality of life and functional outcome. Tech Coloproctol. 2017;21:25–33.
38. Kirat HT, Remzi FH. Technical aspects of ileoanal pouch surgery in patients with ulcerative colitis. Clin Colon Rectal Surg. 2010;23:239–47.
39. Möslein G. Surgical considerations in FAP-related pouch surgery: could we do better? Fam Cancer. 2016;15:457–66.
40. Parks A, Nicholls R. Proctocolectomy without ileostomy for ulcerative colitis. Br Med J. 1978;2:85–8.
41. Heald R, Allen D. Stapled ileo-anal anastomosis: a technique to avoid mucosal proctectomy in the ileal pouch operation. Br J Surg. 1986;73:571–2.
42. Slors J, Ponson A, Taat C, et al. Risk of residual rectal mucosa after proctocolectomy and ileal pouch-anal reconstruction with the double-stapling technique. Dis Colon Rectum. 1995;38:207–10.
43. Von Roon AC, Will OC, Man RF, et al. Mucosectomy with handsewn anastomosis reduces the risk of adenoma formation in the anorectal segment after restorative proctocolectomy for familial adenomatous polyposis. Ann Surg. 2011;253:314–7.
44. Ganschow P, Treiber I, Hinz U, et al. Residual rectal mucosa after stapled vs. handsewn ileal J-pouch-anal anastomosis in patients with familial adenomatous polyposis coli (FAP)—a critical issue. Langenbeck's Arch Surg. 2015;400:213–9.

45. Silva-Velazco J, Stocchi L, Wu X-R, et al. Twenty-year-old stapled pouches for ulcerative colitis without evidence of rectal cancer: implications for surveillance strategy? Dis Colon Rectum. 2014;57:1275–81.
46. Utsunomiya J, Iwama T, Imajo M, et al. Total colectomy, mucosal proctectomy, and ileoanal anastomosis. Dis Colon Rectum. 1980;23:459–66.
47. Hughes JP, Bauer AR, Bauer CM. Stapling techniques for easy construction of an ileal J-pouch. Am J Surg. 1988;155:783–5.
48. Schneider R, Schneider C, Dalchow A, et al. Prophylactic surgery in familial adenomatous polyposis (FAP)—a single surgeon's short-and long-term experience with hand-assisted proctocolectomy and smaller J-pouches. Int J Color Dis. 2015;30:1109–15.
49. Block M, Börjesson L, Lindholm E, et al. Pouch design and long-term functional outcome after ileal pouch–anal anastomosis. Br J Surg. 2009;96:527–32.
50. Campos FG. Surgical treatment of familial adenomatous polyposis: dilemmas and current recommendations. World Journal of Gastroenterology : WJG. 2014;20:16620–9.
51. Carne PWG, Pemberton JH. Technical aspects of ileoanal pouch surgery. Clin Colon Rectal Surg. 2004;17:35–41.
52. Sagar PM, Lewis W, Holdsworth PJ, et al. One-stage restorative proctocolectomy without temporary defunctioning ileostomy. Dis Colon Rectum. 1992;35:582–8.
53. Heuschen UA, Hinz U, Allemeyer EH, et al. Risk factors for ileoanal J pouch-related septic complications in ulcerative colitis and familial adenomatous polyposis. Ann Surg. 2002;235:207–16.
54. Miccini M, Bonapasta SA, Gregori M, et al. Ghost ileostomy: real and potential advantages. Am J Surg. 2010;200:e55–7.
55. Mari FS, Di Cesare T, Novi L, et al. Does ghost ileostomy have a role in the laparoscopic rectal surgery era? A randomized controlled trial. Surg Endosc. 2015;29:2590–7.
56. Hartley J, Church J, Gupta S, et al. Significance of incidental desmoids identified during surgery for familial adenomatous polyposis. Dis Colon Rectum. 2004;47:334–40.
57. Quast DR, Schneider R, Burdzik E, et al. Long-term outcome of sporadic and FAP-associated desmoid tumors treated with high-dose selective estrogen receptor modulators and sulindac: a single-center long-term observational study in 134 patients. Familial Cancer. 2016;15:31–40.
58. Brosens LA, Keller JJ, Offerhaus GJA, et al. Prevention and management of duodenal polyps in familial adenomatous polyposis. Gut. 2005;54:1034–43.
59. Galle TS, Juel K, Bülow S. Causes of death in familial adenomatous polyposis. Scand J Gastroenterol. 1999;34:808–12.
60. Groves C, Saunders B, Spigelman A, et al. Duodenal cancer in patients with familial adenomatous polyposis (FAP): results of a 10 year prospective study. Gut. 2002;50:636–41.
61. Kalady MF, Clary BM, Tyler DS, et al. Pancreas-preserving duodenectomy in the management of duodenal familial adenomatous polyposis. J Gastrointest Surg. 2002;6:82–7.
62. Watanabe Y, Ishida H, Baba H, et al. Pancreas-sparing total duodenectomy for Spigelman stage IV duodenal polyposis associated with familial adenomatous polyposis: experience of 10 cases at a single institution. Fam Cancer. 2017;16:91–8.
63. Samadder NJ, Neklason DW, Boucher KM, et al. Effect of sulindac and erlotinib vs placebo on duodenal neoplasia in familial adenomatous polyposis: a randomized clinical trial. JAMA. 2016;315:1266–75.
64. Møller P, Seppälä T, Bernstein I et al. Incidence of and survival after subsequent cancers in carriers of pathogenic MMR variants with previous cancer: a report from the prospective lynch syndrome database. Gut. 2016.
65. (Nice) TNIOCE. Molecular testing strategies for Lynch syndrome in people with colorectal cancer (DG27): NICE guidance; 2017.
66. Hampel H, Frankel WL, Martin E, et al. Screening for the Lynch syndrome (hereditary nonpolyposis colorectal cancer). N Engl J Med. 2005;66:1657–64.
67. Kastrinos F, Syngal S. Screening patients with colorectal cancer for Lynch syndrome: what are we waiting for? J Clin Oncol. 2012;30:1024–7.

68. Pearlman R, Frankel WL, Swanson B et al. Prevalence and Spectrum of Germline cancer susceptibility gene mutations among patients with early-onset colorectal cancer. JAMA Oncol. 2016.
69. Yurgelun MB, Kulke MH, Fuchs CS et al. (2017) Cancer susceptibility gene mutations in individuals with colorectal cancer. J Clin Oncol 0:JCO.2016.2071.0012.
70. Kumarasinghe AP, De Boer B, Bateman AC, et al. DNA mismatch repair enzyme immunohistochemistry in colorectal cancer: a comparison of biopsy and resection material. Pathology. 2010;42:414–20.
71. Vilkin A, Leibovici-Weissman YA, Halpern M, et al. Immunohistochemistry staining for mismatch repair proteins: the endoscopic biopsy material provides useful and coherent results. Hum Pathol. 2015;46:1705–11.
72. Kim TJ, Kim ER, Hong SN, et al. Survival outcome and risk of metachronous colorectal cancer after surgery in Lynch syndrome. Ann Surg Oncol. 2017;66:1657–64.
73. Fitzgibbons R Jr, Lynch HT, Stanislav GV, et al. Recognition and treatment of patients with hereditary nonpolyposis colon cancer (Lynch syndromes I and II). Ann Surg. 1987;206:289.
74. Stupart DA, Goldberg PA, Baigrie RJ, et al. Surgery for colonic cancer in HNPCC: total vs segmental colectomy. Color Dis. 2011;13:1395–9.
75. Parry S, Win AK, Parry B, et al. Metachronous colorectal cancer risk for mismatch repair gene mutation carriers: the advantage of more extensive colon surgery. Gut. 2010;2010:228056.
76. De Vos Tot Nederveen Cappel WH, Buskens E, Van Duijvendijk P, et al. Decision analysis in the surgical treatment of colorectal cancer due to a mismatch repair gene defect. Gut. 2003;52:1752–5.
77. Syngal S, Weeks JC, Schrag D, et al. Benefits of colonoscopic surveillance and prophylactic colectomy in patients with hereditary nonpolyposis colorectal cancer mutations. Ann Intern Med. 1998;129:787–96.
78. Maeda T, Cannom RR, Beart RW Jr, et al. Decision model of segmental compared with total abdominal colectomy for colon cancer in hereditary nonpolyposis colorectal cancer. J Clin Oncol. 2010;28:1175–80.
79. Elton C, Makin G, Hitos K, et al. Mortality, morbidity and functional outcome after ileorectal anastomosis. Br J Surg. 2003;90:59–65.
80. Haanstra JF, Tot Nederveen WHDV, Gopie JP, et al. Quality of life after surgery for colon cancer in patients with Lynch syndrome: partial versus subtotal colectomy. Dis Colon Rectum. 2012;55:653–9.
81. Cirillo L, Urso ED, Parrinello G, et al. High risk of rectal cancer and of metachronous colorectal cancer in probands of families fulfilling the Amsterdam criteria. Ann Surg. 2013;257:900–4.
82. Kalady MF, Mcgannon E, Vogel JD, et al. Risk of colorectal adenoma and carcinoma after colectomy for colorectal cancer in patients meeting Amsterdam criteria. Ann Surg. 2010;252:507–13.
83. Rodríguez-Bigas MA, Vasen H, Pekka-Mecklin J, et al. Rectal cancer risk in hereditary nonpolyposis colorectal cancer after abdominal colectomy. International Collaborative Group on HNPCC. Ann Surg. 1997;225:202.
84. Habr-Gama A, Perez RO, Nadalin W, et al. Operative versus nonoperative treatment for stage 0 distal rectal cancer following chemoradiation therapy: long-term results. Ann Surg. 2004;240:711–8.
85. Lee JS, Petrelli NJ, Rodriguez-Bigas MA. Rectal cancer in hereditary nonpolyposis colorectal cancer. Am J Surg. 2001;181:207–10.
86. Kalady MF, Lipman J, Mcgannon E, et al. Risk of colonic neoplasia after proctectomy for rectal cancer in hereditary nonpolyposis colorectal cancer. Ann Surg. 2012;255:1121–5.
87. Meagher A, Farouk R, Dozois R, et al. J ileal pouch–anal anastomosis for chronic ulcerative colitis: complications and long-term outcome in 1310 patients. Br J Surg. 1998;85:800–3.
88. HFA V, Blanco I, Aktan-Collan K, et al. Revised guidelines for the clinical management of Lynch syndrome (HNPCC): recommendations by a group of European experts. Gut. 2013;62:812–23.

89. Burn J, Gerdes A-M, Macrae F, et al. Long-term effect of aspirin on cancer risk in carriers of hereditary colorectal cancer: an analysis from the CAPP2 randomised controlled trial. Lancet. 2012;378:2081–7.
90. Burn J, Sheth H. The role of aspirin in preventing colorectal cancer. Br Med Bull. 2016;119:17–24.
91. Jass J, Smyrk TC, Stewart S, et al. Pathology of hereditary non-polyposis colorectal cancer. Anticancer Res. 1993;14:1631–4.
92. Vasen HF, Abdirahman M, Brohet R, et al. One to 2-year surveillance intervals reduce risk of colorectal cancer in families with Lynch syndrome. Gastroenterology. 2010;138:2300–6.
93. Møller P, Seppälä T, Bernstein I, et al. Cancer incidence and survival in Lynch syndrome patients receiving colonoscopic and gynaecological surveillance: first report from the prospective Lynch syndrome database. Gut:gutjnl-2015-309675; 2015.
94. Aarnio M, Mecklin JP, Aaltonen LA, et al. Life-time risk of different cancers in hereditary non-polyposis colorectal cancer (hnpcc) syndrome. Int J Cancer. 1995;64:430–3.
95. Dunlop MG, Farrington SM, Carothers AD, et al. Cancer risk associated with germline DNA mismatch repair gene mutations. Hum Mol Genet. 1997;6:105–10.
96. Quehenberger F, Vasen H, Van Houwelingen H. Risk of colorectal and endometrial cancer for carriers of mutations of the hMLH1 and hMSH2 gene: correction for ascertainment. J Med Genet. 2005;42:491–6.
97. Obermair A, Youlden DR, Young JP, et al. Risk of endometrial cancer for women diagnosed with HNPCC-related colorectal carcinoma. Int J Cancer. 2010;127:2678–84.
98. Faubion S, Kuhle CL, Shuster LT, et al. Long-term health consequences of premature or early menopause and considerations for management. Climacteric. 2015;18:483–91.
99. Schmeler KM, Lynch HT, Chen L-M, et al. Prophylactic surgery to reduce the risk of gynecologic cancers in the Lynch syndrome. N Engl J Med. 2006;354:261–9.
100. Boks DE, Trujillo AP, Voogd AC, et al. Survival analysis of endometrial carcinoma associated with hereditary nonpolyposis colorectal cancer. Int J Cancer. 2002;102:198–200.

Chapter 22
Chemoprevention in Hereditary Colorectal Cancer Syndromes

Reagan M. Barnett, Ester Borras, N. Jewel Samadder, and Eduardo Vilar

Abstract Patients and families diagnosed with hereditary colorectal cancer syndromes present with an accelerated carcinogenesis. In this scenario, screening measures and preventive interventions play a crucial role in modulating the cancer risk by decreasing its incidence and mortality. In this chapter we will provide an overview of the clinical evidence of chemopreventive interventions developed in Familial Adenomatous Polyposis and Lynch Syndrome. Specifically, we will present the use of non-steroidal anti-inflammatory drugs (NSAIDs), which have been the most commonly studied agents in this field. Finally, we will discuss the latest clinical trials deploying targeted agents and modern NSAIDs in the context of prevention of hereditary colorectal cancer syndromes.

Keywords Chemoprevention · Hereditary colorectal cancer syndromes · Nonsteroidal anti-inflammatory drugs · Aspirin · COX-2 inhibitors · Familial adenomatous polyposis · Lynch syndrome

Abbreviations

CIMP	CpG island methylator phenotype
CIN	Chromosomal instability
COX-2	Cyclooxygenase-2
coxib	COX-2 inhibitor
CRC	Colorectal cancer

R. M. Barnett · E. Borras · E. Vilar (✉)
Department of Clinical Cancer Prevention, The University of Texas MD Anderson Cancer Center, Houston, TX, USA
e-mail: EVilar@mdanderson.org

N. Jewel Samadder
Department of Internal Medicine, University of Utah College of Medicine, Salt Lake City, UT, USA

L. Valle et al. (eds.), *Hereditary Colorectal Cancer*,
https://doi.org/10.1007/978-3-319-74259-5_22

DFMO	Difluoromethylornithine
FAP	Familial adenomous polyposis
GI	Gastrointestinal
LS	Lynch syndrome
MMR	Mismatch repair
MSI	Microsatellite instability
NF-κB	Nuclear factor-kappa B
NSAID	Nonsteroidal anti-inflammatory drug
PG	Prostaglandin

1 Introduction

Colorectal cancer (CRC) is the third most common cancer diagnosed in both men and women in the United States and the second leading cause of cancer-related deaths [1]. Overall, the lifetime risk of developing CRC in the general population is approximately 6%, being the average age at diagnosis of 66 years [2]. Approximately 15–30% of patients diagnosed with CRC have a genetic component, given the occurrence of colorectal tumors in first- or second-degree relatives. These cases are termed *familial CRC* [3]. Approximately a fourth of *familial CRC* cases display specific phenotypic features in addition to their family history, thus leading to the diagnosis of a hereditary syndrome. This group of patients is named *hereditary CRC*, with the most prevalent conditions being familial adenomatous polyposis (FAP) and Lynch syndrome (LS). There are also other *hereditary CRC* syndromes that present with polyposis such as Peutz-Jeghers, juvenile polyposis, Cowden's syndrome, hyperplastic polyposis and hereditary-mixed polyposis and without polyposis such as familial colorectal cancer type X. These are however much more rare, and although chemopreventive interventions have been assessed, the level of available evidence is limited for these less common conditions.

Although *hereditary CRC* cases represent a small proportion of all patients diagnosed with colorectal tumors, carcinogenesis is accelerated due to their genetic defects affecting essential pathways involved in intestinal homeostasis, DNA repair, and other mechanisms [4]. Therefore, patients and families present with a higher lifetime risk of cancers and an earlier age of onset. In this scenario, screening measures and preventive interventions play a crucial role in modulating the cancer risk by decreasing its incidence and mortality. In addition, the molecular characteristics of premalignant lesions and tumors arising in these diseases can serve as a model, thus providing an excellent opportunity to understand the carcinogenic process and the activity of preventive interventions that could be later extrapolated to the sporadic setting (i.e., general population; see Fig. 22.1).

In this chapter we will provide an overview of the clinical evidence of chemopreventive interventions developed in FAP and LS. Specifically, we will present the use of nonsteroidal anti-inflammatory drugs (NSAIDs), which have been the most com-

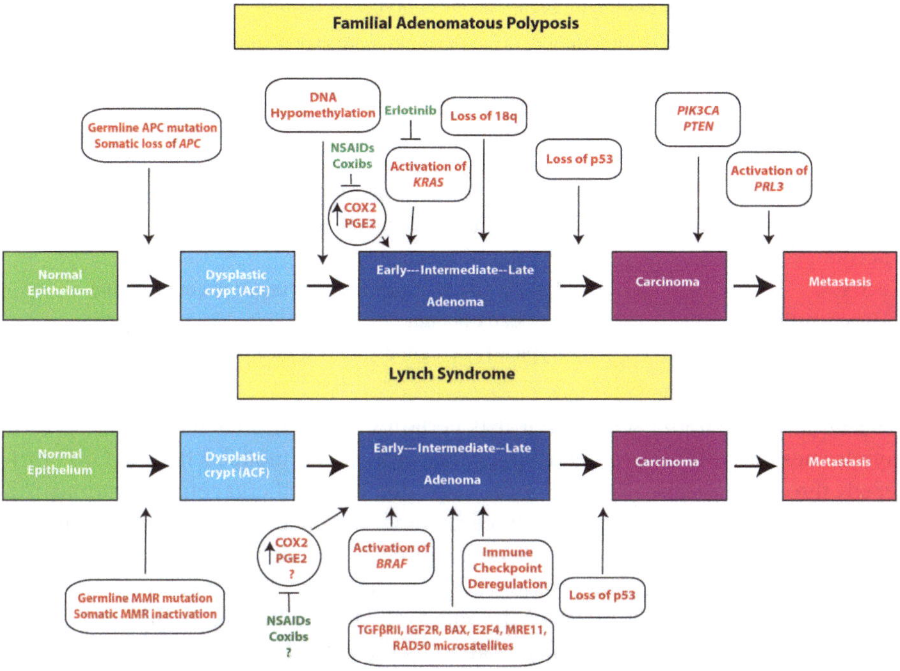

Fig. 22.1 Adenoma-carcinoma sequence. The top of the diagram displays the carcinoma sequence in FAP, while the bottom of the diagram shows the sequence in Lynch syndrome. In each scenario the patient will initially lose their second copy of the gene in which they have a germline mutation (e.g., FAP will experience a somatic loss of their wild-type *APC* gene). Subsequent mutations have been found to occur differently between FAP and LS tumors. COX-2 overexpression is known to be present in FAP tumors; however its status in MMR-deficient LS tumors is still being elucidated. However, NSAIDs have demonstrated benefit in both FAP and LS patients groups

monly studied agents in this field. Finally, we will discuss the latest clinical trials deploying targeted agents and modern NSAIDs in the context of prevention of *hereditary CRC* syndromes. This chapter does not intend to provide a systematic review of all the data developed but to highlight the main accomplishments and put them in the context of the most current research efforts in these two diseases.

2 The Normal Epithelium-Adenoma-Carcinoma Sequence

Cancer chemoprevention was first defined by Michael Sporn in 1976 as the use of natural, synthetic, or biologic chemical agents to reverse, suppress, or prevent carcinogenic progression [5]. It is based on the concepts of multifocal field and multistep carcinogenesis. The development of CRC is a complex process involving multiple molecular pathways from the formation of adenomas to the development of carcinoma in the digestive tract (Fig. 22.1). This process can take up to one

Table 22.1 Pathologic definition of adenoma and subtypes of lesions

Definition of adenoma: a benign tumor formed from glandular structures in epithelial tissues that occasionally becomes malignant	
Type of adenoma	Characteristics
Tubular	Most common adenoma, displaying a tubular structure
Villous	Typically sessile structures with cauliflower-like appearance and more likely to develop into malignancy
Tubulovillous	Less common, with both tubular and villous properties
Sessile	Flat, broad-based polyps
Serrated	Have a saw-tooth appearance under the microscope
Hyperplastic	Typically benign
Hamartoma	Typically benign, containing an abnormal mixture of cells

decade in the sporadic setting, but it is certainly much shorter in *hereditary CRC* syndromes. In 1990 Fearon and Vogelstein proposed a model whereby CRC proceeds through a series of pathological steps due to specific genetic alterations [6]. This model is called the adenoma to carcinoma sequence and emphasizes the central role of adenomas as precursor lesions (Table 22.1), and it provides evidence that in the majority of CRC, the primary event is the aberrant activation of the WNT pathway in the stem-cell niche of the intestinal crypt [7]. This is initiated by the inactivation of *APC*, consequently leading to the activation of B-catenin followed by the activation of RAS/RAF and the loss of *TP53* at later stages [6]. Although genetic alterations have an important role in the development of CRC carcinogenesis, also epigenetic variations in cancer-related genes and noncoding RNAs contribute to malignant progression [8, 9].

This model of CRC development has been recently revised, and, instead of a unique linear progression of events, three distinct pathways have emerged: 1. chromosomal instability (CIN), 2. microsatellite instability (MSI), and 3. CpG island methylator phenotype (CIMP) [10, 11]. The CIN pathway, also called the traditional pathway, is associated with the sequential deregulation of tumor suppressor genes (*APC* and *TP53*) and oncogenes (*KRAS*, *SMAD4*). Also, these tumors present an abnormal karyotype with several chromosomal gains and losses. This pathway has been associated with approximately 80–85% of sporadic CRC and also with inherited syndromes, such as FAP [12]. The MSI pathway is responsible for the 90% of tumors from LS patients and for 7–15% of sporadic CRC cases [13–16]. MSI in LS adenomas and carcinomas is generated by the acquisition of a second somatic hit in one of the DNA MMR genes. The instability introduced in coding microsatellites of target genes causes frameshift mutations and the subsequent functional inactivation of affected proteins, thereby providing a selective growth advantage. These tumors typically have high histological grades, a mucinous phenotype, and are diagnosed at lower pathological stages than CIN tumors [17]. Finally, the CIMP pathway is associated with tumors that show aberrant methylation in CpG sites affecting specific regulatory sites and promoter regions of tumor suppressor genes [18, 19]. The existence of this phenotype has been debated, and a consensus on which markers should be used for its definitions has not been described yet. The CIMP phenotype has been recently validated as an independent pathway using genome-wide methylation approach [20, 21].

The majority of chemopreventive drugs developed to prevent adenomas exert their function by inhibiting cyclooxygenase (COX), which is responsible for the formation of prostaglandins, thromboxane, and prostacyclin. Specifically, prostaglandins (PG) have been shown to play an important role in the transition from normal epithelium to adenoma and later to carcinoma [22, 23]. COX has two isoforms: COX-1 and COX-2. COX-1 is constitutively active, whereas COX-2 is not expressed in most tissues and is inducible at inflammation sites by growth factors and cytokines. In addition, COX-2 has been shown to induce carcinogenesis by inhibiting apoptosis, promoting cellular proliferation, and stimulating angiogenesis. Eberhart et al. first demonstrated that 85% of colorectal tumors displayed an overexpression of COX-2, as well as 50% of adenomas, thus making it an attractive target for treatment and prevention [24]. In addition, it has been shown that COX-2-derived prostaglandins may be acting on surrounding cells to promote tumor growth, either via a cell-autonomous or a cell-nonautonomous effect [25]. COX-2 inhibitors, such as celecoxib and rofecoxib (coxibs), have been developed as chemopreventive strategies and have shown much potential in both preclinical and clinical trials. As NSAIDs appear to exert most of their antineoplastic effects via inhibition of COX-2, these agents have also been extensively assessed for their prevention potential and better safety profile compared to COX-2 inhibitors. However, other evidence suggests that NSAIDs may also have antineoplastic effects that are independent of COX-2 suppression [26]. One such mechanism is through the inhibition of caspases, resulting in a reduction in cell death and pro-inflammatory cytokines, marking a COX-independent anti-inflammatory mechanism [27]. Secondly, NSAIDs have been shown to downregulate nuclear factor-kappa B (NF-κB) [28]. NF-κB is a ubiquitous factor involved in gene regulation, especially as it relates to immune responses. When activated, NF-κB promotes chemoresistance through promoting cell survival. Specifically, NSAIDs have been found to inhibit the I-κB kinase β enzyme responsible for activating NF-κB, resulting in NF-κB's downregulation [29]. Other possible COX-independent mechanisms include alteration of apoptotic proteins and consequently the extrinsic and intrinsic apoptotic pathways, as well as proteasome function and cell cycle checkpoints [28].

3 Chemoprevention in Familial Adenomatous Polyposis

Since FAP patients develop hundreds to thousands of adenomas in the lower gastrointestinal tract (GI) and also in the upper GI tract, there is a high lifetime risk for CRC development in individuals whose adenomas are not removed. Prophylactic surgery is the standard recommendation in this patient population. However, after colectomy, other manifestations of the syndrome continue to put patients at risk of cancer. In fact, those patients that elect rectal-sparing procedures continue developing adenomas and have excessive risk for rectal cancer. Also, duodenal adenomas develop in the vast majority of FAP patients and have the potential to progress into invasive cancer in up to 10%. Therefore, prophylactic colorectal surgery does not completely eliminate the risk of developing cancer, and therefore there is still a need for an exhaustive follow-up and chemoprevention development. Moreover, this type of surgery is normally performed in young individuals and produces strong consequences on their physical and psychological development, thus impacting their quality of life. Therefore, the development of chemopreventive agents is an unmet need, due to their ability to possibly delay the age of prophylactic surgery or potentially eliminate the need of these procedures.

Sulindac Studies Initially, the efficacy of NSAIDs as chemopreventive agents in patients with hereditary CRC syndromes was suggested in families with FAP. In the 1983, the first case report demonstrated a drastic reduction of adenomatous polyps in FAP patients treated with sulindac [30]. After that, multiple randomized controlled trials were designed and executed to test the clinical benefits of this agent [31–33]. The first randomized trial of sulindac versus placebo was published by Labayle in 1991 (Table 22.2) [33]. In this trial, 20 patients, all with colectomy and ileorectal anastomosis, were randomized to receive either placebo or sulindac 300 mg daily for 2 months. A significant reduction in rectal polyps was observed with a complete regression observed in six patients taking sulindac. Subsequently, two studies were published in 1993 and 2002 from the same group analyzing the efficacy of sulindac in reducing the number of polyps in FAP patients without prior prophylactic surgery [31, 32]. In the first study, 22 patients with FAP, including 18 who had not undergone colectomy, were randomized to receive either placebo or sulindac at a dose of 150 mg orally twice a day for 9 months. The number and size of the polyps every 3 months were evaluated. After 9 months of treatment, a significant decrease in the number of polyps (44%, $P = 0.014$) and their diameter (35%, $P < 0.001$) compared with the placebo arm was observed. Although there were not significant demographic differences in the two arms, the placebo group had a greater number of polyps at baseline (53 versus 28). It is noteworthy that the maximal effect of sulindac occurred at 6 months of treatment, while the number and size of the polyps increased after treatment with sulindac ceased at 9 months [31]. In the second study, 41 young FAP patients (8–25 years) with confirmed *APC* germline mutations, but without phenotypical manifestations, were randomized in a double-blind, placebo-controlled study. The subjects received either 75 or 150 mg of sulindac twice a day (according to their body weight) or the placebo for 48 months. No significant differences in the number of polyps between the two arms were observed. In both studies, no adverse events from sulindac were noted [32].

More additional data from small studies have reproduced similar results [34]. While treatment with sulindac appears to induce regression in the number and size of polyps, the effect appears to be restricted to the duration of treatment. The benefits of sulindac are also limited to the large intestine, thus signifying differences in biology between duodenum and colorectal adenomas and also a need for chemopreventive agents that reduced polyp burden in both the large and small GI tract, given

Table 22.2 Summary of clinical trials conducted in FAP patients

References	Syndrome	Drug	Type of study	Trial number	Outcome
Pfizer	FAP	Celecoxib	Clinical trial	NCT00151476	Terminated prior to completion
CHIP trial	FAP	Celecoxib	Clinical trial	NCT00585312	Terminated prior to completion
Labayle (1991)	FAP	Sulindac	Clinical study	N/A	Decrease in rectal polyps
Van Stolk (2000)	FAP	Sulindac sulfone	Clinical trial	N/A	No decrease in polyp number
Steinbach (2000)	FAP	Celecoxib	Clinical study	N/A	Reduction in colorectal polyps
Phillips (2002)	FAP	Celecoxib	Clinical study	N/A	Reduction in duodenal polyps
Giardiello (2002)	FAP	Sulindac	Clinical study	N/A	No decrease in adenoma number
Higuchi (2003)	FAP	Rofecoxib	Clinical study	N/A	Decrease in number and size of polyps
Hallak (2003)	FAP	Rofecoxib	Clinical study	N/A	Inhibition of polyposis
Bertagnolli (2006)	FAP	Celecoxib	Clinical trial	NCT00005094	Not reported
Arber (2006)	FAP	Celecoxib	Clinical trial	N/A	Reduced colorectal polyps
Lynch (2010)	FAP (children)	Celecoxib	Clinical trial (KIM)	NCT00685568	Reduced colorectal polyps
Burn (2011)	FAP	Aspirin	Clinical trial	N/A	Decrease in polyp number and size
Nagengast (2013)	FAP	Celecoxib	Clinical trial	NCT00808743	Not reported

N/A not available

the risks among FAP patients for cancer in both of these organs and more specifically during the past decade in the duodenum [35]. Moreover, long-term use of NSAIDs generates gastrointestinal side effects such as bleeding, ulceration, and cardiovascular effects, which has fostered interest in developing more selective and targeted approaches [36–39]. Currently there are studies being conducted to remedy these limitations and concerns.

Celecoxib Studies The first clinical trial that studied celecoxib as a chemopreventive agent in FAP patients was led by investigators in MD Anderson Cancer Center [40, 41]. Seventy-seven patients, without surgery and with polyps at the baseline colonoscopy, were randomized in a 2:1:1 fashion to receive either 100 or 400 mg of celecoxib twice daily or placebo for 6 months. The study demonstrated that treatment with the two doses reduced the number of polyps and the polyp burden. After 6 months the patients receiving 100 or 400 mg of celecoxib had 11.9% and 28.0%

reduction in the mean number of colorectal polyps, respectively. Also, there is a reduction in the polyp burden of 14.6% in patients treated with 100 mg and 30.7% in those patients treated with 400 mg of celecoxib, respectively. The incidence of side effects was similar among the groups. These results led to the approval of celecoxib by the FDA as chemopreventive agent in families with FAP.

After this clinical trial, additional coxibs were studied. In 2003, two small studies, Hallak et al. and Higuchi et al., were conducted with 8 and 21 patients, respectively, resulting in a significant reduction in the size and number of polyps [42, 43]. In Hallak et al., the patients were treated with rofecoxib 25 mg per day, resulting in a highly significant reduction in the rate of polyp formation (70–100%) in all patients at 1 year and at the end of follow-up (mean 16 months) [43]. Also, a study by Higuchi et al. treated the patients with 25 mg of rofecoxib a day for 9 months [42]. At 9 months, the rofecoxib group showed a significant reduction in polyp number and size of 6.8% and 16.2%, respectively. In 2006, 1561 patients were randomized in a placebo-controlled double-blind study with a daily dose of 400 mg celecoxib for 3 years [44]. The results demonstrated that the use of celecoxib reduced the occurrence of adenomas (RR 0.64; 95% CI, 0.56–0.75) within 3 years after polypectomy. Also, they detected serious cardiovascular events in 2.5% of subjects in the celecoxib group and 1.9% of those in the placebo group.

Furthermore, subsequent clinical trials with celecoxib in the general population of individuals at moderate-high risk for CRC showed that long-term use of coxibs was associated with unacceptable cardiovascular side effects [38, 39, 45]. Based on the safety data developed in sporadic populations, the benefit of regular use of coxibs in terms of delaying the growth of polyps and delaying prophylactic surgery in patients with FAP needs to be weighed against the risk of toxic cardiovascular effects. Since the onset of polyps in patients with FAP begins occurring during the teenage years, the toxicity profile of coxibs in these patients with FAP may be essentially different from that in the general population. In fact, Lynch et al. (2010) demonstrated that celecoxib at a dose of 16 mg/kg/day in children (10–14 years) with FAP is safe, well tolerated, and produced a significant reduction of the number of colorectal polyps [46].

Aspirin and Other NSAIDs Given the potential cardiovascular side effects of coxibs, the focus of efforts to develop chemoprevention drugs for patients with hereditary CRC syndromes has turned into aspirin, which has shown beneficial effects in terms of cardiovascular disease and CRC prevention with long-term use. The concerted action polyp prevention (CAPP) group accomplished an international, multicenter, randomized, placebo-controlled trial (CAPP1 protocol) of aspirin and/or resistant starch in young FAP patients with confirmed *APC* mutations for 1–12 years [47, 48]. In a 2x2 factorial design, a total of 206 FAP patients were randomly assigned to four study arms: aspirin (600 mg daily), resistant starch (30 g daily), aspirin plus resistant starch, and placebo. After 17 months of treatment, the risk of an increased polyp number in the rectum and sigmoid colon was not significantly reduced in either the aspirin or resistant starch group, with relative risks of 0.77 for aspirin (95% CI 0.54–1.10 aspirin versus non-aspirin group and 1.05 for resistant starch; 95% CI 0.73–1.49 resistant starch versus nonresistant starch group).

Noteworthy, the diameter of the largest polyp detected by endoscopy at the end of intervention tended to be smaller in the aspirin group ($P = 0.05$). In addition, the planned subgroup analyses of patients who elected to continue on the study for more than 1 year found a significant reduction in the size of the largest polyps in the aspirin group ($P = 0.02$). In summary, the CAPP1 study found a trend toward reduced polyp load (number and size) with 600 mg of aspirin daily. However, this study does not provide sufficient evidence to recommend long-term use of aspirin in FAP patients, and long-term toxicity studies would still need to be conducted.

Combination Studies: DFMO Combinations Polyamines (putrescine, spermidine, and spermine) are low-molecular-weight, organic cations that are ubiquitous in all higher eukaryotes. Polyamine levels are elevated in neoplastic tissues compared to normal tissues and in presymptomatic patients with FAP. Activity of ornithine decarboxylase (ODC), the first enzyme in the polyamine synthesis, is also significantly elevated in presymptomatic patients with germline *APC* mutations [49].

Difluoromethylornithine (DFMO) is a potent enzyme-activated irreversible inhibitor of ODC and inhibits the promotion and proliferation/progression stages of initiated cancer cells [50–52]. Although DFMO is thought to inhibit proliferation of fast-growing colon adenomas and CRC cells by polyamine depletion, the chemopreventive mechanism of polyamine depletion is not clear. Recently, Witherspoon et al. identified the first shared mechanism for CRC chemoprevention and chemotherapy suggesting a common metabolic target for both premalignant and malignant colon cells [53]. They conducted an untargeted metabolite profiling study of DFMO actions on cancer cell lines and intestinal tumors from *Apc*$^{Min/+}$ mice and found that DFMO has anti-CRC activity that arises from thymidine synthesis.

DMFO is the most studied example of a polyamine-metabolism inhibitor that suppresses cancer development in animal models leading to the design and implementation of prevention clinical trials of DFMO in CRC [54–57]. However, the efficacy of DFMO alone in polyp prevention has not been reported [58–61]. Moreover, the clinical use of DFMO has been limited by side effects found at high doses, including hearing loss, diarrhea, abdominal pain, emesis, anemia, leukopenia, and thrombocytopenia [58]. Studies in rodent models have shown that combination of DFMO and NSAIDs such as sulindac prevents the growth and viability of human colon cancer cells. After that, one phase III clinical chemoprevention trial evaluating the combination of DFMO and sulindac for the prevention of colon polyp recurrence in sporadic patients was published [54]. Three hundred seventy-five patients with history of resected adenomas were randomly assigned to receive DFMO 500 mg and sulindac 150 mg once daily or placebo for 36 months, stratified by use of aspirin (81 mg) at baseline and clinical site. Patients that received DFMO and sulindac had reduced recurrence of all adenomas (70% reduction) and advanced adenomas (92% reduction) and recurrence of more than one adenoma (95% reduction). There was no significant difference between the two arms in regard to serious side effects, but some patients presented hearing changes. Moreover, this study was not designed to have adequate power to identify differences in toxicity rates between two groups, such as cardiovascular toxicity. New trials will help us to determine the risk of cardiovascular events and also the clinical implications of audiological changes. Ultimately, DMFO with an NSAID treatment could be a good chemoprevention strategy in very high-risk populations, such as FAP. In fact, a clinical trial is currently ongoing for patients with FAP (NCT01483144).

Duodenal Adenoma Prevention Duodenal adenomas are also common in FAP patients and present a unique management situation when it comes to prevention, as some agents may act differently in the small intestine versus the large intestine in relation to prevention of adenomas [35]. Specifically, given the lack of effect sulindac has on the small intestine, combination studies have been considered. Recently, a study was published by Samadder et al. detailing their clinical trial with the combinatory treatment of sulindac and erlotinib on preventing duodenal neoplasia in FAP patients [62]. This was a double-blind randomized placebo-controlled study conducted with 92 participants diagnosed with FAP. Participants were given either 150 mg of sulindac twice daily combined with 75 mg of erlotinib once daily ($n = 46$) for 6 months or were placed on the placebo arm ($n = 46$). The end point of the trial was a positive change in duodenal polyp burden at 6 months compared to the baseline at trial initiation. A 71% reduction in duodenal polyp burden was observed between the treatment and placebo groups. In relation to toxicity, 87% of the sulindac-erlotinib group presented with acneiform rash, compared to 20% in the placebo group, and only two participants experienced grade three side effects. Based on this experience, a new clinical trial testing an alternative scheduling of erlotinib has been launched (NCT02961374). In this phase II trial, a dose of erlotinib of 350 mg once weekly will be administered to a total of 70 FAP patients. This study will examine the effects of erlotinib alone in reducing the polyp burden both in the small and the large intestine.

4 Chemoprevention in Lynch Syndrome

Chemoprevention in Lynch syndrome is a more complicated model to develop as endoscopic end points such as adenoma burden are more difficult to assess and the follow-up time required for an adequate clinical trial is longer than would be ideal. There is also a barrier in finding participants willing to participate in a trial with a placebo arm, which is important for separating results from possible psychosomatic influence [63, 64]. The CAPP3 study, which is currently ongoing, contains no placebo arm and has allowed the investigators to quickly obtain over 1000 participants, with the end goal being 3000. Since this trial is looking specifically at dosing of aspirin, withholding a placebo arm is logical, especially given the CAPP2 trial has included a placebo arm and the results have been communicated. However, other studies which require a placebo arm are beginning to offer other effective agents in place of a placebo in order to recruit more patients, who may be disinclined to participate otherwise. This has proved to be a particular problem in Lynch syndrome prevention trials, as well as in some prevention trials in general.

Aspirin Studies Aspirin has thus far been the primary NSAID for chemoprevention in Lynch syndrome patients, including a large clinical trial (CAPP2) that was conducted by Dr. John Burn in Europe (Table 22.3) [65–68]. A total of 861 Lynch syndrome patients were given 600 mg of aspirin or aspirin placebo or 30 mg resistant starch or starch placebo per day for up to 4 years. The end point of the study was development of CRC. At a mean follow-up time of 55.7 months, 18 of 427 participants on the aspirin arm and 30 of 434 in the aspirin placebo arm had developed CRC. They found 600 mg of aspirin given over an average of 25 months was effective in reducing CRC occurrence in LS patients. A total of 27 of 463 participants being given resistant starch and 26 of 455 participants on the starch placebo developed CRC, yielding no significant effect of resistant starch on cancer development in LS patients. A non-inferiority clinical trial (CAPP-3) is now being conducted by the same group to study the long-term effect of aspirin at different doses, including 100, 300, or 600 mg per day in 3000 Lynch syndrome patients [48].

In the CAPP2 study, the team also evaluated the effect of aspirin on obesity in LS patients and how it related to risk reduction [69]. They demonstrated that LS participants who were obese had an increased risk of CRC. Each increase of 1 kg/m2 in BMI resulted in a 7% increase of CRC risk, double what has been seen in the general population. Aspirin use was actually seen to abrogate the excess cancer risk in these patients. Overall, this study demonstrated the further benefits of aspirin chemoprevention but also highlighted the potential benefit for lifestyle interventions in overweight and/or obese patients with LS.

Further Studies A phase I–II multidose safety and efficacy of celecoxib in LS patients was concluded in 2002; however the clinical results related to polyp burden or cancer reduction have not been made available (NCT00001693). The participants were given either 200 mg or 400 mg of celecoxib or a placebo for 12 months. However, a paper by Glebov et al. did report that the trial saw changes in gene expression in healthy colonic samples, suggesting celecoxib may inhibit inflammation [70]. The authors identified 175 genes that showed significant alteration between pre- and posttreatment biopsies from 25 patients, with many of these genes related to immune response. However, more research is needed to determine the clinical relevancy of these results.

A new wave of early phase clinical trials are being conducted with other NSAIDs that show an improved cardiovascular safety profile, such as naproxen [71]. Currently, there is a multicenter phase 1b biomarker trial of naproxen in patients who are at risk for MMR-deficient CRC (NCT02052908). This study includes both mutation-positive and mutation-negative LS patients ($n = 80$) that are randomized to either 440 mg, 220 mg naproxen, or placebo for a total of 6 months. All participants undergo colonoscopy before and after the intervention as well as collection of blood, plasma, tissue, and urine for subsequent biomarker studies with mRNA-seq, miRNA-seq and determination of levels PGE2 in tissue, naproxen in blood and plasma, and PGM in urine. The primary end point of this trial is safety and modulation of PGE2 levels in tissue. This study has completed accrual, and its results are expected for early 2018.

Table 22.3 Summary of clinical trials conducted in LS

References	Syndrome	Drug	Type of study	Trial number	Outcome
NCI (1998)	LS	Celecoxib	Clinical trial	NCT00001693	Results not available
Glebov (2006)	LS	Celecoxib	Clinical trial	NCT27002448	Not reported
Rijcken (2007)	LS	Sulindac	Clinical trial	N/A	Benefit not seen adverse effect of increased cell proliferation observed
Burn (2008)	LS	Aspirin	Clinical trial	ISRCTN59521990	No adenoma or carcinoma reduction seen
Burn (2011)	LS	Aspirin	Clinical trial	ISRCTN59521991	Reduced polyp burden
Burn (2016)	LS	Aspirin	Clinical trial	(trial ID- EudraCT) #2014–000411-14	Ongoing
CAPP3 (2017)	LS	Aspirin	Clinical trial	NCT02497820 (Israel)	Ongoing
Vilar (2017)	LS	Naproxen	Clinical trial	NCT 02052908	Ongoing

N/A not available

5 Limitations

There are several obstacles which need to be overcome when it comes to chemoprevention in *hereditary CRC* syndromes. First, this method of prevention is only a viable option for patients with an identified germline mutation in either *APC* or one of the Lynch syndrome-associated genes (*MLH1*, *MSH2*, *MSH6*, *PMS2*, *EPCAM*). For patients with a variant of uncertain significance (VUS), Lynch-like patients [72], and familial cancer type X patients, the value of chemoprevention is not known [73]. This approach is also limited by individuals who refuse genetic testing as well as those who the medical professional fails to identify as being at risk for these conditions. In short, chemoprevention is limited to those who are identified as being at risk for FAP or LS, are offered genetic testing, accept genetic testing, and receive a mutation-positive test result in one of the relevant genes.

Secondly, willingness of health-care professionals to recommend chemoprevention, especially in the case of Lynch syndrome, can be an obstacle. While sulindac and celecoxib are well established in prevention of adenomas and CRC in FAP patients, the use of aspirin in LS patients is still being evaluated. There are no concrete guidelines for optimal dosage and duration of aspirin in LS, which lends to hesitancy among professionals to recommend it. Chen et al. published a study in

2017 evaluating willingness of medical teams to recommend aspirin for risk reduction among their LS patients [74]. A cohort of 181 professionals responded to their query, including 59 genetics specialists, 49 gastroenterologists, and 73 colorectal surgeons. Seventy-six percent of clinicians believe aspirin was an effective method of risk reduction in this population, and 72% felt comfortable discussing it with their patients. Eighty percent of genetics specialists had discussed aspirin with their patients, compared to 69% of gastroenterologists and 68% of colorectal surgeons. Health-care professionals who were confident in their knowledge of aspirin as a chemopreventive as well as those who saw ten or more LS patients per year were both more likely to recommend this method of risk reduction to their patients. Seventy-eight percent reported they had explicitly recommended aspirin to their patients. Eighty-seven percent believed more patient literature was needed for education about aspirin use. Since geographic location has not been assessed, it is possible that some of these percentages could be drastically reduced in more rural areas where LS is not as well known. More research in this area is warranted for further understanding barriers which either exist or are perceived to exist.

Third, the interest by pharmaceutical companies in developing agents for the field of prevention has been minimal during the last two decades. In fact, the notable failure of celecoxib in FAP has steered many companies away from this field. Also the need for long-term follow-up to observe incidence of cancer as well as the difficulty to mobilize enough number of patients is perceived as a barrier to entry in the field by many companies.

6 Conclusion

The ultimate goal of chemoprevention in groups at high risk for GI cancers is to reduce polyp burden, prolong the need for prophylactic colectomy, prevent cancer development, and potentially decrease the frequency of screening procedures. An ideal and effective chemopreventive agent will accomplish all of the above and also be effective in both the upper and lower GI tract. There has been considerable progress in identifying potential drugs to accomplish this including novel immunotherapy approaches such as checkpoint inhibitors and vaccines [75, 76], but we still have more work to do in order to each of those goals with a single agent. Significant thought must be interjected into future clinical trial designs in order to achieve success, and they should be guided by successful preclinical models. The limitations which have been discovered in previous studies should be taken into consideration when moving forward. If we are critical of our ideas and expectations, thoughtful in our trial design, and impeccable in our execution, then we will find an efficacious method for preventing hereditary colorectal cancers.

Conflict of Interest The authors declare no conflicts of interest.

References

1. Siegel R, Ma J, Zou Z, Jemal A. Cancer statistics, 2014. CA Cancer J Clin. 2014;64(1):9–29.
2. Hawk ET, Levin B. Colorectal cancer prevention. J Clin Oncol. 2005;23(2):378–91.
3. Taylor DP, Burt RW, Williams MS, Haug PJ, Cannon-Albright LA. Population-based family history-specific risks for colorectal cancer: a constellation approach. Gastroenterology. 2010;138(3):877–85.
4. Fearon ER. Molecular genetics of colorectal cancer. Annu Rev Pathol. 2011;6:479–507.
5. Sporn MB, Dunlop NM, Newton DL, Smith JM. Prevention of chemical carcinogenesis by vitamin A and its synthetic analogs (retinoids). Fed Proc. 1976;35(6):1332–8.
6. Fearon ER, Vogelstein B. A genetic model for colorectal tumorigenesis. Cell. 1990;61(5):759–67.
7. Barker N, Ridgway RA, van Es JH, van de Wetering M, Begthel H, van den Born M, et al. Crypt stem cells as the cells-of-origin of intestinal cancer. Nature. 2009;457(7229):608–11.
8. Bonasio R, Tu S, Reinberg D. Molecular signals of epigenetic states. Science. 2010;330(6004):612–6.
9. Pancione M, Remo A, Colantuoni V. Genetic and epigenetic events generate multiple pathways in colorectal cancer progression. Pathol Res Int. 2012;2012:509348.
10. Issa J-P. Colon cancer: it's CIN or CIMP. Clin Cancer Res off J am Assoc Cancer Res. 2008;14(19):5939–40.
11. Hanahan D, Weinberg RA. Hallmarks of cancer: the next generation. Cell. 2011;144(5):646–74.
12. Grady WM, Carethers JM. Genomic and epigenetic instability in colorectal cancer pathogenesis. Gastroenterology. 2008;135(4):1079–99.
13. Aaltonen LA, Peltomäki P, Leach FS, Sistonen P, Pylkkänen L, Mecklin JP, et al. Clues to the pathogenesis of familial colorectal cancer. Science. 1993;260(5109):812–6.
14. Ionov Y, Peinado MA, Malkhosyan S, Shibata D, Perucho M. Ubiquitous somatic mutations in simple repeated sequences reveal a new mechanism for colonic carcinogenesis. Nature. 1993;363(6429):558–61.
15. González-García I, Moreno V, Navarro M, Martí-Ragué J, Marcuello E, Benasco C, et al. Standardized approach for microsatellite instability detection in colorectal carcinomas. J Natl Cancer Inst. 2000;92(7):544–9.
16. Pedroni M, Tamassia MG, Percesepe A, Roncucci L, Benatti P, Lanza G, et al. Microsatellite instability in multiple colorectal tumors. Int J Cancer. 1999;81(1):1–5.
17. Vilar E, Gruber SB. Microsatellite instability in colorectal cancer-the stable evidence. Nat Rev Clin Oncol. 2010;7(3):153–62.
18. Toyota M, Ahuja N, Suzuki H, Itoh F, Ohe-Toyota M, Imai K, et al. Aberrant methylation in gastric cancer associated with the CpG island methylator phenotype. Cancer Res. 1999;59(21):5438–42.
19. Ballestar E, Esteller M. SnapShot: the human DNA methylome in health and disease. Cell. 2008;135(6):1144. e1.
20. Liu Y, Siegmund KD, Laird PW, Berman BP. Bis-SNP: combined DNA methylation and SNP calling for Bisulfite-seq data. Genome Biol. 2012;13(7):R61.
21. Hinoue T, Weisenberger DJ, Lange CPE, Shen H, Byun H-M, Van Den Berg D, et al. Genome-scale analysis of aberrant DNA methylation in colorectal cancer. Genome Res. 2012;22(2):271–82.
22. Tsujii M, DuBois RN. Alterations in cellular adhesion and apoptosis in epithelial cells overexpressing prostaglandin endoperoxide synthase 2. Cell. 1995;83(3):493–501.
23. Sawaoka H, Kawano S, Tsuji S, Tsujii M, Murata H, Hori M. Effects of NSAIDs on proliferation of gastric cancer cells in vitro: possible implication of cyclooxygenase-2 in cancer development. J Clin Gastroenterol. 1998;27(Suppl 1):S47–52.
24. Eberhart CE, Coffey RJ, Radhika A, Giardiello FM, Ferrenbach S, DuBois RN. Up-regulation of cyclooxygenase 2 gene expression in human colorectal adenomas and adenocarcinomas. Gastroenterology. 1994;107(4):1183–8.

25. Gupta RA, Dubois RN. Colorectal cancer prevention and treatment by inhibition of cyclooxygenase-2. Nat Rev Cancer. 2001;1(1):11–21.
26. Fritsche E, Baek SJ, King LM, Zeldin DC, Eling TE, Bell DA. Functional characterization of cyclooxygenase-2 polymorphisms. J Pharmacol Exp Ther. 2001;299(2):468–76.
27. Smith CE, Soti S, Jones TA, Nakagawa A, Xue D, Yin H. Non-steroidal anti-inflammatory drugs are caspase inhibitors. Cell Chem Biol. 2017;24(3):281–92.
28. Jana NR. NSAIDs and apoptosis. Cell Mol Life Sci CMLS. 2008;65(9):1295–301.
29. Yin MJ, Yamamoto Y, Gaynor RB. The anti-inflammatory agents aspirin and salicylate inhibit the activity of I(kappa)B kinase-beta. Nature. 1998;396(6706):77–80.
30. Waddell WR, Loughry RW. Sulindac for polyposis of the colon. J Surg Oncol. 1983;24(1):83–7.
31. Giardiello FM, Hamilton SR, Krush AJ, Piantadosi S, Hylind LM, Celano P, et al. Treatment of colonic and rectal adenomas with sulindac in familial adenomatous polyposis. N Engl J Med. 1993;328(18):1313–6.
32. Giardiello FM, Yang VW, Hylind LM, Krush AJ, Petersen GM, Trimbath JD, et al. Primary chemoprevention of familial adenomatous polyposis with sulindac. N Engl J Med. 2002;346(14):1054–9.
33. Labayle D, Fischer D, Vielh P, Drouhin F, Pariente A, Bories C, et al. Sulindac causes regression of rectal polyps in familial adenomatous polyposis. Gastroenterology. 1991;101(3):635–9.
34. Barry ELR, Baron JA, Grau MV, Wallace K, Haile RW. K-ras mutations in incident sporadic colorectal adenomas. Cancer. 2006;106(5):1036–40.
35. Brosens LAA, Iacobuzio-Donahue CA, Keller JJ, Hustinx SR, Carvalho R, Morsink FH, et al. Increased cyclooxygenase-2 expression in duodenal compared with colonic tissues in familial adenomatous polyposis and relationship to the -765G -> C COX-2 polymorphism. Clin Cancer Res Off J Am Assoc Cancer Res. 2005;11(11):4090–6.
36. Bertoni G, Sassatelli R, Bedogni G, Nigrisoli E. Sulindac-associated ulcerative pouchitis in familial adenomatous polyposis. Am J Gastroenterol. 1996;91(11):2431–2.
37. Lanza LL, Walker AM, Bortnichak EA, Dreyer NA. Peptic ulcer and gastrointestinal hemorrhage associated with nonsteroidal anti-inflammatory drug use in patients younger than 65 years. A large health maintenance organization cohort study. Arch Intern Med. 1995;155(13):1371–7.
38. Patrono C. Cardiovascular effects of nonsteroidal anti-inflammatory drugs. Curr Cardiol Rep. 2016;18(3):25.
39. Anwar A, Anwar IJ, Delafontaine P. Elevation of cardiovascular risk by non-steroidal anti-inflammatory drugs. Trends Cardiovasc Med. 2015;25(8):726–35.
40. Steinbach G, Lynch PM, Phillips RK, Wallace MH, Hawk E, Gordon GB, et al. The effect of celecoxib, a cyclooxygenase-2 inhibitor, in familial adenomatous polyposis. N Engl J Med. 2000;342(26):1946–52.
41. Phillips RKS, Wallace MH, Lynch PM, Hawk E, Gordon GB, Saunders BP, et al. A randomised, double blind, placebo controlled study of celecoxib, a selective cyclooxygenase 2 inhibitor, on duodenal polyposis in familial adenomatous polyposis. Gut. 2002;50(6):857–60.
42. Higuchi T, Iwama T, Yoshinaga K, Toyooka M, Taketo MM, Sugihara K. A randomized, double-blind, placebo-controlled trial of the effects of rofecoxib, a selective cyclooxygenase-2 inhibitor, on rectal polyps in familial adenomatous polyposis patients. Clin Cancer Res Off J Am Assoc Cancer Res. 2003;9(13):4756–60.
43. Hallak A, Alon-Baron L, Shamir R, Moshkowitz M, Bulvik B, Brazowski E, et al. Rofecoxib reduces polyp recurrence in familial polyposis. Dig Dis Sci. 2003;48(10):1998–2002.
44. Arber N, Eagle CJ, Spicak J, Rácz I, Dite P, Hajer J, et al. Celecoxib for the prevention of colorectal adenomatous polyps. N Engl J Med. 2006;355(9):885–95.
45. Garcia Rodriguez LA, Cea-Soriano L, Tacconelli S, Patrignani P. Coxibs: pharmacology, toxicity and efficacy in cancer clinical trials. Recent Results Cancer Res Fortschritte Krebsforsch Progres Dans Rech Sur Cancer. 2013;191:67–93.
46. Lynch PM, Ayers GD, Hawk E, Richmond E, Eagle C, Woloj M, et al. The safety and efficacy of celecoxib in children with familial adenomatous polyposis. Am J Gastroenterol. 2010;105(6):1437–43.

47. Burn J, Mathers J, Bishop DT. Genetics, inheritance and strategies for prevention in populations at high risk of colorectal cancer (CRC). Recent Results Cancer Res Fortschritte Krebsforsch Progres Dans Rech Sur Cancer. 2013;191:157–83.
48. Burn J, Mathers JC, Bishop DT. Chemoprevention in Lynch syndrome. Familial Cancer. 2013;12(4):707–18.
49. Giardiello FM, Hamilton SR, Hylind LM, Yang VW, Tamez P, Casero RA. Ornithine decarboxylase and polyamines in familial adenomatous polyposis. Cancer Res. 1997;57(2):199–201.
50. Celano P, Baylin SB, Casero RA. Polyamines differentially modulate the transcription of growth-associated genes in human colon carcinoma cells. J Biol Chem. 1989;264(15):8922–7.
51. Celano P, Berchtold CM, Giardiello FM, Casero RA. Modulation of growth gene expression by selective alteration of polyamines in human colon carcinoma cells. Biochem Biophys Res Commun. 1989;165(1):384–90.
52. Casero RA. Say what? The activity of the polyamine biosynthesis inhibitor difluoromethylornithine in chemoprevention is a result of reduced thymidine pools? Cancer Discov. 2013;3(9):975–7.
53. Witherspoon M, Chen Q, Kopelovich L, Gross SS, Lipkin SM. Unbiased metabolite profiling indicates that a diminished thymidine pool is the underlying mechanism of colon cancer chemoprevention by alpha-difluoromethylornithine. Cancer Discov. 2013;3(9):1072–81.
54. Meyskens FL, McLaren CE, Pelot D, Fujikawa-Brooks S, Carpenter PM, Hawk E, et al. Difluoromethylornithine plus sulindac for the prevention of sporadic colorectal adenomas: a randomized placebo-controlled, double-blind trial. Cancer Prev Res Phila Pa. 2008;1(1):32–8.
55. Jacoby RF, Seibert K, Cole CE, Kelloff G, Lubet RA. The cyclooxygenase-2 inhibitor celecoxib is a potent preventive and therapeutic agent in the min mouse model of adenomatous polyposis. Cancer Res. 2000;60(18):5040–4.
56. Rao CV, Tokumo K, Rigotty J, Zang E, Kelloff G, Reddy BS. Chemoprevention of colon carcinogenesis by dietary administration of piroxicam, alpha-difluoromethylornithine, 16 alpha-fluoro-5-androsten-17-one, and ellagic acid individually and in combination. Cancer Res. 1991;51(17):4528–34.
57. Erdman SH, Ignatenko NA, Powell MB, Blohm-Mangone KA, Holubec H, Guillén-Rodriguez JM, et al. APC-dependent changes in expression of genes influencing polyamine metabolism, and consequences for gastrointestinal carcinogenesis, in the Min mouse. Carcinogenesis. 1999;20(9):1709–13.
58. Meyskens FL, Gerner EW. Development of difluoromethylornithine (DFMO) as a chemoprevention agent. Clin Cancer Res Off J Am Assoc Cancer Res. 1999;5(5):945–51.
59. Love RR, Jacoby R, Newton MA, Tutsch KD, Simon K, Pomplun M, et al. A randomized, placebo-controlled trial of low-dose alpha-difluoromethylornithine in individuals at risk for colorectal cancer. Cancer Epidemiol Biomark Prev Publ Am Assoc Cancer Res Cosponsored Am Soc Prev Oncol. 1998;7(11):989–92.
60. Meyskens FL, Emerson SS, Pelot D, Meshkinpour H, Shassetz LR, Einspahr J, et al. Dose de-escalation chemoprevention trial of alpha-difluoromethylornithine in patients with colon polyps. J Natl Cancer Inst. 1994;86(15):1122–30.
61. Meyskens FL, Gerner EW, Emerson S, Pelot D, Durbin T, Doyle K, et al. Effect of alpha-difluoromethylornithine on rectal mucosal levels of polyamines in a randomized, double-blinded trial for colon cancer prevention. J Natl Cancer Inst. 1998;90(16):1212–8.
62. Samadder NJ, Neklason DW, Boucher KM, Byrne KR, Kanth P, Samowitz W, et al. Effect of sulindac and erlotinib vs placebo on duodenal neoplasia in familial adenomatous polyposis: a randomized clinical trial. JAMA. 2016;315(12):1266–75.
63. Vrhovac B. Placebo and its importance in medicine. Int J Clin Pharmacol Biopharm. 1977;15(4):161–5.
64. Ricciardiello L, Ahnen DJ, Lynch PM. Chemoprevention of hereditary colon cancers: time for new strategies. Nat Rev Gastroenterol Hepatol. 2016;13(6):352–61.
65. Burn J, Gerdes A-M, Macrae F, Mecklin J-P, Moeslein G, Olschwang S, et al. Long-term effect of aspirin on cancer risk in carriers of hereditary colorectal cancer: an analysis from the CAPP2 randomised controlled trial. Lancet Lond Engl. 2011;378(9809):2081–7.

66. Mathers JC, Movahedi M, Macrae F, Mecklin J-P, Moeslein G, Olschwang S, et al. Long-term effect of resistant starch on cancer risk in carriers of hereditary colorectal cancer: an analysis from the CAPP2 randomised controlled trial. Lancet Oncol. 2012;13(12):1242–9.
67. Burn J, Bishop DT, Mecklin J-P, Macrae F, Möslein G, Olschwang S, et al. Effect of aspirin or resistant starch on colorectal neoplasia in the Lynch syndrome. N Engl J Med. 2008;359(24):2567–78.
68. Liljegren A, Barker G, Elliott F, Bertario L, Bisgaard ML, Eccles D, et al. Prevalence of adenomas and hyperplastic polyps in mismatch repair mutation carriers among CAPP2 participants: report by the colorectal adenoma/carcinoma prevention programme 2. J Clin Oncol Off J Am Soc Clin Oncol. 2008;26(20):3434–9.
69. Movahedi M, Bishop DT, Macrae F, Mecklin J-P, Moeslein G, Olschwang S, et al. Obesity, aspirin, and risk of colorectal cancer in carriers of hereditary colorectal cancer: a prospective investigation in the CAPP2 Study. J Clin Oncol Off J Am Soc Clin Oncol. 2015;33(31):3591–7.
70. Glebov OK, Rodriguez LM, Lynch P, Patterson S, Lynch H, Nakahara K, et al. Celecoxib treatment alters the gene expression profile of normal colonic mucosa. Cancer Epidemiol Biomark Prev Publ Am Assoc Cancer Res Cosponsored Am Soc Prev Oncol. 2006;15(7):1382–91.
71. Nissen SE, Yeomans ND, Solomon DH, Lüscher TF, Libby P, Husni ME, et al. Cardiovascular safety of celecoxib, naproxen, or ibuprofen for arthritis. N Engl J Med. 2016;375(26):2519–29.
72. You YN, Vilar E. Classifying MMR variants: time for revised nomenclature in Lynch syndrome. Clin Cancer Res Off J Assoc Cancer Res. 2013;19(9):2280–2.
73. Boland CR. Recent discoveries in the molecular genetics of Lynch syndrome. Familial Cancer. 2016;15(3):395–403.
74. Chen Y, Peate M, Kaur R, Meiser B, Wong T, Kirk J, et al. Exploring clinicians' attitudes about using aspirin for risk reduction in people with Lynch syndrome with no personal diagnosis of colorectal cancer. Familial Cancer. 2017;16(1):99–109.
75. Spira A, Disis ML, Schiller JT, Vilar E, Rebbeck TR, Bejar R, et al. Leveraging premalignant biology for immune-based cancer prevention. Proc Natl Acad Sci U S A. 2016;113(39):10750–8.
76. Spira A, Yurgelun MB, Alexandrov L, Rao A, Bejar R, Polyak K, et al. Precancer atlas to drive precision prevention trials. Cancer Res. 2017;77(7):1510–41.

Chapter 23
The Immune Biology of Microsatellite Unstable Cancer

Matthias Kloor and Magnus von Knebel Doeberitz

Abstract Lynch syndrome-associated cancers arise through DNA mismatch repair (MMR) deficiency. MMR deficiency boosts the accumulation of insertion/deletion mutations at repetitive microsatellite sequences throughout the cancer cell genome (microsatellite instability, MSI). As microsatellite sequences are common in gene-encoding regions, MMR deficiency can cause gene inactivation through frameshift mutations. These frameshift mutations can trigger the generation of mutant proteins carrying novel amino acid sequences resulting from a shift of the translational reading frame (frameshift *neo*antigens). MSI cancers express a defined set of neoantigens, which are the direct result of functionally relevant driver mutations. The fact that these mutation events not only always affect the same genes but also exactly the same microsatellite loci within these genes leads to the unique situation that most MSI cancers share a precisely defined set of mutational *neo*antigens. MSI cancer patients frequently develop immune responses against these *neo*antigens. Surprisingly, such immune responses were also observed in tumor-free Lynch syndrome carriers, indicating that Lynch syndrome is characterized by lifelong interaction between the immune system and precancerous cells. We discuss the current knowledge about driver mutation-derived neoantigens, immune evasion mechanisms of MSI cancers, and potential clinical approaches to improve the host's immune response against frameshift neoantigens.

Keywords Cancer vaccines · Frameshift peptide neoantigens · Immune evasion · Immune therapy · Lynch syndrome · Microsatellite instability

---

M. Kloor (✉) · M. von Knebel Doeberitz
Department of Applied Tumor Biology, Institute of Pathology, University Hospital Heidelberg, Clinical Cooperation Unit (CCU 105) of the German Cancer Research Center and Molecular Medicine Partner Unit (MMPU) of the European Molecular Biology Laboratory, Heidelberg, Germany
e-mail: matthias.kloor@med.uni-heidelberg.de; Magnus.Knebel-Doeberitz@med.uni-heidelberg.de

L. Valle et al. (eds.), *Hereditary Colorectal Cancer*,
https://doi.org/10.1007/978-3-319-74259-5_23

1 Overview

Lynch syndrome-associated cancers arise through deficiency of the DNA mismatch repair (MMR) system. MMR deficiency boosts the accumulation of insertion/deletion mutations at repetitive sequence stretches throughout the cancer cell genome, a phenotype termed microsatellite instability (MSI). As such repetitive microsatellite sequences are also common in gene-encoding regions, MMR deficiency can directly lead to gene inactivation through frameshift mutations. In addition, frameshift mutations at coding microsatellites can trigger the generation of mutant proteins that carry novel amino acid sequences resulting from a shift of the translational reading frame (frameshift *neo*antigens). MSI cancers typically express a defined set of neoantigens, which are the direct result of functionally relevant driver mutations. The fact that these driver mutation events not only always affect the same genes but also exactly the same microsatellite loci in these genes leads to the unique situation that the majority of MSI cancers share a precisely defined set of mutational neoantigens. MSI cancer patients frequently develop specific immune responses against these neoantigens. Surprisingly, such immune responses were also observed in tumor-free Lynch syndrome mutation carriers, indicating that Lynch syndrome is characterized by a lifelong interaction between the immune system and potential precancerous cell clones. In the following, we outline the current knowledge about driver mutation-derived neoantigens and their role in the natural course of Lynch syndrome. We will discuss immune evasion mechanisms of MSI cancers and potential clinical approaches to improve patients' prognosis by modulating the host's anti-FSP immune responses.

2 Genomic Instability in Lynch Syndrome Cancers

Cancer outgrowth requires enormous phenotypic flexibility, which allows survival in changing conditions through selection of the fittest cancer cell clone [1]. The plasticity of cancer, which manifests in the classical survival-enhancing cancer hallmarks [2], is enabled by instability of the cancer cells' genome, which is a unifying feature of malignant tumors. The most common forms of genomic instability in cancer are chromosomal instability (CIN) [3, 4], genome-wide epigenetic alterations (CpG island methylator phenotype, CIMP) [5, 6], and DNA MMR deficiency, the latter being typical of Lynch syndrome-associated cancers.

Genomic instability provides cancer cells with high adaptability during the process of Darwinian evolution from an initiated cell clone toward large clinically apparent tumors. In addition, genomic instability leads to structural changes in proteins that can lead to the recognition of cancer cells by the immune system. Although structural changes due to genomic alterations are common in all types of malignant cancers, the "visibility" for the immune system is particularly high in MMR-deficient cancers that develop in the context of Lynch syndrome.

The reason for the pronounced immunogenicity of MMR-deficient cancers is rooted in the molecular mechanism that drives their development. In contrast to other types of genomic instability, mutations accumulating in MMR-deficient cancer cells are mostly insertion/deletion mutations. The phenotype of genomic alterations observed in MMR-deficient cancers is in fact dominated by insertion/deletion mutations at microsatellite sequences and therefore termed *microsatellite instability* (*MSI*) or *high-level microsatellite instability* (*MSI-H*).

If these insertion/deletion mutations affect microsatellite sequences in gene-encoding genome regions (coding microsatellites, cMS), they can, unlike missense mutations typically found in oncogenes such as *KRAS* or *BRAF*, lead to shifts of the translational reading frame and to mutational neoantigens that result from these frameshifts (frameshift peptides, FSPs). These FSPs in part encompass very long stretches of entirely novel amino acid sequences, which only occur in MMR-deficient cells harboring the respective frameshift mutation. In this regard, MMR-deficient cancers resemble virally infected cells, as they express a variety of antigens that are entirely foreign to the host's immune system. The link between the mechanisms of genomic instability enabling the outgrowth of Lynch syndrome-associated cancers and the recognition of these cancers by the host's immune system will be discussed in the following. As among Lynch syndrome-associated cancers, the largest body of information is available on colorectal cancer (CRC), which is also the most common and a clinically very relevant manifestation, we will start with this tumor type and its special clinical presentation in frame of Lynch syndrome.

3 Clinical Presentation of Lynch Syndrome Cancers

Lynch syndrome-associated CRCs display the MSI phenotype, which makes them strikingly different from sporadic, non-MSI CRCs. Histologically, typical features of Lynch syndrome-associated CRCs are poor differentiation, often with a mixed appearance containing areas of mucinous or solid growth, and a high number of tumor-infiltrating lymphocytes, which is in line with the favorable prognostic of these cancers [7–10]. In contrast to sporadic CRCs that predominantly develop in the distal colon, Lynch syndrome cancers more frequently grow out in the proximal colon, and they can be accompanied by syn- or metachronous occurrence of additional tumors. Although Lynch syndrome CRCs can grow to large local tumor masses, they rarely develop hematogenous metastases to distant organs [9, 11, 12], which is in line with the concept that the host's immune response may control tumor cell spread and dissemination.

All these clinical observations and histopathology characteristics reflect the fact that the interaction between tumor cells and immune cells is of high relevance for the course of the disease in Lynch syndrome mutation carriers. In fact, rigorous immune surveillance is also a possible reason for the limited penetrance of Lynch syndrome; as despite a very high likelihood of continuously developing multiple MMR-deficient cell clones during life [13], only 50–70% of Lynch syndrome mutation carriers will develop clinically manifest cancers [14]. We will discuss the basic molecular mechanisms behind the immunogenicity of MMR-deficient cells and its potential consequences on immune surveillance in more detail in the following.

4 Coding Microsatellite Instability as a Driver of MSI Tumor Development

The clinical presentation of MSI cancers and their immunological characteristics are all directly or indirectly traceable back to the initial enabling mechanism of genomic instability – DNA MMR deficiency. This is why most of the immunological features typical of Lynch syndrome-associated colorectal cancers are also encountered in MSI colorectal cancers of sporadic origin [8], notably including a high sensitivity toward immune checkpoint blockade [15]. This clearly indicates that the recognition of cancer cells and their antigens by the immune system in Lynch syndrome is not primarily related to the hereditary nature of the disease, but rather a direct consequence of the specific neoantigen-inducing somatic mutations occurring in cancers with a deficient MMR system.

In order to understand the special immunology of MSI cancers, it is important to take a closer look at the steps taking place between tumor initiation and the manifestation of full-blown cancer. MMR-deficient cells have an exceptionally high rate of somatic mutations, which not only but predominantly accumulate as insertion/deletion mutations at repetitive sequence stretches [16, 17]. The majority of these repetitive microsatellites including the ones commonly used for diagnostic purposes are located in noncoding regions; mutations affecting such noncoding microsatellites are commonly regarded, with some exceptions [18], as functionally irrelevant [19]. In stark contrast, single-nucleotide deletions or insertions at microsatellites in gene-encoding regions have immediate functional consequences, as they can induce a shift of the translational reading frame and therefore inactivation of the respective gene.

It is mutations of such coding microsatellites (cMS) that apparently are key factors for promoting MMR-deficient cancer outgrowth [12, 20–22]. In fact, the number of microsatellites in gene-encoding regions is high within the human genome; there are more than 10,000 mononucleotide repeats of a length of 6 or more repeat units located in genomic regions annotated as gene encoding [23]. However, most of these cMS are never or only very rarely found mutant in MSI cancers. This indicates that slippage events occurring at cMS sequences are significantly less frequent than slippage events leading to insertion/deletion mutations at long, noncoding microsatellites that are used for diagnostic purposes [24, 25]. This observation reflects the fact that the rate of spontaneous slippage and consecutive mutation is closely related to the length of a microsatellite, with a steep increase from a mutation rate

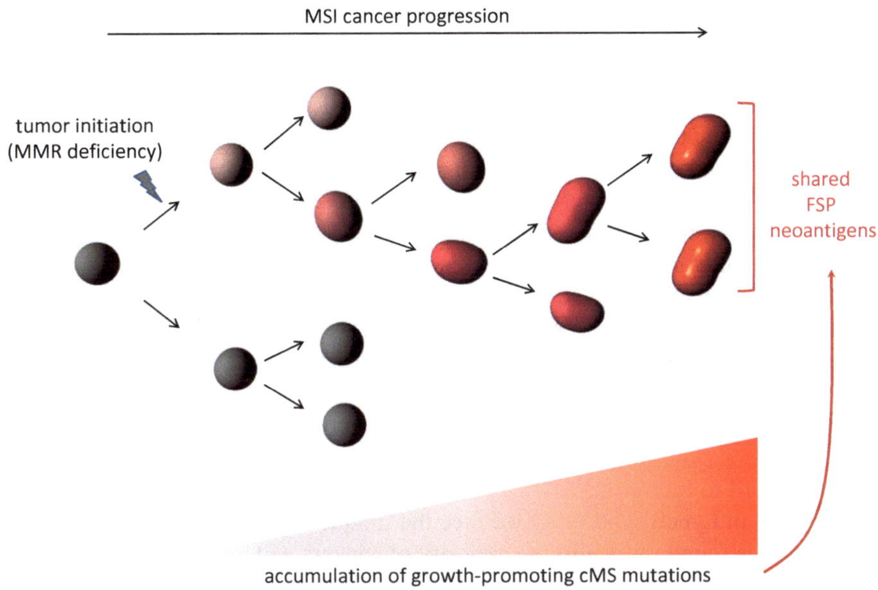

Fig. 23.1 The development of MSI cancers in Lynch syndrome follows a process of Darwinian evolution. During this process, random mutation events at coding microsatellite (cMS) sequences accumulate as a consequence of DNA mismatch repair (MMR) deficiency (left). Though the majority of MMR-deficient cell clones will not progress into a detectable lesion, a very small subset will by chance acquire mutations in cMS that favor proliferation and survival, predominantly mediated by mutations affecting cMS located in tumor suppressor genes such as *TGFBR2* or genes relevant for antigen presentation such as *B2M*. These clones will progress into manifest MSI cancers. As the pattern of cMS mutations found in manifest MSI cancers is shaped by functional relevance and selection, clinically manifest MSI cancers in Lynch syndrome share a set of recurrent cMS mutations that in part occur at frequencies of up to 90% of cancers. From the immunology point of view, this means that MSI cancers share a defined set of frameshift peptide (FSP) neoantigens that directly result from functionally relevant cMS mutations

of close to zero in short microsatellites (4–6 repeat units) to mutation rates of more than 90% in microsatellites with a length of 20 repeat units or longer [21, 26].

From another perspective, if a cMS is recurrently found to be mutant in MSI cancers, it suggests selection and functional relevance (Fig. 23.1). And in fact, MSI cancers do show recurrent cMS mutation patterns that enabled a novel systematic approach, which was entirely based on tracking mutation frequencies of cMS, to identify tumor suppressor genes in the pre-genomic era [20, 22, 23]. These analyses have in the meantime been validated and complemented by whole-genome sequencing and exome sequencing data that also add valuable information about the frequency of MSI and non-MSI mutations in MMR-deficient cancers [17, 27, 28].

The distribution of cMS mutations in the human genome thus influences the spectrum of genes that are inactivated preferentially in MMR-deficient cells. This may explain why MMR-deficient cancers have a characteristic organ distribution: whereas colorectal cancer, one of the most frequent cancers in humans, shows

MMR deficiency in approximately 15% of tumors, MMR deficiency is extremely rare in other common tumor types such as breast cancer and lung cancer [28, 29]. This may reflect the fact that the patterns of cMS target genes that are inactivated by MMR deficiency provide the outgrowing cancer cells a selective growth advantage only under certain conditions and in certain organs. The close relation between target gene mutation patterns and clinical manifestations becomes further apparent through the significant differences between different manifestations of MMR-deficient cancers, for example, colorectal and endometrial cancers [27].

One of the first described target genes containing a cMS (an A10 mononucleotide repeat) frequently affected by mutation in MMR-deficient cancers is the *transforming growth factor beta receptor II* (*TGFBR2*) gene [30]. Underlining the concept of distinct cMS mutation spectra in different types of MMR-deficient cancers, *TGFBR2* mutations are very common in MMR-deficient colorectal cancers (more than 80% carry *TGFBR2* mutations) but rarely observed in MSI endometrial cancer.

With regard to tumor immunology and potential vaccination approaches to prevent cancers in Lynch syndrome, we face the unique situation that a defined set of target genes is found mutant in the majority of cancers and that the observed mutations uniformly affect the same location within these genes. Therefore, all MSI cancers in Lynch syndrome share at least some identical mutation-induced neoantigens that may serve as vaccine agents for a tumor-preventive application. An overview of cMS-containing genes that are of potential relevance as a source of vaccination targets in MSI cancers has been provided in [31].

5 Frameshift Peptide (FSP) Neoantigens in Lynch Syndrome Cancers

As discussed above, mutations of coding microsatellites (cMS) are a major driver of cancer development in Lynch syndrome. Due to their susceptibility toward polymerase slippage, they are frequently hit by insertions and deletions, if those slippage events are not recognized and properly corrected by a functional MMR system.

CMS mutations are not only capable of promoting tumorigenesis by abrogating the function of critical tumor suppressor proteins, but they can also lead to the formation of neoantigens that directly result from shifts of the translational reading frame (frameshift peptides, FSPs) (Fig. 23.2).

FSP neoantigens are similar to viral antigens in the sense that they are completely novel to the host's immune system, as they only occur in MMR-deficient cell clones with a potential to develop into manifest cancers. Frameshift mutations have early been identified as a mechanism to generate powerful tumor-specific neoantigens [32], and their outstanding significance for the recognition of tumor cells by the immune system has been convincingly confirmed by recent studies [33–35]. Whereas point mutation-induced neoantigens only differ from the wild-type protein

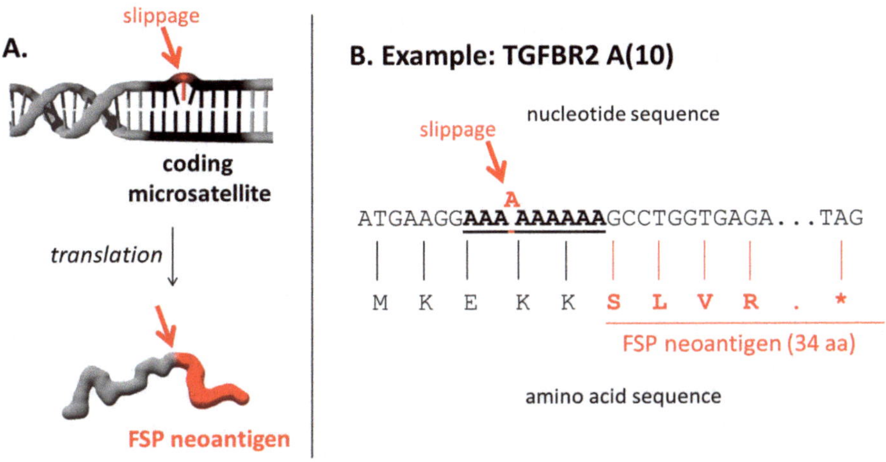

Fig. 23.2 Coding microsatellite mutations lead to the generation of frameshift peptide (FSP) neoantigens. (**a**) Schematic illustration: slippage events during DNA replication lead to insertions or (more frequently) deletions of single nucleotides at repetitive microsatellite sequences. Translation of cMS-mutant sequences results in the generation of FSP neoantigens (lower panel, red). Although the mutation only affects one single nucleotide, the entire carboxy-terminal amino acid sequence is changed because of the shift of the reading frame. (**b**) Example of a single-nucleotide deletion affecting the A10 coding microsatellite located in the *TGFBR2* gene. A change of the microsatellite length from A10–A9 results in a mutational FSP neoantigen that encompasses 34 novel amino acids that can be recognized as foreign by the immune system

by the exchange of single amino acids, FSP neoantigens are often long amino acid stretches at the C-terminus of the mutant protein, and they can contain many immunologically relevant neoepitopes that can be presented by many types of HLA class I and HLA class II molecules [31]. Hence, the high immunogenicity of MSI cancers in Lynch syndrome is not only caused by a defined set of shared neoantigens, but these neoantigens are also entirely different from any human protein sequences and in their sum encompass neopeptide stretches sufficiently long to contain at least a few epitopes that may potentially be presented on the specific HLA class I and II molecules of every patient [31]. Particularly the existence of shared antigens occurring at a high frequency is different from any other types of human cancers [36], and the high risk of developing cancer in Lynch syndrome provides a scenario suitable for evaluating the efficacy of neoantigen-based cancer-preventive vaccines, as effects of a vaccine on the tumor incidence in the vaccinated population in comparison with the control population can potentially be observed in comparatively short follow-up intervals and with realistic study group sizes.

6 Immune Responses Against Predicted FSP Neoantigens in Lynch Syndrome Patients

In 2001, immune responses against FSP neoantigens caused by cMS mutations affecting the *TGFBR2* gene have first been described in the scientific literature [37, 38]. Importantly, these studies also demonstrated the capacity of FSP-specific T cells to specifically lyse MSI tumor cells expressing the respective *TGFBR2*-derived FSP neoantigen [37]. In the following years, immune responses against numerous other FSP neoantigens have been detected [37, 39–42], and it was shown that spontaneous FSP-specific T-cell responses are common in MSI CRC patients and even in tumor-free Lynch syndrome mutation carriers [43]. Such FSP-specific T cells were present in the peripheral blood, but also among tumor-infiltrating lymphocytes, which exhibited cytotoxic activity on MSI cancer cells [43]. We can therefore assume that a significant proportion of lymphocytes infiltrating MSI cancers is specific for FSP neoantigens, which could also be the reason for the observation that MSI CRCs with a very high number of FSP-inducing cMS mutations are particularly densely infiltrated with lymphocytes [44].

One of the surprising findings of the studies addressing immune response patterns in Lynch syndrome was the observation that Lynch syndrome mutation carriers who had never developed a clinically apparent lesion already presented with FSP-specific T-cell responses [43]. Such responses were not observed in patients diagnosed with microsatellite stable (MSS) CRC or in healthy individuals who were not carriers of Lynch syndrome-causing mutations, underlining the specificity of the observation. What, however, is the reason for this finding? How can the immune system "know" neoantigens that evidently only develop in cells that have lost the functionality of the MMR system, as it is the case in MSI cancer cells? The most likely answer came from a histopathology study published in 2012 [13]: The normal-appearing gut mucosa of a 40-year-old Lynch syndrome mutation carrier is estimated to contain thousands of MMR-deficient crypt foci that have lost a functional MMR system as a consequence of somatic second hits. Part of these MMR-deficient crypt foci already express MMR deficiency-induced FSP neoantigens [45], which show that the immune system interacts with non-cancerous and precancerous MMR-deficient cells long before manifest cancers grow out. It is thus conceivable that FSP neoantigen-specific immune surveillance may contribute to the elimination of such early MMR-deficient lesions before they become clinically apparent. Although there is no experimental evidence proving this hypothesis, immune surveillance in Lynch syndrome may very well be a unique example for the existence of the "elimination" and "equilibrium" phases in human cancer development according to the immuno-editing model [46, 47]. Successful immune surveillance and elimination of precancers by the immune system may also explain why Lynch syndrome has a limited penetrance [48].

7 Immune Evasion in MSI Cancer

If immune surveillance in fact controls the outgrowth of MMR-deficient cell clones by T-cell-mediated elimination, the question emerges which mechanisms enable clinically manifest Lynch syndrome-associated cancers to appear. Conceptually, two possible explanations exist: First, the immune system may – transiently or persistently – lose the capacity of controlling tumor outgrowth, and second, outgrowing tumor cell clones can evade a still functional immune surveillance by losing the capacity of presenting neoantigens on their surface (Fig. 23.3).

In fact, the latter variant, i.e., inactivation of HLA antigens, is the most common mechanism that enables MSI cancer cells to grow out in an environment of pronounced neoantigen-specific immune responses [49]. HLA inactivation is frequently observed in a variety of tumor types and particularly common among tumors that are characterized by a high antigen load and pronounced responses of the adaptive immune system [50, 51]. It is known that different cancers use different mechanisms to impair their capacity of presenting antigens, which could lead to their own rejection and elimination, to the immune system [51, 52].

In Lynch syndrome-associated CRCs, the most common molecular alterations associated with a loss of HLA class I antigen presentation are mutations of the *Beta-2-microglobulin* (*B2M*) gene (Fig. 23.3b) [53]. These mutations lead to the inactivation of the HLA class I antigen light chain B2M, so that no functional HLA class I antigen complexes are presented any more on the cell surface. Consequently, HLA class I epitopes derived from FSP neoantigens cannot be presented anymore, and CD8-positive T cells that might lead to cytolytic tumor cell destruction cannot recognize *B2M*-mutant MSI CRC cells.

What are the reasons for the observation that immune evasion of MSI CRCs is typically mediated by *B2M* mutations? First, *B2M* mutations are an "efficient" way of eliminating HLA class I antigen expression from the tumor cell perspective: Only two mutations (one on each *B2M* allele) are required to shut down the cell surface expression of all six possible HLA class I antigens (encoded by *HLA-A*, *HLA-B*, and *HLA-C*, two per each of the three gene loci). Second, the *B2M* gene sequence encompasses four cMS (one (CA)4 dinucleotide repeat in exon 1, two A5, and one C5 mononucleotide in exon 2), which – naturally – are preferred mutational targets in MMR-deficient cells such as Lynch syndrome cancer cells [53]. Hence, the basic mechanism of MMR deficiency-induced microsatellite instability not only leads to the generation of multiple FSP neoantigens enhancing the immunogenicity of Lynch syndrome cancers, but it also enables their outgrowth by facilitating immune evasion through *B2M* mutation-mediated loss of HLA class I antigen expression.

Interestingly, Lynch syndrome-associated MSI CRCs have a higher frequency of *B2M* mutations when compared to MSI CRCs with a sporadic background [54]. This observation may point to an increased immune selection pressure during the development of Lynch syndrome cancers, potentially because the immune system of Lynch syndrome mutation carriers has been pre-sensitized to FSP neoantigens through the recurrent generation of MMR-deficient cell clones during life (Fig. 23.4)

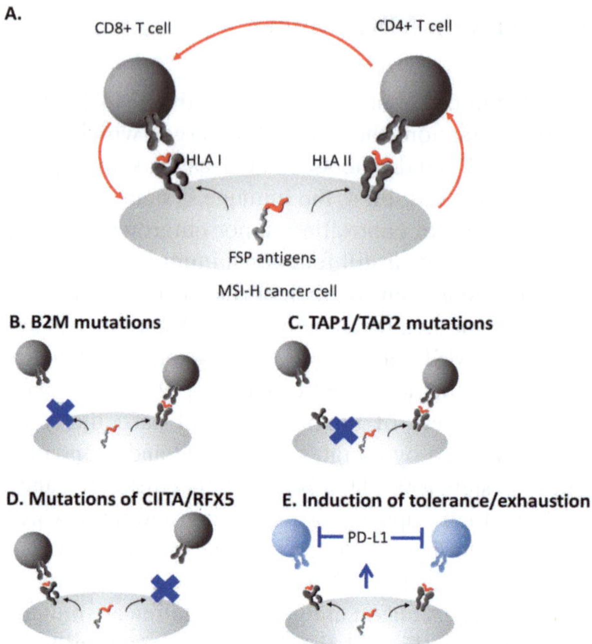

Fig. 23.3 Mechanisms of immune evasion in MSI colorectal cancer. MSI cancers show several alterations that lead to a breakdown of functional recognition and attack by the host's T cells (**a**). (**b**) *Beta2-microglobulin* (*B2M*) mutations are the most common alteration (approximately 30% of MSI colorectal cancers) leading to immune evasion through a complete breakdown of HLA class I-mediated presentation of tumor antigens in MSI cancer. Mutation-induced loss of B2M, the essential light chain of HLA class I antigens, induces a complete lack of assembled HLA class I antigens on the tumor cell surface. As a consequence, CD8-positive T cells cannot attack *B2M*-mutant MSI cancer cells. (**c**) Mutations have also been described in genes encoding essential components of the cellular antigen-processing and presentation machinery, most prominently mutations leading to a loss of the transporters of antigen presentation (TAP1 and TAP2), which are encountered in approximately 10% of MSI colorectal cancers. (**d**) Mutations of the genes *CIITA* and *RFX5*, which are required for functional HLA class II antigen expression on the tumor cell surface, are found in up to 20% of MSI colorectal cancers and associated with a complete loss of HLA class II antigens on the tumor cell surface. (**e**) Additional direct and indirect mechanisms do not structurally interfere with the tumor cells' capacity to present FSP neoantigens, but influence the T-cell activation status. Most importantly, expression of PD-L1, which is induced upon prolonged immune activation, e.g., through IFN-gamma secretion, on tumor-associated macrophages can induce exhaustion of PD-1-positive T cells infiltrating MSI cancers

[13, 45]. Although no data are available currently to support this hypothesis, evidence is strong that *B2M* mutations in fact reflect immune evasion, as it preferentially occurs in cancers that develop in an active local immune environment [55].

The consequences of *B2M* mutations on the clinical appearance of MSI cancers are wide-ranging. Among locally restricted MSI CRCs, *B2M* mutations are associated with a higher stage, i.e., infiltration depth of the tumor and local lymph node metastases [53]. In contrast, *B2M*-mutant cancers are only very rarely associated

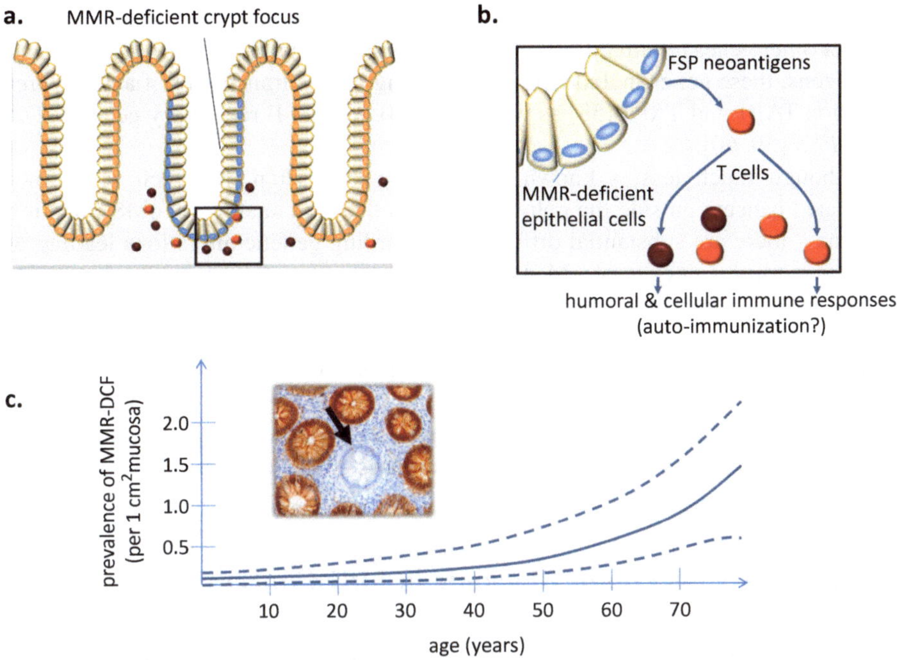

Fig. 23.4 MMR-deficient crypt foci may cause autoimmunization of Lynch syndrome mutation carriers. MMR-deficient crypt foci, which occur at a high frequency in phenotypically normal tissue in Lynch syndrome mutation carriers, may be recognized by the host's immune system (**a**). (**b**) Detailed view. MMR-deficient crypt foci harbor coding microsatellite mutations that can give rise to the generation of FSP neoantigens, even before a clinically manifest tumor develops. Humoral and cellular immune responses against FSP neoantigens have been detected in healthy, tumor-free Lynch syndrome mutation carriers [43]. (**c**) The prevalence of MMR-deficient crypt foci (inlay: immunohistochemical EPCAM staining of an MMR-deficient crypt focus in an *EPCAM* deletion carrier; loss of EPCAM/MSH2 is marked by a black arrow) increases with age (dashed line: 95% confidence interval, derived from Staffa et al. [45]). This may be responsible for the increased incidence of colon cancer with higher age in Lynch syndrome. The precise consequences of MMR-deficient crypts for the induction of immune responses over time in Lynch syndrome are not yet known and require further research

with distant metastases disease relapses in the further course of the disease [53, 56, 57]. *B2M* gene mutations and lack of B2M expression are in fact the strongest favorable prognostic marker in MSI CRC. Though the mechanisms underlying the favorable prognosis of *B2M*-mutant cancers are still not fully resolved, the existing data indicate that they are curable by surgery in almost all cases. This is important to note, as immune evasion through *B2M* mutations does therefore not jeopardize the efficacy of tumor-preventive vaccines in Lynch syndrome: If the immune selection pressure imposed on emerging MSI cancer cell clones can be increased by vaccination with FSP neoantigens or by other immunomodulatory approaches, not only a lower cancer incidence would be expected but also a better prognosis and better treatment options in cancers might still develop.

In addition to *B2M* mutations, MSI CRCs show MMR deficiency-induced mutations of other genes required for functional antigen presentation via HLA class I and II antigens; these genes include the genes coding for the transporter of antigen presentation TAP1 and TAP2 [58] as well as the HLA class II regulatory genes *CIITA* and *RFX5* [59, 60].

Although much less is known about immune evasion of Lynch syndrome-associated cancers outside the colon, it appears that – in analogy to cMS mutation patterns – there are substantial differences regarding genetic alterations leading to immune evasion. For example, MSI endometrial cancers only very rarely show *B2M* mutations but instead present with mutations of the *JAK1* gene in about one-third of tumors. *JAK1* mutations can lead to impaired interferon-gamma-mediated upregulation of antigen presentation components and therefore likely to immune evasion [61]. The reasons for these differences are not known, although one can speculate about a potential influence of different neoantigen patterns resulting from distinct cMS mutation profiles as well as about differences of the local immune milieu.

8 Immune Checkpoint Blockade in MSI Cancers

As already mentioned above, not only loss of functional HLA-mediated antigen presentation can favor cancer outgrowth in Lynch syndrome, but alterations of the local immune environment also seem to play an important role in a subset of cancers.

Generally, the pronounced effector T-cell infiltration typically observed in MSI CRCs is accompanied and balanced by high expression levels of immune checkpoint molecules [62]. The exceptionally high neoantigen load typical of MSI cancers [63, 64] apparently can induce PD-1 (programmed cell death protein 1) receptor expression on tumor-infiltrating T cells upon prolonged stimulation [65]. If such PD-1-positive T cells interact with the ligand PD-L1 (programmed death-ligand 1), which is often expressed by myeloid cells surrounding MSI CRCs, they may become exhausted and, at least transiently, lose their killing capacity [62]. T-cell exhaustion may therefore allow MSI tumor cells to grow out even if they still have functional HLA-mediated antigen presentation capacity.

In such a scenario, it is apparent that reactivation of exhausted T cells may lead to tumor regression and potentially even elimination. In fact, novel immune checkpoint modulators [65] that directly target the exhaustion-related molecules PD-1/PD-L1 have proven to be very effective specifically in tumors displaying the MSI phenotype [15] with an objective response rate of approximately 40%. Clinical responses upon treatment with the anti-PD-1 antibody were detectable in patients with MSI CRCs and extracolonic MSI cancers, including MSI cholangiocellular carcinoma, MSI endometrial cancer, and MSI gastrointestinal cancer [15].

The high response rate of MSI cancer patients toward anti-PD-1 antibody treatment underlines the fact that MSI cancer patients in most cases have pre-existing CD8-positive T-cell responses that can be reactivated by checkpoint blockade [66].

9 Vaccination with FSP Antigens

Immunomodulation through checkpoint blockade has quickly become a very important new treatment column in patients with advanced-stage MSI cancers. It also has increased the need for MSI typing to be performed in patients with metastasized cancers because of the potential availability of a highly effective treatment option in case a positive MSI typing result is found.

However, in tumor-free Lynch syndrome individuals, the immune checkpoint blockade approaches that are currently available in the clinics are not appropriate due to their side effect profiles [15]. Therefore, alternative approaches need to be considered that – in addition to secondary prevention approaches including regular colonoscopy – may help to reduce the tumor incidence in Lynch syndrome mutation carriers. One milestone in this direction has been achieved with the publication of the results of the randomized controlled CAPP2 trial that evaluated aspirin as a chemopreventive agent in Lynch syndrome [67]. The study showed that daily intake of 600 mg aspirin for approximately 2 years leads to a significant reduction of the cancer incidence in Lynch syndrome mutation carriers. Although the mechanisms underlying the cancer-preventive effect of the multivalent drug aspirin are not fully resolved, there are indications that the mechanism of action may involve a shift from a non-specific inflammatory state toward a more active state of the adaptive immune system, which enhance the likelihood of T cells recognizing and potentially eliminating immunogenic early cancer precursor cells [68].

In addition to using aspirin as a chemopreventive agent, more specific approaches are currently discussed. The fact that Lynch syndrome cancers share a broad repertoire of cMS mutations and resulting FSP neoantigens, as described above, opens up the possibility to design entirely novel preventive vaccines that are based on the combination of highly immunogenic FSP neoantigens. Neoantigens that can be used in preventive vaccines should occur in many Lynch syndrome cancers, preferentially already during the early steps of tumor development and ideally before immune evasion phenomena can occur [20, 26, 43, 45].

Following this rationale, a vaccine with three FSP antigens that fulfill these requirements (those derived from the −1 mutant variants of the cMS-containing genes *AIM2*, *HT001*, and *TAF1B*; Micoryx, http://clinicaltrials.gov/show/NCT01461148) has recently been successfully tested in an initial clinical phase I/IIa trial [31]. The strong and specific induction of immune responses against the vaccine antigens observed in this trial nurtures the hope that preventive vaccines that specifically target immunogenic neoantigens derived from early driver mutations may in the future help to prevent tumor formation in Lynch syndrome. Such a success would also serve as a proof of principle that it is possible to sensitize the immune system toward cancer cells before cancer development starts, which may open up the path toward a variety of potential cancer-preventive vaccines beyond the boundaries of Lynch syndrome in the future. The unique high-risk scenario of Lynch syndrome represents, in that sense, the perfect setting to evaluate the concept of anticancer vaccines. In addition to a potential application for cancer prevention, FSP neoantigen-based vaccines may also have beneficial effects in the treatment of MSI cancers, alone or in combination with immune checkpoint blockade.

References

1. Greaves M, Maley CC. Clonal evolution in cancer. Nature. 2012;481(7381):306–13. https://doi.org/10.1038/nature10762.
2. Hanahan D, Weinberg RA. Hallmarks of cancer: the next generation. Cell. 2011;144(5):646–74. https://doi.org/10.1016/j.cell.2011.02.013.
3. Lengauer C, Kinzler KW, Vogelstein B. Genetic instability in colorectal cancers. Nature. 1997;386(6625):623–7. https://doi.org/10.1038/386623a0.
4. Michor F, Iwasa Y, Vogelstein B, Lengauer C, Nowak MA. Can chromosomal instability initiate tumorigenesis? Semin Cancer Biol. 2005;15(1):43–9. https://doi.org/10.1016/j.semcancer.2004.09.007.
5. Toyota M, Ahuja N, Ohe-Toyota M, Herman JG, Baylin SB, Issa JP. CpG island methylator phenotype in colorectal cancer. Proc Natl Acad Sci U S A. 1999;96(15):8681–6.
6. Lao VV, Grady WM. Epigenetics and colorectal cancer. Nat Rev Gastroenterol Hepatol. 2011;8(12):686–700. https://doi.org/10.1038/nrgastro.2011.173.
7. Shia J, Ellis NA, Paty PB, Nash GM, Qin J, Offit K, Zhang XM, Markowitz AJ, Nafa K, Guillem JG, Wong WD, Gerald WL, Klimstra DS. Value of histopathology in predicting microsatellite instability in hereditary nonpolyposis colorectal cancer and sporadic colorectal cancer. Am J Surg Pathol. 2003;27(11):1407–17.
8. Shia J, Holck S, Depetris G, Greenson JK, Klimstra DS. Lynch syndrome-associated neoplasms: a discussion on histopathology and immunohistochemistry. Familial Cancer. 2013;12(2):241–60. https://doi.org/10.1007/s10689-013-9612-4.
9. Buckowitz A, Knaebel HP, Benner A, Blaker H, Gebert J, Kienle P, von Knebel DM, Kloor M. Microsatellite instability in colorectal cancer is associated with local lymphocyte infiltration and low frequency of distant metastases. Br J Cancer. 2005;92(9):1746–53. https://doi.org/10.1038/sj.bjc.6602534.
10. Galon J, Costes A, Sanchez-Cabo F, Kirilovsky A, Mlecnik B, Lagorce-Pages C, Tosolini M, Camus M, Berger A, Wind P, Zinzindohoue F, Bruneval P, Cugnenc PH, Trajanoski Z, Fridman WH, Pages F. Type, density, and location of immune cells within human colorectal tumors predict clinical outcome. Science. 2006;313(5795):1960–4. https://doi.org/10.1126/science.1129139.
11. Jung SB, Lee HI, Oh HK, Shin IH, Jeon CH. Clinico-pathologic parameters for prediction of microsatellite instability in colorectal cancer. Cancer Res Treat Off J Kor Cancer Assoc. 2012;44(3):179–86. https://doi.org/10.4143/crt.2012.44.3.179.
12. Boland CR, Goel A. Microsatellite instability in colorectal cancer. Gastroenterology. 2010;138(6):2073–87. e2073. https://doi.org/10.1053/j.gastro.2009.12.064.
13. Kloor M, Huth C, Voigt AY, Benner A, Schirmacher P, von Knebel Doeberitz M, Blaker H. Prevalence of mismatch repair-deficient crypt foci in lynch syndrome: a pathological study. Lancet Oncol. 2012;13(6):598–606. https://doi.org/10.1016/S1470-2045(12)70109-2.
14. Moller P, Seppala T, Bernstein I, Holinski-Feder E, Sala P, Evans DG, Lindblom A, Macrae F, Blanco I, Sijmons R, Jeffries J, Vasen H, Burn J, Nakken S, Hovig E, Rodland EA, Tharmaratnam K, de Vos Tot Nederveen Cappel WH, Hill J, Wijnen J, Green K, Lalloo F, Sunde L, Mints M, Bertario L, Pineda M, Navarro M, Morak M, Renkonen-Sinisalo L, Frayling IM, Plazzer JP, Pylvanainen K, Sampson JR, Capella G, Mecklin JP, Moslein G. Cancer incidence and survival in Lynch syndrome patients receiving colonoscopic and gynaecological surveillance: first report from the prospective Lynch syndrome database. Gut. 2017;66(3):464–72. https://doi.org/10.1136/gutjnl-2015-309675.
15. Le DT, Uram JN, Wang H, Bartlett BR, Kemberling H, Eyring AD, Skora AD, Luber BS, Azad NS, Laheru D, Biedrzycki B, Donehower RC, Zaheer A, Fisher GA, Crocenzi TS, Lee JJ, Duffy SM, Goldberg RM, de la Chapelle A, Koshiji M, Bhaijee F, Huebner T, Hruban RH, Wood LD, Cuka N, Pardoll DM, Papadopoulos N, Kinzler KW, Zhou S, Cornish TC, Taube JM, Anders RA, Eshleman JR, Vogelstein B, Diaz LA Jr. PD-1 blockade in tumors with mismatch-repair deficiency. N Engl J Med. 2015. https://doi.org/10.1056/NEJMoa1500596.

16. Alexandrov LB, Nik-Zainal S, Wedge DC, Aparicio SA, Behjati S, Biankin AV, Bignell GR, Bolli N, Borg A, Borresen-Dale AL, Boyault S, Burkhardt B, Butler AP, Caldas C, Davies HR, Desmedt C, Eils R, Eyfjord JE, Foekens JA, Greaves M, Hosoda F, Hutter B, Ilicic T, Imbeaud S, Imielinski M, Jager N, Jones DT, Jones D, Knappskog S, Kool M, Lakhani SR, Lopez-Otin C, Martin S, Munshi NC, Nakamura H, Northcott PA, Pajic M, Papaemmanuil E, Paradiso A, Pearson JV, Puente XS, Raine K, Ramakrishna M, Richardson AL, Richter J, Rosenstiel P, Schlesner M, Schumacher TN, Span PN, Teague JW, Totoki Y, Tutt AN, Valdes-Mas R, van Buuren MM, van't Veer L, Vincent-Salomon A, Waddell N, Yates LR, Zucman-Rossi J, Futreal PA, McDermott U, Lichter P, Meyerson M, Grimmond SM, Siebert R, Campo E, Shibata T, Pfister SM, Campbell PJ, Stratton MR. Signatures of mutational processes in human cancer. Nature. 2013;500(7463):415–21. https://doi.org/10.1038/nature12477.
17. Timmermann B, Kerick M, Roehr C, Fischer A, Isau M, Boerno ST, Wunderlich A, Barmeyer C, Seemann P, Koenig J, Lappe M, Kuss AW, Garshasbi M, Bertram L, Trappe K, Werber M, Herrmann BG, Zatloukal K, Lehrach H, Schweiger MR. Somatic mutation profiles of MSI and MSS colorectal cancer identified by whole exome next generation sequencing and bioinformatics analysis. PLoS One. 2010;5(12):e15661. https://doi.org/10.1371/journal.pone.0015661.
18. Dorard C, de Thonel A, Collura A, Marisa L, Svrcek M, Lagrange A, Jego G, Wanherdrick K, Joly AL, Buhard O, Gobbo J, Penard-Lacronique V, Zouali H, Tubacher E, Kirzin S, Selves J, Milano G, Etienne-Grimaldi MC, Bengrine-Lefevre L, Louvet C, Tournigand C, Lefevre JH, Parc Y, Tiret E, Flejou JF, Gaub MP, Garrido C, Duval A. Expression of a mutant HSP110 sensitizes colorectal cancer cells to chemotherapy and improves disease prognosis. Nat Med. 2011;17(10):1283–9. https://doi.org/10.1038/nm.2457.
19. Sammalkorpi H, Alhopuro P, Lehtonen R, Tuimala J, Mecklin JP, Jarvinen HJ, Jiricny J, Karhu A, Aaltonen LA. Background mutation frequency in microsatellite-unstable colorectal cancer. Cancer Res. 2007;67(12):5691–8. https://doi.org/10.1158/0008-5472.CAN-06-4314.
20. Woerner SM, Kloor M, von Knebel DM, Gebert JF. Microsatellite instability in the development of DNA mismatch repair deficient tumors. Cancer Biomark Sect A Dis Markers. 2006;2(1–2):69–86.
21. Alhopuro P, Sammalkorpi H, Niittymaki I, Bistrom M, Raitila A, Saharinen J, Nousiainen K, Lehtonen HJ, Heliovaara E, Puhakka J, Tuupanen S, Sousa S, Seruca R, Ferreira AM, Hofstra RM, Mecklin JP, Jarvinen H, Ristimaki A, Orntoft TF, Hautaniemi S, Arango D, Karhu A, Aaltonen LA. Candidate driver genes in microsatellite-unstable colorectal cancer. Int J Cancer. 2012;130(7):1558–66. https://doi.org/10.1002/ijc.26167.
22. Duval A, Rolland S, Compoint A, Tubacher E, Iacopetta B, Thomas G, Hamelin R. Evolution of instability at coding and non-coding repeat sequences in human MSI-H colorectal cancers. Hum Mol Genet. 2001;10(5):513–8.
23. Woerner SM, Gebert J, Yuan YP, Sutter C, Ridder R, Bork P, von Knebel Doeberitz M. Systematic identification of genes with coding microsatellites mutated in DNA mismatch repair-deficient cancer cells. Int J Cancer. 2001;93(1):12–9.
24. Suraweera N, Duval A, Reperant M, Vaury C, Furlan D, Leroy K, Seruca R, Iacopetta B, Hamelin R. Evaluation of tumor microsatellite instability using five quasimonomorphic mononucleotide repeats and pentaplex PCR. Gastroenterology. 2002;123(6):1804–11. https://doi.org/10.1053/gast.2002.37070.
25. Findeisen P, Kloor M, Merx S, Sutter C, Woerner SM, Dostmann N, Benner A, Dondog B, Pawlita M, Dippold W, Wagner R, Gebert J, von Knebel Doeberitz M. T25 repeat in the 3' untranslated region of the CASP2 gene: a sensitive and specific marker for microsatellite instability in colorectal cancer. Cancer Res. 2005;65(18):8072–8. https://doi.org/10.1158/0008-5472.CAN-04-4146.
26. Woerner SM, Benner A, Sutter C, Schiller M, Yuan YP, Keller G, Bork P, Doeberitz M, Gebert JF. Pathogenesis of DNA repair-deficient cancers: a statistical meta-analysis of putative Real Common Target genes. Oncogene. 2003;22(15):2226–35. https://doi.org/10.1038/sj.onc.1206421.
27. Kim TM, Laird PW, Park PJ. The landscape of microsatellite instability in colorectal and endometrial cancer genomes. Cell. 2013;155(4):858–68. https://doi.org/10.1016/j.cell.2013.10.015.

28. Hause RJ, Pritchard CC, Shendure J, Salipante SJ. Classification and characterization of microsatellite instability across 18 cancer types. Nat Med. 2016;22(11):1342–50. https://doi.org/10.1038/nm.4191.
29. Warth A, Korner S, Penzel R, Muley T, Dienemann H, Schirmacher P, von Knebel-Doeberitz M, Weichert W, Kloor M. Microsatellite instability in pulmonary adenocarcinomas: a comprehensive study of 480 cases. Virchows Archiv Int J Pathol. 2016;468(3):313–9. https://doi.org/10.1007/s00428-015-1892-7.
30. Markowitz S, Wang J, Myeroff L, Parsons R, Sun L, Lutterbaugh J, Fan RS, Zborowska E, Kinzler KW, Vogelstein B, et al. Inactivation of the type II TGF-beta receptor in colon cancer cells with microsatellite instability. Science. 1995;268(5215):1336–8.
31. Kloor M, von Knebel Doeberitz M. The immune biology of microsatellite-unstable cancer. Trends in Cancer. 2016;2(3):121–31.
32. Townsend A, Ohlen C, Rogers M, Edwards J, Mukherjee S, Bastin J. Source of unique tumour antigens. Nature. 1994;371(6499):662. https://doi.org/10.1038/371662a0.
33. Schumacher TN, Schreiber RD. Neoantigens in cancer immunotherapy. Science. 2015;348(6230):69–74. https://doi.org/10.1126/science.aaa4971.
34. Anagnostou V, Smith KN, Forde PM, Niknafs N, Bhattacharya R, White J, Zhang T, Adleff V, Phallen J, Wali N, Hruban C, Guthrie VB, Rodgers K, Naidoo J, Kang H, Sharfman W, Georgiades C, Verde F, Illei P, Li QK, Gabrielson E, Brock MV, Zahnow CA, Baylin SB, Scharpf RB, Brahmer JR, Karchin R, Pardoll DM, Velculescu VE. Evolution of neoantigen landscape during immune checkpoint blockade in non-small cell lung cancer. Cancer Discov. 2017;7(3):264–76. https://doi.org/10.1158/2159-8290.CD-16-0828.
35. Giannakis M, Mu XJ, Shukla SA, Qian ZR, Cohen O, Nishihara R, Bahl S, Cao Y, Amin-Mansour A, Yamauchi M, Sukawa Y, Stewart C, Rosenberg M, Mima K, Inamura K, Nosho K, Nowak JA, Lawrence MS, Giovannucci EL, Chan AT, Ng K, Meyerhardt JA, Van Allen EM, Getz G, Gabriel SB, Lander ES, Wu CJ, Fuchs CS, Ogino S, Garraway LA. Genomic correlates of immune-cell infiltrates in colorectal carcinoma. Cell Rep. 2016;17(4):1206. https://doi.org/10.1016/j.celrep.2016.10.009.
36. Heemskerk B, Kvistborg P, Schumacher TN. The cancer antigenome. EMBO J. 2013;32(2):194–203. https://doi.org/10.1038/emboj.2012.333.
37. Linnebacher M, Gebert J, Rudy W, Woerner S, Yuan YP, Bork P, von Knebel Doeberitz M. Frameshift peptide-derived T-cell epitopes: a source of novel tumor-specific antigens. Int J Cancer. 2001;93(1):6–11.
38. Saeterdal I, Gjertsen MK, Straten P, Eriksen JA, Gaudernack G. A TGF betaRII frameshift-mutation-derived CTL epitope recognised by HLA-A2-restricted CD8+ T cells. Cancer Immunol Immunother CII. 2001;50(9):469–76.
39. Ripberger E, Linnebacher M, Schwitalle Y, Gebert J, von Knebel DM. Identification of an HLA-A0201-restricted CTL epitope generated by a tumor-specific frameshift mutation in a coding microsatellite of the OGT gene. J Clin Immunol. 2003;23(5):415–23.
40. Schwitalle Y, Linnebacher M, Ripberger E, Gebert J, von Knebel Doeberitz M. Immunogenic peptides generated by frameshift mutations in DNA mismatch repair-deficient cancer cells. Cancer Immun. 2004;4:14.
41. Maletzki C, Schmidt F, Dirks WG, Schmitt M, Linnebacher M. Frameshift-derived neoantigens constitute immunotherapeutic targets for patients with microsatellite-instable haematological malignancies: frameshift peptides for treating MSI+ blood cancers. Eur J Cancer. 2013;49(11):2587–95. https://doi.org/10.1016/j.ejca.2013.02.035.
42. Saeterdal I, Bjorheim J, Lislerud K, Gjertsen MK, Bukholm IK, Olsen OC, Nesland JM, Eriksen JA, Moller M, Lindblom A, Gaudernack G. Frameshift-mutation-derived peptides as tumor-specific antigens in inherited and spontaneous colorectal cancer. Proc Natl Acad Sci U S A. 2001;98(23):13255–60. https://doi.org/10.1073/pnas.231326898.
43. Schwitalle Y, Kloor M, Eiermann S, Linnebacher M, Kienle P, Knaebel HP, Tariverdian M, Benner A, von Knebel DM. Immune response against frameshift-induced neopeptides in HNPCC patients and healthy HNPCC mutation carriers. Gastroenterology. 2008;134(4):988–97. https://doi.org/10.1053/j.gastro.2008.01.015.

44. Maby P, Tougeron D, Hamieh M, Mlecnik B, Kora H, Bindea G, Angell HK, Fredriksen T, Elie N, Fauquembergue E, Drouet A, Leprince J, Benichou J, Mauillon J, Le Pessot F, Sesboue R, Tuech JJ, Sabourin JC, Michel P, Frebourg T, Galon J, Latouche JB. Correlation between density of CD8+ T-cell infiltrate in microsatellite unstable colorectal cancers and frameshift mutations: a rationale for personalized immunotherapy. Cancer Res. 2015;75(17):3446–55. https://doi.org/10.1158/0008-5472.CAN-14-3051.
45. Staffa L, Echterdiek F, Nelius N, Benner A, Werft W, Lahrmann B, Grabe N, Schneider M, Tariverdian M, von Knebel DM, Blaker H, Kloor M. Mismatch repair-deficient crypt foci in lynch syndrome – molecular alterations and association with clinical parameters. PLoS One. 2015;10(3):e0121980. https://doi.org/10.1371/journal.pone.0121980.
46. Dunn GP, Bruce AT, Ikeda H, Old LJ, Schreiber RD. Cancer immunoediting: from immunosurveillance to tumor escape. Nat Immunol. 2002;3(11):991–8. https://doi.org/10.1038/ni1102-991.
47. Mittal D, Gubin MM, Schreiber RD, Smyth MJ. New insights into cancer immunoediting and its three component phases – elimination, equilibrium and escape. Curr Opin Immunol. 2014;27:16–25. https://doi.org/10.1016/j.coi.2014.01.004.
48. Quehenberger F, Vasen HF, van Houwelingen HC. Risk of colorectal and endometrial cancer for carriers of mutations of the hMLH1 and hMSH2 gene: correction for ascertainment. J Med Genet. 2005;42(6):491–6. https://doi.org/10.1136/jmg.2004.024299.
49. Kloor M, Michel S, von Knebel Doeberitz M. Immune evasion of microsatellite unstable colorectal cancers. Int J Cancer. 2010;127(5):1001–10. https://doi.org/10.1002/ijc.25283.
50. Rooney MS, Shukla SA, Wu CJ, Getz G, Hacohen N. Molecular and genetic properties of tumors associated with local immune cytolytic activity. Cell. 2015;160(1–2):48–61. https://doi.org/10.1016/j.cell.2014.12.033.
51. Chang CC, Ferrone S. Immune selective pressure and HLA class I antigen defects in malignant lesions. Cancer Immunol Immunother CII. 2007;56(2):227–36. https://doi.org/10.1007/s00262-006-0183-1.
52. Cabrera CM, Jimenez P, Cabrera T, Esparza C, Ruiz-Cabello F, Garrido F. Total loss of MHC class I in colorectal tumors can be explained by two molecular pathways: beta2-microglobulin inactivation in MSI-positive tumors and LMP7/TAP2 downregulation in MSI-negative tumors. Tissue Antigens. 2003;61(3):211–9.
53. Kloor M, Michel S, Buckowitz B, Ruschoff J, Buttner R, Holinski-Feder E, Dippold W, Wagner R, Tariverdian M, Benner A, Schwitalle Y, Kuchenbuch B, von Knebel DM. Beta2-microglobulin mutations in microsatellite unstable colorectal tumors. Int J Cancer. 2007;121(2):454–8. https://doi.org/10.1002/ijc.22691.
54. Dierssen JW, de Miranda NF, Ferrone S, van Puijenbroek M, Cornelisse CJ, Fleuren GJ, van Wezel T, Morreau H. HNPCC versus sporadic microsatellite-unstable colon cancers follow different routes toward loss of HLA class I expression. BMC Cancer. 2007;7:33. https://doi.org/10.1186/1471-2407-7-33.
55. Echterdiek F, Janikovits J, Staffa L, Muller M, Lahrmann B, Fruhschutz M, Hartog B, Nelius N, Benner A, Tariverdian M, von Knebel DM, Grabe N, Kloor M. Low density of FOXP3-positive T cells in normal colonic mucosa is related to the presence of beta2-microglobulin mutations in Lynch syndrome-associated colorectal cancer. Oncoimmunology. 2016;5(2):e1075692. https://doi.org/10.1080/2162402X.2015.1075692.
56. Tikidzhieva A, Benner A, Michel S, Formentini A, Link KH, Dippold W, von Knebel DM, Kornmann M, Kloor M. Microsatellite instability and Beta2-Microglobulin mutations as prognostic markers in colon cancer: results of the FOGT-4 trial. Br J Cancer. 2012;106(6):1239–45. https://doi.org/10.1038/bjc.2012.53.
57. Koelzer VH, Baker K, Kassahn D, Baumhoer D, Zlobec I. Prognostic impact of beta-2-microglobulin expression in colorectal cancers stratified by mismatch repair status. J Clin Pathol. 2012;65(11):996–1002. https://doi.org/10.1136/jclinpath-2012-200742.
58. Kloor M, Becker C, Benner A, Woerner SM, Gebert J, Ferrone S, von Knebel DM. Immunoselective pressure and human leukocyte antigen class I antigen machinery defects in microsatellite unstable colorectal cancers. Cancer Res. 2005;65(14):6418–24. https://doi.org/10.1158/0008-5472.CAN-05-0044.

59. Michel S, Linnebacher M, Alcaniz J, Voss M, Wagner R, Dippold W, Becker C, von Knebel DM, Ferrone S, Kloor M. Lack of HLA class II antigen expression in microsatellite unstable colorectal carcinomas is caused by mutations in HLA class II regulatory genes. Int J Cancer. 2010;127(4):889–98. https://doi.org/10.1002/ijc.25106.
60. Surmann EM, Voigt AY, Michel S, Bauer K, Reuschenbach M, Ferrone S, von Knebel DM, Kloor M. Association of high CD4-positive T cell infiltration with mutations in HLA class II-regulatory genes in microsatellite-unstable colorectal cancer. Cancer Immunol Immunother. 2014. https://doi.org/10.1007/s00262-014-1638-4.
61. Stelloo E, Versluis MA, Nijman HW, de Bruyn M, Plat A, Osse EM, van Dijk RH, Nout RA, Creutzberg CL, de Bock GH, Smit VT, Bosse T, Hollema H. Microsatellite instability derived JAK1 frameshift mutations are associated with tumor immune evasion in endometrioid endometrial cancer. Oncotarget. 2016;7(26):39885–93. https://doi.org/10.18632/oncotarget.9414.
62. Llosa NJ, Cruise M, Tam A, Wick EC, Hechenbleikner EM, Taube JM, Blosser L, Fan H, Wang H, Luber B, Zhang M, Papadopoulos N, Kinzler KW, Vogelstein B, Sears CL, Anders RA, Pardoll DM, Housseau F. The vigorous immune microenvironment of microsatellite instable colon cancer is balanced by multiple counter-inhibitory checkpoints. Cancer Discov. 2014. https://doi.org/10.1158/2159-8290.CD-14-0863.
63. Vogelstein B, Papadopoulos N, Velculescu VE, Zhou S, Diaz LA Jr, Kinzler KW. Cancer genome landscapes. Science. 2013;339(6127):1546–58. https://doi.org/10.1126/science.1235122.
64. Cancer Genome Atlas Network. Comprehensive molecular characterization of human colon and rectal cancer. Nature. 2012;487(7407):330–7. https://doi.org/10.1038/nature11252.
65. Pardoll DM. The blockade of immune checkpoints in cancer immunotherapy. Nat Rev Cancer. 2012;12(4):252–64. https://doi.org/10.1038/nrc3239.
66. Tumeh PC, Harview CL, Yearley JH, Shintaku IP, Taylor EJ, Robert L, Chmielowski B, Spasic M, Henry G, Ciobanu V, West AN, Carmona M, Kivork C, Seja E, Cherry G, Gutierrez AJ, Grogan TR, Mateus C, Tomasic G, Glaspy JA, Emerson RO, Robins H, Pierce RH, Elashoff DA, Robert C, Ribas A. PD-1 blockade induces responses by inhibiting adaptive immune resistance. Nature. 2014;515(7528):568–71. https://doi.org/10.1038/nature13954.
67. Burn J, Gerdes AM, Macrae F, Mecklin JP, Moeslein G, Olschwang S, Eccles D, Evans DG, Maher ER, Bertario L, Bisgaard ML, Dunlop MG, Ho JW, Hodgson SV, Lindblom A, Lubinski J, Morrison PJ, Murday V, Ramesar R, Side L, Scott RJ, Thomas HJ, Vasen HF, Barker G, Crawford G, Elliott F, Movahedi M, Pylvanainen K, Wijnen JT, Fodde R, Lynch HT, Mathers JC, Bishop DT. Long-term effect of aspirin on cancer risk in carriers of hereditary colorectal cancer: an analysis from the CAPP2 randomised controlled trial. Lancet. 2011;378(9809):2081–7. https://doi.org/10.1016/S0140-6736(11)61049-0.
68. Zelenay S, van der Veen AG, Bottcher JP, Snelgrove KJ, Rogers N, Acton SE, Chakravarty P, Girotti MR, Marais R, Quezada SA, Sahai E, Reis e Sousa C. Cyclooxygenase-dependent tumor growth through evasion of immunity. Cell. 2015;162(6):1257–70. https://doi.org/10.1016/j.cell.2015.08.015.

Chapter 24
Hereditary Colorectal Cancer: Immunotherapy Approaches

David J. Hermel and Stephen B. Gruber

Abstract Advances in our understanding of the tumor-immune microenvironment have provided new therapeutic approaches to treat cancer. While first-line medical treatment for colorectal cancer typically involves chemotherapy and biological agents, the clinical efficacy of immune checkpoint inhibitors in microsatellite instability-high colorectal cancer has prompted renewed interest in immunotherapy as a treatment strategy for this tumor type. For patients with hereditary colorectal cancer syndromes characterized by exceptionally high somatic mutational loads, immunotherapy has specifically shown exceptional promise. In this chapter, we explore the rationale for immunotherapy in the treatment of colorectal cancer and focus on various immunotherapeutic strategies attempted thus far, including autologous, peptide, dendritic and viral vector-based vaccines, adoptive cell transfer, chimeric antigen receptor T-cell therapy, and immune checkpoint inhibitors. In addition, we discuss novel combination approaches and innovative techniques under investigation to create a more immune-responsive tumor environment for microsatellite stable colorectal cancer.

Keywords Immunotherapy · Hereditary colorectal cancer · Cancer vaccines · Adoptive cell transfer · Immune checkpoint inhibitors

Compelled by anecdotal evidence of erysipelas predating tumor regression in a subset of patients, William Coley carried out the first clinical study of immunotherapy in 1891 using a killed bacterial suspension as a therapy for patients with inoperable tumors [1]. Since Coley's early foray into the field of cancer immunotherapy, a wealth of unique immunotherapeutic approaches have garnered initial enthusiasm from in vitro and in vivo preclinical experiments, yet controlled clinical trials, on the whole, have failed to

D. J. Hermel
University of Southern California, Los Angeles, CA, USA

S. B. Gruber (✉)
University of Southern California, Norris Comprehensive Cancer Center, Los Angeles, CA, USA
e-mail: sgruber@usc.edu

L. Valle et al. (eds.), *Hereditary Colorectal Cancer*,
https://doi.org/10.1007/978-3-319-74259-5_24

achieve anticipated potential, except in very specific circumstances [2]. Nonetheless, with improved understanding of the complex regulatory mechanisms governing the tumor-immune interface [3] as well as the impressive clinical results achieved with immune checkpoint inhibitors in multiple tumor types [4], renewed interest in the field has spurred innovative strategies aimed at leveraging and augmenting a patient's innate antitumor response in an effort to effectively treat colorectal cancer (CRC).

In direct contrast to melanoma, renal carcinoma, and even non-small cell lung cancer (NSCLC), early benefit of immunotherapy in CRC was not immediately realized [5]. However, accumulating data have revealed that subsets of CRC patients with hypermutated tumor phenotypes – specifically those arising on the basis of Lynch syndrome driven by mutations in the mismatch repair (MMR) system or those hypermutated CRCs attributable to mutations in the DNA polymerase genes *POLE* and *POLD1* [6] – have an unprecedented clinical response to immune checkpoint therapy. In this chapter, we will explore the rationale for immunotherapy in CRC, as well as the success and failures of various immunomodulatory strategies employed by investigators and clinicians to target malignant CRC cells.

1 Rationale for Immune Response

With a clear association to intestinal dysbiosis [7] and inflammatory bowel disease [8], CRC would seem to have an inherent biological predisposition to the effects of immunologics. Moreover, a host of molecular inflammatory mediators, including TGF-β, have been implicated in the pathogenesis of CRC [9], with anti-inflammatory agents, such as nonsteroidal anti-inflammatory drugs, associated with a decreased incidence of CRC [10]. Furthermore, multiple studies have explicitly demonstrated that the extent and location of tumor-infiltrating lymphocytes (TILs) are prognostic and predictive of the metastatic potential of CRC. This suggests that the immune response to CRC has a fundamental role in the pathogenesis and clinical course of the disease.

Numerous studies have investigated the association between TILs and CRC progression and survival. In a study of 959 resected CRC specimens, designation of a strong immune cell infiltrate by histopathologic assessment in 377 samples correlated with the absence of early metastatic processes, including vascular emboli, lymphatic invasion, and perineural inflammation [11]. Further characterization of this infiltrate with flow cytometry identified a predominance of early memory and effector memory CD8+ T cells. Moreover, the extent of CD45RO+ memory T cells using tissue microarray analysis of 415 specimens correlated with clinical outcomes and was an independent prognostic factor [12]. Subsequent genomic and in situ immunostaining of tumors from this patient cohort found that increased immune cell density (CD3, CD8, GZMB, and CD45RO) in both the center and invasive margin could better predict patient survival than the histopathological methods devised by the UICC-TNM classification.

Given the demonstrated prognostic utility of TILs in CRC, a follow-up analysis of 602 stage I and II CRC patients from 2 independent cohorts quantified the survival benefit and tumor recurrence rate in 4 groups of patients stratified based on tumor CD45RO+ and CD8+ cells in the center and invasive margin. Patients with the highest density of immune cells had a 5-year survival rate of 86.2% and a 4.8% tumor recurrence rate, while those with the lowest density of immune cells had a 27.5% 5-year survival rate and a 75% tumor recurrence rate [13]. This immune criterion was found to be an independent prognostic factor in multivariate analysis, which lead to the introduction of an "immunoscore" [14] that was subsequently validated as a prognostic marker in a worldwide consortium-based analysis of 1336 stage I/II/III colon cancer patients [15]. The interplay of other immune cells in the tumor microenvironment, including M1 and M2 tumor-associated macrophages [16], tumor-infiltrating dendritic cells [17], and different T regulatory subsets [18], may aid in the future clinical refinement of this score.

Beyond the prognostic information conferred by TILs, the presence of a Crohn's-like lymphoid reaction (CLR) is an important, independent marker of the host immune response and CRC outcomes. In a population-based study of 2369 incident cases of CRC, patients whose tumors demonstrated a prominent CLR experienced better CRC-specific survival and overall survival (OS) than those patients whose tumors lacked a CLR. This prognostic advantage was evident even after adjustment for the presence of traditional prognostic factors, microsatellite instability (MSI), and the presence of TILs [19].

Representative histopathologic images illustrate the recognizable microscopic features of the host immune response in CRCs. TILs are recognized by their small blue mononuclear cells, typically surrounded by a halo (Fig. 24.1). True TILs need to be directly observed infiltrating between tumor cells, not in the surrounding stroma. The advancing edge of CRCs is the best place to assess the presence of a prominent inflammatory reaction. Standard pathologic criteria consider a minimum of three lymphoid aggregates to be present at the leading edge of the tumor in order to be considered a prominent CLR. Figure 24.2 illustrates the low-power histopathologic appearance of CLR.

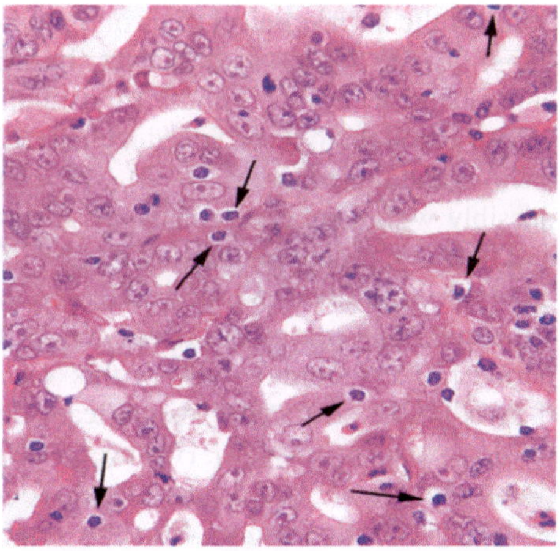

Fig. 24.1 Tumor-infiltrating lymphocytes (TILs) infiltrating between tumor cells are shown with arrows (Photomicrograph courtesy of Dr. Joel Greenson)

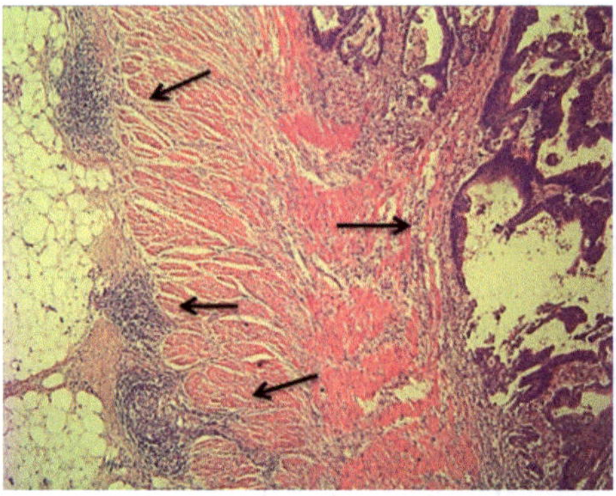

Fig. 24.2 Low-power view of Crohn's-like lymphoid reaction (CLR – shown with left arrows) at the advancing edge of an invasive colorectal cancer (right arrow). These lymphoid aggregates are constituted largely of B cells, with smaller populations of T cells (Photomicrograph courtesy of Dr. Joel Greenson)

2 Therapeutic Strategies for Immune Modulation in CRC

Given the well-delineated evidence for immune cell involvement in the tumorigenesis of CRC, multiple therapeutic strategies have been attempted to specifically augment the host adaptive immune response to hone in on malignant cells. Some of the earliest approaches in this regard include cancer vaccines and autologous adoptive cell transfer, with more recent approaches including immune checkpoint inhibitors and novel combination regimens.

2.1 Autologous Tumor Cell Vaccines

Some of the initial clinical trials of immunotherapy in CRC used autologous whole-tumor vaccines as a way to activate host defenses against a variety of non-specific antigens present in the tumor. Augmentation of the immune response to the tumor cells was sought to be achieved with an adjuvant immunostimulatory agent, such as bacillus Calmette-Guerin (BCG). The results of this approach largely failed, except possibly within subgroup analyses. A randomized phase III study of 412 stage II and III colon cancer patients found no difference in clinical outcomes between surgical resection alone and surgical resection in combination with intradermal vaccine injections of an autologous tumor cell-BCG vaccine at a 7.6-year median follow-up period [20]. A similar study of this vaccine with a booster vaccination given at 6 months demonstrated no significant difference in OS between vaccinated and unvaccinated patients [21]. However, vaccinated patients did have a 44% risk reduction for recurrence at 5.3-year median follow-up, and subgroup analysis of patients with stage II colon cancer did show improved recurrence-free survival (RFS) and OS in vaccinated patients [22]. Subsequent retrospective investigation of banked tumor samples from this study identified improved disease-specific survival and an increased recurrence-free interval in vaccinated patients with MSI irrespective of tumor stage [23].

An alternative strategy using whole-tumor vaccines in CRC made use of a non-lytic, attenuated Newcastle disease virus (NDV) strain rather than BCG to stimulate the immune response [24]. In a prospective, randomized phase III trial of 50 patients with CRC-proven hepatic metastases, there was no significant difference in OS between those vaccinated and those not, yet those with colon primary (vs. rectal) had descreased metastases and improved OS in the intention-to-treat analysis.

Given the technical difficulty with garnering autologous tumor cells, a novel vaccine was developed using irradiated, allogenic CRC cells in combination with GM-CSF-producing cells and showed early promise in a phase I study [25]. In addition, a phase I study of an autologous tumor-based product incorporating a plasmid encoding GM-CSF and a bifunctional short hairpin RNAi targeting the proprotein convertase furin, which normally activates both TGF-β1 and TGF-β2, has shown success in a variety of advanced solid tumors [26]. Future studies are planned with this vaccine in patients with metastatic CRC planning to undergo curative resection.

2.2 *Peptide Vaccines*

In contrast to autologous whole-cell tumor vaccines, which contain a myriad of undefined tumor antigens, peptide vaccines consist of specific antigens that are designed to generate a host tumor-directed immune response. A number of peptide vaccines have been tested in early-phase clinical trials directed against known CRC-associated antigens, including SART3 [27], p53 [28], MUC1 [29], heat shock protein gp96 [30], β-HCG [31], CEA [32], survivin 2b [33], RNF43 and TOMM34 [34]. While many of these studies succeeded in generating a measured host immune response against the various targeted antigens, there were no substantial survival advantages demonstrating clinical benefit.

Other studies have utilized vaccines with multiple antigens combined to trigger a broader immune response. For example, in an HLA-A-status double-blind, phase II clinical trial of 96 chemotherapy-naïve, advanced CRC patients, a vaccine with HLA-A24-restricted peptides RNF43, TOMM34, KOC1, VEGFR1, and VEGFR2 was tested in combination with oxaliplatin-based chemotherapy as first-line therapy [35]. No difference in OS, PFS, or overall response rates (ORR) was observed between the HLA groups; however, HLA-matched patients with a neutrophil/lymphocytic ratio of <3.0 showed a delayed response to therapy.

Similarly, a phase II clinical study evaluated the utility of a personalized peptide vaccination (PPV) in patients with CRC. This vaccine included a range of 2–4 peptides based on preexisting IgG titers to 31 MHC class I epitopes from 15 tumor-associated antigens [36]. In this study, 60 patients with previously treated, advanced CRC were treated with 2 series of 6 vaccinations while receiving standard-of-care therapy. In the interim between the two vaccination series, repeat IgG titer testing was performed, and, based on the IgG titer response, new peptide combinations were selected. Overall, 1- and 2-year survival rates were unimpressive at 53% and 22%, respectively. However, in subgroup analysis, increased peptide-specific cytotoxic response after vaccinations was associated with an improvement in OS.

2.3 Dendritic Cell Vaccines

As an essential intermediary between antigen presentation and the T-cell effector response, dendritic cells (DCs) have been utilized in clinical vaccine trials as a rational approach to elicit an antigen-mediated T-cell response against directed tumor cells. Prior to injection, DCs are loaded with tumor-specific antigens in vitro. In CRC patients, a number of different strategies have been employed to maximize the efficacy of DC vaccines with limited success thus far.

An early straightforward approach involved loading autologous DCs with CEA peptide CAP-1 and administering the cells to 21 patients with advanced CEA-expressing malignancies (11 with CRC) [37]. While no significant toxicities were observed, efficacy of the vaccine was limited, with only one patient experiencing stable disease after vaccination.

In contrast to the previous study, which loaded autologous DCs with only one antigenic peptide, an alternative clinical phase 1/2 trial loaded DCs with six HLA-A*0201 binding peptides derived from CEA, MAGE, HER2/neu, keyhole limpet hemocyanin protein, and pan-DR epitope peptide [38]. Of the 11 evaluable patients with CRC, all had progressive disease despite the increased immune titers to the tumor-associated antigens.

However, some encouraging results have been observed as well. In a phase II clinical study, autologous DCs pulsed with an allogenic melanoma cell lysate containing high expression of MAGE-A3 were tested in a group of 20 patients with MAGE-enriched stage IV CRC [39]. Although median PFS was 2.4 months, five patients (25%) experience greater than 6-month prolonged PFS, showing evidence of durability in a population that initially had progressive disease.

In addition, a phase II, randomized clinical trial explored a vaccine with autologous DCs pulsed with autologous tumor lysate in combination with cytokine-induced killer cell therapy in 54 patients with either gastric or CRC [40]. The 13 CRC patients in the treatment arm showed significant improvement in 5-year disease-free and OS compared to the CRC controls (66% vs. 8% and 75% vs. 15%, respectively). Further studies are exploring this in the adjuvant setting.

The first randomized clinical trial in metastatic CRC patients with autologous DCs was completed in 2016. In this phase II study, 52 patients were randomized to either receive an autologous tumor lysate DC vaccine plus best supportive care (BSC) or BSC [41]. While this vaccine did generate a tumor-specific immune response, there were no benefits seen in PFS and OS, and the study was terminated early due to futility. In general, while a few studies highlight some positive results from DC vaccination, no substantial clinical benefit has been observed in clinical trials with this treatment modality.

2.4 Viral Vector-Based Vaccines

Many viruses have been engineered to express tumor-associated antigens and exert their immunogenicity by directly infecting DCs and facilitating an accelerated T- and B-cell response against cancer-specific cells. Multiple viral vectors have been studied in CRC, including poxvirus, adenovirus, and adeno-associated virus, with various tumor-associated antigens incorporated into the viral architecture for cellular expression, such as CEA, epithelial glycoprotein (Ep-CAM), and guanylyl cyclase 2C (GUCY2C) [42].

An early phase I clinical trial tested a poxvirus expressing CEA and three co-stimulatory molecules (B7–1, ICAM-1, and LFA-3; TRICOM), with a follow-up booster vaccination of a fowl pox virus expressing the same transgenes [43]. In this study, of 58 patients with advanced CEA-expressing cancers, 40% of patients had stable disease for at least 4 months, many with prolonged stable disease for greater than 6 months, and the majority had CEA-specific T-cell responses after vaccination.

In addition, a poxvirus vaccine, OXB-301, expressing oncofetal antigen 5 T4 was studied in a phase II trial of 20 metastatic CRC patients both pre- and postoperatively after resection of CRC liver metastases [44]. Patients with an above-the-median 5 T4 antibody response and a proliferative lymphocytic infiltration in the metastatic lesions had significantly prolonged OS compared to patients that did not have these findings.

Two other open-label, single-arm trials tested this vaccine before, during, and after chemotherapy in patients with metastatic CRC [45, 46]. In both studies, the majority had 5 T4 antibody-specific immune responses, with ORR of 54% and 58%, respectively, yet survival at 2 years was comparable to historic data. Moreover, a randomized, phase II study using a canarypox viral vector expressing CEA and B7–1 in combination with palliative chemotherapy was tested in 118 patients with metastatic CRC [47]. All patients developed anti-canarypox IgG, but increased anti-CEA antibody titers were detected in only three patients. Overall, only 42 (40.4%) of 104 evaluable patients achieved an objective clinical response, which is comparable to chemotherapy alone, casting doubt on the therapeutic efficacy of this approach.

Researchers have also investigated a combination poxvector vaccine encoding CEA and MUC1 plus TRICOM and unique approaches to augment host immunity to this vaccine. For example, a prospective, randomized phase II clinical trial evaluated whether this vaccine in combination with autologous DCs modified ex vivo or the vaccine alone would provide greater clinical benefit and induce more specific antigen-specific immune responses in patients disease-free after CRC surgery and perioperative chemotherapy [48]. There were no differences in clinical outcomes (RFS/OS) between the two strategies.

Alternatively, another viral vector evaluated in clinical trials is the recombinant non-replicating adenovirus serotype 5 (Ad5)-based vector platform with early 1 (E1) and early 2b (E2b) gene deletions and a transgene inserted for CEA. In a completed, phase I/II trial in patients with metastatic CRC who had failed prior chemotherapy, 29-month OS was 20% in the intent-to-treat group with a median OS of 11 months [49]. Further investigation was deemed warranted with a phase III trial planned.

2.5 Adoptive Cell Transfer Therapy

In contrast to vaccines that activate the adaptive immune response, adoptive cell transfer therapy involves the passive infusion of T cells into a patient. The process begins with the extraction of T cells from a patient, ex vivo activation and expansion, and passive reinfusion into a patient, typically after a lymphodepleting preparative regimen. An early open, nonrandomized clinical study investigated the utility of a TIL infusion and modulated doses of IL-2 as adjuvant treatment in 47 patients with liver metastases from CRC [50]. Overall, postoperative administration of this infusion did not lead to a significantly improved long-term survival or reduced risk of cancer recurrence.

A subsequent phase I/II study of 71 metastatic CRC patients who underwent radical or palliative surgery likewise evaluated the efficacy of a TIL infusion. In this study, TILs were extracted from sentinel lymph nodes in 55 patients with stage I–IV disease (9 with stage IV disease) [51]. These lymphocytes were expanded ex vivo and transfused them back into patients without any apparent toxicity. In a 24-month follow-up of the stage IV patients, there was a significant survival benefit in comparison to the control group (55.6 versus 17.5, $p = 0.02$).

While TILs from the previous studies did not undergo T-cell reengineering, a phase I study of three patients with metastatic, treatment-refractory CRC utilized autologous peripheral T cells that were genetically modified to express a high-avidity murine T-cell receptor against CEA [52]. These T cells were adoptively transferred into patients with IL-2 after receiving an immunodepleting regimen of cyclophosphamide and fludarabine. Though all patients had reductions in serum CEA and one patient had a partial objective response, all developed a severe transient inflammatory colitis with early closure of the study secondary to adverse events.

A notable case report as part on an ongoing phase II clinical trial (NCT01174121) identified a patient with metastatic CRC who had regression of all seven of her metastatic CRC lung lesions after receiving adoptive transfer of ex vivo expanded TILs directed against mutant *KRAS* p.G12D [53]. The therapy was preceded by a myeloablative regimen of cyclophosphamide and fludarabine and followed by five doses of IL-2. The highest reacting T-cell clone against *KRAS* p.G12D contained an increasing frequency of CD28 and CD57 markers and had a central memory phenotype (CD45RO + CD62L+). The identification of HLA-C*08:02-restricted T-cell receptors that target *KRAS* p.G12D neoepitopes provides an opportunity to develop T-cell receptor gene therapy directed against a common driver mutation found in multiple cancer types and is an exciting avenue of current research.

A subsequent study by Maoz et al. investigated a large, population-based sample of 4346 colorectal cancer patients that had been studied for the presence of *KRAS* p.G12D and imputed HLA types to better understand the generalizability of this important single case report [54]. The prevalence of any *KRAS* mutation was 33.2% (1441 of 4346 patients), and nearly 38% of the *KRAS*-positive tumors harbored a p.G12D mutation. HLA typing found that 18.4% of patients had the same HLA-C*08:02 type observed in the above case report. Overall, 2.3% of a representative population of CRC cases shared the same combination of *KRAS* mutation and HLA configuration as the patient that responded to the adoptive transfer of TILs.

2.6 *Adoptive CAR-T-Cell Therapy*

Chimeric antigen receptor T (CAR-T)-cell therapy has achieved impressive results in the treatment of CD19+ B-cell hematologic malignancies, but developing CAR-T therapy for solid tumors has been challenging to date. CAR-T cells are genetically modified autologous T cells that express a single-chain variable fragment (scFv) against a tumor-associated antigen and a CD3ζ domain that triggers cell activation upon antigen binding [55]. Despite the success in hematologic malignancy, it has been difficult to replicate that success in solid tumors for a variety of reasons, including the heterogeneity of solid tumors, difficulty in trafficking the cells to the tumor, the challenges of overcoming the inhibitory tumor microenvironment of solid tumors, and the associated systemic toxicity of this therapy [56].

CAR-T-cell therapy has been evaluated in CRC, with, as of yet, no real demonstration of substantial efficacy in early phase trials, with most trials ongoing to date. A case report of significant toxicity in a patient with HER-2-positive colon cancer who received HER-2-targeted CAR-T-cell therapy has led to reconsideration of appropriate antigen targets [57]. This patient developed lethal pulmonary toxicity 5 days after T-cell administration, which was thought to be due to recognition of HER-2 on lung epithelial cells. While no lymphodepletive preconditioning regimen was used in this patient, CAR-T-cell therapy remains in its infancy as a treatment for CRC at the present time.

2.7 *Immune Checkpoint Inhibitors*

Remarkable progress in our understanding of the tumor microenvironment has led to the recognition that tumor immune evasion constitutes a new, independent hallmark of cancer cell biology [58]. One of the fundamental inhibitory mechanisms exploited by tumor cells for immune escape is that of the immune checkpoint receptor/ligand interaction, which physiologically serves to dampen immune overactivation to ensure tissue homeostasis. Antibodies directed against immune checkpoints, cytotoxic T-lymphocyte-associated protein 4 (CTLA-4) and programmed death-1 receptor (PD-1) and its ligand (PD-L1), have demonstrated clinical efficacy in melanoma, NSCLC, and renal cell carcinoma [59]. While they were first thought to be ineffective in CRC based upon the results of early phase trials with inhibitors of CTLA-4 [60], PD-1 [61], and PD-L1 [62], a 3-year follow-up analysis from a trial with PD-1 inhibitor nivolumab [63] interestingly noted one patient with refractory MSI-high (MSI-H) CRC who achieved a complete response that was ongoing at 3 years [64]. The case prompted efforts to identify characteristics of this specific patient conducive to clinical benefit from immune checkpoint inhibitor therapy.

To date, emerging biomarkers of immune checkpoint inhibitor efficacy include MSI, upregulation of PD-L1 on tumor and immune cells, TIL expression, and somatic mutational load. In regard to mutational load, experimental evidence has shown that increased mutational burden directly leads to increased tumor neoantigen formation and facilitates a more robust immune response from checkpoint blockade [65]. Whole exome sequencing of tumor DNA from patients on anti-CTLA-4 and anti-PD-1 therapy have revealed a correlation between response to therapy and non-synonymous mutational load [66–68]. Additionally, studies have shown that efficacy of immune checkpoint inhibitors is significantly associated with neoantigen burden [68]; however, no consensus neoantigen sequences with associated clinical benefit have been identified, and, in some cases, patients with low mutational burden and atypical neoantigen patterns have derived clinical benefit from checkpoint blockade [66, 67].

MSI is present in approximately 15% of all CRCs and arises from dysfunctional DNA replication secondary to either monoallelic germline or, more often sporadic, MMR-deficient (MMR-D) enzyme activity [69]. Indeed, MSI is one of the hallmarks of Lynch syndrome. MSI-H CRCs are characterized by significantly increased mutational load when compared to microsatellite stable (MSS) CRCs. For example, whole exome pyrosequencing of 454 primary CRCs found 8 times more somatic nonsynonymous variations in MSI cancers than in MSS cancers [70]. In addition, a study of 103 MSI CRCs from 2 independent cohorts identified a correlation between CD8+ TIL density and the total number of frameshift mutations [71]. The robust immune response in these tumors is thought to be secondary to a T-cell-driven response to mutation-derived neoepitopes. This reaction, in combination with other elements of tumor environment, including PD-L1 expression, is thought to facilitate the response to immune checkpoint inhibitors.

The first clinical data to show benefit in MSI-H CRC emerged from a multicenter phase II study of PD-1 inhibitor pembrolizumab in patients with chemo-refractory MSI-H or MSS metastatic CRC [72]. Among a total of 32 patients with CRC (10 with dMMR and 18 with pMMR) who were given 10 mg/kg of pembrolizumab every 14 days, 4 patients with dMMR CRC experienced a response and 7 had stable disease. In contrast, patients with pMMR had no responses, and two achieved stable disease at 12 weeks. Updated at ASCO 2017, among a total of 61 patients with MSI-H CRC with a median follow-up of 7.4 months, ORR for MSI-H CRC was 26.2% (95% CI, 15.8–39.1%), with 15 confirmed responses and 1 unconfirmed response [73]. In addition, median duration of response was not reached, and 100% of responses were ongoing. Given these encouraging results, the FDA granted accelerated approval for pembrolizumab in patients with MSI-H metastatic colon cancer in May 2017. This landmark approval was notable since FDA approved pembolizumab for the treatment of any tumor demonstrating the MSI-H phenotype or deficient MMR, regardless of the tumor site of origin. This data have also resulted in efforts to encourage more broad MSI screening, even in those with metastatic disease.

In addition to pembrolizumab, combination checkpoint inhibition with nivolumab (3 mg/kg) and/or ipilimumab (1 mg/kg) is currently being investigated in patients with MSI-H metastatic CRC [74]. With the combination arm still enrolling, an interim analysis of 74 patients in the nivolumab monotherapy arm demonstrated an ORR of 31.1%, and the disease control rate was 68.9%. Median PFS was 9.6 months, and median OS had still not been reached. The majority of patients achieving stable disease at greater than 18 weeks remained on study, and 83% of responses were ongoing at the time of the interim analysis.

In addition to MSI-H CRC, new approaches are under study for patients with MSS CRC. One strategy is to combine immune checkpoint inhibitors with a mitogen-activated protein kinase kinase (MEK) inhibitor, which has been shown in preclinical studies to upregulate PD-L1 tumor expression and foster a more attractive milieu for checkpoint blockade. This was tested in a phase 1b clinical trial using PD-L1 inhibitor atezolizumab in conjunction with the MEK inhibitor cobimetinib in patients with heavily pretreated MMR-proficient (pMMR) metastatic CRC [75]. In this study, 800 mg of atezolizumab was given every 2 weeks in combination with escalating doses of cobimetinib to 23 patients. The ORR was 17%, with tumor shrinkage of at least 30% in four patients and stable disease in five patients (22%). Of the four responders, three had CRCs that were pMMR, and one had a tumor with an unknown MMR status. Responses were ongoing at the data cutoff point and lasted up to 7.7 months.

Overall, PD-1 inhibitors have demonstrated impressive results in patients with MSI CRC. Early clinical trials of immune checkpoint inhibitors in combination with chemotherapy and radiation are accruing data. Finding ways to elicit a substantial response in patients with MSS CRC has been encouraging in preliminary studies.

3 Conclusion

While the diversity of hereditary CRC syndromes suggests that many therapeutic approaches will be required to address the underlying pathophysiology of these distinct entities, some important lessons about immunotherapy are already emerging. First, all of the refractory or relapsing cancers arising in Lynch syndrome are likely to benefit from some type of immunotherapy in the future. Second, immunotherapy holds promise for rare genetic syndromes characterized by exceptionally high somatic mutational loads, such as those related to inherited mutations in *POLD1* or *POLE*. Third, as expertise continues to develop in the manipulation of the adaptive host immune response, it appears likely that targeted therapies for hereditary CRCs with specific mutational profiles will be able to incorporate immune regulation with other types of chemotherapy. The promise of engineered T cells for hematologic malignancies and other forms of immune therapy have special challenges in the setting of the complex tumor microenvironment of CRC, but improved understanding of the role of TILs, CLR, and immune manipulation offers an enticing future for the successful management of patients with hereditary CRCs.

References

1. McCarthy EF. The toxins of William B. Coley and the treatment of bone and soft-tissue sarcomas. Iowa Orthop J. 2006;26:154–8.
2. Sell S. Cancer immunotherapy: breakthrough or "deja vu, all over again"? Tumour Biol. 2017;39:1010428317707764.

3. Santarpia M, Karachaliou N. Tumor immune microenvironment characterization and response to anti-PD-1 therapy. Cancer Biol Med. 2015;12:74–8.
4. Farkona S, Diamandis EP, Blasutig IM. Cancer immunotherapy: the beginning of the end of cancer? BMC Med. 2016;14:73.
5. Xiang B, Snook AE, Magee MS, Waldman SA. Colorectal cancer immunotherapy. Discov Med. 2013;15:301–8.
6. Bourdais R, Rousseau B, Pujals A, et al. Polymerase proofreading domain mutations: new opportunities for immunotherapy in hypermutated colorectal cancer beyond MMR deficiency. Crit Rev Oncol Hematol. 2017;113:242–8.
7. Nistal E, Fernandez-Fernandez N, Vivas S, Olcoz JL. Factors determining colorectal cancer: the role of the intestinal microbiota. Front Oncol. 2015;5:220.
8. Triantafillidis JK, Nasioulas G, Kosmidis PA. Colorectal cancer and inflammatory bowel disease: epidemiology, risk factors, mechanisms of carcinogenesis and prevention strategies. Anticancer Res. 2009;29:2727–37.
9. Hong S, Lee HJ, Kim SJ, Hahm KB. Connection between inflammation and carcinogenesis in gastrointestinal tract: focus on TGF-beta signaling. World J Gastroenterol. 2010;16:2080–93.
10. Ruder EH, Laiyemo AO, Graubard BI, Hollenbeck AR, Schatzkin A, Cross AJ. Non-steroidal anti-inflammatory drugs and colorectal cancer risk in a large, prospective cohort. Am J Gastroenterol. 2011;106:1340–50.
11. Pages F, Berger A, Camus M, et al. Effector memory T cells, early metastasis, and survival in colorectal cancer. N Engl J Med. 2005;353:2654–66.
12. Galon J, Costes A, Sanchez-Cabo F, et al. Type, density, and location of immune cells within human colorectal tumors predict clinical outcome. Science. 2006;313:1960–4.
13. Pages F, Kirilovsky A, Mlecnik B, et al. In situ cytotoxic and memory T cells predict outcome in patients with early-stage colorectal cancer. J Clin Oncol. 2009;27:5944–51.
14. Galon J, Mlecnik B, Bindea G, et al. Towards the introduction of the 'Immunoscore' in the classification of malignant tumours. J Pathol. 2014;232:199–209.
15. Galon J, Mlecnik B, Marliot F, et al. Validation of the immunoscore (IM) as a prognostic marker in stage I/II/III colon cancer: results of a worldwide consortium-based analysis of 1,336 patients. J Clin Oncol. 2016;34. (suppl; abstr 3500).
16. Kwak Y, Koh J, Kim DW, Kang SB, Kim WH, Lee HS. Immunoscore encompassing CD3+ and CD8+ T cell densities in distant metastasis is a robust prognostic marker for advanced colorectal cancer. Oncotarget. 2016;7:81778–90.
17. Sandel MH, Dadabayev AR, Menon AG, et al. Prognostic value of tumor-infiltrating dendritic cells in colorectal cancer: role of maturation status and intratumoral localization. Clin Cancer Res. 2005;11:2576–82.
18. Syed Khaja AS, Toor SM, El Salhat H, Ali BR, Elkord E. Intratumoral FoxP3+Helios+ Regulatory T cells upregulating immunosuppressive molecules are expanded in human colorectal cancer. Front Immunol. 2017;8:619.
19. Rozek LS, Schmit SL, Greenson JK, et al. Tumor-infiltrating lymphocytes, Crohn's-like lymphoid reaction, and survival from colorectal cancer. J Natl Cancer Inst. 2016;108.
20. Harris JE, Ryan L, Hoover HC Jr, et al. Adjuvant active specific immunotherapy for stage II and III colon cancer with an autologous tumor cell vaccine: Eastern Cooperative Oncology Group Study E5283. J Clin Oncol. 2000;18:148–57.
21. Vermorken JB, Claessen AM, van Tinteren H, et al. Active specific immunotherapy for stage II and stage III human colon cancer: a randomised trial. Lancet. 1999;353:345–50.
22. Uyl-de Groot CA, Vermorken JB, Hanna MG Jr, et al. Immunotherapy with autologous tumor cell-BCG vaccine in patients with colon cancer: a prospective study of medical and economic benefits. Vaccine. 2005;23:2379–87.
23. de Weger VA, Turksma AW, Voorham QJ, et al. Clinical effects of adjuvant active specific immunotherapy differ between patients with microsatellite-stable and microsatellite-instable colon cancer. Clin Cancer Res. 2012;18:882–9.
24. Schulze T, Kemmner W, Weitz J, Wernecke KD, Schirrmacher V, Schlag PM. Efficiency of adjuvant active specific immunization with Newcastle disease virus modified tumor cells in

colorectal cancer patients following resection of liver metastases: results of a prospective randomized trial. Cancer Immunol Immunother. 2009;58:61–9.
25. Zheng L, Edil BH, Soares KC, et al. A safety and feasibility study of an allogeneic colon cancer cell vaccine administered with a granulocyte-macrophage colony stimulating factor-producing bystander cell line in patients with metastatic colorectal cancer. Ann Surg Oncol. 2014;21:3931–7.
26. Senzer N, Barve M, Kuhn J, et al. Phase I trial of "bi-shRNAi(furin)/GMCSF DNA/autologous tumor cell" vaccine (FANG) in advanced cancer. Mol Ther. 2012;20:679–86.
27. Miyagi Y, Imai N, Sasatomi T, et al. Induction of cellular immune responses to tumor cells and peptides in colorectal cancer patients by vaccination with SART3 peptides. Clin Cancer Res. 2001;7:3950–62.
28. Speetjens FM, Kuppen PJ, Welters MJ, et al. Induction of p53-specific immunity by a p53 synthetic long peptide vaccine in patients treated for metastatic colorectal cancer. Clin Cancer Res. 2009;15:1086–95.
29. Kimura T, McKolanis JR, Dzubinski LA, et al. MUC1 vaccine for individuals with advanced adenoma of the colon: a cancer immunoprevention feasibility study. Cancer Prev Res (Phila). 2013;6:18–26.
30. Mazzaferro V, Coppa J, Carrabba MG, et al. Vaccination with autologous tumor-derived heat-shock protein gp96 after liver resection for metastatic colorectal cancer. Clin Cancer Res. 2003;9:3235–45.
31. Moulton HM, Yoshihara PH, Mason DH, Iversen PL, Triozzi PL. Active specific immunotherapy with a beta-human chorionic gonadotropin peptide vaccine in patients with metastatic colorectal cancer: antibody response is associated with improved survival. Clin Cancer Res. 2002;8:2044–51.
32. Ullenhag GJ, Frodin JE, Jeddi-Tehrani M, et al. Durable carcinoembryonic antigen (CEA)-specific humoral and cellular immune responses in colorectal carcinoma patients vaccinated with recombinant CEA and granulocyte/macrophage colony-stimulating factor. Clin Cancer Res. 2004;10:3273–81.
33. Kameshima H, Tsuruma T, Torigoe T, et al. Immunogenic enhancement and clinical effect by type-I interferon of anti-apoptotic protein, survivin-derived peptide vaccine, in advanced colorectal cancer patients. Cancer Sci. 2011;102:1181–7.
34. Okuno K, Sugiura F, Hida JI, et al. Phase I clinical trial of a novel peptide vaccine in combination with UFT/LV for metastatic colorectal cancer. Exp Ther Med. 2011;2:73–9.
35. Hazama S, Nakamura Y, Tanaka H, et al. A phase Iotal study of five peptides combination with oxaliplatin-based chemotherapy as a first-line therapy for advanced colorectal cancer (FXV study). J Transl Med. 2014;12:108.
36. Kibe S, Yutani S, Motoyama S, et al. Phase II study of personalized peptide vaccination for previously treated advanced colorectal cancer. Cancer Immunol Res. 2014;2:1154–62.
37. Morse MA, Deng Y, Coleman D, et al. A Phase I study of active immunotherapy with carcinoembryonic antigen peptide (CAP-1)-pulsed, autologous human cultured dendritic cells in patients with metastatic malignancies expressing carcinoembryonic antigen. Clin Cancer Res. 1999;5:1331–8.
38. Kavanagh B, Ko A, Venook A, et al. Vaccination of metastatic colorectal cancer patients with matured dendritic cells loaded with multiple major histocompatibility complex class I peptides. J Immunother. 2007;30:762–72.
39. Toh HC, Wang WW, Chia WK, et al. Clinical benefit of allogeneic melanoma cell lysate-pulsed autologous dendritic cell vaccine in MAGE-positive colorectal cancer patients. Clin Cancer Res. 2009;15:7726–36.
40. Gao D, Li C, Xie X, et al. Autologous tumor lysate-pulsed dendritic cell immunotherapy with cytokine-induced killer cells improves survival in gastric and colorectal cancer patients. PLoS One. 2014;9:e93886.
41. Caballero-Banos M, Benitez-Ribas D, Tabera J, et al. Phase II randomised trial of autologous tumour lysate dendritic cell plus best supportive care compared with best supportive care in pre-treated advanced colorectal cancer patients. Eur J Cancer. 2016;64:167–74.

42. Chaurasiya S, Warner S. Viroimmunotherapy for colorectal cancer: clinical studies. Biomedicine. 2017;5:11.
43. Marshall JL, Gulley JL, Arlen PM, et al. Phase I study of sequential vaccinations with fowlpox-CEA(6D)-TRICOM alone and sequentially with vaccinia-CEA(6D)-TRICOM, with and without granulocyte-macrophage colony-stimulating factor, in patients with carcinoembryonic antigen-expressing carcinomas. J Clin Oncol. 2005;23:720–31.
44. Elkord E, Dangoor A, Drury NL, et al. An MVA-based vaccine targeting the oncofetal antigen 5T4 in patients undergoing surgical resection of colorectal cancer liver metastases. J Immunother. 2008;31:820–9.
45. Harrop R, Drury N, Shingler W, et al. Vaccination of colorectal cancer patients with modified vaccinia ankara encoding the tumor antigen 5T4 (TroVax) given alongside chemotherapy induces potent immune responses. Clin Cancer Res. 2007;13:4487–94.
46. Harrop R, Drury N, Shingler W, et al. Vaccination of colorectal cancer patients with TroVax given alongside chemotherapy (5-fluorouracil, leukovorin and irinotecan) is safe and induces potent immune responses. Cancer Immunol Immunother. 2008;57:977–86.
47. Kaufman HL, Lenz HJ, Marshall J, et al. Combination chemotherapy and ALVAC-CEA/B7.1 vaccine in patients with metastatic colorectal cancer. Clin Cancer Res. 2008;14:4843–9.
48. Morse MA, Niedzwiecki D, Marshall JL, et al. A randomized phase II study of immunization with dendritic cells modified with poxvectors encoding CEA and MUC1 compared with the same poxvectors plus GM-CSF for resected metastatic colorectal cancer. Ann Surg. 2013;258:879–86.
49. Balint JP, Gabitzsch ES, Rice A, et al. Extended evaluation of a phase 1/2 trial on dosing, safety, immunogenicity, and overall survival after immunizations with an advanced-generation Ad5 [E1-, E2b-]-CEA(6D) vaccine in late-stage colorectal cancer. Cancer Immunol Immunother. 2015;64:977–87.
50. Gardini A, Ercolani G, Riccobon A, et al. Adjuvant, adoptive immunotherapy with tumor infiltrating lymphocytes plus interleukin-2 after radical hepatic resection for colorectal liver metastases: 5-year analysis. J Surg Oncol. 2004;87:46–52.
51. Zhen YH, Liu XH, Yang Y, et al. Phase I/II study of adjuvant immunotherapy with sentinel lymph node T lymphocytes in patients with colorectal cancer. Cancer Immunol Immunother. 2015;64:1083–93.
52. Parkhurst MR, Yang JC, Langan RC, et al. T cells targeting carcinoembryonic antigen can mediate regression of metastatic colorectal cancer but induce severe transient colitis. Mol Ther. 2011;19:620–6.
53. Tran E, Robbins PF, Lu YC, et al. T-cell transfer therapy targeting mutant KRAS in cancer. N Engl J Med. 2016;375:2255–62.
54. Maoz A, Rennert G, Gruber SB. T-cell transfer therapy targeting mutant KRAS. N Engl J Med. 2017;376:e11.
55. Yu S, Li A, Liu Q, et al. Chimeric antigen receptor T cells: a novel therapy for solid tumors. J Hematol Oncol. 2017;10:78.
56. Yong CSM, Dardalhon V, Devaud C, Taylor N, Darcy PK, Kershaw MH. CAR T-cell therapy of solid tumors. Immunol Cell Biol. 2017;95:356–63.
57. Morgan RA, Yang JC, Kitano M, Dudley ME, Laurencot CM, Rosenberg SA. Case report of a serious adverse event following the administration of T cells transduced with a chimeric antigen receptor recognizing ERBB2. Mol Ther. 2010;18:843–51.
58. Hanahan D, Weinberg RA. Hallmarks of cancer: the next generation. Cell. 2011;144:646–74.
59. Hermel DJ, Ott PA. Combining forces: the promise and peril of synergistic immune checkpoint blockade and targeted therapy in metastatic melanoma. Cancer Metastasis Rev. 2017;36:43–50.
60. Chung KY, Gore I, Fong L, et al. Phase II study of the anti-cytotoxic T-lymphocyte-associated antigen 4 monoclonal antibody, tremelimumab, in patients with refractory metastatic colorectal cancer. J Clin Oncol. 2010;28:3485–90.
61. Topalian SL, Hodi FS, Brahmer JR, et al. Safety, activity, and immune correlates of anti-PD-1 antibody in cancer. N Engl J Med. 2012;366:2443–54.

62. Brahmer JR, Tykodi SS, Chow LQ, et al. Safety and activity of anti-PD-L1 antibody in patients with advanced cancer. N Engl J Med. 2012;366:2455–65.
63. Brahmer JR, Drake CG, Wollner I, et al. Phase I study of single-agent anti-programmed death-1 (MDX-1106) in refractory solid tumors: safety, clinical activity, pharmacodynamics, and immunologic correlates. J Clin Oncol. 2010;28:3167–75.
64. Lipson EJ, Sharfman WH, Drake CG, et al. Durable cancer regression off-treatment and effective reinduction therapy with an anti-PD-1 antibody. Clin Cancer Res. 2013;19:462–8.
65. Hermel D, Sigal D. "Check"-ing the data: a review of immune checkpoint inhibitor biomarkers. Personalized medicine in. Oncology. 2016;5:234–40.
66. Snyder A, Makarov V, Merghoub T, et al. Genetic basis for clinical response to CTLA-4 blockade in melanoma. N Engl J Med. 2014;371:2189–99.
67. Van Allen EM, Miao D, Schilling B, et al. Genomic correlates of response to CTLA-4 blockade in metastatic melanoma. Science. 2015;350:207–11.
68. Rizvi NA, Hellmann MD, Snyder A, et al. Cancer immunology. Mutational landscape determines sensitivity to PD-1 blockade in non-small cell lung cancer. Science. 2015;348:124–8.
69. Boland CR, Goel A. Microsatellite instability in colorectal cancer. Gastroenterology. 2010;138:2073–87. e3.
70. Timmermann B, Kerick M, Roehr C, et al. Somatic mutation profiles of MSI and MSS colorectal cancer identified by whole exome next generation sequencing and bioinformatics analysis. PLoS One. 2010;5:e15661.
71. Maby P, Tougeron D, Hamieh M, et al. Correlation between density of CD8+ T-cell infiltrate in microsatellite unstable colorectal cancers and frameshift mutations: a rationale for personalized immunotherapy. Cancer Res. 2015;75:3446–55.
72. Le DT, Uram JN, Wang H, et al. PD-1 blockade in tumors with mismatch-repair deficiency. N Engl J Med. 2015;372:2509–20.
73. Diaz LA, Marabelle A, Delord J, et al. Pembrolizumab therapy for microsatellite instability high (MSI-H) colorectal cancer (CRC) and non-CRC. J Clin Oncol. 2017;35. (suppl; abstr 3071).
74. Overman MJ, Lonardi S, Leone F, et al. Nivolumab in patients with DNA mismatch repair deficient/microsatellite instability high metastatic colorectal cancer: update from CheckMate 142. J Clin Oncol. 2017;35. (suppl; abstr 591).
75. Bendell JC, Kim TW, Goh BC, et al. Clinical activity and safety of cobimetinib (cobi) and atezolizumab in colorectal cancer (CRC). J Clin Oncol. 2016;34. (suppl; abstr 3502).

Chapter 25
Medical Oncology Management of Hereditary Colorectal Cancer

Eduardo Vilar, Ramón Salazar, and Josep Tabernero

Abstract Hereditary colorectal cancer syndromes represent approximately 5% of the total of colorectal cancer cases. Although there are a myriad of diseases that are considered rare due to their frequency, there are two conditions that are common enough to be found in the daily medical oncology clinic: Lynch syndrome and Familial Adenomatous Polyposis. In this chapter, we will review the specific aspects of these two conditions from the medical oncology standpoint with particular emphasis to the use of systemic chemotherapy and targeted therapies for the treatment of these cases.

Keywords Colorectal cancer · Chemotherapy · Immunotherapy · Microsatellite instability · Lynch syndrome · Familial adenomatous polyposis

E. Vilar (✉)
Department of Clinical Cancer Prevention, The University of Texas MD Anderson Cancer Center, Houston, TX, USA

GI Medical Oncology, The University of Texas MD Anderson Cancer Center, Houston, TX, USA

Clinical Cancer Genetics Program, The University of Texas MD Anderson Cancer Center, Houston, TX, USA

Graduate School of Biomedical Sciences, The University of Texas MD Anderson Cancer Center, Houston, TX, USA
e-mail: EVilar@mdanderson.org

R. Salazar
Department of Medical Oncology, Catalan Institute of Oncology (ICO), Bellvitge Biomedical Research Institute (IDIBELL), Universitat de Barcelona, L'Hospitalet de Llobregat, Barcelona, Spain

J. Tabernero
Department of Medical Oncology, Vall d'Hebron University Hospital and Vall d'Hebron Institute of Oncology (VHIO), Universitat Autònoma de Barcelona, Barcelona, Spain

L. Valle et al. (eds.), *Hereditary Colorectal Cancer*,
https://doi.org/10.1007/978-3-319-74259-5_25

Abbreviations

CALGB	The Cancer and Leukemia Group B
CMMR-D	Congenital deficiency of mismatch repair
Cox-2	Cyclo-oxygenase-2
CRC	Colorectal cancer
FAP	Familial adenomatous polyposis
FU	5-Fluorouracil
LS	Lynch syndrome
MMR	Mismatch repair
MSI	Microsatellite instable
MSS	Microsatellite stable
NGS	Next-generation sequencing
NSAIDs	Nonsteroidal anti-inflammatory drugs
PPAP	Polymerase proofreading-associated polyposis
TCGA	The Cancer Genome Atlas
TILs	Tumor-infiltrating lymphocytes

1 Introduction

Colorectal cancer (CRC) continues to be the third most common cancer diagnosed in the United States in both men and women [1] in spite of the sustained decline in incidence observed among adults older than 50 years, which has been attributed to an increased uptake of colonoscopy screening with removal of premalignant polyps [1]. In parallel, the incidence rate predicted by 2030 among young patients aged 20–34 years is increasing at a rate of 90–124% [2] due to unclear reasons that most likely include a myriad of factors such as changes in diet, obesity, reduced physical activity, and exposure to carcinogenic agents. While age at diagnosis of cancer is a factor that has been associated with hereditary cancer syndromes, a surge in genetic cases is not expected to be a contributing factor to the increasing rates observed among young adults.

Although the prevalence of hereditary cases among the colorectal cancer population is stable at around 5% [3], several studies have recently reported remarkably higher rates among young-onset cohorts with 16% in CRC patients diagnosed under age 50 [4] and 35% under age 35 [5], which is a reflection of the enrichment of genetic cases among individuals that present with an extreme phenotype and also the nonlinear nature of the association between age and diagnosis of hereditary cancer. Furthermore, the availability of germline next-generation sequencing (NGS) tools paired with the discovery of immunotherapy for patients with hereditary syndromes, such as checkpoint blockade for the treatment of stage IV cases arising in a background of Lynch syndrome (LS) [6], has led medical oncologists to increasingly recognize the presence of hereditary syndromes in patients diagnosed under age 50.

In general, the biology of tumors diagnosed in patients with hereditary syndromes is considered to be identical to those arising in the sporadic setting [7]. In fact, the biology knowledge acquired on colorectal carcinogenesis was derived from the study of premalignant lesions and carcinomas from patients diagnosed with LS as a prototype of sporadic microsatellite instable (MSI) CRC [also known as hypermutant in the post-The Cancer Genome Atlas (TCGA) era], which represents approximately 15% of the total of early stage CRC, and familial adenomatous polyposis (FAP) as the model for microsatellite stable (MSS) tumors harboring chromosomal instability (non-hypermutant), which represents approximately the remaining 85% [8] . Therefore, the medical management of hereditary cases does not defer substantially from the current guidelines developed for sporadic CRC, but there are some specific considerations that medical oncologists need to address involving the diagnostic workup of patients and unaffected family members, the discussion of surgical treatments, updating the prognostic assessment, and the selection of chemotherapeutic agents.

In this chapter, we provide an overview of the prognostic aspects and therapeutic interventions available for the management of patients diagnosed with locally advanced and metastatic CRC arising in a genetic background of mainly LS and FAP.

2 Lynch Syndrome and Microsatellite Instability as a Prognostic and Predictive Biomarker

The controversy on the role of MSI as a prognostic marker has been settled, and the assessment of MSI is now considered standard of care for early stages. Colorectal tumors displaying MSI that are diagnosed at early stages have a better prognosis compared to MSS. This survival advantage matches with the observation that MSI tumors experience lower rates of local tumor recurrence, especially at distant sites, than do MSS tumors [9] although this effect is restricted to stage II [10–13]. This favorable biological effect in early stages contrasts with the poorer prognosis observed in metastatic MSI CRC [14]. *BRAF* mutations are thought to be the main contributor to this worse outcome with dismal overall and progression-free survival compared to wild-type tumors [15–17]. But at the same time, in the early stages of disease, there are conflicting results among studies that point toward a modulatory effect of MSI over *BRAF* mutations in survival [14, 18, 19]. In fact, the PETACC-3 survival analysis stratifying stage II and III patients based on MSI and *BRAF* status did not confirm the prognostic effect of *BRAF* on relapse of the disease, but those patients with tumors harboring *BRAF* mutations had a poorer prognosis once they had relapsed, thus pointing out on the detrimental effect induced by acquisition of *BRAF* alterations in the metastatic disease setting [13].

Regarding the value of MSI as a predictive marker of response to fluorouracil (5-FU), the initial studies performed in the 1990s and early 2000s were not definitive (Table 25.1) [12, 20] due to the retrospective and single-institution nature of most of them as well as the use of different methodologies and criteria to determine MSI

Table 25.1 Clinical studies analyzing the effect of 5-fluorouracil in cohorts of MSI CRC

Reference	Study type	No. of patients	Tumor stage	MSI-H (%)	Follow-up duration (mo)	Effect
5-Fluouracil						
Elsaleh et al. PMID 10832824	R	656	III	8.5	54	Benefit
Hemminki et al. PMID 11040179	P NR	95	III	12	31	Benefit
Liang et al. PMID 12237891	P NR	244	IV	21.3	NA	Benefit
Ribic et al. PMID 12867608	R from RCT	570	II/III	16.7	88.8	Detriment
Carethers et al. PMID 10381918	R	204	II/III	17.6	43.7	None
Benatti et al. PMID 16322293	R	1263	All	20.3	64	None
Jover et al. PMID 16299036	P NR	754	All	8.8	24.3	None
Lamberti et al. PMID 16724208	P NR	416	All	12.5	32.9	None
Kim et al. PMID 17228023	R from RCT	542	II/III	18.1	60	None
Sargent et al. PMID 12867608	R from RCT	1027	II/III	16	60	Detriment
Des Guetz et al. PMID 19443375	MA	3690	II/III	14	NA	None
Sinicrope et al. PMID 20498393	R from RCT	2141	II/III	16.1	96	Benefit for Lynch syndrome None for sporadic MSI
Irinotecan						
Koopman et al. PMID 19165197	R from RCT	515	IV	3.5	43	Inconclusive
Fallik et al. PMID 14522894	R	72	IV	9.7	NA	Benefit
Bertagnolli et al. PMID 19273709	R from RCT	723	III	13.3	79.8	Benefit
Tejpar et al. PMID 25361982	R from RCT	1254	II/III	22–12	68	No benefit

The vast majority of these studies were observational studies, and some had retrospectively reviewed data collected in the context of randomized controlled trials

R retrospective, *P* prospective, *NR* nonrandomized, *RCT* randomized clinical trial, *mo* months, *NA* not assessed, *MA* meta-analysis

status and inadequate statistical interpretation of results. Two large prospective-retrospective analyses collecting data from different randomized trials clarified that the use of adjuvant 5-FU-based chemotherapy was not effective in stage II CRC displaying MSI [21]. However, it seemed that stage III MSI cases did derive some benefit but apparently only if MSI was associated with Lynch syndrome (Table 25.1) [9]. However this must be taken with caution, since it is a result of highly exploratory analysis [9].

The predictive role for irinotecan-based chemotherapy continues lingering in the space of conflicting results, thus not reaching to any definitive conclusion. Some preclinical [22–25] and clinical [13, 26–29] data have suggested a selective sensitivity of MSI tumors to irinotecan (Table 25.1). Although the molecular basis of this increased sensitivity remains partially elusive, different research groups have linked it to a deficiency in the DNA repair mechanism involved in the correction of double-strand breaks induced by irinotecan such as somatic alterations in MRE11 and RADJO [24, 25]. Clinical data derived from retrospective reviews of patients enrolled in clinical trials have generated conflicting results. The post hoc analysis of the Cancer and Leukemia Group B (CALGB) 89,803 trial, which was originally designed to evaluate the efficacy of irinotecan, bolus 5-FU, and folinic acid compared with weekly bolus of 5-FU (IFL) as adjuvant therapy in stage III cases, showed a trend toward greater 5-year disease-free survival for patients with MSI-H tumors treated with the combined regimen, although it did not reach statistical significance [27]. The retrospective analysis of 1254 patients included in the PETACC3 trial, which studied the effect of irinotecan, infusional 5-FU, and folinic acid (FOLFIRI) as adjuvant therapy compared with infusional 5-FU and folinic acid alone in stage II and III cases, failed to demonstrate improved patient disease-free survival (Table 25.1) [13]. Therefore, the role of MSI as a predictive factor for chemotherapy is restricted to avoid the administration of adjuvant 5-FU to patients with stage II CRC. At present MSI should not be considered a validated marker for establishing treatment decisions regarding irinotecan-based regimens.

3 Immuno-oncology in the Treatment of Hereditary CRC Syndromes

Immuno-oncology has recently resurfaced as a therapeutic alternative in the management of patients with MSI/hypermutant CRC. The biology basis for the hyperactivation of the immune system among LS-associated carcinomas has been very well known by pathologists that had described for decades the infiltration by so-called tumor-infiltrating lymphocytes (TILs) of the invasive front of MSI tumors [30]. In fact, after the recognition that MSI/hypermutant CRC was almost exclusively associated with the presence of TILs, it became standard pathology criteria to suspect the presence of a genetic diagnosis of LS [31].

LS tumors display MMR deficiency through the acquisition of a second somatic hit in the alternate allele of the MMR gene that harbors the germline mutation and subsequently will be hypermutated due to the accumulation of base-to-base mismatches and insertion deletions due to the inactivity of one of the functional units of the MMR complex [12]. However, the most relevant alterations are the frame-shift mutations introducing stopgains that will become highly specific peptides (neoantigens) [32, 33]. Some of these neoantigens will be processed, presented on MHC, and recognized as foreign by T-cells and thus fostering the areas with abundant TILs. In fact, the activation of TILs has been already confirmed in a very detailed immunopathology analysis performed by Llosa and colleagues combining immunohistochemistry, laser capture microdissection, and quantitative RT-PCR to profile the immune environment of MSI/hypermutant tumors [34]. These tumors displayed high infiltration with activated CD8-positive cytotoxic T lymphocytes as well as activated Th1 cells characterized by IFNγ production. Then, as a consequence to counterbalance this immune environment, MSI tumors upregulated the expression of multiple immune checkpoints such as PD-1, PD-L1, CTLA-4, and others, thus making them particularly susceptible to immune checkpoint inhibitors [35]. Simultaneously to this observation, a phase II clinical trial reported a high level of activity of the PD-1 immune checkpoint inhibitor pembrolizumab, which is a humanized IgG4 monoclonal antibody against PD-L1 and PD-L2, as a single agent for the treatment of metastatic MSI/hypermutant tumors. In the study cohort that was integrated by sporadic MSI/hypermutant and LS cases, the immune-related objective response rate was 40% (4 of 10 patients; 95% confidence interval [CI], 12–74), and the immune-related progression-free survival rate at 20 weeks was 78% (7 of 9 patients; 95% CI, 40–97). A total of seven patients with CRC were LS carriers, and four of them showed stable disease [6]. Nivolumab, which is another IgG4 PD-1 blocking antibody, has also showed antitumoral activity by itself or combined with ipilimumab, an anti-CTLA4 agent that provides double checkpoint blockade, in a preliminary report of the initial 59 patients with MSI tumors treated in a larger metastatic colorectal trial showing confirmed response rates of 27 and 15% and 4-month progression-free survival rates of 55% and 80% for the single agent and the combination arms, respectively [36]. In an update of this study, additional data was presented on the cohort of patients treated with nivolumab as single agent. A total of 74 patients have been treated with 31% achieving a response and 69% of disease control rate. Overall, there were no differences in terms of response when patients were stratified by Lynch syndrome status [37]. These interventions are in general well tolerated, but potential adverse events have been reported among 21–41% of the patients including immune-related reactions involving the gastrointestinal tract (colitis), lung (pneumonitis), liver, skin, and endocrine system (hypophysitis, thyroid deregulation, and diabetes mellitus type 1). Although the development of checkpoint inhibitors is still at its infancy, the remarkable antitumoral activity reported in the two available studies has generated great promise in the CRC community, thus leading the expert panel in colorectal cancer of the National Comprehensive Cancer Network to include pembrolizumab and nivolumab among the recommended agents for the treatment of stage IV CRC patients displaying MSI [38] in its guidelines. This recommendation has paved the road for a rapid implementation of checkpoint inhibitors in the United States, although is not yet approved by the regulatory agencies (FDA) for this indication.

In terms of biomarkers, although the expressions of PD-L1 and CD8-positive lymphocytes are important factors in the recognition of neoantigens, they have not demonstrated a predictive value for checkpoint blockade. However, mutation rates and numbers of mutation-associated neoantigens itself have showed an association with clinical response that need to be confirmed in subsequent analysis [6], thus putting NGS and systems biology tools for their detection at the center of biomarker development in immune-oncology [39].

Similarly to the mechanisms described for hypermutant tumors displaying MSI, there are two other hereditary syndromes that predispose to the development of premalignant polyps and CRC that accumulate thousands of mutations (named ultramutators): congenital deficiency of mismatch repair (CMMR-D) [40] and polymerase proofreading-associated polyposis (PPAP), both displaying a phenotype that overlaps with both Lynch syndrome and MYH-associated polyposis [41]. The former is secondary to a bi-allelic germline inactivation of the MMR system and the latter to the inactivation of polymerase ε (*POLE*) or δ (*POLD1*). The molecular basis for these two syndromes has been already discussed in other chapters of this book. Although there are no reports on the activity of checkpoint blockade for the treatment of GI tumors in these two conditions, it has been already observed an overexpression of immune checkpoints and infiltration by TILs in endometrial and brain tumors arising in the context of a somatic inactivation of POLE [41], thus making the proposal to expand the use of checkpoint blockade to GI tumors in these two diseases a logical expansion of the same concept. In parallel, GI tumors in CMMR-D patients have shown an elevated mutational rate and neoantigen proportion as well as a high level of activity of nivolumab for the treatment of pediatric brain tumors, thus also making the case for the same approach in CRC cases with CMMR-D [40, 42].

4 Targeted Therapies in Prevention and Treatment of Hereditary Colorectal Cancers

Many targeted agents have been tested in animal models that resemble the phenotype of hereditary CRC syndromes and have demonstrated encouraging antitumor activity. However, only three targeted agents have been translated into clinical trials for treatment and prevention of GI and extraintestinal manifestations: erlotinib, rapamycin, and everolimus (Table 25.2). It is out of the scope of this chapter to discuss the medical oncology management of extraintestinal tumors. Other agents with known targets have been developed, but their mechanism was discovered after their development or simultaneously to it, therefore not being considered "targeted" during their development, such as the case of nonsteroidal anti-inflammatory drugs (NSAIDs) and cyclo-oxygenase-2 (COX-2) inhibitors (also known as coxibs). The targeted chemopreventive use of NSAIDs and coxibs is already discussed in detail in another chapter of this book. We will briefly describe the recent promising results showed by EGFR inhibitors (erlotinib) for the treatment of advanced duodenal lesions in FAP and also the proof-of-concept testing of mTOR inhibitors in patients diagnosed with Peutz-Jeghers syndrome and Cowden disease.

Table 25.2 Targeted therapies tested in hereditary colorectal cancer syndromes

Hereditary cancer syndrome tumor type	Genetic defect	Drug	Target	Level of evidence
FAP – polyps	*APC*	Celecoxib, sulindac	COX-2	RCT RCT
FAP – desmoid tumors	*APC*	Sulindac Imatinib SERMs	COX-2 PDGFRα ER	Case series
Lynch syndrome – polyps	*MLH1, MSH2, MSH6, PMS2, TACSTD1*	Aspirin	COX?	Phase III
Lynch syndrome – colon cancer	*MLH1, MSH2, MSH6, PMS2, TACSTD1*	5-FU Irinotecan PARPi	DPD Topo MRE11	Retrospective Retrospective Preclinical
Peutz-Jeghers syndrome	*LKB1, STK11*	Rapamycin Everolimus	mTOR	Phase II (terminated) Preclinical
Cowden syndrome	*PTEN*	Rapamycin	mTOR	Phase II Preclinical

For a long time, the management of small intestine adenomas and duodenal carcinomas in patients with FAP has been defaulted to the same approaches tested and implemented for colorectal lesions. However, clinical observations pointed out to a different biology between the large and small intestine with notable differences even in the expression of COX-2 [43]. Although, they are microscopically and phenotypically similar (i.e., tubular adenomas), duodenal lesions do not present a uniform response to NSAIDs and coxibs compared to colorectal adenomas [44, 45]. Also, patients with advanced duodenal adenomatosis have a 36% relative risk of developing duodenal carcinoma, which has now become the leading cause of cancer mortality among FAP patients. Therefore, prophylactic pancreaticoduodenectomy is recommended for patients with advanced adenomatosis that are not responding to increased surveillance and chemoprevention [46]. These observations prompted the preclinical assessment and study of the differences in expression and pathway activation between duodenal and colorectal polyps and highlighted the activation of the epidermal growth factor receptor as a critical difference. In fact, the use of erlotinib in the *Apc*$^{Min/+}$ mice showed high levels of activity inducing regression of small intestinal lesions [47]. Therefore, as a logical extension of this preclinical finding, the cancer genetics group at the University of Utah launched a single-institution phase I clinical trial testing the activity of the combination of sulindac (150 mg twice daily) and erlotinib (75 mg daily) during 6 months for the management of duodenal polyposis. This study recruited a total of 92 patients, and, although the initial dose of 75 mg daily needed to be reduced in the vast majority of participants, the activity showed by the treatment was very encouraging and had a reasonable tolerance level with skin toxicity as the main side effect [48]. In fact, the results from this trial have motivated a follow-up study to identify a more reasonable weekly schedule for administration of erlotinib (NCT02961374). It is worth to mention that a proportion of patients with advanced duodenal adenomatosis do not have access to surgical resection of the disease due to the presence of intra-abdominal desmoids, thus leaving pharmacological modulation of the growth of these lesions as the only resource available to avoid progression into duodenal cancer.

A very different course has followed the development of mTOR inhibitors (sirolimus and everolimus) for treatment and prevention in Cowden and Peutz-Jeghers disease. Patients with Cowden disease harbor a germline mutation in *PTEN* and patients with Peutz-Jeghers in the *LKB1* and *STK11* gene, all of them encoding proteins that are involved in the PI3K-AKT-mTOR pathway. *PTEN* is in charge of regulating AKT, which is a mediator of PI3K signaling. Similarly, inactivation of *STK11* leads to activation of mTOR, which will increase protein synthesis by phosphorylating and inhibiting the mRNA translational repressor, eIF-4E binding protein 1, and phosphorylating and activating ribosomal p70S6 kinases. Two clinical trials were launched to explore the activity in these two conditions: Peutz-Jeghers (NCT00811590) [49] and Cowden syndrome (NCT00971789) [50]. The former was halted due to slow accrual as it could only enroll two patients, and the later demonstrated therapeutic activity and modulation of the main biomarker in GI polyps with manageable toxicity; however, the course of the treatment was shorter than 2 months.

Therefore, we can conclude that translational drug development of targeted therapies in hereditary CRC syndromes has not made prime time, mainly due to slow trial accrual secondary to the involvement of centers that do not have large registries of these patients. The success demonstrated by erlotinib trial demonstrates that focused efforts involving large referral genetics clinics can successfully complete clinical studies repurposing targeted agents for these orphan diseases.

5 Practical Notes for the Practicing Medical Oncologist

The care of patients with suspected or confirmed hereditary colorectal cancer syndromes requires the attention of the medical oncologist to several clinical issues that are not common in the daily clinical practice of sporadic individuals. The first one is the age factor, as hereditary cases are usually diagnosed at earlier ages with the majority of patients being diagnosed earlier than 50 years [5]. Therefore, patients coming for treatment recommendations are still at fertile age, and they want to be attentive to reproductive issues that may arise after the completion of treatment planning to form a family. Therefore, before proceeding with chemotherapy or radiation treatment, the patient will require to have discussions on fertility preservation and offer a consultation with a specialist. The second one pertains to the coordination of care with surgical oncologists. Either before primary resection, total or subtotal colectomy, or after primary resection completion colectomy with rectal-sparing procedures will need to be discussed with the patient as a preventive intervention to decrease the risk of metachronous tumors or as an alternative to yearly colonoscopy screening. The third consideration pertains to the genetic workup of patients suspected to have a hereditary syndrome based on the presentation and phenotype.

In this case, genetic counseling should be offered during the initial consultation. At the present time, the process of genetic diagnosis has been expedited and simplified due to the implementation of germline sequencing panels that allow ruling out a myriad of syndromes in just one step. In addition, tumor testing, which before was a crucial step in the initial genetic evaluation to rule out Lynch syndrome, is now mandatory due to the potential indication of immunotherapy for metastatic disease. Therefore, providers need to become familiar with the ordering and interpretation of these results to trigger specific immunotherapy interventions and also refer them to genetic counseling. In those cases that genetic testing is positive, then there is an obligation to inform the patient on the need to disseminate the results among family members in order to activate the testing of other at-risk individuals that may require enhance surveillance if they are confirmed to be carriers. The fourth consideration pertains to the surveillance that hereditary patients will need upon completion of the standard treatment. These patients are going to need enhanced endoscopic screening beyond the recommendation of colonoscopy at 1 year after the surgical resection. In addition, additional surveillance tests will be required to screen for extra-GI malignancies such as the referral to gynecology oncology for ovarian and endometrial screening in Lynch syndrome patients or urine test to screen for urinary tract tumors, although both of these two procedures are not endorsed by all expert panels. Finally, oncologists should pay special attention for hints of the presence of germline mutations in the mutation reports of somatic profiling that are obtained in stage IV patients that are looking for clinical trial options. Although genes involved in cancer susceptibility can also harbor somatic mutations, it should raise a red flag the fact of identifying alterations with high allelic frequencies (around the 50% cutoff, therefore from 40 to 60%) in genes linked to hereditary predisposition (such as the MMR genes, *APC*, *MUTYH*, *TP53*, *PTEN*, *STK11*, *SMAD4*, etc.), as this fact can be indicative of the presence of underlying genetic diseases.

Conflict of Interest The authors declare no conflicts of interest.

References

1. Siegel RL, Miller KD, Jemal A. Cancer statistics, 2017. CA Cancer J Clin. 2017;67(1):7–30.
2. Bailey CE, CY H, You YN, Bednarski BK, Rodriguez-Bigas MA, Skibber JM, et al. Increasing disparities in the age-related incidences of colon and rectal cancers in the United States, 1975–2010. JAMA Surg. 2015;150(1):17–22.
3. Jasperson KW, Tuohy TM, Neklason DW, Burt RW. Hereditary and familial colon cancer. Gastroenterology. 2010;138(6):2044–58.
4. Pearlman R, Frankel WL, Swanson B, Zhao W, Yilmaz A, Miller K, et al. Prevalence and spectrum of germline cancer susceptibility gene mutations among patients with early-onset colorectal cancer. JAMA Oncol. 2017;3(4):464–471.
5. Mork ME, You YN, Ying J, Bannon SA, Lynch PM, Rodriguez-Bigas MA, et al. High prevalence of hereditary cancer syndromes in adolescents and young adults with colorectal cancer. J Clin Oncol. 2015;33(31):3544–9.
6. Le DT, Uram JN, Wang H, Bartlett BR, Kemberling H, Eyring AD, et al. PD-1 blockade in tumors with mismatch-repair deficiency. N Engl J Med. 2015;372(26):2509–20.

7. Fearon ER. Molecular genetics of colorectal cancer. Annu Rev Pathol. 2011;6:479–507.
8. Vilar E, Tabernero J. Molecular dissection of microsatellite instable colorectal cancer. Cancer Discov. 2013;3(5):502–11.
9. Sinicrope FA, Foster NR, Thibodeau SN, Marsoni S, Monges G, Labianca R, et al. DNA mismatch repair status and colon cancer recurrence and survival in clinical trials of 5-fluorouracil-based adjuvant therapy. J Natl Cancer Inst. 2011;103(11):863–75.
10. Popat S, Hubner R, Houlston RS. Systematic review of microsatellite instability and colorectal cancer prognosis. J Clin Oncol. 2005;23(3):609–18.
11. Roth AD, Tejpar S, Delorenzi M, Yan P, Fiocca R, Klingbiel D, et al. Prognostic role of KRAS and BRAF in stage II and III resected colon cancer: results of the translational study on the PETACC-3, EORTC 40993, SAKK 60-00 trial. J Clin Oncol. 2010;28(3):466–74.
12. Vilar E, Gruber SB. Microsatellite instability in colorectal cancer-the stable evidence. Nat Rev Clin Oncol. 2010;7(3):153–62.
13. Tejpar S, Bosman F, Delorenzi M, Fiocca R, Yan P, Klingbiel D, et al. Microsatellite instability (MSI) in stage II and III colon cancer treated with 5FU-LV or 5FU-LV and irinotecan (PETACC 3-EORTC 40993-SAKK 60/00 trial). ASCO Meet Abstr. 2009;27(15S):4001.
14. Tran B, Kopetz S, Tie J, Gibbs P, Jiang ZQ, Lieu CH, et al. Impact of BRAF mutation and microsatellite instability on the pattern of metastatic spread and prognosis in metastatic colorectal cancer. Cancer. 2011;117(20):4623–32.
15. Tol J, Nagtegaal ID, Punt CJA. BRAF mutation in metastatic colorectal cancer. N Engl J Med. 2009;361(1):98–9.
16. Van Cutsem E, Köhne C-H, Láng I, Folprecht G, Nowacki MP, Cascinu S, et al. Cetuximab plus irinotecan, fluorouracil, and leucovorin as first-line treatment for metastatic colorectal cancer: updated analysis of overall survival according to tumor KRAS and BRAF mutation status. J Clin Oncol. 2011;29(15):2011–9.
17. Price TJ, Hardingham JE, Lee CK, Weickhardt A, Townsend AR, Wrin JW, et al. Impact of KRAS and BRAF gene mutation status on outcomes from the phase III AGITG MAX trial of capecitabine alone or in combination with bevacizumab and mitomycin in advanced colorectal cancer. J Clin Oncol. 2011;29(19):2675–82.
18. Ogino S, Shima K, Meyerhardt JA, McCleary NJ, Ng K, Hollis D, et al. Predictive and prognostic roles of BRAF mutation in stage III colon cancer: results from intergroup trial CALGB 89803. Clin Cancer Res. 2012;18(3):890–900.
19. Phipps AI, Buchanan DD, Makar KW, Burnett-Hartman AN, Coghill AE, Passarelli MN, et al. BRAF mutation status and survival after colorectal cancer diagnosis according to patient and tumor characteristics. Cancer Epidemiol Biomark Prev. 2012;21(10):1792–8.
20. Des Guetz G, Schischmanoff O, Nicolas P, Perret GY, Morere JF, Uzzan B. Does microsatellite instability predict the efficacy of adjuvant chemotherapy in colorectal cancer? A systematic review with meta-analysis. Eur J Cancer. 2009;45(10):1890–6.
21. Sargent DJ, Marsoni S, Thibodeau SN, Labianca R, Hamilton SR, Torri V, et al. Confirmation of deficient mismatch repair (dMMR) as a predictive marker for lack of benefit from 5-FU based chemotherapy in stage II and III colon cancer (CC): a pooled molecular reanalysis of randomized chemotherapy trials. J Clin Oncol (Meet Abstr). 2008;26(15 Suppl):4008.
22. Magrini R, Bhonde MR, Hanski ML, Notter M, Scherubl H, Boland CR, et al. Cellular effects of CPT-11 on colon carcinoma cells: dependence on p53 and hMLH1 status. Int J Cancer. 2002;101(1):23–31.
23. Jacob S, Aguado M, Fallik D, Praz F. The role of the DNA mismatch repair system in the cytotoxicity of the topoisomerase inhibitors camptothecin and etoposide to human colorectal cancer cells. Cancer Res. 2001;61(17):6555–62.
24. Vilar E, Scaltriti M, Balmana J, Saura C, Guzman M, Arribas J, et al. Microsatellite instability due to hMLH1 deficiency is associated with increased cytotoxicity to irinotecan in human colorectal cancer cell lines. Br J Cancer. 2008;99(10):1607–12.
25. Rodriguez R, Hansen LT, Phear G, Scorah J, Spang-Thomsen M, Cox A, et al. Thymidine selectively enhances growth suppressive effects of camptothecin/irinotecan in MSI+ cells and tumors containing a mutation of MRE11. Clin Cancer Res. 2008;14(17):5476–83.

26. Fallik D, Borrini F, Boige V, Viguier J, Jacob S, Miquel C, et al. Microsatellite instability is a predictive factor of the tumor response to irinotecan in patients with advanced colorectal cancer. Cancer Res. 2003;63(18):5738–44.
27. Bertagnolli MM, Niedzwiecki D, Compton CC, Hahn HP, Hall M, Damas B, et al. Microsatellite instability predicts improved response to adjuvant therapy with irinotecan, fluorouracil, and leucovorin in stage III colon cancer: cancer and leukemia group B protocol 89803. J Clin Oncol. 2009;27(11):1814–21.
28. Koopman M, Kortman GA, Mekenkamp L, Ligtenberg MJ, Hoogerbrugge N, Antonini NF, et al. Deficient mismatch repair system in patients with sporadic advanced colorectal cancer. Br J Cancer. 2009;100(2):266–73.
29. Des Guetz G, Uzzan B, Nicolas P, Schischmanoff O, Perret GY, Morere JF. Microsatellite instability does not predict the efficacy of chemotherapy in metastatic colorectal cancer. A systematic review and meta-analysis. Anticancer Res. 2009;29(5):1615–20.
30. Smyrk TC, Watson P, Kaul K, Lynch HT. Tumor-infiltrating lymphocytes are a marker for microsatellite instability in colorectal carcinoma. Cancer. 2001;91(12):2417–22.
31. Greenson JK, Huang SC, Herron C, Moreno V, Bonner JD, Tomsho LP, et al. Pathologic predictors of microsatellite instability in colorectal cancer. Am J Surg Pathol. 2009;33(1):126–33.
32. Xiao Y, Freeman GJ. The microsatellite instable subset of colorectal cancer is a particularly good candidate for checkpoint blockade immunotherapy. Cancer Discov. 2015;5(1):16–8.
33. The Cancer Genome Atlas Network. Comprehensive molecular characterization of human colon and rectal cancer. Nature. 2012;487(7407):330–7.
34. Llosa NJ, Cruise M, Tam A, Wicks EC, Hechenbleikner EM, Taube JM, et al. The vigorous immune microenvironment of microsatellite instable colon cancer is balanced by multiple counter-inhibitory checkpoints. Cancer Discov. 2015;5(1):43–51.
35. Spira A, Disis ML, Schiller JT, Vilar E, Rebbeck TR, Bejar R, et al. Leveraging premalignant biology for immune-based cancer prevention. Proc Natl Acad Sci U S A. 2016;113:10750–8.
36. Overman MJ, Kopetz S, McDermott RS, Leach J, Lonardi S, Lenz HJ, et al. Nivolumab ± ipilimumab in treatment (tx) of patients (pts) with metastatic colorectal cancer (mCRC) with and without high microsatellite instability (MSI-H): CheckMate-142 interim results. J Clin Oncol. 2016;34(suppl; abstr 3501).
37. Overman MJ, Lonardi S, Leone F, McDermott RS, Morse MA, Wong KYM, et al. Nivolumab in patients with DNA mismatch repair deficient/microsatellite instability high metastatic colorectal cancer: update from CheckMate 142. J Clin Oncol. 2017;35(suppl 4S; abstract 519).
38. National Comprehensive Cancer Network. Colon Cancer (Version 1.2017). 2017. Available from: https://www.nccn.org/professionals/physician_gls/pdf/colon.pdf
39. Hackl H, Charoentong P, Finotello F, Trajanoski Z. Computational genomics tools for dissecting tumour-immune cell interactions. Nat Rev Genet. 2016;17(8):441–58.
40. Shlien A, Campbell BB, de Borja R, Alexandrov LB, Merico D, Wedge D, et al. Combined hereditary and somatic mutations of replication error repair genes result in rapid onset of ultra-hypermutated cancers. Nat Genet. 2015;47(3):257–62.
41. Rayner E, van Gool IC, Palles C, Kearsey SE, Bosse T, Tomlinson I, et al. A panoply of errors: polymerase proofreading domain mutations in cancer. Nat Rev Cancer. 2016;16(2):71–81.
42. Bouffet E, Larouche V, Campbell BB, Merico D, de Borja R, Aronson M, et al. Immune checkpoint inhibition for hypermutant glioblastoma multiforme resulting from germline biallelic mismatch repair deficiency. J Clin Oncol. 2016;34(19):2206–11.
43. Brosens LA, Iacobuzio-Donahue CA, Keller JJ, Hustinx SR, Carvalho R, Morsink FH, et al. Increased cyclooxygenase-2 expression in duodenal compared with colonic tissues in familial adenomatous polyposis and relationship to the -765G -> C COX-2 polymorphism. Clin Cancer Res. 2005;11(11):4090–6.
44. Groves CJ, Saunders BP, Spigelman AD, Phillips RK. Duodenal cancer in patients with familial adenomatous polyposis (FAP): results of a 10 year prospective study. Gut. 2002;50(5):636–41.
45. Kim B, Giardiello FM. Chemoprevention in familial adenomatous polyposis. Best Pract Res Clin Gastroenterol. 2011;25(4–5):607–22.

46. Gallagher MC, Phillips RK, Bulow S. Surveillance and management of upper gastrointestinal disease in familial adenomatous polyposis. Familial Cancer. 2006;5(3):263–73.
47. Roberts RB, Min L, Washington MK, Olsen SJ, Settle SH, Coffey RJ, et al. Importance of epidermal growth factor receptor signaling in establishment of adenomas and maintenance of carcinomas during intestinal tumorigenesis. Proc Natl Acad Sci. 2002;99(3):1521–6.
48. Samadder NJ, Neklason DW, Boucher KM, Byrne KR, Kanth P, Samowitz W, et al. Effect of sulindac and erlotinib vs placebo on duodenal neoplasia in familial adenomatous polyposis: a randomized clinical trial. JAMA. 2016;315(12):1266–75.
49. Kuwada SK, Burt R. A rationale for mTOR inhibitors as chemoprevention agents in Peutz-Jeghers syndrome. Familial Cancer. 2011;10(3):469–72.
50. Komiya T, Blumenthal GM, Ballas MS, Dechowdhury R, Manu M, Fioravanti S, et al. A pilot study of sirolimus (S) in subjects with Cowden syndrome (CS) with germ-line mutations in PTEN. J Clin Oncol. 2013;31(15_suppl):2532.

Part IV
Registries and Databases

Chapter 26
Databases: Intentions, Capabilities, and Limitations

Pål Møller, Sigve Nakken, and Eivind Hovig

Abstract Computers may be used to hold, retrieve, and manipulate data. However, for each task they have to be instructed exactly what to do, and many tasks, such as interpreting human language, still await perfection. To be analyzed by computers, the data require formatting as required for efficient computation. This is often achieved in the form of a database. Also, computer instructions for computations are often provided by dedicated computer languages for increased efficiency in converting human instructions into computation, based on ready access to the data on which computations are to be performed. In principle, the design of a database to a purpose (intention) by definition declares the capabilities and limitations of the database. This chapter is meant as a general comment for the biologist, as to some use of database principles within the field of heritable cancer and mentions some relevant principles, strengths, and weaknesses in the design and use of such databases.

Keywords Database · Research · Structure · Capabilities · Limitations · Relational database · Typecasting · Formatting

---

P. Møller (✉)
Research Group on Inherited Cancer, Department of Medical Genetics, The Norwegian Radium Hospital, Oslo University Hospital, Oslo, Norway

Department of Tumor Biology, Institute of Cancer Research, The Norwegian Radium Hospital, Part of Oslo University Hospital, Oslo, Norway

Surgical Center for Hereditary Tumors, HELIOS University Clinic Wuppertal, University Witten-Herdecke, Wuppertal, Germany

S. Nakken
Department of Tumor Biology, Institute of Cancer Research, The Norwegian Radium Hospital, Part of Oslo University Hospital, Oslo, Norway

E. Hovig
Institute of Cancer Genetics and Informatics, The Norwegian Radium Hospital, Part of Oslo University Hospital, Oslo, Norway

Department of Informatics, University of Oslo, Oslo, Norway

Department of Tumor Biology, Institute of Cancer Research, The Norwegian Radium Hospital, Part of Oslo University Hospital, Oslo, Norway

L. Valle et al. (eds.), *Hereditary Colorectal Cancer*,
https://doi.org/10.1007/978-3-319-74259-5_26

1 What Is a Database?

A database may be defined as an organized collection of information referred to here as "data" (https://en.wikipedia.org/wiki/Database). To be useful, a database should have a way to import and export the data stored for efficient retrieval and computation. To manage these operations, an interface between the human and the database is useful. How these separate functions are organized in different solutions may vary from a simple spreadsheet available as an all-in-one package to the most advanced systems where each single functional unit may be separately manipulated according to potentially very complex instructions. An allegoric example of the basic concept may be that a blood sample from one person may be considered a database holding all genetic information on that person, and our activities to read this information are to establish an export system to make the information available in a different format. Having learned to read the code, we are now trying to understand how the human DNA data are organized to which purposes. A database on inherited cancers may typically include information on the patients' phenotypes (in our case cancers), the patients' environment (carcinogens, preventive and treatment modalities), and results of genetic testing (results of reading the patients' DNA codes). The research goal may be to describe associations between the pieces of information (variables) filed.

2 Intentions

A practical way to make a database may be to precisely declare the purpose, which will implicitly provide the description on what should be included in the solution. This may be straightforward when testing one single hypothesis. Research may, however, be to describe what is not known. What is an optimal way to structure a database for discovery of the unknown? One approach may be to enter all available data, hoping to get something out. The day may soon come, however, in a world of limited resources; it may become relevant to use power calculations to consider what you will give priority with your resources at hand. Which means you will have to consider the number of data points needed, and the quality metrics of each piece of information entered, to arrive at an answer to the research question of highest priority. This implies to determine in advance what to look for. Further, it will be beneficial to have data structures allowing additional information to be entered later to address more problems, without the need to redo the original database structure. If a precise intention exists, put it in writing. If it is difficult to write it down, the intention may not be sufficiently precise for implementation, and thus a refinement of the intention will serve the final solution well. If you are a scientist without programming skills, the programmer to implement your concepts may not know what to do if the concepts cannot be conceptualized for the computer in the form of instructions. Thus, it is necessary to speak a language the programmer understands.

Similarly, if the programmer does not understand the scientific question at hand, while the scientist does not understand what programmers do, then communication toward a useful result may be difficult. Thus, some level of understanding the strengths and limitation of databases and how to utilize them will clearly be important for any scientist approaching heritable cancer databases.

3 Statistics

In principle, database design and programming are not statistics. Databases exist to store and retrieve information. Statistical analyses may be built-in functions in the database; on the other hand, statistics is a separate area of knowledge of how to analyze data (https://en.wikipedia.org/wiki/Statistics); and databases may be constructed to output data preformatted to advanced statistical analyses. The output of a query to a database may serve as input to analyses by statistical software. Statistical software may have internal requirements for preformatted/specified database structures exactly meeting the needs of each analysis to be executed. Frequently, databases may come with built-in functions for statistical analyses or may provide functionality for development for statistical routines within the database software. How to separate the statistical analyses from the database is a matter of convenience: if the statistical requirements are limited, and the competence is in hand, then the statistical analysis may be developed within the framework of the database. If both a programmer and a statistical expert are at hand, an initial negotiation on how to solve the research questions with reference to what is in principle and practice achievable inside and outside different software may be useful.

4 Spreadsheet

A spreadsheet may be seen as a simple database having two dimensions: rows and columns (https://en.wikipedia.org/wiki/Spreadsheet). Each spreadsheet table cell, or database field, may be defined as the combination of one row and one column. Each field may be assigned a value. The values in each field are the single pieces of information which combined are the content of the spreadsheet database. Typically, the columns serve as the pieces of information to include, where for each column a declaration of the class of information a given information element belongs to (figures, dates, text, etc.). Each row may represent an object (patient), and the values given in each column in each row are the information elements held in the database for the given patient. No information that is not predefined as a column to hold that information can be entered, nor is it possible to enter information on any other objects than those initially determined to be the rows. In principle, three steps are required: first the decision on exactly what the spreadsheet is to address and next information is entered into the required number of rows to hold the values in the predesigned column fields (commonly denoted to "populate" the table). As the third step, some kind of statistical analysis is performed on content. No information besides the initial conception can be entered, and consequently, nothing but what is allowed with the data that were initially decided to be included can be calculated.

The above comments refer to one alone-standing spreadsheet. Collections of spreadsheets may be organized to become complex relational databases as discussed below. A spreadsheet may be a convenient format for import and export for each table in a relational database but with the formatting problems discussed below.

5 Objects, Fields, and Formats

To interpret the values given in each field, the database must be instructed how to do so, providing restrictions on what is allowed to enter according to field formats. This will predefine what later can be achieved with the contents. If a word is entered as a text string, which is a defined format, this text string cannot later be multiplied by the number 2, because that will have no meaning. But two text strings may be joined together to a longer string, concatenated, to contain both. In contrast, the numbers 2 and 3 may be mathematically added to become 5, or multiplied to become 6, not 23 as would be the result if concatenating them as text strings. There are many classes of objects which require different handling strategies. The computer languages are constructed to handle the different classes of objects appropriately, and to do so, each variable is to be formatted according to be what the computer language required. If not, the system stops – or worse: misleading output may be the result.

6 Typecasting and Some Specific Problems

Changing the type of the format (class) of a variable (a field) to something else may be denoted "typecasting" (https://www.tutorialspoint.com/cprogramming/c_type_casting.htm). Any database will come with built-in functions for typecasting. Typecasting will be automatically done in the most used spreadsheets, and this may be very convenient for an unexperienced user. There is no strict requirement to declare the format of a field in the most used spreadsheets: it will assume a number to be a number, a text string to be text, a date to be a date, etc., and permission will be granted to sum the numbers in a column containing nothing but numbers without telling the spreadsheet that they actually are numbers. In research, this may create problems and data corruption, because the database may without further notice make incorrect assumptions on data type. It may be difficult – sometimes impossible – to turn off such built-in functions. The typical example is a spreadsheet converting the content of a variable to something else when exporting it to another database.

How the different system handles dates is difficult and time-consuming to control. Mathematical defaults on how to handle numbers may lead to problems: If rounded off to an integer, 44.75 will by mathematical standards usually become 45. If calculating annual incidence in 5-year age cohorts, a patient who died 44 years and 9 months old should be included in the 40–44 year cohort, not the 45–49 year cohort, because a human is 44 years of age until the day he/she becomes 45.

An example which may seem sophisticated at first glance but which may become critical to a scientist is the difference between a blank space, the figure zero, and no information. No information is often in database language denoted NULL and is different from zero, which is a quantity (https://en.wikipedia.org/wiki/Null). In the computer, a blank space and zero are stored with their different numeric ASCII values (http://www.asciitable.com/). NULL means that there is no value stored in the field in question, and this is actually an ASCII code, because all binary fields in the computer storage are zero until manipulated to become something else. With the consequence that if NULL is included in data manipulation, there may be no answer (an error message which the programmer usually will hide from the end user to see). A short mathematical explanation is that when an argument in a calculation is unknown, the result is unknown, whatever the value of all the other arguments may be. Any advanced database will discriminate between NULL, zero, and blank, but spreadsheets usually do not. The built-in functions in spreadsheets will consider both NULL and blank to be zero. If a summation is attempted, the risk exists that it may be allowed to enter a blank space into a column assumed to hold numbers without it being realized – as the display shows nothing (blank) despite the computer actually has stored a piece of information (the ASCII code for a space in a text string) in the field. And worse, it may not be allowed to control these problems if exporting the spreadsheet content to a more sophisticated database.

The data format can in this way cause trouble: The cheap and easy-to-use systems to be handled by anyone are by and large working nicely for simple problems but may cause serious trouble if exporting the content from simple structures to more complex and demanding database solutions.

In addition, the researcher often may like to identify missing values. To do so, a value to denote "missing value" is required, which should be neither blank, zero, nor NULL. It may also be of relevance to discriminate between a question not asked and a question asked, but not answered, etc., for which purpose a definition of two or more different values to be stored and declared in the database structure for allowed options for stored values.

Another specific class is logical operators – often reflecting options not overlapping and where the sum of all valid options together will categorize the whole material. A typical example may be a field "dead" to give the user the opportunity to enter "yes" or "no." Such data are specifically designed to be used for special forms of algebra, logic, etc., and are often presented to the user by a graphical user interface, where he/she has to choose one out of two or more options.

The problems related to the data format are that when using simple databases, the options will always be restricted to the original definition, and it may be very time-consuming – if at all possible – to update the database to discriminate between different classes of data not having been declared initially.

7 One Piece of Information Should Be Entered Once Only

If two fields appear to include the same information, which one is correct if they differ? Synchronizing databases expected to hold the same information is a major challenge. To which end there is but one solution: one piece of information should be entered once and once only and together with the metadata information of who entered it and when. Information on the quality of the information entered may also be valuable. From there, this piece of information should be copied whenever needed, but never stored anywhere else in the database. If the information is to be updated, it will best be performed in the one place where it is stored and when notifying who did so and when. Doing it this way, the whole database, and any output including this piece of information, will be updated by updating one field only. Any doctor will recognize this as how to file medical information. They will also know that it is forbidden to delete information previously filed – it is to be marked as no longer valid, but cannot be erased. These rules are making databases for filing medical information complex. The complexity of a database structure is, in principle, independent of how many objects on which the database holds information: The complexity is given by the structure, and the capability to handle large data sets is a separate issue. The combination of complex structure and large number of entries will, however, require higher performance of the database.

8 Assumption-Free, Unbiased Information

Information entered into a database should, in principle, be assumption-free. If not, the information includes the assumption. If two pieces of information include the same assumption, it will be in conflict with the principle that one piece of information should be entered once only. Also, if a piece of information includes an assumption (or many assumptions), it may be misleading, because when retrieving this piece of information, the assumption will also be retrieved, while not necessarily visible to the user: The output may have hidden assumptions/restrictions, which may invalidate an interpretation of the results of a query. A typical assumption potentially invalidating the output from a medical research registry is ascertainment biases when collecting the data. A practical example of such is that if all families subjected to genetic testing for Lynch syndrome are selected because they meet the Amsterdam clinical criteria, all families demonstrated to have pathogenic genetic variants causing Lynch syndrome will meet the Amsterdam clinical criteria. Another example is that if two or more pieces of information actually reflect the same underlying cause, degrees of freedom in statistical analyses may be incorrectly estimated. Also, the two pieces of information may be associated because they include the same assumption while the information assumed to be provided may not be associated: The association is false.

9 How to Create a Database

The arguments mentioned leads to a limited selection of good options of useful database solutions, among which we briefly discuss two:

- A simple spreadsheet for a simple task
- A relational database which may initially be simple but constructed for expansion

10 A Simple Spreadsheet for a Simple Task

If there is a clear-cut and simple question to which an answer may be obtained with a limited set of arguments, a simple spreadsheet may be suitable. Typically, the name of the columns in the spreadsheet will be the variables for the study, and population of the spreadsheet may be performed with one row per patient studied. The commonly used spreadsheets may include sufficient statistical functions to answer the relevant research question, or the spreadsheet data may be entered into dedicated statistical software packages for more refined calculations. If the latter option is used, the spreadsheet data are to be formatted to meet the specification for data import to the statistical software.

Typically, such a spreadsheet may not be expanded to include more research data/questions of interest and may not be expanded to include repeated observations of the same patient.

11 A Relational Database

A relational database is a way to organize data in potentially more complex structures (https://en.wikipedia.org/wiki/Relational_database). The construction of a relational database with the capacity to later be expanded for different purposes will have to at least meet all the requirements discussed in this chapter. A failure to meet these will result in a predictable eventual collapse, due to the inability to handle a more complex research question. Following the basic rules may at first glance seem simple, but it is not, because the complexity will soon grow and the systems for analyzing the database (the queries) will become complicated. Such databases may include stored queries providing result sets which may be further manipulated by other stored queries as if the result sets of the first queries were tables in the database. The complexity will be a function of the problems addressed, not the number of objects (patients) included. Each single piece of argument to be entered requires an exact logically description in advance, including any assumption underlying the argument. If there is an assumption to an argument, the assumption should preferably be a separate variable. As humans, we have used our whole life to define and use conceptions which are the underlying cognitive systems for language and communication. These conceptions are often not clearly defined, and two persons may interpret the same words differently. In contrast, databases do not have a cognitive system interpreting the content – they have to be told the exact definitions of each single piece of information as a prerequisite for interpretation of the data to be stored.

Examples of ill-defined objects in cancer genetics are "family," "gene," and "mutation." A logical definition of a concept is not only to describe what it is; it includes the description of what it is not: the delineation of the object from other objects. A concept without delineation means nothing, because it includes everything. The examples mentioned are not delineated: There is no universal definition of a "family," exactly which DNA bases to be referred to as a "gene" has no universal definition, and "mutation" has more than one definition. With the consequence that if such terms are used, then it is necessary to define exactly what they do not mean and what they do mean in the database. If not, what is stored in the database will be undeclared assumptions, and the output of a query to the database will reflect the (unconscious) assumptions when entering the data. This is not only a problem when different persons are entering data into the database. Looking back, it may become clearly visible how perceptions of a term may have changed over time. Two examples from breast cancer genetics may be illustrative: What is the difference between invasive cancer and microinvasive carcinoma in situ and exactly where is the cutoff point between receptor negative and positive? If there is a need to examine such issues in the database, exact definitions are required of what the stored information means. The typical solution for scoring a (quasi)continuous variable as "low or high" is to score it in three options: high, intermediate, and low – offering the option of excluding the intermediate group to look for differences between the extremes (cfr. Histopathological grade scored as 1, 2, or 3).

Typically, a database for medical research will have a person/patient as the main object. This object has to have a unique identifier – the name will not do, because the name may change and because more than one person may have the same name. So it is customary to use a unique number – the patient's social security number may be used. If the social security number is used as the main object, a known person with unknown social security number cannot be included – with the consequence that the generation of a pedigree of a family without consent from all family members would not be possible because it is not allowed to file persons in this way without consent. Consent from dead or emigrated relatives will not be available, and relatives dead generations ago may never have had a social security number. The simple solution is to generate a distinct unique identifier to all persons included – such as a sequential number when entered – and later relate social security code, name, and similar to the internal identifier.

Some registries are based on diagnoses which may be incorrect and later changed, new diagnostic systems may be incompatible with older systems, and there may be more than one patient with the same diagnosis. Diagnostic codes should not be used as the primary object in a relational database.

The main object in the main table is referred to as the primary key in the parent table. In principle, as many pieces of information as required may be entered as columns in the main table, but only if the information will never change. Typically, inclusion of date of birth, date of death, and gender is entered in the main table. If a suitable number of columns in the main table are exceeded, the establishment of a new free-standing table with new columns may be initiated. The new table will use the patient's ID (the primary key) in the parent table, and this will be used to relate the information in the two tables (cfr. the name relational database).

If there is repeated information of the same sort (like result of two colonoscopies of the same patient), this may be included in another table containing the results of the colonoscopies. If two colonoscopies, the same patient will have two rows populated: both rows will include the patient's ID (primary key in the parent table), and when the colonoscopy was undertaken: The patient's ID will be the same in both rows, but the date of the colonoscopies will differ. In principle, as many tables as required may be established for different purposes, and as many rows as required can be entered for the same patient in any such Table. A correctly constructed relational database will have no limit for expansions in these directions.

12 Structured Query Language (SQL)

SQL is the commonly used method to design, maintain, and query a relational database (https://en.wikipedia.org/wiki/Relational_database). To analyze a relational database, a question is asked – a query. The query is formatted in a language designed for the task – a mathematically structured language to relate the different pieces of information with their relationships to typically provide a two-dimensional result table as an answer to the query (the return value of the query). This return value may be used as input to a new query, etc., to build complex analytical systems. The return value of the query may be formatted to meet the input format for the statistical software of choice for further statistical analyses as mentioned above. What can and what cannot be achieved in this way is decided by the exact definitions and formatting of the objects in the given database as discussed above. Whether or not the return value has a meaning is the responsibility of the person deciding the question. The question may be given by a scientist, and then it is the responsibility of the programmer that the programmed query actually is the question to be asked – if not, the return value is not an answer to the question asked by the scientist. There is no output from a database besides return values of queries.

Whether or not the return value of the query has a meaning and is a valid answer to the question is a function of to which degree the logical requirements are met to objects included as discussed above. The latter is critical: If the data include assumptions, any return value of a query to the database will reflect the assumptions. The often cited slogan "garbage in–garbage out" will thus hold. If patients are followed over time, there will be a need to correct typos and misunderstandings. In a medical file, it will not be allowed to delete previously entered information. Typically, a row in a table is "flagged" to be incorrect, with information on who decided this to be so, and a new row is inserted with the correct information and flag in that row who did so and when. "Flag" means adding the information in a separate variable in the row.

The ordinary user will see only the correct information at a given time, but it will be possible to backtrack all information entered and all changes done by whom and when. Implementing such capacity for all variables in a medical file makes it very complex both in design and to be maintained.

Establishing a relational database following the principle rules may this way become very complex, and doing such is often referred to as "normalization" – making it right. Starting a research project and obtaining a result may be time-critical, and the resources to do everything right may not be available. Then the decision on where to start, while ensuring that while starting in a simple way, all the basic rules are adhered to, will be important. If this is achieved, the database may be expanded to any further research questions. The alternative is to violate some of the basic rules, because they make the start too complex and resource-demanding. Doing so is often referred to as "de-normalizing" the database to the task at hand. Doing so may in advance predict exactly which limitations to include and which tasks the database in the future cannot perform.

13 Conclusions

It follows from the above, and which the examples are meant to illustrate, that a research database has to be constructed to the declared need of the research project. Also, SQL queries may be preprogrammed before the data are entered into the database – they may be your research goals declared in your research protocol reformatted into the programming language you use. If you are a scientist needing a programmer to establish and handle your database, you possibly have to engage in database capabilities and limitations to avoid misunderstanding and be sure to reach your research goals. If you have a statistical expert in your group as well, all three should preferably communicate when planning the database design.To have the possibility to expand your database for additional purposes, you may select to establish a relational database meeting all the principle requirements among which a few are discussed above. If you because of lack of time and resources make some shortcuts, you can predict in advance what future limitations your database will have. Both the old statement "Divide each difficulty into as many parts as is feasible and necessary to resolve it" (https://www.brainyquote.com/quotes/quotes/r/renedescar154431.html) and the more recent version "every problem should be made as simple as possible, but not simpler" (http://quoteinvestigator.com/2011/05/13/einstein-simple/) still hold true.

References

1. All websites mentioned were downloaded February 2017.

Chapter 27
The Colon Cancer Family Registry Cohort

Mark A. Jenkins, Aung K. Win, and Noralane M. Lindor

Abstract The Colon Cancer Family Registry Cohort (CCFRC) was established in 1997 for NIH stated purposes of research on the genetic and environmental aetiology of colorectal cancer and the identification of individuals who, because of their high risk, could benefit from preventive strategies. A case-control-family design was utilised to enhance genetic as well as environmental research, including gene discovery and characterisation, and to evaluate modifiers of genetic risk. The 42,489 study participants from 15,049 families were recruited between 1998 and 2012 in the USA, Canada, Australia and New Zealand including recently diagnosed colorectal cancer cases from population-based cancer registries, controls from population-based sources, patients from family cancer clinics with a strong family history of colorectal cancer or young-onset disease and their relatives, both those affected and those unaffected by cancer. At baseline, participants provided a blood/buccal wash sample and access to medical records and tumour specimens and completed a detailed risk factor questionnaire (height, weight, alcohol use, smoking, physical activity, medication use, diet, screening, cancer diagnoses, detailed family history

M. A. Jenkins (✉)
Centre for Epidemiology and Biostatistics, Melbourne School of Population and Global Health, Faculty of Medicine, Dentistry and Health Sciences, The University of Melbourne, Parkville, VIC, Australia

University of Melbourne Centre for Cancer Research, Victorian Comprehensive Cancer Centre, Parkville, VIC, Australia
e-mail: m.jenkins@unimelb.edu.au

A. K. Win
Centre for Epidemiology and Biostatistics, Melbourne School of Population and Global Health, Faculty of Medicine, Dentistry and Health Sciences, The University of Melbourne, Parkville, VIC, Australia

University of Melbourne Centre for Cancer Research, Victorian Comprehensive Cancer Centre, Parkville, VIC, Australia

Genetic Medicine and Familial Cancer Centre, The Royal Melbourne Hospital, Parkville, VIC, Australia

N. M. Lindor
Department of Health Science Research, Mayo Clinic Arizona, Scottsdale, AZ, USA

L. Valle et al. (eds.), *Hereditary Colorectal Cancer*,
https://doi.org/10.1007/978-3-319-74259-5_27

of cancer). Every 4–5 years after baseline, all population-based case-families and clinic-based families were followed up for updates on their personal and family history of cancer as well as history of surgery, cancer screening and some risk factors. The total follow-up of 37,436 participants covers 339,000 person-years (277,000 via direct survey of participants and 62,000 via interview of participating relatives). During follow-up, 824 (2.2%) participants were diagnosed with a colorectal cancer and 3582 (9.5%) were diagnosed with a non-colorectal cancer. Participants have had germline testing for major colorectal cancer genetic syndromes (Lynch syndrome and *MUTYH*) and undergone genome-wide SNP genotyping. Colorectal cancer cases were tested for major somatic alterations, for clinically relevant molecular subtypes, including tumour microsatellite instability, mismatch repair protein loss in immunohistochemistry, the common somatic *KRAS* and *BRAF* variants, *MLH1* methylation and CpG island methylator phenotype (CIMP). Data and biospecimens are available for collaborative research and have been utilised for over 400 publications and approximately 300 projects (53% are external investigator-driven projects) – see http://www.coloncfr.org/.

Keywords Colorectal cancer · Family study · Lynch syndrome · Risk factors · Cohort · Family history

1 Rationale and Structure of the Colon Cancer Family Registry Cohort

Colorectal cancer has long been one of the most frequently diagnosed cancers in the world with an estimated 1.4 million new cases diagnosed each year (9.8% of worldwide cancer diagnoses) and the cause of 694,000 deaths (8.5% of all worldwide cancer deaths) in 2012 [1].

In 1996, as a commitment to reduce morbidity and mortality from this disease, the National Cancer Institute (NCI) of the US National Institutes of Health invited investigators to apply for funding to establish a "Cooperative Family Registry for Colorectal Cancer Studies" (RFA: CA-96-011). The main NIH stated aims were to collect pedigree information, epidemiologic data and related biologic specimens from participants with and without colorectal cancer and with and without a family history of the disease as a resource for interdisciplinary studies on the aetiology of colorectal cancer and to identify a population at high risk of colorectal cancer that could benefit from preventive strategies. This cohort profile provides an update of the Colon Cancer Family Registry, described in detail in Newcomb et al. [2].

The basic premise of this initiative is that family-based designs across the spectrum of risk, in which cases, controls and their relatives are all recruited into a single research infrastructure, would enable efficient study of genetic aetiology, gene penetrance, gene-gene interaction, and interaction with lifestyle factors.

Thus, in 1997, the Colon Cancer Family Registry was established with funding support from the NCI. For Phase-I (1998–2002), 5 years of funding was awarded to six Colon Cancer Family Registry sites:

- Cancer Care Ontario (Toronto, Ontario, Canada)
- Fred Hutchinson Cancer Research Center (Seattle, Washington, USA)
- Mayo Clinic (Rochester, Minnesota, USA)
- University of Hawaii (Honolulu, Hawaii, USA)
- University of Southern California Consortium (comprised of Universities of Southern California, Minnesota, North Carolina, Colorado and Arizona, Dartmouth University and the Cleveland Clinic Foundation, USA)
- The University of Queensland (Brisbane, Queensland, Australia)

The Colon Cancer Family Registry received funding renewals for Phase-II (2003–2007) and Phase-III (2008–2012) with the addition of:

- The University of Melbourne (Melbourne, Victoria, Australia) substituting the University of Queensland
- Memorial University (Newfoundland, Canada) as a collaborative site within the Cancer Care Ontario

In 2004–2011, the ethnic/racial minority component of the Colon Cancer Family Registry was expanded through the recruitment of additional African American and Japanese American families with a separate NCI grant that included the University of Hawaii, the University of Southern California, the University of North Carolina, the Fred Hutchinson Cancer Research Center and the Cancer Prevention Institute of California.

Phase-IV (2013–2018) of the Colon Cancer Family Registry was funded by the NCI as a Cancer Epidemiology Cohort and consequently renamed as the Colon Cancer Family Registry Cohort (CCFRC). This phase saw the changes of Stanford University (California, USA) as the administering site for the CCFRC and Mayo Clinic (Scottsdale, Arizona, USA) as the administering site for the Mayo Clinic.

2 Recruitment and Follow-Ups

Recruitment By design, recruitment sampling schemes and inclusion and exclusion criteria varied by the CCFRC sites and funding phase. Details of the recruitment methods at each institution of the CCFRC have been published previously [2]. Recruitment protocols fall broadly into two main categories: population-based and clinic-based. The CCFRC recruited 42,489 participants – from 15,049 families – who completed a baseline questionnaire between 1998 and 2012 (Table 27.1). Recruitment within clinic-based families was, on average, twice that for population-based families (5.3 vs. 2.6 relatives per family, respectively). The majority of participants self-reported as Caucasian (86%) followed by Asian ethnicities (5.5%), African American (5%), Native American (1%) and others (Pacific Islander, more than one race, or not reported). Of all participants, ~55% were female.

Table 27.1 Number of families and participants of the Colon Cancer Family Registry Cohort by sex and colorectal cancer (CRC) status at baseline recruitment

	Males *N* (%)	Females *N* (%)	Total *N* (%)
Population-based families[a]			13,190
Probands with CRC (case-probands)	4321 (29.2)	4419 (24.6)	8740 (26.7)
Relatives with CRC	332 (2.2)	372 (2.1)	704 (2.1)
Relatives without CRC	7769 (52.5)	10,516 (58.5)	18,285 (55.8)
Probands without CRC (control-probands)	2071 (14.0)	2205 (12.3)	4276 (13.0)
Relatives of control-probands[b]	310 (2.1)	467 (2.6)	777 (2.4)
Total population-based individuals	*14,803*	*17,979*	*32,782*
Clinic-based families[c]			1859
Probands and relatives with CRC	1139 (26.1)	1108 (20.7)	2247 (23.1)
Probands and relatives without CRC	3221 (73.9)	4239 (79.3)	7460 (76.9)
Total clinic-based individuals	*4360*	*5347*	*9707*
Total families			*15,049*
Total participants	*19,163*	*23,326*	*42,489*

[a]Probands recruited from a population-based source
[b]Only the University of Melbourne recruited relatives of control-probands
[c]Probands recruited from a family cancer clinic source

Active Follow-Up Efforts have been made to follow up all participants from all population-based case families (but not controls) and clinic-based families approximately every 4–5 years after completing their baseline questionnaire. At follow-up, all participants were asked, either by telephone interview or self-completed questionnaire (mailed or online), to update their personal and family history of cancer as well as their history of surgery, cancer screening and selected risk factors.

Of the 37,436 participants who completed baseline questionnaires and were approached for follow-up, 27,918 completed the first follow-up questionnaire (response proportion or response "rate" of those alive = 83%), 3549 died before being approached for the first follow-up, and 5969 could not be contacted or refused follow-up. Of the 27,918 participants who had completed the first follow-up, 18,958 completed their second follow-up questionnaire (response = 87%), 1934 died, 2824 were either uncontactable or refused and 4202 are still in process. Of the 18,958 participants who had completed the second follow-up, 8371 had completed their third follow-up questionnaire (response = 95%), 1536 had died, 368 were either uncontactable or refused and 8683 are still in progress (Fig. 27.1).

The total number of person-years of follow-up by participants who completed questionnaires is 276,762 person-years. As this is a family study, the vital status and cancer diagnoses of participants were also ascertained, even if they did not participate in the follow-up themselves, based on interviews of any relatives who were also participants. Including the reports by relatives, the total number of person-years of follow-up of all participants who completed a baseline questionnaire was 338,970 person-years, an average of 9.1 years per participant. These comprise

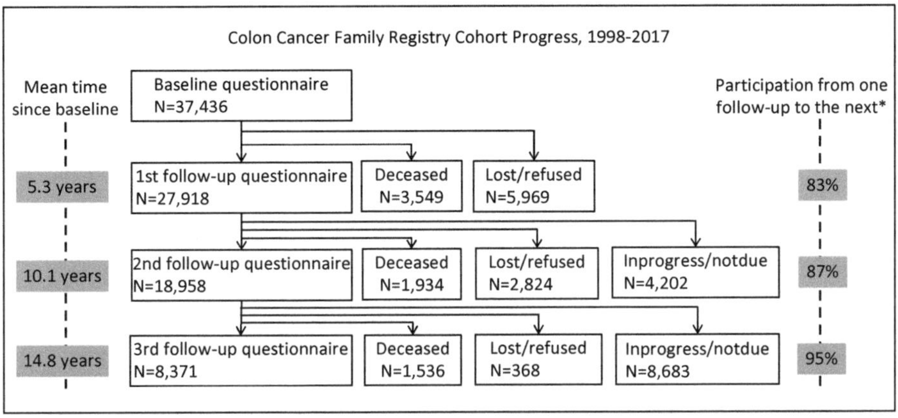

Fig. 27.1 Progress of follow-up of participants of the Colon Cancer Family Registry Cohort (as of June 2017). Participation is defined as the percentage of those who were alive at contact attempt who completed the questionnaire

approximately: 49,000 person-years for those recruited within 2 years after colorectal cancer diagnosis (thus relevant for studies of colorectal cancer survival and risk of metachronous cancer); 39,000 person-years for those recruited more than 2 years after colorectal cancer diagnosis (thus relevant for studies of survivors of colorectal cancer); and 251,000 person-years for those with no previous diagnosis of colorectal cancer (thus relevant for studies of colorectal cancer risk and aetiology) – Table 27.2.

Passive Follow-Up One or more of the following passive follow-up activities have been conducted at each site of the CCFRC – data linkage with local and national death files, population-based cancer registries and electoral rolls, annual newsletters, reviews by genetic counsellors, obituary notices and other mailings to participants. Passive follow-up was regularly conducted on all participants – at intervals that varied by CCFRC site, type of follow-up activity and cost – to obtain information on new cancers, vital status and cause of death and to update contact information.

Incident Cancers and deaths during Follow-Up During active and passive follow-up, all new reports of colorectal polyps and all new cancers were recorded. Attempts were made to verify cancers using medical records, cancer registry data and confirmatory reports from relatives. To date, 824 (2.2%) participants have been diagnosed with a colorectal cancer since baseline (Table 27.2). 3582 (9.5%) participants have been diagnosed with an incident non-colorectal cancer since baseline – total 4164 incident non-colorectal cancers as follows: 772 skin, 568 breast, 599 prostate, 97 gastric, 52 small bowel, 103 hepatobiliary, 102 pancreas, 147 renal, 40 ureteric, 150 urinary bladder, 76 brain, 355 lung, 27 bone, 219 blood, 163 endometrial, 73 ovarian and 35 cervical cancers and 586 in other organs. A total of 7019 (19%) participants (including those with and without colorectal cancer at baseline) are known to have died since baseline – Fig. 27.1.

Table 27.2 Numbers of incident colorectal cancer diagnosis and deaths occurring in study participants (except controls) of the Colon Cancer Family Registry Cohort since baseline recruitment by different cohort types, as of June 2017

	Number of participants	Number of incident colorectal cancer at any age (%)	Number of incident colorectal cancer under age 50 years (%)	Number of deaths (%)	Average follow-up (years)[d]
Colorectal cancer within 2 years prior to recruitment[a]	6765	144 (2.1)	31 (0.5)	2694 (39.8)	7.5
Colorectal cancer over 2 years prior to recruitment[b]	4623	202 (4.4)	25 (0.5)	1411 (30.5)	8.8
No history of colorectal cancer prior to recruitment[c]	26,048	478 (1.8)	114 (0.4)	2914 (11.2)	10.0
Total	37,436	824 (2.2)	170 (0.5)	7019 (18.7)	9.4

[a]Cohort useful for studies of colorectal cancer survival and risk of metachronous cancer
[b]Cohort useful for studies of survivors of colorectal cancer
[c]Cohort useful for studies of colorectal cancer risk and aetiology
[d]Based on follow-up interview or report from participating relative

3 Data

At the *baseline recruitment*, CCFRC participants were asked to complete a detailed family history of cancer, a risk factor questionnaire, permission to access medical records pertaining to any colorectal cancer diagnoses and permission to access colorectal cancer tumours and, depending on the degree of relationship to the proband, to provide a blood (or buccal wash) sample – Table 27.3.

Baseline Risk Factor Questionnaires All participants (probands and their participating relatives) were asked to complete the same detailed baseline risk factor survey using standardised questionnaires via personal or telephone interviews or mailed questionnaires. Items included demography, lifestyle factors, screening, treatment and family history. Four CCFRC sites also asked participants to complete a self-administered food frequency dietary questionnaire. Three CCFRC sites (University of Hawaii, Cancer Care Ontario and University of Southern California consortium) used the questionnaire developed by the Multiethnic Cohort study in Hawaii and California [3]. The University of Melbourne used the questionnaire developed by the Melbourne Collaborative Cohort Study [4].

Follow-Up Risk Factor Questionnaires At each follow-up, participants were asked for the following events that occurred since the previous contact, including cancer diagnoses, bowel and gynaecological surgery, screening for colorectal cancer, polyps and cancer diagnoses and deaths in relatives. Some CCFRC sites opted to include additional questions pertaining to colorectal cancer risk factors.

Table 27.3 Resources available for the Colon Cancer Family Registry Cohort, as of June 2017

			Males N (%)	Females N (%)	Total N (%)
Population-based case families[a]	Probands	Baseline questionnaire	4321 (22.5)	4419 (18.9)	8740 (20.6)
		Food frequency questionnaire	2096 (22.7)	2409 (20.5)	4505 (21.5)
		Blood/buccal samples	3759 (27.3)	3886 (22.8)	7645 (24.8)
		Polyp material	14 (7.9)	8 (4.0)	22 (5.8)
		Cancer material	3561 (73.6)	3447 (70.2)	7008 (71.9)
		Diagnosis and treatment	1563 (84.2)	1526 (85.7)	3089 (85.0)
	Relatives[b]	Baseline questionnaire	7740 (40.4)	10,328 (44.3)	18,068 (42.5)
		Food frequency questionnaire	3323 (36.0)	4700 (40.0)	8023 (38.3)
		Blood/buccal samples	4751 (34.4)	6731 (39.5)	11,482 (37.2)
		Polyp material	7 (3.9)	8 (4.0)	15 (3.9)
		Cancer material	265 (5.5)	325 (6.6)	590 (6.1)
		Diagnosis and treatment	40 (2.2)	44 (2.5)	84 (2.3)
	Spouse controls[c]	Baseline questionnaire	361 (1.9)	560 (2.4)	921 (2.2)
		Food frequency questionnaire	135 (1.5)	197 (1.7)	332 (1.6)
		Blood/buccal samples	149 (1.1)	225 (1.3)	374 (1.2)
Population-based control families[d]	Probands	Baseline questionnaire	2071 (10.8)	2205 (9.5)	4276 (10.1)
		Food frequency questionnaire	1142 (12.4)	1023 (8.7)	2165 (10.3)
		Blood/buccal samples	1399 (10.1)	1497 (8.8)	2896 (9.4)
	Relatives[b]	Baseline epi data	310 (1.6)	467 (2.0)	777 (1.8)
		Food frequency questionnaire	260 (2.8)	383 (3.3)	643 (3.1)
		Blood/buccal samples	6 (0.0)	5 (0.0)	11 (0.0)
Clinic-based case families[e]	Probands with CRC[a]	Baseline questionnaire	699 (3.6)	644 (2.8)	1343 (3.2)
		Food frequency questionnaire	247 (2.7)	270 (2.3)	517 (2.5)
		Blood/buccal samples	645 (4.7)	625 (3.7)	1270 (4.1)
		Polyp material	24 (13.5)	29 (14.4)	53 (13.9)
		Cancer material	561 (11.6)	526 (10.7)	1087 (11.2)
		Diagnosis and treatment	239 (12.9)	204 (11.5)	443 (12.2)
	Probands w/o CRC[c]	Baseline questionnaire	137 (0.7)	304 (1.3)	441 (1.0)
		Food frequency questionnaire	62 (0.7)	164 (1.4)	226 (1.1)
		Blood/buccal samples	101 (0.7)	250 (1.5)	351 (1.1)
		Polyp material	13 (7.3)	27 (13.4)	40 (10.5)
		Cancer material	20 (0.4)	67 (1.4)	87 (0.9)
		Diagnosis and treatment	0 (0.0)	0 (0.0)	0 (0.0)
	Relatives[b]	Baseline questionnaire	3524 (18.4)	4399 (18.9)	7923 (18.6)
		Food frequency questionnaire	1953 (21.2)	2596 (22.1)	4549 (21.7)
		Blood/buccal samples	2983 (21.6)	3814 (22.4)	6797 (22.0)
		Polyp material	120 (67.4)	130 (64.4)	250 (65.8)
		Cancer material	429 (8.9)	542 (11.0)	971 (10.0)
		Diagnosis and treatment	14 (0.8)	6 (0.3)	20 (0.6)

(continued)

Table 27.3 (continued)

			Males N (%)	Females N (%)	Total N (%)
Total	All population and clinic-based probands and relatives				
		Baseline questionnaire	19,163	23,326	42,489
		Food frequency questionnaire	9218	11,742	20,960
		Blood/buccal samples	13,793	17,033	30,826
		Polyp material	178	202	380
		Cancer material	4836	4907	9743
		Diagnosis and treatment	1856	1780	3636

[a]Proband has a history of colorectal cancer (CRC) at baseline interview
[b]Affected or unaffected with colorectal cancer at baseline interview
[c]Spouse of proband. Has no history of colorectal cancer at baseline interview
[d]Proband has no history of colorectal cancer at baseline interview
[e]Proband is recruited from a family cancer clinic

All baseline and follow-up questionnaires used by each CCFRC sites can be accessed at http://www.coloncfr.org/questionnaires.

Family History One or more participants from each family was asked to provide their family history of cancer by answering a standard set of questions for each of their relatives including sex and date of birth, cancer sites (except nonmelanoma skin cancer) and ages or dates at diagnoses, vital status and, if deceased, date of death. All CCFR sites recorded detailed family history information for each first- and second-degree relative, and some sites expanded to third-degree relatives, depending on site-specific protocols (detail in Newcomb et al. [2]). Extensive efforts were made to verify the anatomical site, extent of disease, age at diagnosis and pathology of tumours. Sources of verification used included pathology reports, medical and surgical records, cancer registry information and death certificates.

Blood/Mouthwash Samples Participants were asked to provide a blood or mouthwash sample. Of those who agreed, 93% provided a blood sample – Table 27.3 [5]. DNA was extracted from blood and mouthwash samples under CCFRC quality-control protocols to maximise target DNA concentration and fragment size. To provide an unlimited supply of DNA and RNA for probands and selected relatives, lymphoblastoid cell lines of case-probands were immortalised on a subset of participants using Epstein-Barr virus [6].

Tumours and Pathology Paraffin-embedded colorectal cancer tumours – as well as diagnostic pathology reports – were obtained from treating facilities with the consent of the participant or the next of kin if the participant was deceased. In addition, some CCFRC sites also obtained polyps and non-colorectal tumours, especially cancers commonly identified as part of Lynch syndrome. Multiple sections were cut from each tumour (for immunohistochemistry and nucleic acid extraction) and normal tissue block, one of which was stained with haematoxylin and eosin (H&E) and reviewed by pathologists. For each colorectal cancer, a pathology review was completed (either by examination of the H&E slides or extraction of relevant data from available pathology reports) to obtain the following standardised set of tumour features: grade, histological type, stage (depth of infiltration in large bowel wall and spread to regional lymph nodes), lymphovascular invasion and perineural invasion. Sections were stored for future research at each CCFRC site. When allowed by outside institutions, tumour blocks were also stored for future studies. Two sites (Ontario and University of Southern California consortium) have made tumour microarrays (TMAs) from colorectal cancers ($n = 1278$).

Virtual Tissue Repository CCFRC has created a digitised library of pathology slides (electronic representations of traditional glass slides). A total of 4510 H&E stained slides of histological sections of colorectal tumours from the probands were scanned using either the NanoZoomer Digital Pathology Scanner (Hamamatsu Corp.) or the Aperio ScanScope digital slide scanner. Each image is stored as a series of 752 × 480 pixel JPEG image tiles that are reconstructed with relevant software. Typical size of these images is between 200mb and 1.5gb per slide. All images were archived on five image servers: one for short-term storage and four for long-term storage. This process can facilitate morphology-based studies and allows sharing of H&E sections without jeopardising the resource due to possible unreturned original slides.

Clinical Records Clinical treatment and outcome records were requested from 3830 case-probands and 111 relatives with an incident colorectal cancer diagnosed since baseline and have been abstracted into standardised items for analysis.

Molecular Characterisation of Tumours Probands' colorectal cancers were characterised for DNA mismatch repair (MMR) deficiency by PCR-based microsatellite instability (MSI) tests and/or by immunohistochemistry (IHC) for the four DNA MMR proteins [7]. Colorectal cancer tumour DNA was tested for the *BRAF* V600E somatic point mutation [8, 9] and somatic mutations in codons 12 and 13 of *KRAS* [8, 9]. Tumours were also tested for methylation of the *MLH1* gene promoter (an epigenetic phenotype that can be used to indicate that tumour MMR deficiency is more likely to have been caused by somatic epigenetic event in *MLH1* than by a germline mutation in *MLH1*) [11]. Characterisation of the CpG island methylator phenotype (CIMP) was also performed by assessing quantitative methylation across five gene promoters (*CACNA1G*, *IGF2*, *NEUROG1*, *RUNX3* and *SOCS1*) [10] – Table 27.4.

Molecular Characterisation of Germline DNA Screening for germline mutations in *MLH1*, *MSH2*, *MSH6*, *PMS2* and *EPCAM* was performed for all population-based probands who had a colorectal tumour displaying a MSI-high or a loss of expression of one or more of the MMR protein expression by IHC and for the youngest-onset colorectal cancer case participant from each clinic-based family, regardless of MSI or MMR protein expression status. All case-probands were genotyped for specific

Table 27.4 Molecular characterisations of participants (probands and relatives) at the Colon Cancer Family Registry Cohort, as of June 2017

Molecular test	Number of participants tested	Number of colorectal cancer tumours tested	Test results
Tumour			
DNA MSI	5147	5305	1065 high 665 low 3575 stable
IHC for MMR proteins	8036	8338	1671 loss 6667 present
CIMP[a]	3877	4502	506 positive 3996 negative
MLH1 methylation	3041	3412	465 methylated 2947 normal
BRAF V600E mutation	7080	7322	679 positive 6643 negative
KRAS mutation	4014	4154	1299 positive 2855 negative
Blood			
MMR gene[b]	2895 probands 4106 relatives		710 mutations 1408 mutations
MUTYH[b]	10649 probands 3571 relatives		47 biallelic, 195 monoallelic 12 biallelic, 197 monoallelic

MSI microsatellite instability, IHC immunohistochemistry, MMR mismatch repair, CIMP CpG island methylator phenotype

[a]Tumours were classified as CIMP-positive if ≥3 of 5 genes gave percent of methylated reference value ≥10

[b]sequencing (probands) or predictive testing (relatives)

germline mutations in *MUTYH*. DNA from the participating and consented relatives of probands with a pathogenic mutation were tested for the specific mutation (MMR gene or *MUTYH*) identified in the proband (predictive testing). Of the CCFRC participants, 2118 carry a mutation in one of the MMR genes (761 in *MLH1*, 976 in *MSH2*, 243 in *MSH6*, 109 in *PMS2*, 29 in *EPCAM*), and 451 carry either a monoallelic ($n = 392$) or biallelic mutation ($n = 59$) in *MUTYH*. Since baseline, these mutation carriers have contributed a total of 18,514 MMR-mutation person-years and 3732 *MUTYH*-mutation person-years.

In addition, targeted sequencing was conducted of 36 known or putative colorectal cancer susceptibility genes (including the MMR genes) for 1231 cases including cases with familial colorectal cancer type X [12], early-onset (age < 50 years at colorectal cancer diagnosis) or suspected Lynch syndrome and cases for which no tumour was available to triage by tumour MMR deficiency status. CCFRC has genome-wide SNP genotyping data for 10,716 participants (6732 cases and 2435 controls) by various platforms, all now imputed to the 1000 Genomes Project [13].

4 Research Summary

CCFRC resource has been used for more than 400 original peer-reviewed publications – see http://coloncfr.org/publications. Here, we highlight a few findings that illustrate the power of this cohort to understand genetic and environmental risk factors for colorectal cancer.

1. *Lynch syndrome*: Research utilising the CCFRC has significantly refined and advanced multiple aspects of our understanding and approach to this cancer-predisposing genetic syndrome, specifically, in the following major studies which have:
   (i) Estimated age-specific cumulative risk of cancer (penetrance) for carriers of germline mutations in *MLH1* and *MSH2* [14], *MSH6* [15] and *PMS2* [16].
   (ii) Conducted the first prospective cohort study of Lynch syndrome carriers [17].
   (iii) Described MMR gene mutation spectrum and estimated penetrance for African American carriers [18] and estimated the risk of metachronous colorectal cancer following colon cancer [19] or rectal cancer [20] and subsequent cancers following colorectal cancer [21, 22] or endometrial cancer [23].
   (iv) Estimated the risk of childhood cancers in Lynch syndrome families [24].
   (v) Investigated modifiers on cancer risks including environmental (body mass index [25, 26]; smoking [27]; alcohol drinking [28]; aspirin and ibuprofen use [29]; multivitamin, calcium and folic acid supplements use [30]; and female hormonal factors [31]) and genetic (*TERT* [32], *MUTYH* [33] and other common genetic variants [34]) factors.
   (vi) Investigated whether fertility was associated with Lynch syndrome [35, 36].
   (vii) Described the clinical phenotypes associated with Lynch syndrome [37].
   (viii) Provided evidence that people with Lynch syndrome have modestly increased risks of breast [17, 21, 23, 38], cervical [14, 39] and prostate [21, 40] cancers.
   (ix) Shown the role of tumour *BRAF* mutation [41] and *MLH1* promoter methylation [42] testing in the detection of MMR gene mutation carriers.
   (x) Described recurrent and founder mutations in the *PMS2* gene [43].
   (xi) Determined the frequency of de novo mutations for MMR genes [44].
   (xii) Provided essential data for MMR gene variant classification in collaboration with InSiGHT. This was possible because of the extensive

Table 27.5 Population prevalence of Lynch syndrome. Estimated proportion (and 95% confidence interval) of the general population carrying a pathogenic germline mutation in a DNA mismatch repair gene

Gene	Estimate	95%CI
MLH1	1 in 1900	1 in 1500–2500
MSH2	1 in 2800	1 in 2100–3800
MSH6	1 in 760	1 in 510–1100
PMS2	1 in 710	1 in 640–1050
Any mismatch repair gene	1 in 280	1 in 190–400

Note: Adapted from Win et al. [48]. Copyright 2017 by American Association for Cancer Research

descriptions of the CCFRC participants including tumour characteristics and detailed family history for the incorporating probabilities based on sequence bioinformatics and tumour characteristics [45–47].

(xiii) Provided the first evidence-based prevalence of Lynch syndrome in the general population (1 in 280 people is estimated to carry mutations in any MMR gene, see Table 27.5) [48]. This research has contributed to national and international clinical guidelines and is being incorporated in future cancer prevention efforts by the Cancer Moonshot initiative.

(xiv) Defined a new classification for colorectal cancer, familial colorectal cancer type X, the phenotype of approximately 50% of MMR-proficient colorectal cancer cases who fulfilled the Amsterdam Criteria-I for hereditary non-polyposis colorectal cancer [12].

2. *MUTYH studies*: CCFRC resource has been used for estimating age-specific cumulative risk (penetrance) of colorectal cancer [49, 50] as well as non-colorectal cancers [51, 52] for biallelic (mutation inherited from each parent) and monoallelic (mutation inherited from only one parent) mutation carriers. This research has direct impact on the genetic testing and clinical management for *MUTYH* mutation carriers.
3. *Prognosis*: Using both baseline and follow-up data of the CCFRC, there have been many publications on multiple aspects of colorectal cancer survival possible given in-depth person and tumour characterisation efforts, including:

(i) Tumour molecular features including MSI status [53, 54], *BRAF* mutation [55], CIMP status [56], molecular subtypes (combining all these features) [57], *KRAS* mutation [58], *PIK3CA* mutation [59] and genome-wide copy number alterations[60]

(ii) Genetic variations in *SMAD7* [61], C-reactive protein [62], inflammatory pathways [63], catechol-O-methyltransferase [64] and oestrogen receptor beta promoter [65]

(iii) Pre-diagnostic factors including family history [66], inflammatory bowel disease [67], obesity [68], smoking [69], alcohol consumption [70], NSAID use [71], postmenopausal hormone use [72] and physical activity [73]

(iv) Metachronous colorectal cancer – we recently reported, for the first time, the risk factors associated with metachronous colorectal cancer including personal, tumour and lifestyle factors [74]

4. *Aetiology studies*: Often as an international collaboration, CCFRC has contributed data to the studies of environmental and lifestyle risk factors for colorectal cancer, with emphasis of the interactions with candidate genes or pathways:

   (i) Cigarette smoking [75], obesity and height [76], parity [77], family history [78], gender of the affected parent [79], alcohol consumption and smoking [80], NSAID use [81–85], exogenous hormone use [86–88], dietary folate [89–91], calcium and vitamin D [92–96], meat intake [97], cooking method [98], leptin levels [99], dietary phytoestrogen [100] and other nutrients [101]
   (ii) Mendelian randomisation studies on height [102], body mass index [103] and adiposity [104]

5. *New gene discoveries*: CCFRC GWAS data has been utilised for colorectal cancer research which have:

   (i) Discovered new colorectal cancer susceptibility loci (SNPs) for Caucasians [105–114], East Asians [115] and African Americans [116] as well as new pan-ethnic colorectal cancer susceptibility locus at 10q25 [117]
   (ii) Shown the cumulative impact of common genetic variants and other risk factors on colorectal cancer risk [118]
   (iii) Shown a new serrated neoplasia, Jass syndrome, linked to chromosome 2 [119]
   (iv) Described germline mutations in *EPHB2* in familial colorectal cancer [120]
   (v) Shown serrated pathway involvement in colorectal cancers with somatic *BRAF* mutations [121–123]
   (vi) Investigated the association with genetic variations in *SMAD7* [124], inflammation and innate immunity pathways [125, 126] and phospholipase A2G1B polymorphisms [127]
   (vii) Shown the association between germline *HOXB13* p.Gly84Glu mutation and colorectal cancer risk [128]
   (viii) Shown the association between germline *TP53* mutations and early-onset colorectal cancer [129]

6. *Epigenetics*: CCFRC has contributed extensively to understanding of epigenetics related to colorectal cancer including its role in MSI [130], the relationship with ethnicity [131], somatic *BRAF* mutations in MSI tumours and the confirmation of CIMP [132], DNA methylation in serrated polyps [133], the possibility that some epigenetic change may be inherited in Lynch syndrome [134], the role of age in association with MSI prevalence [135] and *MLH1*

expression [136], methylation in the promoter region of *MLH1* [56] and *ITF2* [137], association between hypermethylation in white blood cell DNA and colorectal cancer [138] and associations between colorectal CIMP phenotype and tumour molecular features and other risk factors [10].

7. *Risk prediction*: We published a study [139] explaining the familial aggregation by taking into account all known and unknown major genes and polygenic component, which is an essential step in the development of a risk prediction model for colorectal cancer. Further, in collaborations with other investigators, we validated MMR gene mutation prediction models including MMRpro and PREMM [140–142].
8. *Molecular pathology*: CCFRC has contributed in various aspects of colorectal cancer molecular pathology, from basic science to clinical studies – the relationship between MSI and IHC phenotyping of tumours [7], MMR gene mutation detection by use of diploid to haploid conversion analysis [143], the significance of missense mutations in *APC* [144, 145], discovery of deletion-related monoallelic drop-out of *BAT26* in MSI testing [146], determining the sensitivity and specificity of pathology features in Bethesda Guidelines for MSI-H tumours [147], copy number variants in germline DNA [148], detection of *PMS2* mutations in colorectal tumours [149, 150], telomere length variation by DNA extraction method [151] and age of colorectal cancer diagnosis [152], *MGMT* methylation in colorectal cancer tumours [153], genome-wide copy number alteration [60, 154] and association between tumour molecular subtypes and colorectal cancer risk in the relatives [155].
9. *Behavioural studies*: CCFRC has contributed to psychosocial and behavioural studies in the area of genetic information about Lynch syndrome [156, 157], communication of genetic results [158], genetic information and uptake of screening [159, 160] and quality of life and lifestyle changes in colorectal cancer survivors [161–163]. We also conducted a randomised controlled trial on the effectiveness of a telephone-based counselling intervention to increase colonoscopy screening [164].
10. *Research on non-colorectal cancers*: CCFRC has also enabled a broad range of research on other cancers beyond colorectal cancer because of our extended recruitment on the family members. CCFRC has contributed to identify genetic and environmental risk factors for endometrial [111, 165], breast [166] and pancreatic [167–171] cancers.

5 Research Focus: Identification of Lynch Syndrome

One of the major contributions to Lynch syndrome research that the CCFRC is contributing to is the identification of Lynch syndrome carriers in the population. Once identified, relatives of the mutation carriers can undergo predictive testing for the mutation found in the family, but there are many possible strategies for identifying families carrying a mutation, each with their own advantages and disadvantages. The CCFRC can contribute a substantial amount of important data to assess these strategies.

Before considering any strategy, some estimates of the number or proportion of the population that have Lynch syndrome. There have been previous attempts to estimate this based on the observed proportion of colorectal cancer cases that are Lynch syndrome, the proportion that have colorectal cancer and the estimated prevalence by age of Lynch syndrome for colorectal cancer. The CCFRC has sufficient *family* data to calculate this prevalence based on observed data. By analysing the families of 5744 colorectal cancer cases recruited from population cancer registries in the USA, Canada and Australia, the estimated proportion of the population with Lynch syndrome was approximately 1 in 280 (0.35%) [48]. For a population of 320 million people in the USA, this equates to over one million people with Lynch syndrome. The estimated prevalence varied considerably by DNA MMR gene (Table 27.5). Approximately three times as many of the population are estimated to carry mutations in *MSH6* or *PMS2* compared with *MLH1* or *MSH2*. This may first appear counter-intuitive given the majority of colorectal cancer cases with Lynch syndrome are *MLH1* or *MSH2*, but these are the higher penetrant genes and therefore more likely to be observed in colorectal cancer cases and do not reflect the expected number in the general population, the vast majority of whom do not have colorectal cancer.

The primary question then becomes how to best identify the people in the population with Lynch syndrome. Most efficiently, this will be done by first identifying the carriers in those with a previous diagnosis of colorectal cancer, given the proportion of colorectal cancer cases with Lynch syndrome (approximately 3%) is approximately ten times greater than the general population. However, this 3% prevalence is an average over all colorectal cancer cases and certainly not uniformly distributed.

Family history was one of the first criteria for identifying families to test for Lynch syndrome. For example, Amsterdam Criteria-I [172] and the Amsterdam Criteria-II [173] specified definitions of strong family history, thought to be more commonly due to Lynch syndrome than other cases. Data from the CCFRC suggest that family history is not an effective way to identify which colorectal cancer cases have Lynch syndrome. In Fig. 27.2, the rectangles represent the number of colorectal cancer cases in the population with the area of each of the rectangles being directly proportional to the number of colorectal cancer diagnoses in the population. Each rectangle represents a different definition of family history. The thin red vertical rectangle represents the number of colorectal cancer cases with Lynch syndrome, again with the area of each of the rectangles being directly proportional to the number of Lynch syndrome cases with colorectal cancer in the population. Using this representation, it can be seen that while those with two or more first-degree relatives with colorectal cancer or those meeting Amsterdam Criteria-I [172] are enriched for Lynch syndrome (one in six has Lynch syndrome), the majority of Lynch syndrome cases are in those with no first-degree relatives with colorectal cancer. Only 2% of this category will have a mutation but because of the size of this group, it will contain 58% of colorectal cancer cases that have Lynch syndrome.

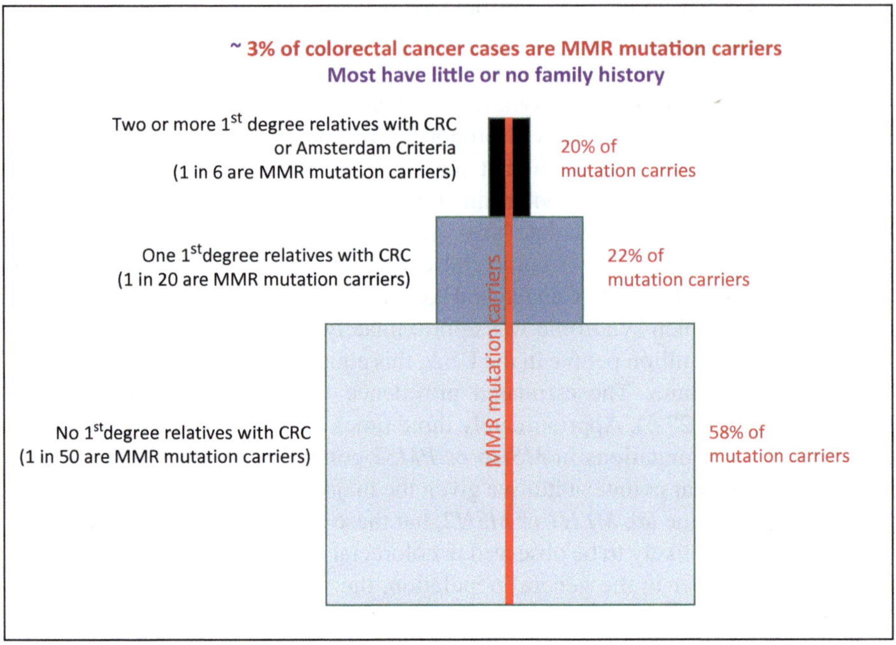

Fig. 27.2 Estimate distribution of Lynch syndrome (pathogenic mutation in a DNA mismatch repair gene) in colorectal cancer cases by family history

Another method which is commonly used by almost all clinical services is to test the colorectal cancer tumours for evidence of MMR deficiency, either by testing for high-MSI or loss of expression of any of the MMR proteins by IHC. Data from the CCFRC show that there is a U-shaped relationship between colorectal cancer MMR deficiency and age of diagnosis, with the proportions of tumours having MMR deficiency for those diagnosed in their 30s and 70s (approximately 20%) being twice as high compared with tumours in cases diagnosed in their 50s (approximately 9%) (Fig. 27.3a). For early-onset cases, tumour MMR deficiency is ten times more likely to be due to inherited MMR gene mutations (~50%) compared with late-onset cases (~5%) (Fig. 27.3b) which is more likely to be due to age-related methylation of *MLH1*. About 9% of cases diagnosed in their 30s are due to Lynch syndrome compared with about 1% of late-onset cases (Fig. 27.3c).

The CCFRC has conducted a molecular study of the colorectal tumours for the causes for the MMR deficiency. There were marked differences by age of diagnosis (Fig. 27.4). For colorectal cancers diagnosed before age 50, the majority (57%) were Lynch syndrome compared with only 10% of those diagnosed over age 50. In contrast *MLH1* methylation occurred in only 4% of tumours diagnosed before age 50 but was present in the 69% of those diagnosed at ages 50 years or over. In both age categories, a substantial proportion of tumours exhibited somatic mutation in both alleles of MMR genes, 1 in 8 early-onset and 1 in 16 late-onset. These represent the most challenging cases for Lynch syndrome diagnosis as the tumours exhibit MMR deficiency, and there is no *MLH1* methylation suggesting a germline mutation is the

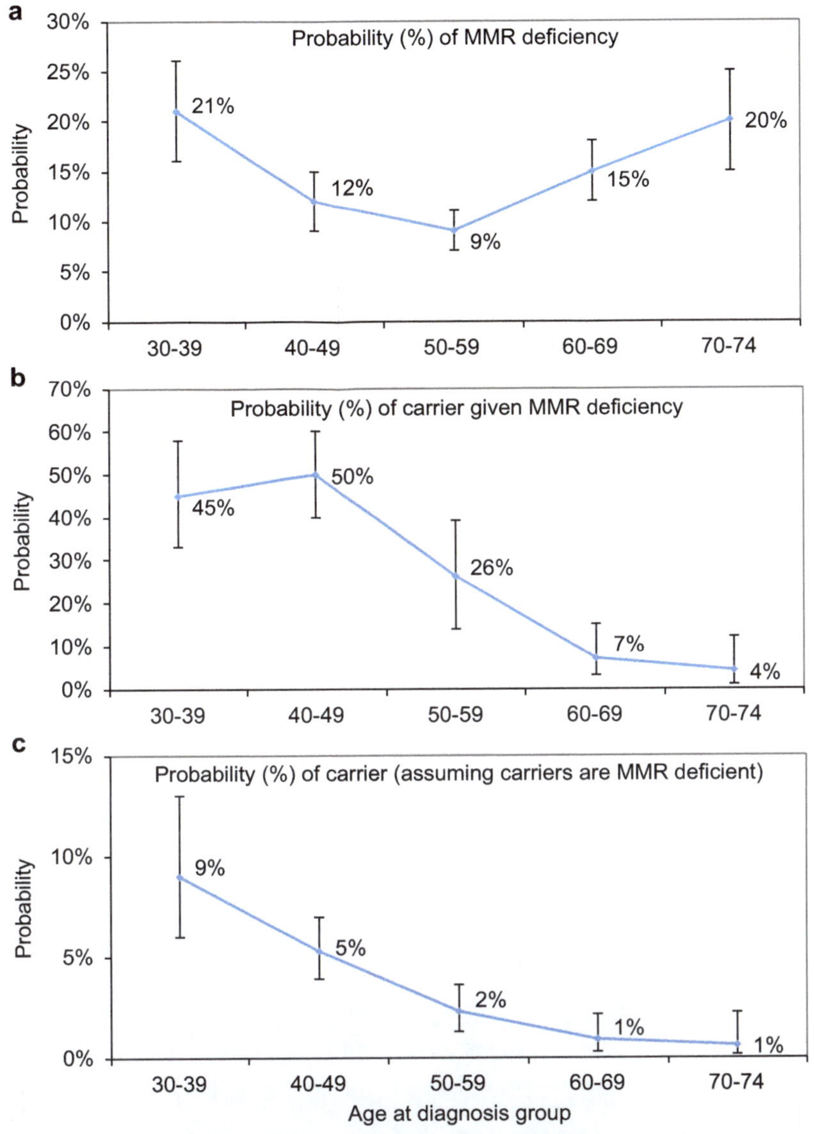

Fig. 27.3 Distribution of colorectal cancers by age of diagnosis from population-based sources between the ages of 18 and 74 years at diagnosis: (**a**) probability that a colorectal cancer has tumour MMR deficiency defined by high-MSI or loss of expression of MMR proteins by IHC; (**b**) probability that a colorectal cancer case has Lynch syndrome (carrier of a mutation in a MMR gene) given they have a MMR-deficient colorectal cancer; and (**c**) probability that a colorectal cancer case is Lynch syndrome

culprit even though it cannot be identified. Under this scenario, relatives would be expected to be potential carriers of an undetected mutation in a Lynch syndrome gene and therefore recommended to undergo intensive colonoscopy screening, when in fact, they are highly unlikely to carry a germline mutation.

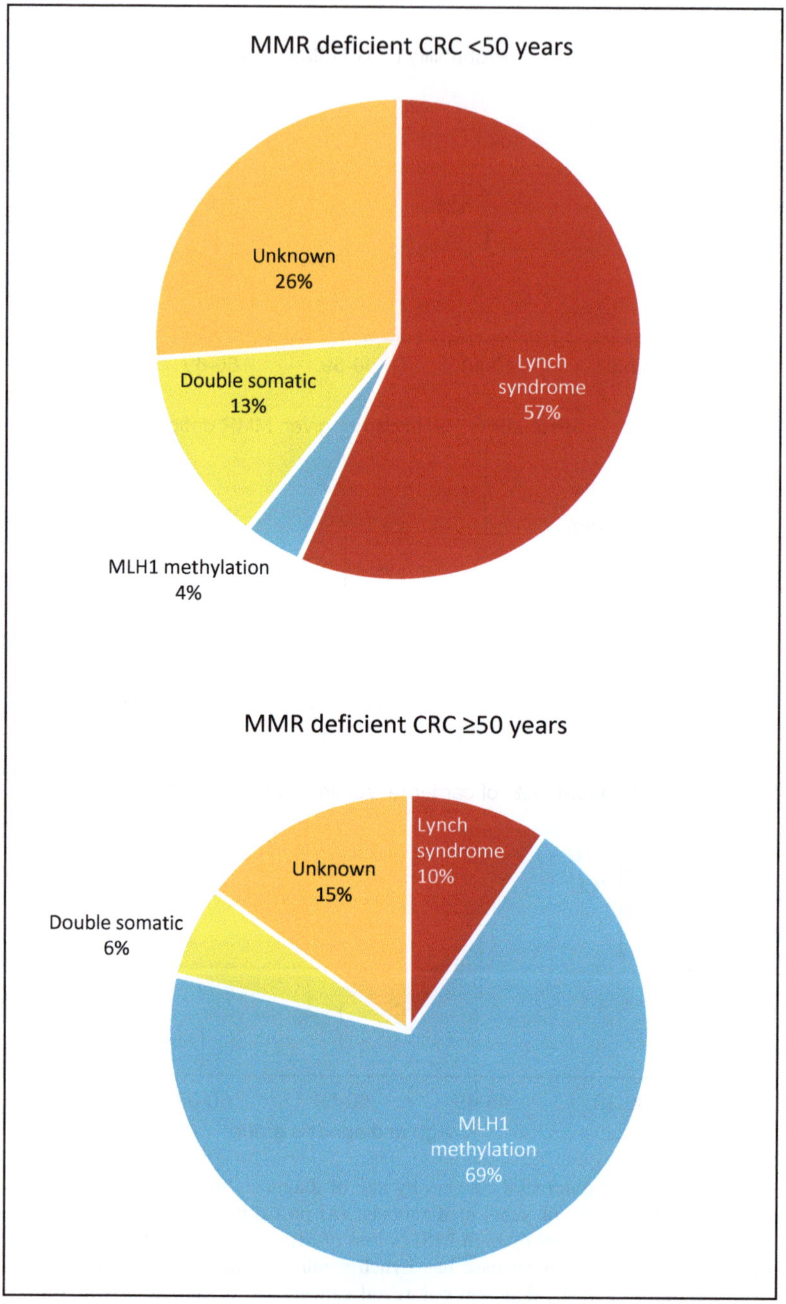

Fig. 27.4 Distribution of genetic characterisation of the probable cause of mismatch repair (MMR) deficiency in colorectal cancer tumours for cases diagnosed under the age of 50 years and for cases diagnosed at ages 50 years and over

Based on the data presented in Fig. 27.3. in combination with the population prevalence of Lynch syndrome (approximately 1 in 280), it is possible to estimate the expected proportions of carriers that would be identified if only colorectal cancer cases were tested. If population testing for Lynch syndrome was conducted for all people at age 50 years, more than 95% of all identified people with Lynch syndrome will have never been diagnosed with colorectal cancer. If the population of 70-year-olds were tested, less than 10% will ever have had colorectal cancer. Therefore, although much less efficient, Lynch syndrome testing of the whole population, will identify 10–20 times more carriers than testing colorectal cancer cases alone.

Identification of people with Lynch syndrome is important so they can receive intensive risk reduction measures including colorectal cancer screening [174] and chemoprevention such as aspirin use [29, 175]. This is because the average risk of colorectal cancer is considered high enough to warrant such measures. We estimated the penetrance of colorectal cancer in Lynch syndrome, and, using a sophisticated statistical methodology, we have identified that the *distribution* is not described well by the average risk [14]. Figure 27.5 shows that while the average

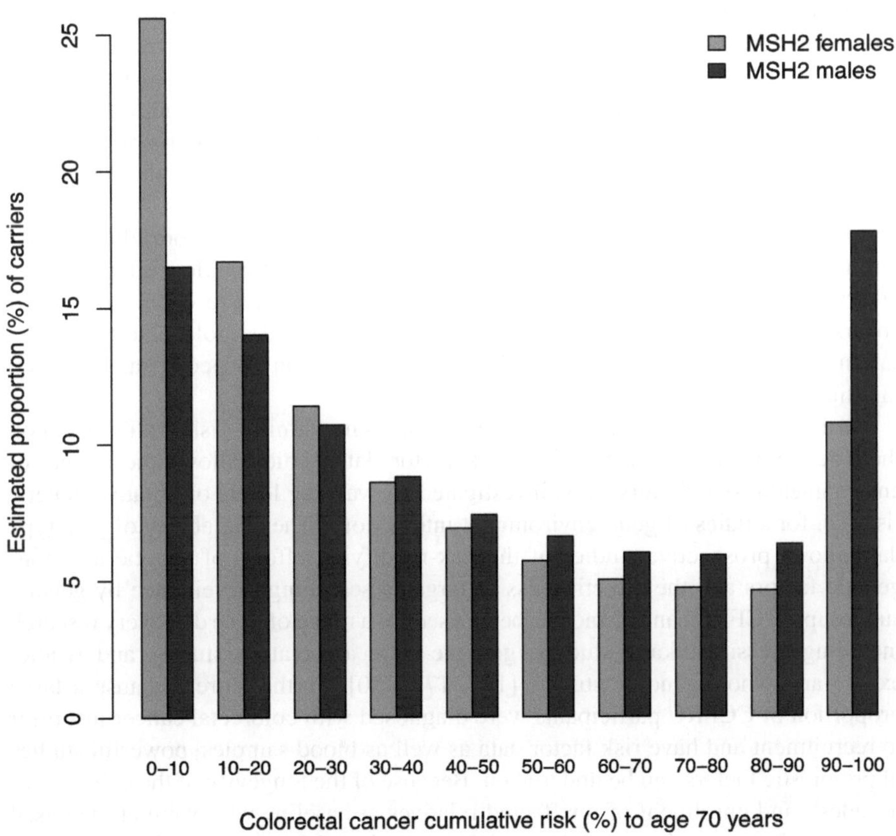

Fig. 27.5 Distribution of lifetime risk of colorectal cancer (up to age 70 years) for carriers of a germline mutation in the Lynch syndrome gene, *MSH2*. The patterns for *MLH1* males and females resembled a similar U-shape. *Note*: Adapted from Dowty et al. [14]. Copyright 2012 by Wiley Periodicals, Inc.

risk of colorectal cancer for carries of mutations in DNA MMR genes might be on average 30–40%, this is not the most likely risk. Rather than being a bell-shaped Gaussian distribution, a high proportion of people with Lynch syndrome have only moderately increased risk of colorectal cancer (<10%), and, at the other extreme, a high proportion are very likely to get colorectal cancer (>80%). Penetrance in Lynch syndrome is complex. This distribution of cancer risks is consistent with the existence of important modifiers of risk (genetic or environmental) that could, if identified, be used to reduce the risk of Lynch syndrome. The CCFRC has been very active in searching for these modifiers of risk (see Chapter 5 Genetic and Environmental Modifiers of Risk in Lynch syndrome).

5.1 What Are the Main Strengths and Weaknesses of the CCFRC?

The unique strength of the CCFRC is its prospective, observational design, with familial enrichment and molecular characterisation. The consenting process allowed for conduct of multiple studies of many types that did not require re-consent unless recontact was required. Participants have deliberately been oversampled for both young age at diagnosis (in Phase-II) and for familial risk in some recruitment site and consisted of consecutively ascertained cases in one site. Because the design was intentional, proband weights are known and can be used for analysis of the population-based cases to apply back to the general population. Therefore, the CCFRC differs from the usual cancer research cohort in novel ways that allow inferences not otherwise possible [176]. This facilitates a deeper and broader research agenda that covers aetiological factors (both genetic and environmental), molecular characterisation, behavioural issues and clinical research relevant to people at increased familial risk.

Participants can be categorised on their underlying familial risk profile based on their genotype, family history and risk factor data, which allows the effects of environmental risk factors to be investigated for varying levels of putative genetic risk, i.e. for studies of gene-environment interactions. The availability of genotype data allows prospective studies of the risk-modifying effects of genetic and non-genetic factors and the effectiveness of targeted screening/surveillance by genetic subgroups. CCFRC can be, and has been, used for a range of gene discovery research including classic linkage studies, genome-wide association studies and whole-exome and whole-genome studies [119, 177–180]. Furthermore, because a large proportion of CCFRC participants were diagnosed with colorectal cancer just prior to recruitment and have risk factor data as well as blood samples, powerful studies of prognostic factors can be undertaken. Because of the longevity of the cohort (two decades), and enrolment of unaffected relatives at baseline who were at increased risk due to being in a known colorectal cancer-affected family, the CCFRC now has almost 800 new colorectal cancer cases that "converted" from being unaffected to affected (despite screening advice) during their follow-up period, which has enabled prospective study of multiple factors. CCFRC also facilitates novel behavioural, psychosocial and health utilisation research for clinical translation as genetic results were disclosed and recontact is feasible.

From a practical perspective, conducting family studies can be challenging because of the often-complex nature of familial relationships, as well as the additional layers of protocol that need to be incorporated to protect privacy within families (e.g. procedures to ensure that sensitive information is not inadvertently passed to other family members). We have demonstrated that these issues, however, can be managed through carefully designed study protocols and training. We strongly believe the benefits of a family cohort far outweigh its limitations and that more epidemiologists should consider this design when conducting aetiologic research focused on environmental risk factors across the risk spectrum.

5.2 *Can I Use the Data? Where Can I Find Out More?*

From its inception, the CCFRC has functioned under the principle that it is a resource for research on the aetiology, risk and prognosis of colorectal cancer for all researchers, including those not affiliated with CCFRC. To this end, CCFRC welcomes collaborative applications to access and analyse both electronic data (questionnaire, genotypes, medical records, family history, etc.) and biospecimens (DNA, blood, serum, tumour specimens, etc.). Of total 294 approved applications to use CCFRC resources, 157 (53%) have come from external investigators and nearly every application submitted has been approved only except for those directly and completely overlapping with prior applications or those requesting something that CCFRC cannot provide. It is the CCFRC's mission to facilitate advancement of knowledge about all aspects of colorectal cancer, and this mission has driven all policy and prioritisation decisions.

CCFRC provides internal and external researchers fair and equitable access to this unique resource. Collaborating investigators have established numerous funded projects. For information on how to collaborate and access data for the CCFRC, including cohort data described here, please see http://coloncfr.org/.

Acknowledgements This work was supported by grant UM1 CA167551 from the National Cancer Institute and through cooperative agreements with the following CCFRC sites: Australasian Colorectal Cancer Family Registry (U01 CA074778 and U01/U24 CA097735), Mayo Clinic Cooperative Family Registry for Colon Cancer Studies (U01/U24 CA074800), Ontario Familial Colorectal Cancer Registry (U01/U24 CA074783), Seattle Colorectal Cancer Family Registry (U01/U24 CA074794), University of Hawaii Colorectal Cancer Family Registry (U01/U24 CA074806) and USC Consortium Colorectal Cancer Family Registry (U01/U24 CA074799). The targeted minority recruitment was supported by grant R01 CA104132. The genome-wide association studies (GWAS) were supported by grants U01 CA 122839, R01 CA143237 and U19 CA148107. The CIMP and *KRAS* mutation testing was supported by R01 CA118699.

Additional support for case ascertainment was provided from the Surveillance, Epidemiology, and End Results (SEER) Program of the National Cancer Institute to Fred Hutchinson Cancer Research Center (Control Nos. N01-CN-67009 and N01-PC-35142 and Contract No.

HHSN2612013000121), the Hawaii Department of Health (Control Nos. N01-PC-67001 and N01-PC-35137 and Contract No. HHSN26120100037C) and the California Department of Public Health (contracts HHSN261201000035C awarded to the University of Southern California and HHSN261201000140C awarded to the Cancer Prevention Institute of California), by the following US state cancer registries, AZ, CO, MN, NC, and NH, and by the Victorian Cancer Registry, Australia and the Ontario Cancer Registry, Canada. AKW is an Australian National Health and Medical Research Council (NHMRC) Early Career Fellow. MAJ is an NHMRC Senior Research Fellow.

References

1. Ferlay J, Soerjomataram I, Dikshit R, Eser S, Mathers C, Rebelo M, et al. Cancer incidence and mortality worldwide: sources, methods and major patterns in GLOBOCAN 2012. Int J Cancer. 2015;136(5):E359–86. https://doi.org/10.1002/ijc.29210.
2. Newcomb PA, Baron J, Cotterchio M, Gallinger S, Grove J, Haile R, et al. Colon Cancer Family Registry: an international resource for studies of the genetic epidemiology of colon cancer. Cancer Epidemiol Biomark Prev. 2007;16(11):2331–43. https://doi.org/10.1158/1055-9965.epi-07-0648.
3. Kolonel LN, Henderson BE, Hankin JH, Nomura AM, Wilkens LR, Pike MC, et al. A multiethnic cohort in Hawaii and Los Angeles: baseline characteristics. Am J Epidemiol. 2000;151(4):346–57.
4. Ireland P, Jolley D, Giles G, O'Dea K, Powles J, Rutishauser I, et al. Development of the Melbourne FFQ: a food frequency questionnaire for use in an Australian prospective study involving an ethnically diverse cohort. Asia Pac J Clin Nutr. 1994;3(1):19–31.
5. Lum A, Le Marchand L. A simple mouthwash method for obtaining genomic DNA in molecular epidemiological studies. Cancer Epidemiol Biomark Prev. 1998;7(8):719–24.
6. Miller G. Immortalization of human lymphocytes by Epstein-Barr virus. Yale J Biol Med. 1982;55(3–4):305–10.
7. Lindor NM, Burgart LJ, Leontovich O, Goldberg RM, Cunningham JM, Sargent DJ, et al. Immunohistochemistry versus microsatellite instability testing in phenotyping colorectal tumors. J Clin Oncol. 2002;20(4):1043–8. https://doi.org/10.1200/jco.20.4.1043.
8. Buchanan DD, Sweet K, Drini M, Jenkins MA, Win AK, English DR, et al. Risk factors for colorectal cancer in patients with multiple serrated polyps: a cross-sectional case series from genetics clinics. PLoS One. 2010;5(7):e11636. https://doi.org/10.1371/journal.pone.0011636
9. Buchanan DD, Win AK, Walsh MD, Walters RJ, Clendenning M, Nagler BN, et al. Family history of colorectal cancer in BRAF p.V600E mutated colorectal cancer cases. Cancer Epidemiol Biomark Prev. 2013;22(5):917–26. https://doi.org/10.1158/1055-9965.epi-12-1211.
10. Weisenberger DJ, Levine AJ, Long TI, Buchanan DD, Walters R, Clendenning M, et al. Association of the colorectal CpG island methylator phenotype with molecular features, risk factors, and family history. Cancer Epidemiol Biomark Prev. 2015;24(3):512–9. https://doi.org/10.1158/1055-9965.EPI-14-1161.
11. Levine AJ, Win AK, Buchanan DD, Jenkins MA, Baron JA, Young JP, et al. Cancer risks for the relatives of colorectal cancer cases with a methylated MLH1 promoter region: data from the Colorectal Cancer Family Registry. Cancer Prev Res. 2012;5(2):328–35. https://doi.org/10.1158/1940-6207.CAPR-11-0419.
12. Lindor NM, Rabe K, Petersen GM, Haile R, Casey G, Baron J, et al. Lower cancer incidence in Amsterdam-I criteria families without mismatch repair deficiency: familial colorectal cancer type X. JAMA. 2005;293(16):1979–85. https://doi.org/10.1001/jama.293.16.1979.
13. The 1000 Genomes Project Consortium. An integrated map of genetic variation from 1,092 human genomes. Nature. 2012;491(7422):56–65. https://doi.org/10.1038/nature11632.

14. Dowty JG, Win AK, Buchanan DD, Lindor NM, Macrae FA, Clendenning M, et al. Cancer risks for MLH1 and MSH2 mutation carriers. Hum Mutat. 2013;34(3):490–7. https://doi.org/10.1002/humu.22262.
15. Baglietto L, Lindor NM, Dowty JG, White DM, Wagner A, Gomez Garcia EB, et al. Risks of Lynch syndrome cancers for MSH6 mutation carriers. J Natl Cancer Inst. 2010;102(3):193–201. https://doi.org/10.1093/jnci/djp473.
16. Senter L, Clendenning M, Sotamaa K, Hampel H, Green J, Potter JD, et al. The clinical phenotype of Lynch syndrome due to germ-line PMS2 mutations. Gastroenterology. 2008;135(2):419–28. https://doi.org/10.1053/j.gastro.2008.04.026.
17. Win AK, Young JP, Lindor NM, Tucker KM, Ahnen DJ, Young GP, et al. Colorectal and other cancer risks for carriers and noncarriers from families with a DNA mismatch repair gene mutation: a prospective cohort study. J Clin Oncol. 2012;30(9):958–64. https://doi.org/10.1200/jco.2011.39.5590.
18. Guindalini RS, Win AK, Gulden C, Lindor NM, Newcomb PA, Haile RW, et al. Mutation spectrum and risk of colorectal cancer in African American families with Lynch syndrome. Gastroenterology. 2015;149(6):1446–53. https://doi.org/10.1053/j.gastro.2015.07.052.
19. Parry S, Win AK, Parry B, Macrae FA, Gurrin LC, Church JM, et al. Metachronous colorectal cancer risk for mismatch repair gene mutation carriers: the advantage of more extensive colon surgery. Gut. 2011;60(7):950–7. https://doi.org/10.1136/gut.2010.228056.
20. Win AK, Parry S, Parry B, Kalady MF, Macrae FA, Ahnen DJ, et al. Risk of metachronous colon cancer following surgery for rectal cancer in mismatch repair gene mutation carriers. Ann Surg Oncol. 2013;20(6):1829–36. https://doi.org/10.1245/s10434-012-2858-5.
21. Win AK, Lindor NM, Young JP, Macrae FA, Young GP, Williamson E, et al. Risks of primary extracolonic cancers following colorectal cancer in Lynch syndrome. J Natl Cancer Inst. 2012;104(18):1363–72. https://doi.org/10.1093/jnci/djs351.
22. Obermair A, Youlden DR, Young JP, Lindor NM, Baron JA, Newcomb P, et al. Risk of endometrial cancer for women diagnosed with HNPCC-related colorectal carcinoma. Int J Cancer. 2010;127(11):2678–84. https://doi.org/10.1002/ijc.25501.
23. Win AK, Lindor NM, Winship I, Tucker KM, Buchanan DD, Young JP, et al. Risks of colorectal and other cancers after endometrial cancer for women with Lynch syndrome. J Natl Cancer Inst. 2013;105(4):274–9. https://doi.org/10.1093/jnci/djs525.
24. Heath JA, Reece JC, Buchanan DD, Casey G, Durno CA, Gallinger S, et al. Childhood cancers in families with and without Lynch syndrome. Fam Cancer. 2015;14(4):545–51. https://doi.org/10.1007/s10689-015-9810-3.
25. Win AK, Dowty JG, Antill YC, English DR, Baron JA, Young JP, et al. Body mass index in early adulthood and endometrial cancer risk for mismatch repair gene mutation carriers. Obstet Gynecol. 2011;117(4):899–905. https://doi.org/10.1097/AOG.0b013e3182110ea3.
26. Win AK, Dowty JG, English DR, Campbell PT, Young JP, Winship I, et al. Body mass index in early adulthood and colorectal cancer risk for carriers and non-carriers of germline mutations in DNA mismatch repair genes. Br J Cancer. 2011;105(1):162–9. https://doi.org/10.1038/bjc.2011.172.
27. Pande M, Lynch PM, Hopper JL, Jenkins MA, Gallinger S, Haile RW, et al. Smoking and colorectal cancer in Lynch syndrome: results from the Colon Cancer Family Registry and the University of Texas M.D. Anderson Cancer Center. Clin Cancer Res. 2010;16(4):1331–9. https://doi.org/10.1158/1078-0432.ccr-09-1877.
28. Dashti SG, Buchanan DD, Jayasekara H, Ait Ouakrim D, Clendenning M, Rosty C, et al. Alcohol consumption and the risk of colorectal cancer for mismatch repair gene mutation carriers. Cancer Epidemiol Biomark Prev. 2017;26(3):366–75. https://doi.org/10.1158/1055-9965.epi-16-0496.
29. Ait Ouakrim D, Dashti SG, Chau R, Buchanan DD, Clendenning M, Rosty C, et al. Aspirin, ibuprofen, and the risk of colorectal cancer in Lynch syndrome. J Natl Cancer Inst. 2015;107(9). https://doi.org/10.1093/jnci/djv170.
30. Chau R, Dashti SG, Ait Ouakrim D, Buchanan DD, Clendenning M, Rosty C, et al. Multivitamin, calcium and folic acid supplements and the risk of colorectal cancer in Lynch syndrome. Int J Epidemiol. 2016;45(3):940–53. https://doi.org/10.1093/ije/dyw036.

31. Dashti SG, Chau R, Ouakrim DA, Buchanan DD, Clendenning M, Young JP, et al. Female hormonal factors and the risk of endometrial cancer in Lynch syndrome. JAMA. 2015;314(1):61–71. https://doi.org/10.1001/jama.2015.6789.
32. Win AK, Clendenning M, Crawford W, Rosty C, Preston SG, Southey MC, et al. Genetic variants within the hTERT gene and the risk of colorectal cancer in Lynch syndrome. Genes Cancer. 2015;6(11–12):445–51. https://doi.org/10.18632/genesandcancer.85.
33. Win AK, Reece JC, Buchanan DD, Clendenning M, Young JP, Cleary SP, et al. Risk of colorectal cancer for people with a mutation in both a MUTYH and a DNA mismatch repair gene. Fam Cancer. 2015;14(4):575–83. https://doi.org/10.1007/s10689-015-9824-x.
34. Win AK, Hopper JL, Buchanan DD, Young JP, Tenesa A, Dowty JG, et al. Are the common genetic variants associated with colorectal cancer risk for DNA mismatch repair gene mutation carriers? Eur J Cancer. 2013;49(7):1578–87. https://doi.org/10.1016/j.ejca.2013.01.029.
35. Stupart D, Win AK, Jenkins M, Winship IM, Goldberg P, Ramesar R. Fertility and apparent genetic anticipation in Lynch syndrome. Fam Cancer. 2014;13(3):369–74. https://doi.org/10.1007/s10689-014-9714-7.
36. Stupart D, Win AK, Winship IM, Jenkins M. Fertility after young-onset colorectal cancer: a study of subjects with Lynch syndrome. Colorectal Dis. 2015;17(9):787–93. https://doi.org/10.1111/codi.12940.
37. Shiovitz S, Copeland WK, Passarelli MN, Burnett-Hartman AN, Grady WM, Potter JD, et al. Characterisation of familial colorectal cancer Type X, Lynch syndrome, and non-familial colorectal cancer. Br J Cancer. 2014;111(3):598–602. https://doi.org/10.1038/bjc.2014.309.
38. Walsh MD, Cummings MC, Pearson SA, Clendenning M, Walters RJ, Nagler B, et al. Lynch syndrome-associated breast cancers do not overexpress chromosome 11-encoded mucins. Modern Pathol. 2013;26(7):944–54. https://doi.org/10.1038/modpathol.2012.232.
39. Antill YC, Dowty JG, Win AK, Thompson T, Walsh MD, Cummings MC, et al. Lynch syndrome and cervical cancer. Int J Cancer. 2015;137(11):2757–61. https://doi.org/10.1002/ijc.29641.
40. Rosty C, Walsh MD, Lindor NM, Thibodeau SN, Mundt E, Gallinger S, et al. High prevalence of mismatch repair deficiency in prostate cancers diagnosed in mismatch repair gene mutation carriers from the Colon Cancer Family Registry. Fam Cancer. 2014;13(4):573–82. https://doi.org/10.1007/s10689-014-9744-1.
41. Toon CW, Walsh MD, Chou A, Capper D, Clarkson A, Sioson L, et al. BRAFV600E immunohistochemistry facilitates universal screening of colorectal cancers for Lynch syndrome. Am J Surg Pathol. 2013;37(10):1592–602. https://doi.org/10.1097/PAS.0b013e31828f233d.
42. Newton K, Jorgensen NM, Wallace AJ, Buchanan DD, Lalloo F, RF MM, et al. Tumour MLH1 promoter region methylation testing is an effective prescreen for Lynch Syndrome (HNPCC). J Med Genet. 2014;51(12):789–96. https://doi.org/10.1136/jmedgenet-2014-102552.
43. Tomsic J, Senter L, Liyanarachchi S, Clendenning M, Vaughn CP, Jenkins MA, et al. Recurrent and founder mutations in the PMS2 gene. Clin Genet. 2013;83(3):238–43. https://doi.org/10.1111/j.1399-0004.2012.01898.x.
44. Win AK, Jenkins MA, Buchanan DD, Clendenning M, Young JP, Giles GG, et al. Determining the frequency of de novo germline mutations in DNA mismatch repair genes. J Med Genet. 2011;48(8):530–4. https://doi.org/10.1136/jmedgenet-2011-100082.
45. Thompson BA, Spurdle AB, Plazzer JP, Greenblatt MS, Akagi K, Al-Mulla F, et al. Application of a 5-tiered scheme for standardized classification of 2,360 unique mismatch repair gene variants in the InSiGHT locus-specific database. Nat Genet. 2014;46(2):107–15. https://doi.org/10.1038/ng.2854.
46. Thompson BA, Greenblatt MS, Vallee MP, Herkert JC, Tessereau C, Young EL, et al. Calibration of multiple in silico tools for predicting pathogenicity of mismatch repair gene missense substitutions. Hum Mutat. 2013;34(1):255–65. https://doi.org/10.1002/humu.22214.
47. Thompson BA, Goldgar DE, Paterson C, Clendenning M, Walters R, Arnold S, et al. A multifactorial likelihood model for MMR gene variant classification incorporating probabilities based on sequence bioinformatics and tumor characteristics: a report from the Colon Cancer Family Registry. Hum Mutat. 2013;34(1):200–9. https://doi.org/10.1002/humu.22213.

48. Win AK, Jenkins MA, Dowty JG, Antoniou AC, Lee A, Giles GG, et al. Prevalence and penetrance of major genes and polygenes for colorectal cancer. Cancer Epidemiol Biomarkers Prev. 2017;26(3):404–12. https://doi.org/10.1158/1055-9965.epi-16-0693.
49. Win AK, Dowty JG, Cleary SP, Kim H, Buchanan DD, Young JP, et al. Risk of colorectal cancer for carriers of mutations in MUTYH, with and without a family history of cancer. Gastroenterology. 2014;146(5):1208–11. e1-5. https://doi.org/10.1053/j.gastro.2014.01.022.
50. Jenkins MA, Croitoru ME, Monga N, Cleary SP, Cotterchio M, Hopper JL, et al. Risk of colorectal cancer in monoallelic and biallelic carriers of MYH mutations: a population-based case-family study. Cancer Epidemiol Biomark Prev. 2006;15(2):312–4. https://doi.org/10.1158/1055-9965.epi-05-0793.
51. Win AK, Reece JC, Dowty JG, Buchanan DD, Clendenning M, Rosty C, et al. Risk of extra-colonic cancers for people with biallelic and monoallelic mutations in MUTYH. Int J Cancer. 2016;139(7):1557–63. https://doi.org/10.1002/ijc.30197.
52. Win AK, Cleary SP, Dowty JG, Baron JA, Young JP, Buchanan DD, et al. Cancer risks for monoallelic MUTYH mutation carriers with a family history of colorectal cancer. Int J Cancer. 2011;129(9):2256–62. https://doi.org/10.1002/ijc.25870.
53. Phipps AI, Lindor NM, Jenkins MA, Baron JA, Win AK, Gallinger S, et al. Colon and rectal cancer survival by tumor location and microsatellite instability: the Colon Cancer Family Registry. Dis Colon Rectum. 2013;56(8):937–44. https://doi.org/10.1097/DCR.0b013e31828f9a57.
54. Lynch PM. Colorectal cancer survival by location and microsatellite status: data from the Colon Cancer Family Registries and their implications. Dis Colon Rectum. 2013;56(8):935–6. https://doi.org/10.1097/DCR.0b013e31828f9954.
55. Phipps AI, Buchanan DD, Makar KW, Burnett-Hartman AN, Coghill AE, Passarelli MN, et al. BRAF mutation status and survival after colorectal cancer diagnosis according to patient and tumor characteristics. Cancer Epidemiol Biomark Prev. 2012;21(10):1792–8. https://doi.org/10.1158/1055-9965.epi-12-0674.
56. Levine AJ, Phipps AI, Baron JA, Buchanan DD, Ahnen DJ, Cohen SA, et al. Clinicopathologic risk factor distributions for *MLH1* promoter region methylation in CIMP-positive tumors. Cancer Epidemiol Biomark Prev. 2016;25(1):68–75. https://doi.org/10.1158/1055-9965.epi-15-0935.
57. Phipps AI, Limburg PJ, Baron JA, Burnett-Hartman AN, Weisenberger DJ, Laird PW, et al. Association between molecular subtypes of colorectal cancer and patient survival. Gastroenterology. 2015;148(1):77–87. e2. https://doi.org/10.1053/j.gastro.2014.09.038.
58. Phipps AI, Buchanan DD, Makar KW, Win AK, Baron JA, Lindor NM, et al. KRAS-mutation status in relation to colorectal cancer survival: the joint impact of correlated tumour markers. Br J Cancer. 2013;108(8):1757–64. https://doi.org/10.1038/bjc.2013.118.
59. Phipps AI, Ahnen DJ, Cheng I, Newcomb PA, Win AK, Burnett T. PIK3CA somatic mutation status in relation to patient and tumor factors in racial/ethnic minorities with colorectal cancer. Cancer Epidemiol Biomark Prev. 2015;24(7):1046–51. https://doi.org/10.1158/1055-9965.epi-15-0204.
60. Loo LW, Tiirikainen M, Cheng I, Lum-Jones A, Seifried A, Church JM, et al. Integrated analysis of genome-wide copy number alterations and gene expression in microsatellite stable, CpG island methylator phenotype-negative colon cancer. Genes Chromosomes Cancer. 2013;52(5):450–66. https://doi.org/10.1002/gcc.22043.
61. Passarelli MN, Coghill AE, Hutter CM, Zheng Y, Makar KW, Potter JD, et al. Common colorectal cancer risk variants in SMAD7 are associated with survival among prediagnostic nonsteroidal anti-inflammatory drug users: a population-based study of postmenopausal women. Genes Chromosomes Cancer. 2011;50(11):875–86. https://doi.org/10.1002/gcc.20913.
62. Slattery ML, Curtin K, Poole EM, Duggan DJ, Samowitz WS, Peters U, et al. Genetic variation in C-reactive protein in relation to colon and rectal cancer risk and survival. Int J Cancer. 2011;128(11):2726–34. https://doi.org/10.1002/ijc.25721.

63. Coghill AE, Newcomb PA, Poole EM, Hutter CM, Makar KW, Duggan D, et al. Genetic variation in inflammatory pathways is related to colorectal cancer survival. Clin Cancer Res. 2011;17(22):7139–47. https://doi.org/10.1158/1078-0432.ccr-11-1134.
64. Passarelli MN, Newcomb PA, Makar KW, Burnett-Hartman AN, Phipps AI, David SP, et al. No association between germline variation in catechol-O-methyltransferase and colorectal cancer survival in postmenopausal women. Menopause. 2014;21(4):415–20. https://doi.org/10.1097/GME.0b013e31829e498d.
65. Passarelli MN, Phipps AI, Potter JD, Makar KW, Coghill AE, Wernli KJ, et al. Common single-nucleotide polymorphisms in the estrogen receptor beta promoter are associated with colorectal cancer survival in postmenopausal women. Cancer Res. 2013;73(2):767–75. https://doi.org/10.1158/0008-5472.can-12-2484.
66. Phipps AI, Ahnen DJ, Campbell PT, Win AK, Jenkins MA, Lindor NM, et al. Family history of colorectal cancer is not associated with colorectal cancer survival regardless of microsatellite instability status. Cancer Epidemiol Biomark Prev. 2014;23(8):1700–4. https://doi.org/10.1158/1055-9965.epi-14-0533.
67. Adams SV, Ahnen DJ, Baron JA, Campbell PT, Gallinger S, Grady WM, et al. Survival after inflammatory bowel disease-associated colorectal cancer in the Colon Cancer Family Registry. World J Gastroenterol. 2013;19(21):3241–8. https://doi.org/10.3748/wjg.v19.i21.3241.
68. Campbell PT, Newton CC, Newcomb PA, Phipps AI, Ahnen DJ, Baron JA, et al. Association between body mass index and mortality for colorectal cancer survivors: overall and by tumor molecular phenotype. Cancer Epidemiol Biomark Prev. 2015;24(8):1229–38. https://doi.org/10.1158/1055-9965.epi-15-0094.
69. Phipps AI, Baron J, Newcomb PA. Prediagnostic smoking history, alcohol consumption, and colorectal cancer survival: the Seattle Colon Cancer Family Registry. Cancer. 2011;117(21):4948–57. https://doi.org/10.1002/cncr.26114.
70. Phipps AI, Robinson JR, Campbell PT, Win AK, Figueiredo JC, Lindor NM, et al. Prediagnostic alcohol consumption and colorectal cancer survival: the Colon Cancer Family Registry. Cancer. 2016. https://doi.org/10.1002/cncr.30446.
71. Coghill AE, Newcomb PA, Campbell PT, Burnett-Hartman AN, Adams SV, Poole EM, et al. Prediagnostic non-steroidal anti-inflammatory drug use and survival after diagnosis of colorectal cancer. Gut. 2011;60(4):491–8. https://doi.org/10.1136/gut.2010.221143.
72. Coghill AE, Newcomb PA, Chia VM, Zheng Y, Wernli KJ, Passarelli MN, et al. Pre-diagnostic NSAID use but not hormone therapy is associated with improved colorectal cancer survival in women. Br J Cancer. 2011;104(5):763–8. https://doi.org/10.1038/sj.bjc.6606041.
73. Hardikar S, Newcomb PA, Campbell PT, Win AK, Lindor NM, Buchanan DD, et al. Prediagnostic physical activity and colorectal cancer survival: overall and stratified by tumor characteristics. Cancer Epidemiol Biomark Prev. 2015;24(7):1130–7. https://doi.org/10.1158/1055-9965.epi-15-0039.
74. Jayasekara H, Reece JC, Buchanan DD, Rosty C, Dashti SG, Ait Ouakrim D, et al. Risk factors for metachronous colorectal cancer following a primary colorectal cancer: a prospective cohort study. Int J Cancer. 2016;139(5):1081–90. https://doi.org/10.1002/ijc.30153.
75. Cleary SP, Cotterchio M, Shi E, Gallinger S, Harper P. Cigarette smoking, genetic variants in carcinogen-metabolizing enzymes, and colorectal cancer risk. Am J Epidemiol. 2010;172(9):1000–14. https://doi.org/10.1093/aje/kwq245.
76. Campbell PT, Jacobs ET, Ulrich CM, Figueiredo JC, Poynter JN, JR ML, et al. Case–control study of overweight, obesity, and colorectal cancer risk, overall and by tumor microsatellite instability status. J Natl Cancer Inst. 2010;102(6):391–400. https://doi.org/10.1093/jnci/djq011.
77. Wernli KJ, Wang Y, Zheng Y, Potter JD, Newcomb PA. The relationship between gravidity and parity and colorectal cancer risk. J Women's Health. 2009;18(7):995–1001. https://doi.org/10.1089/jwh.2008.1068.
78. Boardman LA, Morlan BW, Rabe KG, Petersen GM, Lindor NM, Nigon SK, et al. Colorectal cancer risks in relatives of young-onset cases: is risk the same across all first-degree relatives? Clin Gastroenterol Hepatol. 2007;5(10):1195–8. https://doi.org/10.1016/j.cgh.2007.06.001.

79. Lindor NM, Rabe KG, Petersen GM, Chen H, Bapat B, Hopper J, et al. Parent of origin effects on age at colorectal cancer diagnosis. Int J Cancer. 2010;127(2):361–6. https://doi.org/10.1002/ijc.25037.
80. Gong J, Hutter CM, Newcomb PA, Ulrich CM, Bien SA, Campbell PT, et al. Genome-wide interaction analyses between genetic variants and alcohol consumption and smoking for risk of colorectal cancer. PLoS Genet. 2016;12(10):e1006296. https://doi.org/10.1371/journal.pgen.1006296.
81. Makar KW, Poole EM, Resler AJ, Seufert B, Curtin K, Kleinstein SE, et al. COX-1 (PTGS1) and COX-2 (PTGS2) polymorphisms, NSAID interactions, and risk of colon and rectal cancers in two independent populations. Cancer Causes Control. 2013;24(12):2059–75. https://doi.org/10.1007/s10552-013-0282-1.
82. Nan H, Hutter CM, Lin Y, Jacobs EJ, Ulrich CM, White E, et al. Association of aspirin and NSAID use with risk of colorectal cancer according to genetic variants. JAMA. 2015;313(11):1133–42. https://doi.org/10.1001/jama.2015.1815.
83. Resler AJ, Makar KW, Heath L, Whitton J, Potter JD, Poole EM, et al. Genetic variation in prostaglandin synthesis and related pathways, NSAID use and colorectal cancer risk in the Colon Cancer Family Registry. Carcinogenesis. 2014;35(9):2121–6. https://doi.org/10.1093/carcin/bgu119.
84. Scherer D, Koepl LM, Poole EM, Balavarca Y, Xiao L, Baron JA, et al. Genetic variation in UGT genes modify the associations of NSAIDs with risk of colorectal cancer: Colon Cancer Family Registry. Genes Chromosomes Cancer. 2014;53(7):568–78. https://doi.org/10.1002/gcc.22167.
85. Seufert BL, Poole EM, Whitton J, Xiao L, Makar KW, Campbell PT, et al. IkappaBKbeta and NFkappaB1, NSAID use and risk of colorectal cancer in the Colon Cancer Family Registry. Carcinogenesis. 2013;34(1):79–85. https://doi.org/10.1093/carcin/bgs296.
86. Campbell PT, Newcomb P, Gallinger S, Cotterchio M, McLaughlin JR. Exogenous hormones and colorectal cancer risk in Canada: associations stratified by clinically defined familial risk of cancer. Cancer Causes Control. 2007;18(7):723–33. https://doi.org/10.1007/s10552-007-9015-7.
87. Campbell PT, Cotterchio M, Klar N, JR ML, Gallinger S. Colorectal cancer risk among postmenopausal hormone users in a population-based familial case-control study. Ann Epidemiol. 2003;13(8):562. https://doi.org/10.1016/S1047-2797(03)00144-3.
88. Garcia-Albeniz X, Rudolph A, Hutter C, White E, Lin Y, Rosse SA, et al. CYP24A1 variant modifies the association between use of oestrogen plus progestogen therapy and colorectal cancer risk. Br J Cancer. 2016;114(2):221–9. https://doi.org/10.1038/bjc.2015.443.
89. Figueiredo J, Levine A, Lee W, Conti D, Poynter J, Campbell P, et al. Genes involved with folate uptake and distribution and their association with colorectal cancer risk. Cancer Causes Control. 2010;21(4):597–608. https://doi.org/10.1007/s10552-009-9489-6.
90. Levine AJ, Figueiredo JC, Lee W, Poynter JN, Conti D, Duggan DJ, et al. Genetic variability in the MTHFR gene and Colorectal cancer risk using the Colorectal Cancer Family Registry. Cancer Epidemiol Biomark Prev. 2010;19(1):89–100. https://doi.org/10.1158/1055-9965.epi-09-0727.
91. Levine AJ, Figueiredo JC, Lee W, Conti DV, Kennedy K, Duggan DJ, et al. A candidate gene study of folate-associated one carbon metabolism genes and colorectal cancer risk. Cancer Epidemiol Biomark Prev. 2010;19(7):1812–21. https://doi.org/10.1158/1055-9965.EPI-10-0151.
92. Kim HS, Newcomb PA, Ulrich CM, Keener CL, Bigler J, Farin FM, et al. Vitamin D receptor polymorphism and the risk of colorectal adenomas. Cancer Epidemiol Biomark Prev. 2001;10(8):869–74.
93. Poynter JN, Jacobs ET, Figueiredo JC, Lee WH, Conti DV, Campbell PT, et al. Genetic variation in the vitamin D receptor (VDR) and the vitamin D-binding protein (GC) and risk for colorectal cancer: results from the Colon Cancer Family Registry. Cancer Epidemiol Biomark Prev. 2010;19(2):525–36. https://doi.org/10.1158/1055-9965.EPI-09-0662.

94. Sun Z, Wang PP, Roebothan B, Cotterchio M, Green R, Buehler S et al. Calcium and vitamin D and risk of colorectal cancer: results from a large population-based case-control study in Newfoundland and Labrador and Ontario. Can J Public Health. 2011;102(5):382-9.
95. Hiraki LT, Qu C, Hutter CM, Baron JA, Berndt SI, Bezieau S, et al. Genetic predictors of circulating 25-hydroxyvitamin d and risk of colorectal cancer. Cancer Epidemiol Biomark Prev. 2013;22(11):2037–46. https://doi.org/10.1158/1055-9965.epi-13-0209.
96. Du M, Zhang X, Hoffmeister M, Schoen RE, Baron JA, Berndt SI, et al. No evidence of gene-calcium interactions from genome-wide analysis of colorectal cancer risk. Cancer Epidemiol Biomark Prev. 2014;23(12):2971–6. https://doi.org/10.1158/1055-9965.epi-14-0893.
97. Joshi AD, Corral R, Siegmund KD, Haile RW, Le Marchand L, Martinez ME, et al. Red meat and poultry intake, polymorphisms in the nucleotide excision repair and mismatch repair pathways and colorectal cancer risk. Carcinogenesis. 2009;30(3):472–9. https://doi.org/10.1093/carcin/bgn260.
98. Cotterchio M, Boucher BA, Manno M, Gallinger S, Okey AB, Harper PA. Red meat intake, doneness, polymorphisms in genes that encode carcinogen-metabolizing enzymes, and colorectal cancer risk. Cancer Epidemiol Biomark Prev. 2008;17(11):3098–107. https://doi.org/10.1158/1055-9965.epi-08-0341.
99. Chia VM, Newcomb PA, Lampe JW, White E, Mandelson MT, McTiernan A, et al. Leptin concentrations, leptin receptor polymorphisms, and colorectal adenoma risk. Cancer Epidemiol Biomark Prev. 2007;16(12):2697–703. https://doi.org/10.1158/1055-9965.EPI-07-0467.
100. Cotterchio M, Boucher BA, Manno M, Gallinger S, Okey A, Harper P. Dietary phytoestrogen intake is associated with reduced colorectal cancer risk. J Nutr. 2006;136(12):3046–53.
101. Sun Z, Zhu Y, Wang PP, Roebothan B, Zhao J, Dicks E, et al. Reported intake of selected micronutrients and risk of colorectal cancer: results from a large population-based case-control study in Newfoundland, Labrador and Ontario, Canada. Anticancer Res. 2012;32(2):687–96.
102. Thrift AP, Gong J, Peters U, Chang-Claude J, Rudolph A, Slattery ML, et al. Mendelian randomization study of height and risk of colorectal cancer. Int J Epidemiol. 2015;44(2):662–72. https://doi.org/10.1093/ije/dyv082.
103. Thrift AP, Gong J, Peters U, Chang-Claude J, Rudolph A, Slattery ML, et al. Mendelian randomization study of body mass index and colorectal cancer risk. Cancer Epidemiol Biomark Prev. 2015;24(7):1024–31. https://doi.org/10.1158/1055-9965.epi-14-1309.
104. Jarvis D, Mitchell JS, Law PJ, Palin K, Tuupanen S, Gylfe A, et al. Mendelian randomisation analysis strongly implicates adiposity with risk of developing colorectal cancer. Br J Cancer. 2016;115(2):266–72. https://doi.org/10.1038/bjc.2016.188.
105. Houlston RS, Webb E, Broderick P, Pittman AM, Di Bernardo MC, Lubbe S, et al. Meta-analysis of genome-wide association data identifies four new susceptibility loci for colorectal cancer. Nat Genet. 2008;40(12):1426–35. https://doi.org/10.1038/ng.262.
106. Tenesa A, Farrington SM, Prendergast JG, Porteous ME, Walker M, Haq N, et al. Genome-wide association scan identifies a colorectal cancer susceptibility locus on 11q23 and replicates risk loci at 8q24 and 18q21. Nat Genet. 2008;40(5):631–7. https://doi.org/10.1038/ng.133.
107. Poynter JN, Figueiredo JC, Conti DV, Kennedy K, Gallinger S, Siegmund KD, et al. Variants on 9p24 and 8q24 are associated with risk of colorectal cancer: results from the Colon Cancer Family Registry. Cancer Res. 2007;67(23):11128–32. https://doi.org/10.1158/0008-5472.can-07-3239.
108. Schumacher FR, Schmit SL, Jiao S, Edlund CK, Wang H, Zhang B, et al. Genome-wide association study of colorectal cancer identifies six new susceptibility loci. Nat Commun. 2015;6:7138. https://doi.org/10.1038/ncomms8138.
109. Al-Tassan NA, Whiffin N, Hosking FJ, Palles C, Farrington SM, Dobbins SE, et al. A new GWAS and meta-analysis with 1000Genomes imputation identifies novel risk variants for colorectal cancer. Sci Rep. 2015;5:10442. https://doi.org/10.1038/srep10442.

110. Cheng I, Kocarnik JM, Dumitrescu L, Lindor NM, Chang-Claude J, Avery CL, et al. Pleiotropic effects of genetic risk variants for other cancers on colorectal cancer risk: PAGE, GECCO and CCFR consortia. Gut. 2014;63(5):800–7. https://doi.org/10.1136/gutjnl-2013-305189.
111. Cheng TH, Thompson D, Painter J, O'Mara T, Gorman M, Martin L, et al. Meta-analysis of genome-wide association studies identifies common susceptibility polymorphisms for colorectal and endometrial cancer near SH2B3 and TSHZ1. Sci Rep. 2015;5:17369. https://doi.org/10.1038/srep17369.
112. Lemire M, Qu C, Loo LW, Zaidi SH, Wang H, Berndt SI, et al. A genome-wide association study for colorectal cancer identifies a risk locus in 14q23.1. Hum Genet. 2015;134(11–12):1249–62. https://doi.org/10.1007/s00439-015-1598-6.
113. Whiffin N, Hosking FJ, Farrington SM, Palles C, Dobbins SE, Zgaga L, et al. Identification of susceptibility loci for colorectal cancer in a genome-wide meta-analysis. Hum Mol Genet. 2014;23(17):4729–37. https://doi.org/10.1093/hmg/ddu177.
114. Zeng C, Matsuda K, Jia WH, Chang J, Kweon SS, Xiang YB, et al. Identification of susceptibility loci and genes for colorectal cancer risk. Gastroenterology. 2016;150(7):1633–45. https://doi.org/10.1053/j.gastro.2016.02.076.
115. Jia WH, Zhang B, Matsuo K, Shin A, Xiang YB, Jee SH, et al. Genome-wide association analyses in east Asians identify new susceptibility loci for colorectal cancer. Nat Genet. 2013;45(2):191–6. https://doi.org/10.1038/ng.2505.
116. Wang H, Haiman CA, Burnett T, Fortini BK, Kolonel LN, Henderson BE, et al. Fine-mapping of genome-wide association study-identified risk loci for colorectal cancer in African Americans. Hum Mol Genet. 2013;22(24):5048–55. https://doi.org/10.1093/hmg/ddt337.
117. Wang H, Burnett T, Kono S, Haiman CA, Iwasaki M, Wilkens LR, et al. Trans-ethnic genome-wide association study of colorectal cancer identifies a new susceptibility locus in VTI1A. Nat Commun. 2014;5:4613. https://doi.org/10.1038/ncomms5613.
118. Dunlop MG, Tenesa A, Farrington SM, Ballereau S, Brewster DH, Koessler T, et al. Cumulative impact of common genetic variants and other risk factors on colorectal cancer risk in 42,103 individuals. Gut. 2013;62(6):871–81. https://doi.org/10.1136/gutjnl-2011-300537.
119. Roberts A, Nancarrow D, Clendenning M, Buchanan DD, Jenkins MA, Duggan D, et al. Linkage to chromosome 2q32.2-q33.3 in familial serrated neoplasia (Jass syndrome). Fam Cancer. 2011;10(2):245–54. https://doi.org/10.1007/s10689-010-9408-8.
120. Zogopoulos G, Jorgensen C, Bacani J, Montpetit A, Lepage P, Ferretti V, et al. Germline EPHB2 receptor variants in familial colorectal cancer. PLoS One. 2008;3(8):e2885. https://doi.org/10.1371/journal.pone.0002885.
121. Young J, Jass JR. The case for a genetic predisposition to serrated neoplasia in the colorectum: hypothesis and review of the literature. Cancer Epidemiol Biomark Prev. 2006;15(10):1778–84. https://doi.org/10.1158/1055-9965.epi-06-0164.
122. Young J, Jenkins M, Parry S, Young B, Nancarrow D, English D, et al. Serrated pathway colorectal cancer in the population: genetic consideration. Gut. 2007;56(10):1453–9. https://doi.org/10.1136/gut.2007.126870.
123. Yeoman A, Young J, Arnold J, Jass J, Parry S. Hyperplastic polyposis in the New Zealand population: a condition associated with increased colorectal cancer risk and European ancestry. N Z Med J. 2007;120(1266):U2827.
124. Jiang X, Castelao JE, Vandenberg D, Carracedo A, Redondo CM, Conti DV, et al. Genetic variations in *SMAD7* are associated with colorectal cancer risk in the Colon Cancer Family Registry. PLoS One. 2013;8(4):e60464. https://doi.org/10.1371/journal.pone.0060464.
125. Chang CM, Chia VM, Gunter MJ, Zanetti KA, Ryan BM, Goodman JE, et al. Innate immunity gene polymorphisms and the risk of colorectal neoplasia. Carcinogenesis. 2013;34(11):2512–20. https://doi.org/10.1093/carcin/bgt228.
126. Wang H, Taverna D, Stram DO, Fortini BK, Cheng I, Wilkens LR, et al. Genetic variation in the inflammation and innate immunity pathways and colorectal cancer risk. Cancer Epidemiol Biomark Prev. 2013;22(11):2094–101. https://doi.org/10.1158/1055-9965.epi-13-0694.

127. Abbenhardt C, Poole EM, Kulmacz RJ, Xiao L, Curtin K, Galbraith RL, et al. Phospholipase A2G1B polymorphisms and risk of colorectal neoplasia. Int J Mol Epidemiol Genet. 2013;4(3):140–9.
128. Akbari MR, Anderson LN, Buchanan DD, Clendenning M, Jenkins MA, Win AK, et al. Germline HOXB13 p.Gly84Glu mutation and risk of colorectal cancer. Cancer Epidemiol. 2013;37(4):424–7. https://doi.org/10.1016/j.canep.2013.03.003.
129. Yurgelun MB, Masciari S, Joshi VA, Mercado RC, Lindor NM, Gallinger S, et al. Germline *TP53* mutations in patients with early-onset colorectal cancer in the Colon Cancer Family Registry. JAMA Oncol. 2015;1(2):214–21. https://doi.org/10.1001/jamaoncol.2015.0197.
130. Bapat B, Lindor NM, Baron J, Siegmund K, Li L, Zheng Y, et al. The association of tumor microsatellite instability phenotype with family history of colorectal cancer. Cancer Epidemiol Biomark Prev. 2009;18(3):967–75. https://doi.org/10.1158/1055-9965.EPI-08-0878.
131. English DR, Young JP, Simpson JA, Jenkins MA, Southey MC, Walsh MD, et al. Ethnicity and risk for colorectal cancers showing somatic BRAF V600E mutation or CpG island methylator phenotype. Cancer Epidemiol Biomark Prev. 2008;17(7):1774–80. https://doi.org/10.1158/1055-9965.EPI-08-0091.
132. Weisenberger DJ, Siegmund KD, Campan M, Young J, Long TI, Faasse MA, et al. CpG island methylator phenotype underlies sporadic microsatellite instability and is tightly associated with BRAF mutation in colorectal cancer. Nat Genet. 2006;38(7):787–93. https://doi.org/10.1038/ng1834.
133. Kambara T, Simms LA, VLJ W, Spring KJ, CVA W, Walsh MD, et al. BRAF mutation is associated with DNA methylation in serrated polyps and cancers of the colorectum. Gut. 2004;53(8):1137–44. https://doi.org/10.1136/gut.2003.037671.
134. Hitchins M, Williams R, Cheong K, Halani N, Lin VAP, Packham D, et al. MLH1 Germline Epimutations as a factor in hereditary nonpolyposis colorectal cancer. Gastroenterology. 2005;129(5):1392–9. https://doi.org/10.1053/j.gastro.2005.09.003.
135. Coolbaugh-Murphy MI, Xu J, Ramagli LS, Brown BW, Siciliano MJ. Microsatellite instability (MSI) increases with age in normal somatic cells. Mech Ageing Dev. 2005;126(10):1051–9. https://doi.org/10.1016/j.mad.2005.06.005.
136. Kakar S, Burgart LJ, Thibodeau SN, Rabe KG, Petersen GM, Goldberg RM, et al. Frequency of loss of hMLH1 expression in colorectal carcinoma increases with advancing age. Cancer. 2003;97(6):1421–7. https://doi.org/10.1002/cncr.11206.
137. Savio AJ, Daftary D, Dicks E, Buchanan DD, Parfrey PS, Young JP, et al. Promoter methylation of ITF2, but not APC, is associated with microsatellite instability in two populations of colorectal cancer patients. BMC Cancer. 2016;16:113. https://doi.org/10.1186/s12885-016-2149-9.
138. Walters RJ, Williamson EJ, English DR, Young JP, Rosty C, Clendenning M, et al. Association between hypermethylation of DNA repetitive elements in white blood cell DNA and early-onset colorectal cancer. Epigenetics. 2013;8(7):748–55. https://doi.org/10.4161/epi.25178.
139. Win AK, Jenkins MA, Dowty JG, Antoniou AC, Lee A, Giles GG, et al. Prevalence and penetrance of major genes and polygenes for colorectal cancer. Cancer Epidemiol Biomarkers Prev. 2016. https://doi.org/10.1158/1055-9965.EPI-16-0693.
140. Kastrinos F, Ojha RP, Leenen C, Alvero C, Mercado RC, Balmana J, et al. Comparison of prediction models for Lynch syndrome among individuals with colorectal cancer. J Natl Cancer Inst. 2016;108(2). https://doi.org/10.1093/jnci/djv308.
141. Kastrinos F, Steyerberg EW, Balmana J, Mercado R, Gallinger S, Haile R, et al. Comparison of the clinical prediction model PREMM(1,2,6) and molecular testing for the systematic identification of Lynch syndrome in colorectal cancer. Gut. 2013;62(2):272–9. https://doi.org/10.1136/gutjnl-2011-301265.
142. Kastrinos F, Steyerberg EW, Mercado R, Balmana J, Holter S, Gallinger S, et al. The PREMM(1,2,6) model predicts risk of MLH1, MSH2, and MSH6 germline mutations based on cancer history. Gastroenterology. 2011;140(1):73–81. https://doi.org/10.1053/j.gastro.2010.08.021.

143. Casey G, Lindor NM, Papadopoulos N, Thibodeau SN, Moskow J, Steelman S, et al. Conversion analysis for mutation detection in MLH1 and MSH2 in patients with colorectal cancer. JAMA. 2005;293(7):799–809. https://doi.org/10.1001/jama.293.7.799.
144. Cleary SP, Kim H, Croitoru ME, Redston M, Knight JA, Gallinger S, et al. Missense polymorphisms in the adenomatous polyposis coli gene and colorectal cancer risk. Dis Colon Rectum. 2008;51(10):1467–73; discussion 1473-74. https://doi.org/10.1007/s10350-008-9356-7.
145. Hahnloser D, Petersen GM, Rabe K, Snow K, Lindor NM, Boardman L, et al. The APC E1317Q variant in adenomatous polyps and colorectal cancers. Cancer Epidemiol Biomark Prev. 2003;12(10):1023–8.
146. Jaskowski L, Young J, Jackson L, Arnold S, Barker MA, Walsh MD, et al. Stability of BAT26 in Lynch syndrome colorectal tumours. Eur J Hum Genet. 2007;15(2):139–41; author reply 41-2. https://doi.org/10.1038/sj.ejhg.5201740.
147. Jenkins MA, Hayashi S, O'Shea AM, Burgart LJ, Smyrk TC, Shimizu D, et al. Pathology features in Bethesda guidelines predict colorectal cancer microsatellite instability: a population-based study. Gastroenterology. 2007;133(1):48–56. https://doi.org/10.1053/j.gastro.2007.04.044.
148. Zogopoulos G, Ha KC, Naqib F, Moore S, Kim H, Montpetit A, et al. Germ-line DNA copy number variation frequencies in a large North American population. Hum Genet. 2007;122(3–4):345–53. https://doi.org/10.1007/s00439-007-0404-5.
149. Clendenning M, Macrae FA, Walsh MD, Walters RJ, Thibodeau SN, Gunawardena SR, et al. Absence of *PMS2* mutations in Colon-CFR participants whose colorectal cancers demonstrate unexplained loss of MLH1 expression. Clin Genet. 2013;83(6):591–3. https://doi.org/10.1111/cge.12011.
150. Clendenning M, Walsh MD, Gelpi JB, Thibodeau SN, Lindor N, Potter JD, et al. Detection of large scale 3′ deletions in the PMS2 gene amongst Colon-CFR participants: have we been missing anything? Fam Cancer. 2013;12(3):563–6. https://doi.org/10.1007/s10689-012-9597-4.
151. Cunningham JM, Johnson RA, Litzelman K, Skinner HG, Seo S, Engelman CD, et al. Telomere length varies by DNA extraction method: implications for epidemiologic research. Cancer Epidemiol Biomark Prev. 2013;22(11):2047–54. https://doi.org/10.1158/1055-9965.epi-13-0409.
152. Boardman LA, Litzelman K, Seo S, Johnson RA, Vanderboom RJ, Kimmel GW, et al. The association of telomere length with colorectal cancer differs by the age of cancer onset. Clinical and Translat Gastroenterol. 2014;5:e52. https://doi.org/10.1038/ctg.2014.3.
153. Kuroiwa-Trzmielina J, Wang F, Rapkins RW, Ward RL, Buchanan DD, Win AK, et al. SNP rs16906252C>T is an expression and methylation quantitative trait locus associated with an increased risk of developing MGMT-methylated colorectal cancer. Clin Cancer Res. 2016;22(24):6266–77. https://doi.org/10.1158/1078-0432.ccr-15-2765.
154. Uddin M, Thiruvahindrapuram B, Walker S, Wang Z, Hu P, Lamoureux S, et al. A high-resolution copy-number variation resource for clinical and population genetics. Genet Med. 2015;17(9):747–52. https://doi.org/10.1038/gim.2014.178.
155. Win AK, Buchanan DD, Rosty C, RJ MI, Dowty JG, Dite GS, et al. Role of tumour molecular and pathology features to estimate colorectal cancer risk for first-degree relatives. Gut. 2015;64(1):101–10. https://doi.org/10.1136/gutjnl-2013-306567.
156. Kim JS, Coyte PC, Cotterchio M, Keogh LA, Flander LB, Gaff C, et al. The impact of receiving predictive genetic information about Lynch syndrome on individual colonoscopy and smoking behaviors. Cancer Epidemiol Biomark Prev. 2016;25(11):1524–33. https://doi.org/10.1158/1055-9965.epi-16-0346.
157. Esplen MJ, Wong J, Aronson M, Butler K, Rothenmund H, Semotiuk K, et al. Long-term psychosocial and behavioral adjustment in individuals receiving genetic test results in Lynch syndrome. Clin Genet. 2015;87(6):525–32. https://doi.org/10.1111/cge.12509.
158. Graves KD, Sinicrope PS, Esplen MJ, Peterson SK, Patten CA, Lowery J, et al. Communication of genetic test results to family and health-care providers following disclosure of research results. Genet Med. 2014;16(4):294–301. https://doi.org/10.1038/gim.2013.137.
159. Patel SG, Ahnen DJ, Kinney AY, Horick N, Finkelstein DM, Hill DA, et al. Knowledge and uptake of genetic counseling and colonoscopic screening among individuals at increased risk

for Lynch syndrome and their endoscopists from the Family Health Promotion Project. Am J Gastroenterol. 2016;111(2):285–93. https://doi.org/10.1038/ajg.2015.397.
160. Flander L, Speirs-Bridge A, Rutstein A, Niven H, Win AK, Ait Ouakrim D, et al. Perceived versus predicted risks of colorectal cancer and self-reported colonoscopies by members of mismatch repair gene mutation-carrying families who have declined genetic testing. J Genet Couns. 2014;23(1):79–88. https://doi.org/10.1007/s10897-013-9614-2.
161. Steel EJ, Trainer AH, Heriot AG, Lynch C, Parry S, Win AK, et al. The experience of extended bowel resection in individuals with a high metachronous colorectal cancer risk: a qualitative study. Oncol Nurs Forum. 2016;43(4):444–52. https://doi.org/10.1188/16.onf.444-452.
162. Adams SV, Ceballos R, Newcomb PA. Quality of life and mortality of long-term colorectal cancer survivors in the Seattle Colorectal Cancer Family Registry. PLoS One. 2016;11(6):e0156534. https://doi.org/10.1371/journal.pone.0156534.
163. Howell LA, Brockman TA, Sinicrope PS, Patten CA, Decker PA, Ehlers SL, et al. Receptivity and preferences in cancer risk reduction lifestyle programs: a survey of colorectal cancer family members. J Behav Health. 2013;2(4):279–90. https://doi.org/10.5455/jbh.20130921013627.
164. Lowery JT, Horick N, Kinney AY, Finkelstein DM, Garrett K, Haile RW, et al. A randomized trial to increase colonoscopy screening in members of high-risk families in the Colorectal Cancer Family Registry and Cancer Genetics Network. Cancer Epidemiol Biomark Prev. 2014;23(4):601–10. https://doi.org/10.1158/1055-9965.epi-13-1085.
165. Bharati R, Jenkins MA, Lindor NM, Le Marchand L, Gallinger S, Haile RW, et al. Does risk of endometrial cancer for women without a germline mutation in a DNA mismatch repair gene depend on family history of endometrial cancer or colorectal cancer? Gynecol Oncol. 2014;133(2):287–92. https://doi.org/10.1016/j.ygyno.2014.03.011.
166. Ahsan H, Halpern J, Kibriya MG, Pierce BL, Tong L, Gamazon E, et al. A genome-wide association study of early-onset breast cancer identifies PFKM as a novel breast cancer gene and supports a common genetic spectrum for breast cancer at any age. Cancer Epidemiol Biomark Prev. 2014;23(4):658–69. https://doi.org/10.1158/1055-9965.epi-13-0340.
167. Anderson LN, Cotterchio M, Knight JA, Borgida A, Gallinger S, Cleary SP. Genetic variants in vitamin D pathway genes and risk of pancreas cancer; results from a population-based case-control study in Ontario, Canada. PLoS One. 2013;8(6):e66768. https://doi.org/10.1371/journal.pone.0066768.
168. Bosetti C, Lucenteforte E, Bracci PM, Negri E, Neale RE, Risch HA, et al. Ulcer, gastric surgery and pancreatic cancer risk: an analysis from the international pancreatic cancer case-control consortium (PanC4). Ann Oncol. 2013;24(11):2903–10. https://doi.org/10.1093/annonc/mdt336.
169. Jang JH, Cotterchio M, Borgida A, Liu G, Gallinger S, Cleary SP. Interaction of polymorphisms in mitotic regulator genes with cigarette smoking and pancreatic cancer risk. Mol Carcinog. 2013;52(Suppl 1):E103–9. https://doi.org/10.1002/mc.22037.
170. Olson SH, Hsu M, Satagopan JM, Maisonneuve P, Silverman DT, Lucenteforte E, et al. Allergies and risk of pancreatic cancer: a pooled analysis from the pancreatic cancer case-control consortium. Am J Epidemiol. 2013;178(5):691–700. https://doi.org/10.1093/aje/kwt052.
171. Bosetti C, Rosato V, Li D, Silverman D, Petersen GM, Bracci PM, et al. Diabetes, antidiabetic medications, and pancreatic cancer risk: an analysis from the international pancreatic cancer case-control consortium. Ann Oncol. 2014;25(10):2065–72. https://doi.org/10.1093/annonc/mdu276.
172. Vasen HF, Mecklin JP, Khan PM, Lynch HT. The International Collaborative Group on Hereditary Non-Polyposis Colorectal Cancer (ICG-HNPCC). Dis Colon Rectum. 1991;34(5):424–5.
173. Vasen HF, Watson P, Mecklin JP, Lynch HT. New clinical criteria for hereditary nonpolyposis colorectal cancer (HNPCC, Lynch syndrome) proposed by the International Collaborative Group on HNPCC. Gastroenterology. 1999;116(6):1453–6.

174. Jarvinen HJ, Aarnio M, Mustonen H, Aktan-Collan K, Aaltonen LA, Peltomaki P et al. Controlled 15-year trial on screening for colorectal cancer in families with hereditary nonpolyposis colorectal cancer. Gastroenterology 2000;118(5):829–834.
175. Burn J, Gerdes AM, Macrae F, Mecklin JP, Moeslein G, Olschwang S, et al. Long-term effect of aspirin on cancer risk in carriers of hereditary colorectal cancer: an analysis from the CAPP2 randomised controlled trial. Lancet. 2011;378(9809):2081–7. https://doi.org/10.1016/S0140-6736(11)61049-0.
176. Hopper JL. Disease-specific prospective family study cohorts enriched for familial risk. Epidemiol Perspect Innov. 2011;8(1):2. https://doi.org/10.1186/1742-5573-8-2.
177. Cicek MS, Cunningham JM, Fridley BL, Serie DJ, Bamlet WR, Diergaarde B et al. Colorectal cancer linkage on chromosomes 4q21, 8q13, 12q24, and 15q22. PLoS One. 2012;7(5):e38175. https://doi.org/10.1371/journal.pone.0038175.
178. Neklason DW, Kerber RA, Nilson DB, Anton-Culver H, Schwartz AG, Griffin CA et al. Common familial colorectal cancer linked to chromosome 7q31: a genome-wide analysis. Cancer Res. 2008;68(21):8993–7. https://doi.org/10.1158/0008-5472.can-08-1376.
179. Gray-McGuire C, Guda K, Adrianto I, Lin CP, Natale L, Potter JD et al. Confirmation of linkage to and localization of familial colon cancer risk haplotype on chromosome 9q22. Cancer Res. 2010;70(13):5409–18. https://doi.org/10.1158/0008-5472.can-10-0188.
180. DeRycke MS, Gunawardena SR, Middha S, Asmann YW, Schaid DJ, McDonnell SK et al. Identification of novel variants in colorectal cancer families by high-throughput exome sequencing. Cancer Epidemiol Biomarkers Prev. 2013;22(7):1239-51. https://doi.org/10.1158/1055-9965.epi-12-1226.

Chapter 28
The Prospective Lynch Syndrome Database

Pål Møller, Sigve Nakken, and Eivind Hovig

Abstract The aim of the Prospective Lynch Syndrome Database (PLSD) is to store prospectively obtained information on Lynch syndrome (LS) patients to provide knowledge on the natural course of the disease and effects of interventions. Information is currently entered in spreadsheet format and manipulated in Oracle© but may in principle be entered in any suitable format and analysed by any suitable methods. The PLSD outputs annual incidences of cancer in 5-year cohorts in categories. These incidence data are exported as the underlying data for the website www.lscarisk.org, where the user interactively may calculate the lifetime risk for which cancer for any Lynch syndrome patient when indicating the patient's age, gender and genetic variant. The PLSD may be expanded to include any prospective information on a Lynch syndrome patient. Further functionality may be added for data to be manipulated and output tailored for additional purposes/research projects. The original data stored, or results obtained through manipulating these data inside the PLSD, may be exported for further studies.

P. Møller (✉)
Research Group on Inherited Cancer, Department of Medical Genetics, The Norwegian Radium Hospital, Oslo University Hospital, Oslo, Norway

Department of Tumor Biology, Institute of Cancer Research, The Norwegian Radium Hospital, Part of Oslo University Hospital, Oslo, Norway

Surgical Center for Hereditary Tumors, HELIOS University Clinic Wuppertal, University Witten-Herdecke, Wuppertal, Germany

S. Nakken
Department of Tumor Biology, Institute of Cancer Research, The Norwegian Radium Hospital, Part of Oslo University Hospital, Oslo, Norway

E. Hovig
Institute of Cancer Genetics and Informatics, The Norwegian Radium Hospital, Part of Oslo University Hospital, Oslo, Norway

Department of Informatics, University of Oslo, Oslo, Norway

Department of Tumor Biology, Institute of Cancer Research, The Norwegian Radium Hospital, Part of Oslo University Hospital, Oslo, Norway

L. Valle et al. (eds.), *Hereditary Colorectal Cancer*,
https://doi.org/10.1007/978-3-319-74259-5_28

Keywords Prospective · Lynch syndrome · PLSD · *MMR* · *MLH1* · *MSH2* · *MSH6* · *PMS2* · Penetrance · Cancer · Incidence rate · Cumulative risk · Survival · European Hereditary Tumour Group · InSiGHT

1 Intention

The PLSD was established with the intention to describe incidence rates of tumours in carriers of pathogenic variants of the *MMR* genes causing Lynch syndrome, survival when cancer and effects of interventions [1, 2, 3, 4].

2 Development

The decision to make the PLSD was taken by the Mallorca group (current name European Hereditary Tumour Group) (www.mallorca-group.org) in 2012 and later endorsed by InSiGHT (www.insigth-group.org). Contributions from genetic centres in Finland, Denmark, the UK, Norway, Spain, Germany, Holland, Italy, Sweden and Australia were compiled in 2015. Version1 of the PLSD underlying the first reports included 24,475 prospective observation years for 3119 Lynch syndrome patients. A substantial increase of numbers contributed and update of first series contributed are in process. As of January 2018 the PLSD includes 51,646 prospective observation years in 6,350 carriers of pathogenic *MMR* gene variants.

3 Governance

At present the PLSD according to the collaborative guidelines agreed by all contributors is a research project owned by the contributors. All centres having suitable series are welcomed to join (see https://ehtg.org/; PI: moller.pal@gmail.com).

4 Data Structure

The PLSD is currently designed as an Oracle© relational database (see separate chapter describing relational databases). Pathogenic genetic variant, gender, age at inclusion for prospective observation, age at last observation and age of death if dead are fields included in the parent table. In separate tables, information on each single cancer diagnosed at which age, age at prophylactic surgical removal of organs and information on precancers (details are given in Table 28.1).

Table 28.1 Information filed in the PLSD at present. Patient ID is the relational key. All patients included must have one row in Table A, and all variables in Table A must be populated. Age at last update must be higher than age at inclusion. If no relevant information, there may be no row for an included patient in any of the other tables. If relevant information, one patient will have one row only in Table C. Tables B, C2 and D may have more than one row for one patient: one row for each event (cancer, polyp or organectomy, respectively)

Table	Variables	Comments
Table A	Patient ID, contributor, year birth, sex, gene, pathogenic variant HGVS description, age inclusion, age last update, age death	Parent table. One row per patient. All variables must be populated
Table B	Patient ID, ICD cancer diagnoses, age at cancer, stage at diagnosis, surgical treatment if CRC	One row per cancer for each patient. NB: all cancers also including cancers prior to inclusion must be noted
Table C	Patient ID, number of polyps in the colon/rectum categorized by histopathology	One row per patient having had polyps. Censored at first CRC/last update – whatever comes first
Table C2	Patient ID, histopathological description of polyps in the colon/rectum at last colonoscopy before CRC and time between last colonoscopy and CRC	One row per polyp for each patient
Table D	Patient ID, organs completely removed, age at removal	One row for each organ removed for each patient

One information element is entered once only, and reuse of information in data manipulations for different purposes is obtained through the stored queries by copying the information from its storage place whenever needed, but not stored anywhere else. In this way, conflicting information is avoided, and updating made easy: when one piece of information is stored one place only, all outputs from the PLSD using that information are updated when that single piece of information is updated.

Information stored is whenever possible assumption free, and all events scored are accompanied by age at event (e.g. cancer diagnosed and age at diagnosis). If data entered are based on assumptions, the assumptions will be reflected in the results when analysing the data entered. Results are always to be interpreted based on the assumptions included in the data entered. An example may be that for clinical trials, one assumption to consider when interpreting the results will be the inclusion criteria to the study: all patients reported to the PLSD have been subjected to follow-up with colonoscopy, and incidences of colorectal cancer are to be interpreted accordingly. The two inclusion criteria used by the PLSD (age at first prospectively planned and carried out colonoscopy and a demonstrated pathogenic *MMR* variant) are robust. This is not in conflict with later examining for strata in the included patients with respect to how they came to meet the inclusion criteria. An example of such is the first report considering LS patients without previous and/or prevalent cancer at inclusion [1], compared to the second report considering LS patients with previous and/or prevalent cancer at inclusion [2].

5 Inclusion Criteria and Follow-Up

All included patients are selected and included the same way: age at first prospectively planned and carried out colonoscopy due to assumed increased risk for inherited colorectal cancer. By which method the assumed increased risk for colorectal cancer was established is irrelevant. In addition, all patients included are by the contributor demonstrated to carry a pathogenic *MMR* variant. From January 2018 onwards only carriers of pathogenic MMR gene variants verified in the LOVD database (http://chromium.lovd.nl/LOVD2/colon_cancer/home.php) are included in the PLSD. When and why genetic testing demonstrated the pathogenic *MMR* variant, is irrelevant, but all patients included are by the contributor declared to carry a pathogenic *MMR* variant. Because there is no centre observing LS patients without offering follow-up aiming at prevention or early diagnosis and treatment of cancer and because all patients are followed-up in the healthcare system, the information stored is an open prospective trial without control group. In principle, therefore, colorectal cancer incidence monitored is the combined function of both natural course of disease and the preventive effect of colonoscopic follow-up to prevent colorectal cancer. Early diagnosis and treatment of extra-colonic or extra-rectal cancers are not currently considered preventive, while general cancer awareness may impact on survival when any cancer.

The germline genetic variants causing LS are inherited. When the pathogenic germline variant was demonstrated, is irrelevant, it may be before inclusion, at inclusion or after inclusion. The early prospective observations in LS families were undertaken before genetic testing was available, and such patients may be included based on genetic testing done years after follow-up was instituted. In this way, we may use the already existing observations filed through decades in those centres having provided follow-up for LS families prior to genetic testing becoming available.

Those having had cancer at an earlier age than inclusion will be scored as previously having had cancer. Those having any cancer at the same age as when included will be scored as having prevalent cancer. Cancer diagnosed in those having no cancer before or at inclusion will be scored as prospectively diagnosed (incident) cancer in patients healthy (with respect to cancer) at inclusion.

6 Power Calculations

Stratifying the material on four genes, two genders, and nine 5-year age cohorts from 25 to 70 years, there will be 72 groups. Assuming an average annual incidence rate (penetrance) about 2% and an average of 300 follow-up years in each group, one would have on average 6 cancer cases in each group, for which one would need 21,600 follow-up years if the number in each cohort was to be evenly distributed on the 72 groups. It was decided that a minimum of an expected average of six events (cancers) in each categorized group was reasonable before starting analysing the database. As mentioned above, we froze version1 of the database when 24,475 observation years were filed and produced the first reports. At present, new contributors have joined, and we are about to double the number of observation years included, and we are aiming of establishing a new version2 of the database to validate the first reports in a new independent series. If the findings in the first reports are to be confirmed, we may combine all entries into one larger series for additional reports. Also, we may add more observations to the patients already filed to make more detailed reports, including the added information. This process may continue as long as one may wish. The larger number of LS patients and observation years included, the more categorized groups may become sufficiently large to have the power to reach statistically significant results if examined. From January 2018 the PLSD includes follow-up years sufficient to calculate incidences of cancer in any separate organ by age and gene in each gender separately in forthcoming reports.

7 Analytical Methods and Outputs

The main analytical system initially implemented provides output similar to standard output from cancer registries and may use such as control groups for population incidences to estimate relative risk for cancers in LS patients.

The strategy used escapes most of the biases in retrospective studies, like selection biases, survivor bias, time-trends, etc.

The output migrates knowledge on LS from retrospective studies (class C and D) to empirical data prospectively observed (class B). There still are ascertainment problems, however, because inclusion is not from birth. No ascertainment strategy is bias-free. We do have what is commonly denoted as survivor bias when including adult patients (not at birth). Also, inclusion may be considered similar to a cross-sectional study, but in principle, it is not, because the patients were included at different years, which includes a possible time trend bias. A prospective study is, however, in general better than retrospective studies.

An ideal study design is unsuitable, unreachable and unethical. It is unsuitable because inclusion from birth would need 70 years follow-up to estimate cumulative incidences of cancers at 70 years, and we would like to see the best possible estimates sooner. It is unreachable because patients would not like to be randomized to non-intervention and/or not to be treated when experiencing cancer, and the control group will seek appropriate health care elsewhere and violate the study design. Also, we are monitoring health care provided over many years in different countries to get sufficiently high numbers for statistical significance, and we do not have the power to instruct the various health services to be uniform between countries and not to change over time. It will be unethical not to provide adequate health service to the high-risk groups for preventable and curable cancers – none of us will seek allowance to do such a trial, and, if we did, it may not be approved. In sum, an open observational trial aiming at class B evidence is possibly the best we may do. This is not in conflict with the aim of providing a platform for randomized trials to explore improved preventive and treatment modalities according to general ethical and oncological standards.

The PLSD was designed to describe varying annual incidences by age, by gender and by genetic variants. The first report validated the annual incidence to vary and to be correlated to these parameters. The often used Kaplan-Meier survival function is invalid for describing the annual incidence rate (penetrance of the genetic variants), because the Kaplan-Meier function does not include age as a parameter. In retrospective (family) studies, incidences of cancers are usually considered from birth onwards, and the Kaplan-Meier function left censoring study time at birth may be appropriate. PLSD does not include and observe patients from birth onwards, and Kaplan-Meir estimates based on observations from birth onwards will be invalid. Because incidence of cancer in LS syndrome is age dependent, applying the Kaplan-Meier algorithm with left censoring patients included at different ages will be invalid as well. The LS syndrome may no longer be described as one homogenous group without categorizing on gene, age and gender. The method needed to describe this heterogeneity led us to implement the methods currently used in the PLSD, which requires the large number of observation years as discussed. Using the first results published as a platform to address additional questions may make it suitable to include different methods to describe other ends.

The lower number of *path_MSH6* and especially *path_PMS2* carriers included in version1 of the PLSD most probably reflected an ascertainment bias: Because of their lower penetrance, such families did not meet the clinical selection criteria to be genetically tested. This may as well, however, be considered results: The lower number included because lack of adherence to clinical criteria to be genetically tested was predicted and might be considered validation of our previous observations [5]. A larger number of observation years are needed to more precisely describe incidence rates of cancers in *path_MSH6* and *path_PMS2* carriers. If there are differences in penetrance between different pathogenic variants in the same gene, which may be likely, one would need an even larger data set to arrive at numbers needed in the different categories – see discussion on power calculations above.

7.1 Technical Details

In the current format, the primary object in the PLSD is the individual patient (see https://en.wikipedia.org/wiki/Relational_database#Keys for description of primary key in a relational database). The patient is identified by an alias (a code) given by the contributor. No one besides the contributor has the key to determine which patient the alias identifies. This makes the PLSD a de-identified (pseudonymized) database but with the capability of updating and adding more data derived from the same patient later through the original contributor. All entries will have a unique internal identifier in the PLSD when the (telephone) country code and institution code within country (decided by database administrator) are added as prefix to the alias given by contributor. The legal permissions to hold the named data and export the de-identified data are kept by the contributors.

The current structure of the PLSD respects the basic requirements for a relational database as discussed separately. The information is currently stored in an Oracle© database and manipulated by approximately 300 stored queries (views) programmed in TOAD©. The views compile the data to outputs to be exported to statistical software including SYSTAT10© and Excel©. Input and output data may be formatted at wish by use of structured query language (SQL) and functions available in TOAD©. Annual incidence rates in 5-year cohorts are exported to a free-standing visualization tool which may be interactively manipulated on the web (www.lscarisk.org) to calculate any patient's lifetime risk for cancer based on pathogenic variant, age and gender. The interactive analyses offered at www.lscarisk.org are powered by Shiny©, which is a web application framework for the R© language. Utilizing the computational power of R©, Shiny© facilitates rapid integration of core PLSD output data (e.g. cancer incidence rates across age, gender and genotype) with the interactivity of the modern web.

The PLSD is designed to include the capability of adding new tables with additional information. For practical purposes Oracle© has no limit neither with respect to future complexity of the database structure and queries nor with respect to numbers to be included. In principle, data stored in the PLSD may be manipulated by any suitable tool to output wanted for any specific task and/or to be further analysed by other tools. Current limitations include lack of some relevant information to address more complicated research problems and the limited number of patients and observation years included.

The current Oracle© structure inside PLSD may be expanded similar to CGEN (https://www.ncbi.nlm.nih.gov/pubmed/21387464), which has the capacity of a comprehensive medical filing system for a genetic clinic, both with respect to database structure, capabilities and interactive user interface. CGEN has an object-oriented graphical user interface programmed in Pascal/Delphi (Embarcadero©), which in principle modify SQL queries to the Oracle© database with the result that nothing but the SQL query and the return set are transmitted between client and server, and nothing but the return set is stored at the client and only temporarily so. In this way the PLSD is designed to be expanded or to be part of more complex systems to be run interactively if desired. Or the data formatted in spreadsheets or similar may be made available through the web to any user as to be analysed independently by different means, given the permission to do so. The other way around, any medical filing system with capabilities similar to CGEN may be programmed to provide output to contribute to the PLSD.

7.2 *Conclusions*

The methods necessary to describe the results of interests need large numbers of included follow-up years. No centre has sufficient follow-up years to undertake such studies alone, for which reason a broad international collaboration is necessary. The European Hereditary Tumour Group and possibly additional continental bodies, together with the intercontinental body InSiGHT, are the obvious frameworks at hand to organize the activities. The best strategy is to build a core structure with the capacity to be expanded later to whatever additional task one may want to undertake and to invite all with suitable series to participate. In this way we may arrive at the first results within reasonable time and without having to invest too many resources before seeing the first results. A stepwise approach, where not all steps are defined at the outset, but where the later steps are decided upon observing the first results, is scientifically sound. Also, this will ensure the best possible allocation of available resource at any given time.

References

1. Møller P, Seppälä T, Bernstein I, Holinski-Feder E, Sala P, Evans DG, et al. Cancer incidence and survival in Lynch syndrome patients receiving colonoscopic and gynaecological surveillance: first report from the prospective Lynch syndrome database. Gut. 2017;66(3):464–472.
2. Møller P, Seppälä T, Bernstein I, Holinski-Feder E, Sala P, Evans DG, et al. Incidence of and survival after subsequent cancers in carriers of pathogenic MMR variants with previous cancer: a report from the prospective Lynch syndrome database. Gut. 2017;66(9):1657–1664.
3. Møller P, Seppälä TT, Bernstein I, Holinski-Feder E, Sala P, Gareth Evans D, et al. Cancer risk and survival in path_MMR carriers by gene and gender up to 75 years of age: a report from the Prospective Lynch Syndrome Database. Gut. 2017 Jul 28. https://doi.org/10.1136/gutjnl-2017-314057
4. Seppälä T, Pylvänäinen K, Evans DG, Järvinen H, Renkonen-Sinisalo L, Bernstein I, et al. Colorectal cancer incidence in path_MLH1 carriers subjected to different follow-up protocols: a Prospective Lynch Syndrome Database report. Hered Cancer Clin Pract. 2017; 10;15:18.
5. Sjursen W, Haukanes BI, Grindedal EM, Aarset H, Stormorken A, Engebretsen LF, et al. Current clinical criteria for Lynch syndrome are not sensitive enough to identify MSH6 mutation carriers. J Med Genet. 2010;47(9):579–85. https://doi.org/10.1136/jmg.2010.077677. Epub 2010 Jun 28. PubMed PMID: 20587412; PubMed Central PMCID: PMC2976029.

Chapter 29
The InSiGHT Database: An Example LOVD System

John Paul Plazzer, Johan den Dunnen, and Finlay Macrae

Abstract The International Society for Gastrointestinal Hereditary Tumours (InSiGHT) operates a database with an important function in medical genetics – the sharing of clinical and genetic variant data for genes associated with inherited colorectal cancer. The Leiden Open Variation Database (LOVD) technology used for this task has been updated to handle genomic data that is increasingly being generated, often for patients or individuals with diverse clinical phenotypes. The issue of variant interpretation is a high priority, and InSiGHT's approach is detailed here, as well as other technical challenges and possible solutions.

Keywords Variants · Phenotypes · Database · Genomics · Colorectal cancer

1 Introduction

This chapter will examine InSiGHT's role in the databasing of genetic variants relating to inherited gastrointestinal tumours. The approach taken by InSiGHT may provide inspiration to other organisations as part of a wider effort of sharing genetic data for all genes and diseases. DNA diagnostics is based on sharing data on genes, variants and phenotypes. When data is not shared, it is not possible to provide optimal healthcare to patients and their families. Although obvious, the main challenge in this field is still 'sharing'. Since many do not actively share data, there is a lack

J. P. Plazzer (✉)
Colorectal Medicine & Genetics, The Royal Melbourne Hospital, Melbourne, VIC, Australia
e-mail: johnpaul@variome.org

J. den Dunnen
Human Genetics & Clinical Genetics, Leiden University Medical Center, Leiden, the Netherlands

F. Macrae
Colorectal Medicine & Genetics, The Royal Melbourne Hospital, Melbourne, VIC, Australia

Department of Medicine, The University of Melbourne, Melbourne, VIC, Australia

L. Valle et al. (eds.), *Hereditary Colorectal Cancer*,
https://doi.org/10.1007/978-3-319-74259-5_29

of clinical and genetic information which hampers efficient variant classification and has direct negative consequences for patients or individuals and their families.

While ongoing efforts are underway to make healthcare systems interoperable, these often fall short, and in genetics or genomics, there are even more barriers due to the nature of the data. Therefore, InSiGHT utilises the LOVD platform to store and share variant and clinical information and to classify variants and notify relevant parties. Additional to the database system, there are organisational structures that make this endeavour possible.

The InSiGHT database is focused on storing variants associated with Lynch syndrome, familial adenomatous polyposis and other gastrointestinal cancers. The genes involved include *MLH1*, *MSH2*, *MSH6*, *PMS2*, *APC*, *EPCAM*, *MUTYH*, *STK11*, *POLD1*, *POLE* and others. The InSiGHT model is to organise domain expertise around a public database of curated information. InSiGHT formed out of the merger of Leeds Castle Polyposis Group and International Collaborative Group on Hereditary Non-Polyposis Colorectal Cancer (ICG-HNPCC) and is incorporated in England and Wales as a charity. The InSiGHT database was launched on the LOVDv2 system with the merger of three existing databases. Today, the InSiGHT database continues on LOVDv3 at www.insight-database.org.

2 LOVD Software

LOVD (www.lovd.nl) [1] is open-source software that may be freely downloaded and installed by any person or organisation. The purpose of LOVD is to store clinical and variant information from one or more sources and display it either publicly or for private use. It runs on standard web servers (available in free or commercial options). Alternatively, there is a global instance of the database hosted by LUMC which accepts clinical and variant submissions for any gene or phenotype. However, this is primarily designated for genes where other LOVD databases may not exist. A listing of all public LOVD databases is available [2].

3 Main Features

LOVD features a consistent user interface (irrespective of gene, disease or database instance), user management via roles, easy setup and customisation and the use of established standards. LOVDv3 stores variants in two formats: HGVS standard for describing gene-level variants ('c.' description) and also genomic DNA coordinates ('g.' description). Before the advent of MPS technology, variants would typically be described using gene-level coordinates. LOVD offers the flexibility to search for variants using either genomic or coding DNA reference sequence values. The variants are linked to individuals (or patients) via screenings (how the variant was detected and the genes that were screened). Individuals are linked to phenotypes

Table 29.1 Custom columns specific for Lynch syndrome on the InSiGHT database

Column name	Type	Description
Family history	Individual (patient)	Amsterdam criteria met or family history summary
Selection criteria	Individual (patient)	Reason for proband testing
Protein expression	Phenotype	Immunohistochemistry (IHC)
Microsatellite instability (MSI)	Phenotype	Tumour MSI result: High, low or stable
BRAF status/method	Phenotype	*BRAF* mutation detected in tumour
Methylation status/method	Phenotype	*MLH1* methylation status
Protein_test/result/type	Phenotype	Results of in vitro functional assays
Method	Screening	Additional information about screening method
Splicing/transcript expression	Variant	Information about transcript expression or splicing defects
InSiGHT_class	Variant	InSiGHT classification with link to evidence summary

(diseases), and each can be linked to specific phenotypic features. Genes and diseases covered by the database can be specified by the database manager. Various user roles are supported: submitter/colleague, collaborator/curator and manager, with increasing levels of permissions to view or edit data. Custom columns can be added to the variant, screening, individual or phenotype tables to allow for gene or disease specific information to be included. Customisation can be tailored differently depending on disease or gene. InSiGHT has customised LOVD to focus on specific information related to gastrointestinal cancer syndromes. Specific columns for InSiGHT Lynch syndrome and mismatch repair genes are listed in Table 29.1.

4 LOVD and External Web Services

External web services enhance the operation and usability of LOVD. Variant nomenclature and transcript information are dynamically sourced from Mutalyzer (https://mutalyzer.nl/) and gene names from HGNC (http://www.genenames.org), respectively. Allele frequency annotation is automatically provided by LOVD's own web service with frequency data from large genomic studies. LOVD can also provide information to external systems. API access is available to bioinformatics software which allows automated searching of variants. This service can include any instance of LOVD which has enabled 'global listing variants' in its system settings. On the global LOVD shared database alone, there are a reported 549,140 variants from 285,424 individuals [2]. The LOVD API is useful for checking many variants across the network of LOVD systems, with upwards of 39,000,000 API queries performed annually [2]. The InSiGHT database, as well as any other instance of LOVD, is able to leverage these built-in connections for sharing of variant data - primarily to determine whether a variant is in the database and its classification.

5 Transition to Genomic Era

Over the last decade, clinical diagnostic sequencing has transitioned from Sanger sequencing technology to genomic sequencing methods using MPS (NGS) technology. The latter technology can sequence more genes per individual sample via a targeted panel approach or by screening the whole exome or genome. This development has implications for the way that variant databases are designed and operated. LOVDv3 has the capability to store data generated from such genomic sequencing.

However, the aim of the InSiGHT database is to house data from gastrointestinal cancer panels, rather than whole exomes or genomes. Mainly, this is for practical reasons and to avoid potential privacy concerns. Therefore, the InSiGHT database accepts variants only from the genes relevant for inherited gastrointestinal cancer regardless of sequencing method. To enable genomic data import for InSiGHT, the database was updated to the latest version 3 of the database. The migration of all data from LOVDv2 to LOVDv3 format took place in 2016. The LOVDv2 formatted data required processing with a combination of manual and automated procedures for all variants and individual entries. Variants were converted from gene coordinates into genomic coordinates. New records for phenotype data were created from existing free-text disease information. Thirty-one disease codes were created from existing free text disease descriptions and are listed in Table 29.2. Where possible, these have been linked to OMIM numbers. In future, HPO terms may also be used. For mismatch repair genes, the database (as of April 2017) holds 15,284 variant entries covering an estimated 3373 unique variants. Of these, 6241 are missense variant entries (990 unique missense variants). The process of converting variants to genomic format may be required for other genes and diseases, as there is a large amount of historical data in non-genomic format, for example, in published articles.

Table 29.2 Current list of diseases on the InSiGHT Lynch syndrome database (April 2017). General disease types or syndromes, e.g. cancer as well as specific types of cancer are available for users to enter

Lynch syndrome	Muir-Torre syndrome	Adenomatous polyposis, familial	Cancer, pancreatic
Cancer, colorectal	Cancer, rectal	Neoplasia, colorectal, early onset	Neoplasia, colorectal
Cancer, bladder	Cancer, breast	Cancer, ovarian	Cancer, endometrial
Neurofibromatosis, type 1	Cancer, brain	Glioma, malignant	Cancer, kidney
Cancer, prostate	Leukaemia, myeloid, acute	Leukaemia, myeloid, chronic	Cancer, skin, squamous cell carcinoma
Medulloblastoma	Cancer, gastric	Oesophageal cancer	Polyposis/polyp
Adenoma	Cancer	Unknown/not specified/other	Healthy/control

6 Integrating LSDBs into a Global System

There is a need to balance the aims of the InSiGHT database with the benefits of whole genome or exome data. Public sharing of whole genome or whole exome is possible when the data is aggregated (see ExAC http://exac.broadinstitute.org and GnomAD http://gnomad.broadinstitute.org databases). However, the sharing of detailed phenotype data typically occurs on locus-specific/gene-variant databases (LSDBs) [3]. This disparity between detailed clinical information in LSDBs and aggregated genomic data is likely to persist. Indeed, NGS technology may lead to reduced public sharing of clinical data as the issues of having more genetic information per individual creates more privacy and ethical concerns. There is support for a single global system to provide tiered (public and restricted) access to data [4]. However, such a centralised system will encounter difficult obstacles such as competition, national regulations, lack of trust in database or web security among others. For these reasons, decentralised genomic databases using common APIs are the most promising candidate for sharing data globally and between different systems. One such API is under development by GA4GH. If different systems adopt the same API, a global and distributed resource may emerge. It may be hoped that current LSDBs will be retrofitted into a future system.

7 Submitter Rights and Patient Privacy

InSiGHT has enacted a policy which requires submitter approval for external research use. This stems from the notion that submitters retain rights to their data. As such, they have a say on the research that is performed on their public data. This policy is maintained in order to encourage data submissions from prospective submitters. Commercial use of the public data is generally not permitted – although this overlaps with diagnostic use in commercial organisations. The InSiGHT database exists primarily for clinical diagnostic use. Patient privacy is enforced with only de-identified data allowed to be stored on the database. Submitters are expected to adhere to their institutional and national regulations and submit consented and de-identified information only [5]. This is in contrast to databases which store identifying patient information and require high levels of security to protect privacy. With any genetic information, there is a risk that someone could de-identify using advanced data-matching techniques [6]. It should be noted that genetic data can never be anonymous. It will usually be possible to link single variants to specific populations/subpopulations, and some (rare) variants will be unique to families or even one specific individual. However, the risk is in comparison to the benefits from sharing of variant information. The disclaimer text of the database is derived from the Human Variome Project database disclaimer template [7] and summarises the policies of InSiGHT:

All contents of this database are protected by local and international copyright laws. The information is submitted for the purpose of sharing genetic and clinical information. Genetic variants listed may or may not have a causal association with disease phenotypes, irrespective of stated classifications or other information presented in the database. All information in this database, including variant classifications, is subject to change and there is no warranty, express or implied, as to its accuracy, completeness, or fitness for a particular purpose. Use of this database and information is subject to User responsibility and discretion. Clinical decisions regarding individual patient care should be carried out in conjunction with a healthcare professional with expertise in the relevant genes and diseases. We do not accept any liability for any injury, loss or damage incurred by use of or reliance on the information provided by this database. Database submitters are required to adhere to their institution's rules for data sharing, and local and national laws. Personal identifiers should not be submitted. Submitters retain the rights to use and edit their data. Database curators may curate data to ensure that database formatting and quality standards are met. They may also share their submitted data with external parties for research purposes or for sharing with other databases. Use of the data is for clinical diagnostic purposes. Use for research requires permission from the curator in conjunction with submitters' approval. InSiGHT expects that use of the data for commercial operations should be accompanied by payment commensurate to this use.

8 InSiGHT Variant Interpretation Committee

Discordant classification of variants from different organisations remains a major challenge in genomics. Obtaining a consensus classification means people have to share variants found and their initial classification even when the available evidence is limited. Ultimately, by pulling all data together, the community can then come to a better, evidence-based classification. However, even when data is centralised, this does not resolve discordant classifications – ideally a consensus classification or an overriding classification would be assigned. InSiGHT has approached this issue through the formation of its Variant Interpretation Committee (VIC). The VIC is recognised as an expert panel by ClinGen [8] for the mismatch repair genes. InSiGHT variant classifications are included in clinical reports, thereby assisting genetic counselling and patient management. Other organisations can still classify variants differently given their knowledge of patients and using their own classification criteria. The InSiGHT VIC has over 40 experts from multiple disciplines and is overseen by a Governance Committee which is responsible to the InSiGHT Council. Members of the InSiGHT VIC must be a member of InSiGHT for medicolegal reasons.

The establishment of an internationally recognised classification committee provides these advantages:

- A single web location to find classifications, in this case www.insight-database.org/classifications. This can reduce the analysis time often required when a variant is discovered.

- Access to a network of multidisciplinary experts to collaborate on developing classification criteria and assigning variant classifications. Through this network, unpublished information is often made available on the database.
- Classification that can carry more confidence than a classification reported by a single laboratory, especially when discordant classifications exist.

InSiGHT employs dual methods of classification: qualitative and quantitative. Qualitative criteria were developed by the VIC based on existing Colon Cancer Family Registry classification system for mismatch repair genes. The refined criteria were validated on presumed pathogenic variants [9]. The advantage of qualitative criteria is the use of data that has not yet been calibrated for use in quantitative analysis. Quantitative methods involve multifactorial calculation of Bayesian likelihood ratios to produce a posterior probability of pathogenicity. The InSiGHT classification criteria depend on information about patient tumours, family history, segregation, variant type, co-observed variants, in vitro functional assays, allele frequency, transcript expression and other data. Because the criteria are designed for specific genes and diseases, they are more accurate and have greater capacity to reach a definitive classification than general criteria [10].

The variant interpretation process takes place approximately every 3 months on average in the form of a teleconference with committee members from a number of countries. An invitation to participate in each teleconference is sent, and a group of 10 or more participants are assigned to review variants. Occasionally, variants may be classified by email instead of teleconference on a case-by-case basis. The key to successful variant interpretation is clear guidelines on how to determine a classification. This ensures the variants are classified consistently, across time and from multiple different independent reviewers. A final classification must be confirmed by a majority decision of the committee. Each variant is classified by multiple reviewers. Unpublished information available to the committee such as during the teleconference may be taken into consideration. If there is consensus across all reviewers who are nominated to review specific variants, that variant classification is afforded rapid passage for approval by the committee; if there is a discrepancy, these variants are considered in detail to reach consensus. If no consensus is reached, the variant remains in the VUS class. Changes to the classification criteria may be proposed or discussed during a teleconference. The committee must be notified and approve all changes. The InSiGHT VIC has classified 200 unique missense variants as clinically insignificant or actionable (Class 1, 2, 4 or 5). Another 790 missense variants are of uncertain significance.

9 Engaging Data Submissions from Major Sources

Research projects have collected detailed datasets about patients with Lynch syndrome. However, the data is generally not available to the public due to research data privacy rules and limitations around the consent provided at the time of entry into those research projects. InSiGHT has engaged with some projects to obtain their data for publication on the InSiGHT database. The Prospective Lynch Syndrome Database (PLSD) is a research project to determine the risk of developing specific Lynch syndrome cancers based on mutated gene, gender of individual, age of individual and type of cancer. This project has collected data from bowel cancer surveillance programmes which were prospectively done; hence, this mitigates the sources of bias that impacts retrospective studies. The mutation data that was collected was made available, with the agreement of submitters, to the InSiGHT database. The Colon Cancer Family Registry (CCFR) has submitted some data previously to the InSiGHT database to support the interpretation of variants already held on the database. An agreement to submit all mismatch repair gene data has been made, with transfer of data expected to begin in 2018. This will provide a large source of detailed information on variants, patient demographic, family history and tumour assays.

Where possible, InSiGHT seeks data from national repositories. The advantage of this approach is reduction of resources required to negotiate with many smaller organisations, and the effort to centralise data at a national level can be managed at that level. While there have been notable efforts at national data centralisation, only a small number of submissions have so far resulted. In 2016, a collection of all variants discovered in Iceland were transferred to InSiGHT database. In Australia, a network of familial cancer clinics has submitted data. InSiGHT has also accepted other large datasets that do not fall into national programmes but may represent regional, commercial or research datasets. Other large sources of information are not incorporated into InSiGHT database but are otherwise useful for the interpretation of variants. Examples include the Universal Mutation Database (UMD: http://www.umd.be) in France and ClinVar (https://www.ncbi.nlm.nih.gov/clinvar/) in the United States.

10 Funding for Database Curation

Funding is limited for database curation. Hence, many databases are supported by voluntary work or are updated only during research projects. There are opportunities for students to add information to the databases from published literature and/or research projects. Other potential sources of funding include commercial companies, either via donations or a more formal commercial arrangement. However, this raises issues for what is ostensibly a free and public database. There are possible arrangements that may satisfy the variety of stakeholders in a gene/disease-specific database. One possibility is for the commercial arrangement to not include direct association with the database, for example, to provide assistance with variant interpretation. This approach will keep the database free from commercial control or influence while still supporting one of the core activities of database curation and benefiting the wider community. The InSiGHT Governance Committee has determined that under certain circumstances the commercial funding of variant interpretation process could be beneficial for the broader healthcare community, offsetting the negative attributes of a commercial arrangement. Accessing a substantial source of variants and associated clinical phenotype can be part of the arrangements, especially where such data assists in more definitive classification of a variant. Commercial support to academic laboratories conducting functional analyses of variants of uncertain significance is another important reason to consider such arrangements. The conditions would include that the variant classification outcome of any commercially linked interpretation would be made public. This also prevents the situation where a variant receives multiple different interpretations.

11 Conclusion

InSiGHT has worked in collaboration with the Human Variome Project to present a viable model of variant data sharing and interpretation. There have been considerable successes - merging of databases, implementation of the interpretation committee and classification criteria, but much more work remains to be done.

Glossary of Terms

API Application Programming Interface, a technology to allow systems to communicate or share data with other systems, with or without human interaction.

CCFR Colon Cancer Family Registry http://www.coloncfr.org.

GA4GH Global Alliance for Genomics and Health https://genomicsandhealth.org.

HGNC HUGO Gene Nomenclature Committee http://www.genenames.org/. HUGO is the HUman Genome Organisation http://www.hugo-international.org/.

HGVS Human Genome Variation Society http://www.hgvs.org/.

HPO Human Phenotype Ontology http://human-phenotype-ontology.github.io/.

HVP Human Variome Project http://www.humanvariomeproject.org/.

Individual A record in the database that could represent a patient with a disease or an otherwise healthy person.

InSiGHT International Society for Gastrointestinal Hereditary Tumours https://www.insight-group.org.

Instance A specific database in operation. For example, InSiGHT operates its own instance of LOVD.

LOVD Leiden Open Variation Database www.lovd.nl.

LOVDv2 The previous version of LOVD software.

LOVDv3 The latest version of LOVD software, with genomic variant storage and other advanced features.

LSDB Locus-Specific Database, also referred to as gene/disease-specific database.

LUMC Leiden University Medical Center https://www.lumc.nl/.

MPS Massively Parallel Sequencing, also known as NGS.

NGS Next-Generation Sequencing.
OMIM Online Mendelian Inheritance in Man https://www.omim.org/.
PLSD Prospective Lynch Syndrome Database http://www.lscarisk.org.
VIC Variant Interpretation Committee.
VUS Variant of Uncertain Significance.

References

1. Fokkema IF, Taschner PE, Schaafsma GC, et al. LOVD v. 2.0: the next generation in gene variant databases. Hum Mutat. 2011;32(5):557–63.
2. Announcement of LOVD statistics. http://www.lovd.nl/3.0/home. Accessed 22 Feb 2018.
3. Brookes AJ, Robinson PN. Human genotype-phenotype databases: aims, challenges and opportunities. Nat Rev Genet. 2015;16(12):702–15.
4. Bean L, Hegde MR. Gene variant databases and sharing: creating a global genomic variant database for personalized medicine. Hum Mutat. 2016;37(6):559–63.
5. Povey S, Al Aqeel AI, Cambon-Thomsen A, et al. Practical guidelines addressing ethical issues pertaining to the curation of human locus-specific variation databases (LSDBs). Hum Mutat. 2010;31(11):1179–84.
6. Rodriguez LL, Brooks LD, Greenberg JH, Green ED. The complexities of genomic identifiability. Science. 2013;339(6117):275–6.3.
7. Plazzer JP, Bernstein IT, Devereau A. Disclaimer statements for gene/disease specific databases. Human Variome Project. http://www.humanvariomeproject.org/assets/hvp-guidelines/HVP-GL-002-01-EN-Disclaimer_Statements_for_GDSDBs.pdf. Accessed 12 Apr 2017.
8. Rehm HL, Berg JS, Brooks LD, et al. ClinGen—the clinical genome resource. N Engl J Med. 2015;372(23):2235–42.
9. Thompson BA, Spurdle AB, Plazzer JP, et al. Application of a 5-tiered scheme for standardized classification of 2,360 unique mismatch repair gene variants in the InSiGHT locus-specific database. Nat Genet. 2014;46(2):107–15.
10. Velde KJ, Kuiper J, Thompson BA, et al. Evaluation of CADD scores in curated mismatch repair gene variants yields a model for clinical validation and prioritization. Hum Mutat. 2015;36(7):712–9.

Chapter 30
The International Mismatch Repair Consortium

Mark A. Jenkins, Jeanette C. Reece, and Aung K. Win

Abstract The International Mismatch Repair Consortium (IMRC) is a collaboration of clinicians and scientists who have agreed to pool and analyse data on Lynch syndrome, a genetic predisposition to cancer caused by germline mutations in DNA mismatch repair genes or *EPCAM* deletion, with the rationale that research on this hereditary syndrome will benefit from large datasets from many countries. As of October 2017, the IMRC includes approximately 273 members from 122 centres/clinics in 29 countries throughout Africa, Asia, Australasia, Europe, and North and South America, who are involved in research or treatment of people with Lynch syndrome and their families. To date, there are six research projects registered at the IMRC: cancer risks for Lynch syndrome, classification of mismatch repair variants, genetic testing and screening practices, environmental and lifestyle modifiers of cancer risk, inherited methylation and cancer risks for family members of constitutional mismatch repair deficiency (CMMR-D) patients. The most significant project, in terms of data accrued, is the study of cancer risks for Lynch syndrome which mainly asks whether age-specific cumulative risk (penetrance) of cancers differs by country or geographic region. As of October 2017, almost 6200 pedigrees from investigators from approximately 24 countries have been submitted for penetrance analysis – see http://www.sphinx.org.au/imrc.

Keywords Colorectal cancer · Lynch syndrome · Penetrance · *MLH1* · *MSH2* · *MSH6* · *PMS2* · *EPCAM* · International · Risk factors · Cohort · Family history

M. A. Jenkins (✉) · A. K. Win
Centre for Epidemiology and Biostatistics, Melbourne School of Population and Global Health, Faculty of Medicine, Dentistry and Health Sciences, The University of Melbourne, Parkville, VIC, Australia

University of Melbourne Centre for Cancer Research, Victorian Comprehensive Cancer Centre, Parkville, VIC, Australia
e-mail: m.jenkins@unimelb.edu.au

J. C. Reece
Centre for Epidemiology and Biostatistics, Melbourne School of Population and Global Health, Faculty of Medicine, Dentistry and Health Sciences, The University of Melbourne, Parkville, VIC, Australia

L. Valle et al. (eds.), *Hereditary Colorectal Cancer*,
https://doi.org/10.1007/978-3-319-74259-5_30

1 Establishment of the IMRC

The International Mismatch Repair Consortium (IMRC) was formed in 2010 to bridge critical research gaps in the understanding of Lynch syndrome, cancer predisposition caused by inherited heterozygous mutations in DNA mismatch repair genes *MLH1*, *MSH2*, *MSH6*, *PMS2* or *EPCAM* deletions. It comprises research and clinical groups around the world researching and treating Lynch syndrome. The co-founders are Mark Jenkins (University of Melbourne, Victoria, Australia), Robert Haile (Cedars-Sinai Medical Center, California, USA), Finlay Macrae (Royal Melbourne Hospital, Victoria, Australia) and Gabriela Möslein (Helios Clinic, Dusseldorf, Germany) and are coordinated by Allyson Templeton (Fred Hutchinson Cancer Research Center, Seattle, USA).

The establishment of the IMRC was facilitated by the International Society for Gastrointestinal Hereditary Tumours (InSiGHT) and the Collaborative Group of the Americas on Inherited Colorectal Cancer (CGA) via invitation to their respective memberships. IMRC membership is open to anyone involved in research or treatment of people with Lynch syndrome and their families. As of October 2017, the IMRC includes approximately 273 members from 122 centres/clinics in 29 countries throughout Africa, Asia, Australasia, Europe, and North and South America. IMRC member can contribute to the consortium by contributing data or analysis expertise to existing projects (see below) or proposing a new project.

2 Currently Registered Projects

2.1 Worldwide Study of Cancer Risks for Lynch Syndrome

Principal Investigator: Mark A. Jenkins, The University of Melbourne, Victoria, Australia.

Accurate cancer risk estimates are critical to guide and inform genetic counselling and the clinical management of high-risk families. However, we currently lack accurate age-specific estimates of risk of colorectal and other cancers for mismatch repair gene mutation carriers by individual's characteristics (e.g. sex, mismatch repair gene, type of mutation, country, etc.). The only way to address this knowledge gap is to conduct comprehensive penetrance analyses on large, ethnically heterogeneous samples of persons/families segregating mutations in mismatch repair genes. To achieve this, investigators are: (i) establishing a combined dataset of pedigree, cancer and mutation data from around the world for thousands of Lynch syndrome families; and (ii) analysing this data to estimate the age-specific cumulative risk (penetrance) of cancers at each anatomical site by sex, mismatch repair gene, type of mutation and country/geographic region.

2.2 *Mismatch Repair Variant Classification*

Principal Investigators: Marcus Greenblatt, University of Vermont, USA; Sean Tavtigian, University of Utah, USA.

In clinical cancer genetics, molecular diagnostic testing is now commonly performed looking for pathogenic mutations in cancer susceptibility genes. A critical challenge in the field is interpreting whether a genetic variant causes disease or not. About 20–30% of the variants identified in mismatch repair genes and other cancer susceptibility genes are missense or non-coding changes that may or may not be pathogenic but whose effects on function and disease cannot be interpreted easily. They are designated "variants of unknown significance". Classifying variants as pathogenic and neutral significantly improves the management of LS and other hereditary cancer syndromes by identifying which individuals carry a harmful genetic variant and thus benefit from screening and therapeutic measures. To address these needs, investigators are: (i) generating a list of mismatch repair missense variants and how they are classified using available data and criteria; (ii) validating and quantifying the classification ability of in vitro, in silico and clinic-pathologic data; and (iii) creating qualitative and quantitative models to classify variants.

2.3 *Worldwide Study of Genetic Testing and Cancer Screening in Lynch Syndrome*

Principal Investigator: Robert Haile, Cedars-Sinai Medical Center, California, USA.

Development of successful programmes to increase the use of colonoscopy screening within Lynch syndrome family members depends on the availability and uptake of genetic testing of relatives in families with documented Lynch syndrome mutations. Therefore, an understanding of the variables underlying the choice of individual family members to be tested is important for reducing the burden of colorectal cancer screening in Lynch syndrome families. Colonoscopy screening has been demonstrated to significantly decrease both colorectal cancer incidence and mortality in Lynch syndrome. Additional studies in more racial/ethnic groups and in more countries and with longer follow-up are needed to better understand current compliance with screening guidelines and the reasons for lack of screening among those who harbour a pathogenic mutation in a mismatch repair gene. Such information is a prerequisite to design methods to increase compliance with screening guidelines in this very high-risk population. To address these needs, investigators are: (i) clarifying the country-specific guidelines for genetic counselling and testing for Lynch syndrome families and then collecting data on the uptake of genetic counselling/testing by members of Lynch syndrome families; (ii) clarifying country-specific guidelines for cancer screening in Lynch syndrome and then collecting data on compliance with screening guidelines by members of Lynch syndrome families; and (iii) conducting focus groups to better understand "local", country-specific barriers to compliance.

2.4 Collaborative Study on the Role of Lifestyle Factors/Diet/ Body Fatness in the Development of Tumours in Lynch Syndrome

Principal Investigators: Franzel van Duijnhoven and Ellen Kampan, Wageningen University, Netherlands.

Lifestyle factors have a pronounced effect in those at a very high lifetime risk of cancer due to an inherited mutation: for example, being overweight and smoking strongly increase the risk of colorectal tumours in people with Lynch syndrome. Other lifestyle factors such as diet as well as other outcomes such as endometrial cancer in Lynch syndrome have not or only scarcely been studied. To further elucidate the role of lifestyle factors in the development of tumours in people with Lynch syndrome, large populations with a variety in lifestyle habits are needed. Therefore, we propose to cooperate internationally and set up a worldwide collaborative study on the role of lifestyle factors/diet/body fatness in the development of tumours in Lynch syndrome. To do this, investigators are: (i) studying the role of smoking and overweight in relation to cancer risk in those cohorts that already have this information available; and (ii) collecting and analysing data on lifestyle/diet/body fatness for all cohorts in a worldwide collaborative study. The ultimate goal is to develop evidence-based lifestyle recommendations to decrease the risk of cancers for people with Lynch syndrome.

2.5 MLH1 *Epimutations in Predisposing to the Development of Lynch-Like Tumours*

Principal Investigator: Megan Hitchins, Cedars-Sinai Medical Center, California, USA.

MLH1 epimutations manifest high levels of *MLH1* methylation throughout normal tissues and, though comparatively rare, may account for a significant fraction of colorectal cancer cases whose tumours demonstrate *MLH1* absence but who have no germline mutation in *MLH1*. Given its rarity, meaningful comprehensive studies will benefit from collaboration on an international scale. To address these needs, investigators are: (i) establishing the frequency *of MLH1* epimutations in cases with a clinical suspicion of Lynch syndrome by testing the colorectal cancer cases clinically suspected of Lynch syndrome, but for whom no pathogenic mutation can be identified; (ii) measuring the clinical phenotype of epimutation carriers to gain a more detailed clinical profile; (iii) measuring the molecular profiling of tumours in epimutation-positive cases to determine the "second hit" plus more detailed TGCA-type analysis to elucidate the tumour molecular phenotype; and (iv) determining the inheritance patterns associated with *MLH1* epimutations and the mechanisms underlying them by studying family members of epimutation carriers.

2.6 Cancer Risk for Family Members of Constitutional Mismatch Repair-Deficiency (CMMR-D) Patients

Principal Investigator: Maartje Nielsen, Leiden University Medical Center, Netherlands.

Risk of cancer is high for people who have inherited a mutation in a mismatch repair gene from both parents and therefore have constitutional mismatch repair-deficiency (CMMR-D). However very little is known about the risks of cancer for their relatives on both sides of their family who carry a mutation, most often in the *PMS2* gene. Understanding these risks is important for the clinical care of family members of CMMR-D patients. Studying such relatives provides an unbiased estimate of cancer risk for heterozygous mismatch repair gene mutation carriers in general. This is because in principal CMMR-D families are ascertained because of the distinct phenotype of the index case, not because of family history of cancer. Due to the increased use of detection methods for Lynch syndrome, such as standardised tumour testing for immunohistochemistry or microsatellite instability analysis in all colorectal cancer cases and next-generation sequencing, there will be an increase in the detection of Lynch syndrome cases with no or little family history. For these patients, knowledge on unbiased cancer risk is important to provide justified screening protocols. To address this gap, investigators are: (i) determining retrospectively the cancer risk for family members (up to third degree) of patients with CMMR-D; and (ii) conducting a follow-up study of family members with an identified heterozygous mismatch repair gene mutation to prospectively estimate risk of cancer.

3 Detailed Description of IMRC Project: Worldwide Study of Cancer Risks for Lynch Syndrome

Principal Investigator: Mark A. Jenkins; *Co-Principal Investigator*: Aung K. Win; *Coordinator*: Jeanette C. Reece; *Data Manager*: Grant Lee, Centre for Epidemiology and Biostatistics, The University of Melbourne, Victoria, Australia.

3.1 Rationale

3.1.1 Cancer Risks Vary by Sex, Gene and Type of Mutation

While over 25 studies have estimated the *age-specific risks of cancer* in Lynch syndrome (penetrance), many have had major drawbacks, resulting in limited usefulness of the findings.

There is substantial evidence for significant variation in cancer risk by sex and gene. For example, the risk of colorectal cancer is higher for male carriers compared with female carriers and is higher for carriers of *MLH1* and *MSH2* mutations than for carriers of *MSH6* and *PMS2* mutations [1–11]. Larger studies are required to verify these findings, especially for the relatively understudied mutations in *MSH6* and *PMS2*.

Decreasing costs of sequencing of mismatch repair genes has resulted in: (a) increased range of variants detected, many of which have not been classified with respect to penetrance; and (b) increased testing of population-based cases unselected for family history and therefore potentially identifying mutations with, on average, a lower penetrance than those identified in clinic-based families. Several proposed methodologies to classify these variants by clinical significance are being developed [12–14]. These algorithms generally assume penetrance for all mutations is equivalent to truncating mutations, though data from quantitative functional assays suggest likely variability. Different mutation types may result in differences in cancer risks. For example, a particular *MSH2* missense variant appears to be associated with greater risk of pancreatic cancer than truncating mutations [15], and transitional cell cancers are particularly frequent in the common *MSH2* exon 8 deletion families [16].

3.1.2 Current Penetrance Estimates Are Imprecise and Distribution of Risk Is Complex

Current penetrance estimates are imprecise and virtually unknown for some cancers, thereby limiting their clinical utility. This imprecision is predominantly due to the insufficient sample size of most studies only analysing the Lynch families available at their clinics, and even the existing larger collaborative studies have not overcome this limitation. For example, in our recent study of 166 *MLH1* and 224 *MSH2* families, from the Colon Cancer Family Registry, the 95% confidence intervals for colorectal cancer for *MLH1* carriers ranged from 25% to 50% and for endometrial cancer for *MSH2* carriers ranged from 19% to 45% [1]. For less common Lynch syndrome cancers, risk estimates are even less informative. For example, in the same study, we observed that anywhere between 2 and 170 per 1000 carriers of an *MLH1* mutation would be diagnosed with stomach cancer by age 70. A large French consortium was equally challenged, as despite recruiting 248 *MLH1* and 256 *MSH2* Lynch syndrome families (the most families in a single study), estimates of ovarian cancer for *MLH1* mutation carriers ranged between 1% and 65% [3]. A large European consortium study of 1942 people with Lynch syndrome estimated the risk of upper gastrointestinal cancers for *MLH1* carriers to range from 7% to 27% [11].

This lack of precision is also partly due to large variability in risk, even between carriers of same sex with the same mismatch repair gene mutated. We estimated that the lifetime cancer risk (from birth to age 70 years) followed a U-shaped distribution (*not* a normal distribution) with most carriers *either* having a high or low risk. For every 100 *MLH1 and MSH2* mutation carriers, 41 were unlikely (less than 20%

risk) to be diagnosed with colorectal cancer, and 17 were very likely (more than 80%) to be diagnosed [1]. If this large variability in risks can be confirmed, it suggests major potential for stratifying carriers by risk.

3.1.3 Penetrance Estimates May Differ by Geographic Regions

A major gap in assessing penetrance is whether cancer risks depend on geographic region. For the general population, most of whom are noncarriers, there is a well-recognised significant variability in cancer incidence by country (e.g. ten-fold difference internationally for colorectal cancer) [17]. These differences are suggestive of environmental, rather than genetic, risk factors for colorectal cancer, as cancer rates in migrants approach that of the host country within one or two generations [18]. If cancer risks for mismatch repair gene mutation carriers were also found to differ by geographic region, this would: (1) provide further clues as to potential modifiers of cancer risk for carriers, which has obvious potential translational relevance for cancer prevention; and (2) enable generation of geographic region-specific cancer probabilities for mutation carriers that are more relevant for genetic counselling.

However, Lynch syndrome studies have almost exclusively involved carriers of Caucasian ethnicity from Australasia, Europe and the USA. Therefore, cancer risks for carriers from other racial/ethnic or geographical populations are unknown. In support of variability by such heterogeneity, one study observed that stomach cancer risks were higher and endometrial cancer rates were lower for mutation carriers in 18 South Korean Lynch syndrome families compared with those for 17 Dutch Lynch syndrome families [19]. While this may be due to a myriad of environmental and even genetic modifiers of risk that differ by country, the fact that the actual risks differ is, in itself, support for larger and more thorough studies.

3.1.4 Penetrance Might Depend on the Parent of Origin of the Mutation

Penetrance is further complicated by potential non-Mendelian inheritance of risk, as three studies reported that the risk of colorectal cancer in carriers might depend on the parent from whom the mutation was inherited [20, 21]. Confirmation of this in a larger study would have important clinical implications, with recommendations for screening based on the parent from whom the mutation was inherited.

3.1.5 Closing the Knowledge Gap Is Clinically Important

Accurate penetrance estimates are a critical component of public health guidelines, such as those for screening, as well as guidelines for the clinical management of high-risk patients/families, such as recommendations for prophylactic surgery. Understanding how these estimates differ is important to provide for appropriate genetic counselling and risk management advice to mismatch repair mutation carriers. The wider the confidence interval, the less helpful are the estimates in counselling, to the point of potentially not being helpful at all.

There is substantial evidence that the risk of colorectal cancer can be reduced in carriers of mismatch repair gene mutations, and therefore, it is important to know the risks of cancers to facilitate recommendation of preventive measures appropriate to risk which can be recommended. Screening carriers with frequent colonoscopies (and consequent polypectomy) more than halves the risk of colorectal cancer diagnosis and mortality [22]. We have also shown that of mutation carriers who had extensive colon resection for a colon cancer diagnosis, none had a metachronous colorectal cancer in the following 10 years compared with 16% of those who only had segmental resection [23]. Two years of aspirin intake reduces the risk of colorectal cancer for people with Lynch syndrome by 60% [24]. Other modifiers of risk are also likely to be important for counselling [25–30].

However, there is room for improvement in preventing colorectal cancer. Despite preliminary evidence suggesting that penetrance for colorectal cancer may be lower in females than males, current screening guidelines recommend identical screening irrespective of sex, and this could be modified with confirmatory evidence [31].

The use of screening and other preventive methods for cancers other than colorectal cancer varies between and within countries partly due to limited knowledge of cancer risk. Endometrial cancer risks are high for carriers, but there is disagreement about whether screening by transvaginal ultrasound is warranted as no clinical trial data has supported its effectiveness. Some clinical and national guidelines recommend prophylactic hysterectomy and oophorectomy after completion of pregnancies. If there is a high degree of heterogeneity in endometrial cancer risk for carriers, as suggested by our research [1], then such prophylactic surgery may only be warranted for high-risk women. More precise estimates of risk, from large studies, are needed to inform this important debate.

Precise penetrance estimates are also needed to inform efficient use of screening and prophylactic surgery. Guidelines for endoscopy screening for gastric cancer remain imprecise, despite a 15–20% lifetime risk of this cancer for Lynch syndrome carriers. This is particularly pertinent for geographic regions with high rates of gastric cancer which have endoscopists experienced in effective upper gastrointestinal screening, e.g. Japan and Korea. For female mutation carriers at increased risk of ovarian cancer, prophylactic oophorectomy is often undertaken, although the optimal timing of this intervention remains unclear and could be clarified by increased precision of penetrance estimates. Studies have additionally provided preliminary evidence that mutation carriers are at increased risk of prostate cancer [32–35], and precise definition of this risk, if high enough, may justify PSA testing in mutation carriers. Finally, we and others have suggested that carriers could be at increased risk for breast cancer [36–39], but this conclusion is controversial, and confirmation and more precise information on this risk are needed before breast screening practices can be enhanced, such as using MRI to avoid radiation exposure in an already vulnerable population.

3.2 Data Collection

All IMRC members were invited to contribute anonymised pedigree data for penetrance analysis.

3.2.1 Inclusion Criteria

To be included, families needed to have at least one confirmed carrier of a pathogenic mutation in one of the DNA mismatch repair genes *MLH1*, *MSH2*, *MSH6* and *PMS2* or *EPCAM* deletion. Pathogenic mutation is defined as any variant that: (a) causes a protein truncation, is a large deletion or insertion or is a mutation in the consensus splice sites predicted to alter splicing; or (b) is a rare nucleotide change that causes a missense substitution or a small in-frame insertion or deletion or a sequence change located near (but not within) consensus splice sites that has been classified previously as pathogenic. All variants submitted are checked for pathogenicity using the In SiGHT Variant Interpretation Committee's classifications (http://www.insight-database.org/classifications).

As the aim is to estimate cancer risks for mutation carriers, the subjects in this analysis are the known carriers and the possible carriers (untested). Probands are defined as the first person in the family who tested positive for a mismatch repair gene mutation. "Population-based" families are defined as those for which the probands were ascertained from population-based or hospital-based series either irrespective of family history of cancer or using some sampling fraction on family history. Clinic-based families are defined as having attended clinics/hospitals based on referral because of a family history of cancer, and all identified relatives will be included. Where possible, families who were recruited through separate probands but found to contain members in common are combined.

3.2.2 Data Collection

The following information was requested:

(i) For each family: an id number, the gene that is mutated in the family and description of the change to the DNA of each mutation; the method of ascertainment of the family (via a population-based source, e.g. a colorectal cancer case from a cancer registry, from a family cancer clinic, from a hospital-based series); the date the family was ascertained; and the person in the family first found to have the mutation (the proband) and the date they were tested.

(ii) For each family member: id number, mother's and father's id numbers (needed to determine genetic relatedness between all family members), age and sex, mutation status (carrier/noncarrier/untested); cancer diagnoses (anatomical site, age at and year of diagnosis); ages and years of polypectomies and bowel surgery; age and year and details of hysterectomy and oophorectomy; and age at last contact or death.

3.2.3 Data Storage

The group at the Centre for Epidemiology and Biostatistics, the University of Melbourne, is responsible for collecting data from IMRC members, checking data quality and organising a data cleaning process to maximise data quality. A data management system is used to check data quality and to raise queries to the IMRC member if any incomplete or incorrect data are identified. The database is hosted on dedicated servers to ensure maximal availability for the project and integrated in existing computer and network infrastructures to guarantee optimal data safety (backup, firewall, restricted access).

3.2.4 Calculation of Risk

Age-specific hazard ratios (HRs), i.e. the ratio of age-specific cancer incidence for carriers to incidence for the population, are estimated using modified segregation analysis [40], a technique we have successfully used previously [1, 4, 5]. Models are fitted by maximum likelihood using the statistical package MENDEL version 3.2 [41] and adjusted for ascertainment (described in more detail below). Unlike association studies and survival analyses, this analytical method is not subject to population stratification, adjusts for ascertainment and uses data on all study participants, whether genotyped or not, thereby maximising statistical power.

HRs are estimated for each cancer type, sex, gene, mutation type and geographic region (and for various combinations of these). For each anatomical site, the age at cancer diagnosis is modelled as a random variable whose hazard is the relevant population incidence rate multiplied by a site-specific HR. Parent-of-origin effects are estimated using a model we developed [20] which has been independently validated [42].

To adjust for ascertainment, each pedigree is conditioned on the proband's genotype, cancer status and age of onset (for families ascertained from population-based sources) or on the proband's genotype and the affected statuses and ages of onset of all family members at the time the proband was found to be a mismatch repair gene mutation carrier (for families ascertained from clinic-based sources) [43].

To model residual familial aggregation of cancer risk, a genetic mixed model is employed which incorporates an unmeasured polygenic factor in addition to the mismatch repair genes [44]. This is necessary since models that attribute all familial aggregation to the major gene being studied are likely to be biased [45]. The polygenic part of this model approximates the effect of a large number of genes that individually have very small effects on cancer susceptibility [46].

Age-, sex-, gene-, mutation type- and geographical location-specific cumulative risk estimates are calculated from the HR estimates as $1 - e^{(-\int \lambda(t)dt)}$, where $\lambda(t)$ is the HR multiplied by the relevant population incidence. Corresponding confidence intervals (CIs) are calculated using a parametric bootstrap [1].

3.2.5 Current State of Data Collection

As of October 2017, 5965 families have been received (Table 30.1). In this context, families are defined as having at least two individuals of known genetic relationship, at least one of which was a known carrier of a pathogenic mutation in a DNA mismatch repair gene. The majority of these were from Europe and North America but also include families from Australasia, Asia and South America (Fig. 30.1a–c). Family size ranged from 1 member (304 families) to 333 members (1 family), and number of confirmed mutation carriers ranged from 1 member (3011 families) to 41 members (1 family) (Fig. 30.2a, b). It should be noted that all families with at least one mutation carrier can be utilised for penetrance analysis, as the modified segregation analysis models the probability of each untested relative being a

Table 30.1 Accural of Lynch syndrome families to the International Mismatch Repair Consortium, as of October 2017

Countries	*MLH1*	*MSH2*	*MSH6*	*PMS2*	*EPCAM*	Total
South America	**42**	**27**	**5**	**2**	**0**	**76**
Argentina	1	2	0	0	0	3
Brazil	9	10	3	0	0	22
Chile	19	8	0	2	0	29
Uruguay	13	7	2	0	0	22
Australasia	**119**	**134**	**51**	**24**	**2**	**330**
Australia	109	125	46	22	1	303
New Zealand	10	9	5	2	1	27
North America	**687**	**865**	**378**	**290**	**22**	**2242**
Canada	78	95	21	10	2	206
USA	609	770	357	280	20	2036
Asia[a]	**63**	**83**	**14**	**1**	**1**	**162**
Hong Kong	35	61	4	0	1	101
Japan	24	17	7	1	0	49
Singapore	4	5	3	0	0	12
Europe[a]	**1171**	**1371**	**454**	**144**	**15**	**3155**
Denmark	92	150	95	18	1	356
France	247	256	32	0	0	535
Germany	443	529	102	46	0	1120
Italy	4	12	3	0	0	19
Netherlands	33	43	86	27	3	192
Norway	16	48	0	15	1	80
Spain	150	102	58	18	6	334
Switzerland	5	3	1	0	0	9
United Kingdom	181	228	77	20	4	510
Total[a]	**2082**	**2480**	**902**	**461**	**40**	**5965**

[a]Sites from Sweden (157 families), Malaysia (15 families), India (24 families) and Turkey (27 families) have also submitted data – but singletons only (not family data)

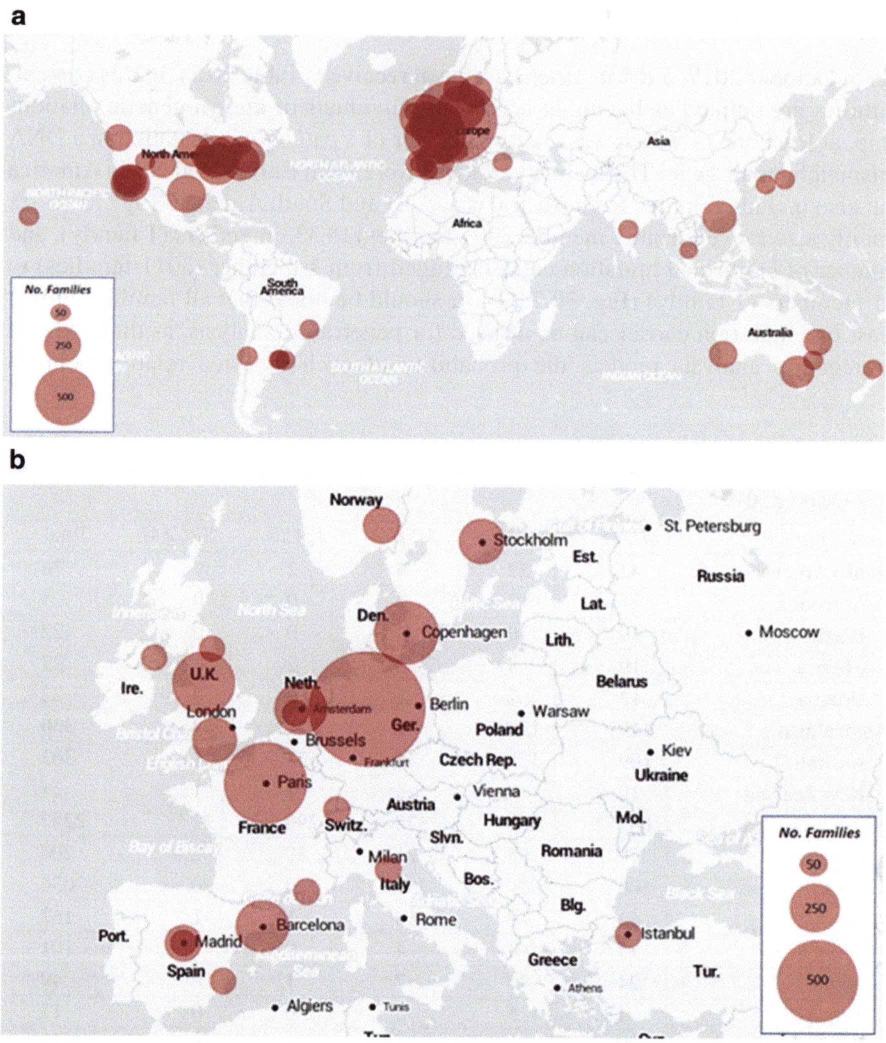

Fig. 30.1 Source and number of Lynch syndrome pedigrees (at least one family member known to carry a pathogenic mutation in a mismatch repair gene) that have been submitted to the International Mismatch Repair Consortium from (**a**) worldwide, (**b**) Europe and (**c**) the USA, as of October 2017

c

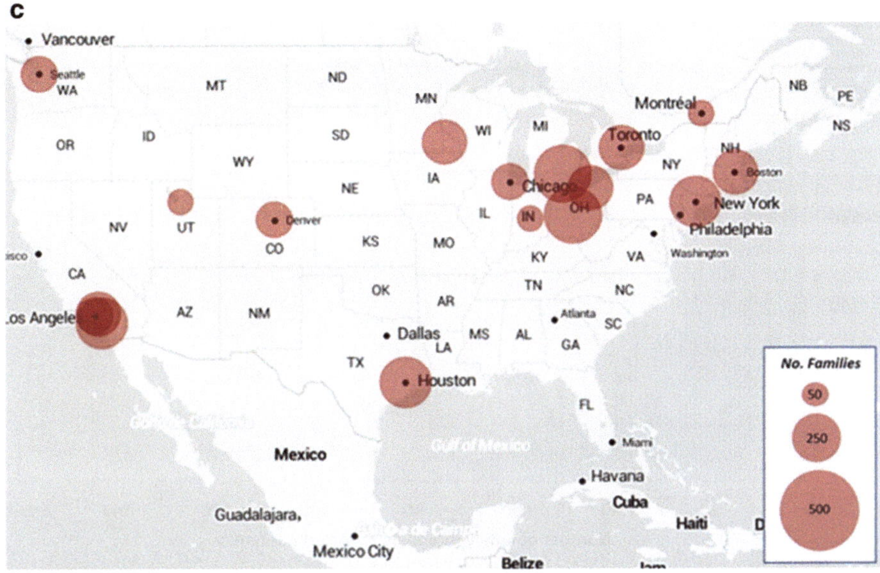

Fig. 30.1 (continued)

mutation carrier given their genetic relationship to known carriers and their disease status and then weights their contribution to the penetrance analysis based on this probability – a strength of modified segregation analysis – although the more confirmed mutation carriers in the family are, the more precise the estimates of the penetrance will be.

4 Data Sharing

From its inception, the IMRC has functioned under the principle that it is a resource for research on the aetiology, risk and prognosis of colorectal cancer for all researchers. However, no data submitted for any project will be made available for any other project without express permission of the contributor of the data. Submission of data to the IMRC has no impact on the submitter's rights to analyse their own data, nor does it imply they will not analyse their own data. Further information on the IMRC can be found on the website: https://sphinx.org.au/imrc.

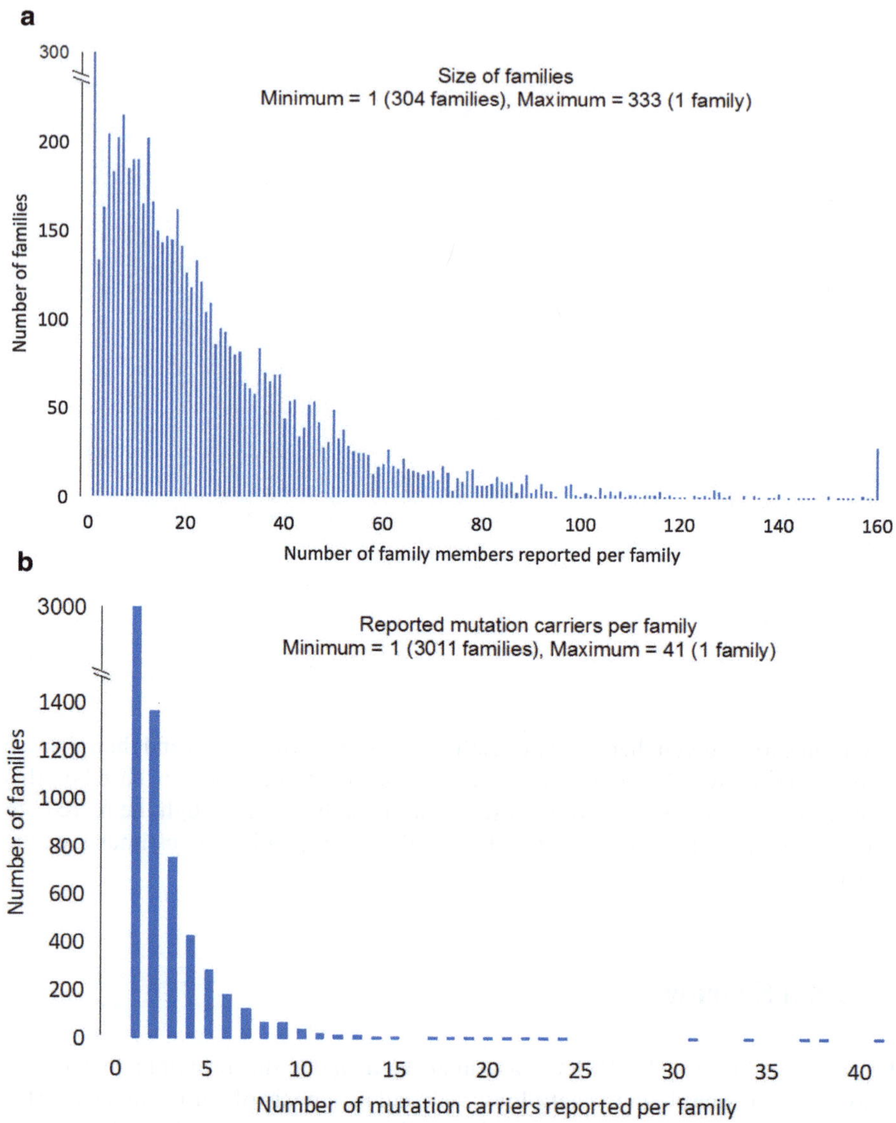

Fig. 30.2 Number of submitted family members per Lynch syndrome family (**a**) and number of confirmed mutation carriers per Lynch syndrome family (**b**) not including obligate carriers, as of October 2017

Acknowledgement The National Health and Medical Research Council, Australia, has supported this research via a project grant and via research fellowships. We thank all researchers, clinicians and genetic counsellors at participating centres who have given their time and resources and the Lynch syndrome families.

References

1. Dowty JG, Win AK, Buchanan DD, Lindor NM, Macrae FA, Clendenning M, et al. Cancer risks for MLH1 and MSH2 mutation carriers. Hum Mutat. 2013;34(3):490–7. https://doi.org/10.1002/humu.22262.
2. Quehenberger F, Vasen HF, van Houwelingen HC. Risk of colorectal and endometrial cancer for carriers of mutations of the hMLH1 and hMSH2 gene: correction for ascertainment. J Med Genet. 2005;42(6):491–6. https://doi.org/10.1136/jmg.2004.024299.
3. Bonadona V, Bonaiti B, Olschwang S, Grandjouan S, Huiart L, Longy M, et al. Cancer risks associated with germline mutations in MLH1, MSH2, and MSH6 genes in Lynch syndrome. JAMA. 2011;305(22):2304–10. https://doi.org/10.1001/jama.2011.743.
4. Baglietto L, Lindor NM, Dowty JG, White DM, Wagner A, Gomez Garcia EB, et al. Risks of Lynch syndrome cancers for MSH6 mutation carriers. J Natl Cancer Inst. 2010;102(3):193–201. https://doi.org/10.1093/jnci/djp473.
5. Senter L, Clendenning M, Sotamaa K, Hampel H, Green J, Potter JD, et al. The clinical phenotype of Lynch syndrome due to germ-line PMS2 mutations. Gastroenterology. 2008;135(2):419–28.e1. https://doi.org/10.1053/j.gastro.2008.04.026.
6. Stoffel E, Mukherjee B, Raymond VM, Tayob N, Kastrinos F, Sparr J, et al. Calculation of risk of colorectal and endometrial cancer among patients with Lynch syndrome. Gastroenterology. 2009;137(5):1621–7. https://doi.org/10.1053/j.gastro.2009.07.039.
7. Choi Y-H, Cotterchio M, McKeown-Eyssen G, Neerav M, Bapat B, Boyd K, et al. Penetrance of colorectal cancer among *MLH1*/ *MSH2* carriers participating in the colorectal cancer familial registry in Ontario. Hered Cancer Clin Prac. 2009;7:14. https://doi.org/10.1186/1897-4287-7-14.
8. Dunlop MG, Farrington SM, Carothers AD, Wyllie AH, Sharp L, Burn J, et al. Cancer risk associated with germline DNA mismatch repair gene mutations. Hum Mol Genet. 1997;6(1):105–10.
9. Hampel H, Stephens JA, Pukkala E, Sankila R, Aaltonen LA, Mecklin JP, et al. Cancer risk in hereditary nonpolyposis colorectal cancer syndrome: later age of onset. Gastroenterology. 2005;129(2):415–21. https://doi.org/10.1016/j.gastro.2005.05.011.
10. ten Broeke SW, Brohet RM, Tops CM, van der Klift HM, Velthuizen ME, Bernstein I, et al. Lynch syndrome caused by germline PMS2 mutations: delineating the cancer risk. J Clin Oncol. 2015;33(4):319–25. https://doi.org/10.1200/jco.2014.57.8088.
11. Moller P, Seppala T, Bernstein I, Holinski-Feder E, Sala P, Evans DG, et al. Cancer incidence and survival in Lynch syndrome patients receiving colonoscopic and gynaecological surveillance: first report from the prospective Lynch syndrome database. Gut. 2017;66(3):464–72. https://doi.org/10.1136/gutjnl-2015-309675.
12. Arnold S, Buchanan DD, Barker M, Jaskowski L, Walsh MD, Birney G, et al. Classifying MLH1 and MSH2 variants using bioinformatic prediction, splicing assays, segregation, and tumor characteristics. Hum Mutat. 2009;30(5):757–70. https://doi.org/10.1002/humu.20936.
13. Thompson BA, Goldgar DE, Paterson C, Clendenning M, Walters R, Arnold S, et al. A multifactorial likelihood model for MMR gene variant classification incorporating probabilities based on sequence bioinformatics and tumor characteristics: a report from the Colon Cancer Family Registry. Hum Mutat. 2013;34(1):200–9. https://doi.org/10.1002/humu.22213.
14. Spurdle AB. Clinical relevance of rare germline sequence variants in cancer genes: evolution and application of classification models. Curr Opin Genet Dev. 2010;20(3):315–23. https://doi.org/10.1016/j.gde.2010.03.009.
15. Lindor N, Peterson G, Spurdle A, Thompson B, Goldgar D, Thibodeau S. Pancreatic cancer and a novel *MSH2* germline alteration. Pancreas. 2011;40(7):1138–40. https://doi.org/10.1097/MPA.0b013e318220c217.
16. Stuckless S, Parfrey PS, Woods MO, Cox J, Fitzgerald GW, Green JS, et al. The phenotypic expression of three *MSH2* mutations in large Newfoundland families with Lynch syndrome. Fam Cancer. 2007;6(1):1–12. https://doi.org/10.1007/s10689-006-0014-8.

17. Ferlay J, Shin HR, Bray F, Forman D, Mathers C, Parkin DM. Estimates of worldwide burden of cancer in 2008: GLOBOCAN 2008. Int J Cancer. 2010;127(12):2893–917. https://doi.org/10.1002/ijc.25516.
18. Le Marchand L. Combined influence of genetic and dietary factors on colorectal cancer incidence in Japanese Americans. J Natl Cancer Inst Monogr. 1999;26:101–5.
19. Park JG, Park YJ, Wijnen JT, Vasen HF. Gene-environment interaction in hereditary nonpolyposis colorectal cancer with implications for diagnosis and genetic testing. Int J Cancer. 1999;82(4):516–9.
20. van Vliet CM, Dowty JG, van Vliet JL, Smith L, Mead LJ, Macrae FA, et al. Dependence of colorectal cancer risk on the parent-of-origin of mutations in DNA mismatch repair genes. Hum Mutat. 2011;32(2):207–12. https://doi.org/10.1002/humu.21408.
21. Green J, O'Driscoll M, Barnes A, Maher ER, Bridge P, Shields K, et al. Impact of gender and parent of origin on the phenotypic expression of hereditary nonpolyposis colorectal cancer in a large Newfoundland kindred with a common MSH2 mutation. Dis Colon Rectum. 2002;45(9):1223–32. https://doi.org/10.1097/01.DCR.0000027034.98952.85.
22. Jarvinen HJ, Aarnio M, Mustonen H, Aktan-Collan K, Aaltonen LA, Peltomaki P, et al. Controlled 15-year trial on screening for colorectal cancer in families with hereditary nonpolyposis colorectal cancer. Gastroenterology. 2000;118(5):829–34.
23. Parry S, Win AK, Parry B, Macrae FA, Gurrin LC, Church JM, et al. Metachronous colorectal cancer risk for mismatch repair gene mutation carriers: the advantage of more extensive colon surgery. Gut. 2011;60(7):950–7. https://doi.org/10.1136/gut.2010.228056.
24. Burn J, Gerdes AM, Macrae F, Mecklin JP, Moeslein G, Olschwang S, et al. Long-term effect of aspirin on cancer risk in carriers of hereditary colorectal cancer: an analysis from the CAPP2 randomised controlled trial. Lancet. 2011;378(9809):2081–7. https://doi.org/10.1016/S0140-6736(11)61049-0.
25. Win AK, Dowty JG, English DR, Campbell PT, Young JP, Winship I, et al. Body mass index in early adulthood and colorectal cancer risk for carriers and non-carriers of germline mutations in DNA mismatch repair genes. Br J Cancer. 2011;105(1):162–9. https://doi.org/10.1038/bjc.2011.172.
26. Botma A, Nagengast FM, Braem MGM, Hendriks JCM, Kleibeuker JH, Vasen HFA, et al. Body mass index increases risk of colorectal adenomas in men with Lynch syndrome: the GEOLynch cohort study. J Clin Oncol. 2010;28(28):4346–53. https://doi.org/10.1200/jco.2010.28.0453.
27. Watson P, Ashwathnarayan R, Lynch HT, Roy HK. Tobacco use and increased colorectal cancer risk in patients with hereditary nonpolyposis colorectal cancer (Lynch syndrome). Arch Intern Med. 2004;164(22):2429–31. https://doi.org/10.1001/archinte.164.22.2429.
28. Pande M, Lynch PM, Hopper JL, Jenkins MA, Gallinger S, Haile RW, et al. Smoking and colorectal cancer in Lynch syndrome: results from the Colon Cancer Family Registry and the University of Texas M.D. Anderson Cancer Center. Clin Cancer Res. 2010;16(4):1331–9. https://doi.org/10.1158/1078-0432.ccr-09-1877.
29. Chau R, Dashti SG, Ait Ouakrim D, Buchanan DD, Clendenning M, Rosty C, et al. Multivitamin, calcium and folic acid supplements and the risk of colorectal cancer in Lynch syndrome. Int J Epidemiol. 2016;45(3):940–53. https://doi.org/10.1093/ije/dyw036.
30. Dashti SG, Buchanan DD, Jayasekara H, Ait Ouakrim D, Clendenning M, Rosty C, et al. Alcohol consumption and the risk of colorectal cancer for mismatch repair gene mutation carriers. Cancer Epidemiol Biomark Prev. 2017;26(3):366–75. https://doi.org/10.1158/1055-9965.epi-16-0496.
31. Ferlitsch M, Reinhart K, Pramhas S, Wiener C, Gal O, Bannert C, et al. Sex-specific prevalence of adenomas, advanced adenomas, and colorectal cancer in individuals undergoing screening colonoscopy. JAMA. 2011;306(12):1352–8. https://doi.org/10.1001/jama.2011.1362.
32. Bauer CM, Ray AM, Halstead-Nussloch BA, Dekker RG, Raymond VM, Gruber SB, et al. Hereditary prostate cancer as a feature of Lynch syndrome. Fam Cancer. 2011;10(1):37–42. https://doi.org/10.1007/s10689-010-9388-8.

33. Grindedal EM, Moller P, Eeles R, Stormorken AT, Bowitz-Lothe IM, Landro SM, et al. Germline mutations in mismatch repair genes associated with prostate cancer. Cancer Epidemiol Biomark Prev. 2009;18(9):2460–7. https://doi.org/10.1158/1055-9965.EPI-09-0058.
34. Barrow PJ, Ingham S, O'Hara C, Green K, McIntyre I, Lalloo F, et al. The spectrum of urological malignancy in Lynch syndrome. Fam Cancer. 2013;12(1):57–63. https://doi.org/10.1007/s10689-012-9573-z.
35. Ryan S, Jenkins MA, Win AK. Risk of prostate cancer in Lynch syndrome: a systematic review and meta-analysis. Cancer Epidemiol Biomark Prev. 2014;23(3):437–49. https://doi.org/10.1158/1055-9965.epi-13-1165.
36. Win AK, Lindor NM, Jenkins MA. Risk of breast cancer in Lynch syndrome: a systematic review. Breast Cancer Res. 2013;15(2):R27. https://doi.org/10.1186/bcr3405.
37. Win AK, Lindor NM, Winship I, Tucker KM, Buchanan DD, Young JP, et al. Risks of colorectal and other cancers after endometrial cancer for women with Lynch syndrome. J Natl Cancer Inst. 2013;105(4):274–9. https://doi.org/10.1093/jnci/djs525.
38. Win AK, Lindor NM, Young JP, Macrae FA, Young GP, Williamson E, et al. Risks of primary extracolonic cancers following colorectal cancer in Lynch syndrome. J Natl Cancer Inst. 2012;104(18):1363–72. https://doi.org/10.1093/jnci/djs351.
39. Win AK, Young JP, Lindor NM, Tucker KM, Ahnen DJ, Young GP, et al. Colorectal and other cancer risks for carriers and noncarriers from families with a DNA mismatch repair gene mutation: a prospective cohort study. J Clin Oncol. 2012;30(9):958–64. https://doi.org/10.1200/JCO.2011.39.5590.
40. Elston RC, Stewart J. A general model for the genetic analysis of pedigree data. Hum Hered. 1971;21(6):523–42.
41. Lange K, Weeks D, Boehnke M. Programs for pedigree analysis: MENDEL, FISHER, and dGENE. Genet Epidemiol. 1988;5(6):471–2. https://doi.org/10.1002/gepi.1370050611.
42. Bonaiti B, Bonadona V, Perdry H, Andrieu N, Bonaiti-Pellie C. Estimating penetrance from multiple case families with predisposing mutations: extension of the 'genotype-restricted likelihood' (GRL) method. Eur J Hum Genet. 2011;19(2):173–9. https://doi.org/10.1038/ejhg.2010.158.
43. Carayol J, Bonaiti-Pellie C. Estimating penetrance from family data using a retrospective likelihood when ascertainment depends on genotype and age of onset. Genet Epidemiol. 2004;27(2):109–17. https://doi.org/10.1002/gepi.20007.
44. Antoniou AC, Pharoah PD, McMullan G, Day NE, Ponder BA, Easton D. Evidence for further breast cancer susceptibility genes in addition to BRCA1 and BRCA2 in a population-based study. Genet Epidemiol. 2001;21(1):1–18. https://doi.org/10.1002/gepi.1014.
45. Gong G, Hannon N, Whittemore AS. Estimating gene penetrance from family data. Genet Epidemiol. 2010;34(4):373–81. https://doi.org/10.1002/gepi.20493.
46. Cannings C, Thompson EA, Skolnick MH. Probability functions on complex pedigrees. Adv Appl Probab. 1978;10(1):26–61. https://doi.org/10.2307/1426718.

Index

L. Valle et al. (eds.), *Hereditary Colorectal Cancer*,
https://doi.org/10.1007/978-3-319-74259-5

J

L

MIX
Papier aus verantwortungsvollen Quellen
Paper from responsible sources
FSC® C105338

If you have any concerns about our products,
you can contact us on
ProductSafety@springernature.com

In case Publisher is established outside the EU,
the EU authorized representative is:
Springer Nature Customer Service Center GmbH
Europaplatz 3, 69115 Heidelberg, Germany

Printed by Libri Plureos GmbH
in Hamburg, Germany